Statistical Methods
in Diagnostic Medicine

Statistical Methods in Diagnostic Medicine

Second Edition

Xiao-Hua Zhou

Department of Biostatistics
University of Washington
Seattle, WA

Northwest HSR&D Center of Excellence
VA Puget Sound Health Care System

Nancy A. Obuchowski

Department of Quantitative Health Sciences
Cleveland Clinic Foundation
Cleveland, OH

Donna K. McClish

Department of Biostatistics
Virginia Commonwealth University
Richmond, VA

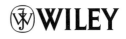

A JOHN WILEY & SONS, INC., PUBLICATION

For general information on our other products and services or for technical support, please contact our Customer Care Department within the United States at (800) 762-2974, outside the United States at (317) 572-3993 or fax (317) 572-4002.

Wiley also publishes its books in a variety of electronic formats. Some content that appears in print may not be available in electronic formats. For more information about Wiley products, visit our web site at www.wiley.com.

Library of Congress Cataloging-in-Publication Data is available.

ISBN 978-0470-18314-4

Printed in the United States of America.

10 9 8 7 6 5 4 3 2 1

*This book is dedicated to
Yea-Jae, Ralph, and
Tom*

CONTENTS IN BRIEF

CONTENTS

PART II   ADVANCED METHODS

LIST OF FIGURES

LIST OF TABLES

0.1 PREFACE

Diagnostic tests play a pivotal role in medicine, often determining what additional diagnostic tests, treatments, and interventions are needed and ultimately affecting patients' outcomes. Given the importance of this role, it is critical that clinicians are given reliable data about the accuracy of the diagnostic tests they order. These clinicians need well-designed diagnostic accuracy studies and they need to understand how the results of these studies apply to their patients. The purpose of this book, then, is two-fold: to provide a comprehensive approach to designing and analyzing diagnostic accuracy studies and to aid clinicians in understanding these studies and in generalizing study results to their patient populations.

Since the first edition, we have updated each chapter with recently published methods. These updates include new methods for tests designed to detect and locate lesions (see Chapters 2, 3, and 9), recommendations for the type of covariate-adjustment needed (Chapter 3) along with new methods for covariate-adjustment (Chapter 8), estimating and comparing predictive values (Chapters 4 and 5) and calculating sample size for studies using predictive values (Chapter 6), sample size calculation for multiple reader studies when pilot data are available (Chapter 6), new methods for correcting for verification bias in estimation of ROC curves of continuous-scale tests (Chapter 10), and new methods for correcting for imperfect standard bias in estimation of ROC curves of ordinal-scale or continuous-scale tests (Chapter 11).

We have also added three case studies: a positron emission tomography (PET) study comparing the accuracy of three tests for detecting diseased parathyroid glands, a computer-aided detection (CAD) study of colon polyps, and a magnetic resonance imaging study of atherosclerosis in the carotid arteries (see Chapter 1). The data from these case studies are provided in the Appendix and are used throughout the book as illustrations of various statistical methods.

The book is organized such that the more basic material about measures of test accuracy and study design appear first (Chapters 2 and 3, respectively), followed by chapters on statistical methods of data analysis with real data examples to illustrate these methods. Chapters 4 and 5 illustrate methods for estimating accuracy and comparing tests' accuracies under a variety of study designs. Calculating the sample size required for a study is described in Chapter 6. Chapters 7 and 12 focus on the design and analysis of meta-analyses of diagnostic test accuracy. Chapters 8 and 9 look at models of diagnostic test accuracy for various patient subgroups and for multiple-reader studies, respectively. Corrections for estimates of test accuracy in studies with verification bias and imperfect gold standards are illustrated in Chapters 10 and 11. Chapters 1-3 are accessible to readers with a basic knowledge of statistical and medical terminology. Chapters 4-7 are geared to the data analyst with basic training in biostatistics. In Chapters 8-12 we provide more detailed statistical methodology for readers with more statistical training, but the examples in these chapters are accessible to all readers. The only needed change is to add mention of the books related Web site to the Preface. The authors have prepared a Web site (http://faculty.washington.edu/azhou/books/diagnostic.html) that contains links to some useful software.

0.2 ACKNOWLEDGEMENTS

We are thankful to many colleagues for supporting us during the writing and publication of both the first (2002) and second (2011) edition of this book. Their helpful critiques and suggestions about the first edition have led to this improved second edition. Particularly, we would like to thank Danping Liu and Zheyu Wang for their helpful comments on the manuscript and their computational assistance in implementing some of methods discussed in the book. We would like to thank Dr. Thomas D. Koepsell for his helpful comments on the manuscript.

We would also like to thank our families for their understanding and encouragement. Dr. Xiao-Hua (Andrew) Zhou thanks his wife, Yea-Jae, and their children, Vanessa and Joshua. Dr. Nancy Obuchowski thanks her husband, Dr. Ralph Harvey, and their children, Tucker, Eli, and Scout. Dr. Donna McClish thanks her husband, Tom, and their daughter Amanda.

PART I

BASIC CONCEPTS AND METHODS

CHAPTER 1

INTRODUCTION

1.1 DIAGNOSTIC TEST ACCURACY STUDIES

Diagnostic medicine is the process of identifying the disease, or condition, that a patient has, and ruling out conditions that the patient does not have, through assessment of the patient's signs, symptoms, and results of various diagnostic tests. *Diagnostic accuracy studies* are research studies which examine the ability of diagnostic tests to discriminate between patients with and without the condition; these studies are the focus of this book.

A diagnostic test has several purposes: (1) to provide reliable information about the patient's condition, (2) to influence the health care provider's plan for managing the patient (Sox et al., 1989), and possibly, (3) to understand disease mechanism and natural history through research (e.g., the repeated testing of patients with chronic conditions) (McNeil and Adelstein, 1976). A test can serve these purposes only if the health care provider knows how to interpret it. Diagnostic test studies are conducted to tell us how diagnostic tests perform and, thus, how they should be interpreted. There are several measures of diagnostic test performance. Fryback and Thornbury (1991) described a hierarchical model for studying diagnostic performance for imaging

Statistical Methods in Diagnostic Medicine,
Second Edition. By Xiao-Hua Zhou, Nancy A. Obuchowski, Donna K. McClish
Copyright © 2011 John Wiley & Sons, Inc.

tests. The model starts with image quality and progresses to diagnostic accuracy, effect on treatment decisions, impact on patient outcome, and finally costs to society. A key feature of the model is that for a diagnostic test to be efficacious at a higher level, it must be efficacious at all lower levels. The reverse is not true; for example, a new test may have better accuracy than a standard test but may be too costly (in terms of monetary expense and/or patient morbidity due to complications) to be efficacious. In this book, we deal exclusively with the assessment of diagnostic *accuracy* (level 2 of the hierarchical model), recognizing that it is only one step in the complete assessment of a diagnostic test.

Diagnostic test accuracy is simply the ability of the test to discriminate among alternative states of health (Zweig and Campbell, 1993). If a test's results do not differ between alternative states of health, then the test has negligible accuracy; if the results do not overlap for the different health states, then the test has perfect accuracy. Most test accuracies fall between these two extremes. It's important to recognize that a test result is not a true representation of the patient's condition (Sox et al., 1989). Most diagnostic information is imperfect; it may influence the health care provider's thinking, but uncertainty remains about the patient's true condition. If the test is negative for the condition, should the health care provider assume that the patient is disease-free and thus send him or her home? If the test is positive, should the health care provider assume the patient has the condition and thus begin treatment? Finally, if the test result requires interpretation by a trained reader (e.g., a radiologist), should the health care provider seek a second interpretation?

To answer these critical questions, the health care provider needs to have information on the test's absolute and relative capabilities and an understanding of the complex interactions between the test and the trained readers who interpret the imaging data (Beam, 1992). The health care provider must ask: How does the test perform among patients with the condition (i.e., the test's sensitivity)? How does the test perform among patients without the condition (i.e., the test's specificity)? Does the test serve as a replacement for an older test or should multiple tests be performed? If multiple tests are performed, how should they be executed (i.e., sequentially or in parallel)? How reproducible are interpretations by different readers? These sorts of questions are addressed in diagnostic test accuracy studies.

Diagnostic test accuracy studies have three common features: a sample of subjects who have, or will, undergo one or more of the diagnostic medical tests under evaluation; some form of interpretation or scoring of the test's findings; and a reference, or *gold standard*, to which the test findings are compared. This may sound simple enough, but diagnostic accuracy studies are difficult to design. Here are three common misperceptions about diagnostic test accuracy.

The first misperception involves the interpretation of diagnostic tests. Investigators of new diagnostic tests sometimes develop criteria for interpreting their tests based only on the findings from healthy volunteers. For example, in a new test to detect pancreatitis, investigators measure the amount of a certain enzyme in healthy volunteers. A typical decision criterion, or *cutpoint*, is three standard deviations (SDs) below the mean of the normals. New patients with an enzyme level of three SDs below the mean of the healthy volunteers are labeled "positive " for pancreatitis; patients with enzyme levels above this cutpoint are labeled "negative". In proposing such a criterion, investigators fail to recognize (1) the relevance of the natural distributions of the test results (i.e. are they really Gaussian [normal]?); (2) the magnitude of any overlap between the test results of patients with and without pancreatitis (i.e. are the test results from most pancreatitis patients 3 SDs below the mean?); (3) the clinical significance of diagnostic errors (i.e. falsely labeling a patient without pancreatitis as "positive" for the condition and falsely labeling a patient with pancreatitis as "negative"); and (4) the poor generalization of results from studies based on healthy volunteers (i.e. healthy volunteers may have very different enzyme levels than sick patients without pancreatitis who might undergo the test). In Chapter 2, we discuss factors involved in determining optimal cutpoints for diagnostic tests; in Chapter 4, we discuss methods of finding optimal cutpoints and estimating diagnostic errors associated with them.

Another common misperception in diagnostic test studies is the notion that a rigorous assessment of a patient's true condition - with the exclusion of patients for whom a less rigorous assessment was made - allows for a scientifically sound study. An example comes from literature on the use of ventilation-perfusion lung scans for diagnosing pulmonary emboli. The ventilation-perfusion lung scan is a noninvasive test used to screen high-risk patients for pulmonary emboli; its accuracy in various populations is unknown. Pulmonary angiography, on the other hand, is a highly accurate but invasive test. It is often used as a reference for assessing the accuracy of other tests. (See Chapter 2 for the definition and examples of *gold standards*.) To assess the accuracy of ventilation-perfusion lung scans, patients who have undergone both a ventilation-perfusion lung scan and a pulmonary angiogram are recruited, while patients who did not undergo the angiogram are excluded. Such a design usually leads to biased estimates of test accuracy. The reason is that the study sample is not representative of the patient population undergoing ventilation-perfusion lung scans - rather, patients with a positive scan are often recommended for angiograms, while patients with a negative scan are often not sent for an angiogram because of the risk of complications with it. In Chapter 3, we define *work-up bias*, and its most common form, *verification bias*, as well as strategies to avoid them. In Chapter 10, we present statistical methods developed specifically to correct for verification bias.

A third error common in diagnostic test accuracy studies involves confusion between accuracy and agreement. Investigators sometimes draw incorrect conclusions about a new test's diagnostic accuracy because it agrees well with a conventional test; however, what if the new and conventional tests do not agree? We cannot simply conclude that the new test has inferior accuracy. In fact, a new test with superior accuracy will definitely disagree sometimes with the conventional test. Similarly, the two tests may have the same accuracy but make mistakes on different patients, resulting in poor agreement. A more valid approach to assessing a new test's diagnostic accuracy is to compare both tests against a gold standard reference. Assessment of diagnostic accuracy is usually more difficult than assessment of agreement, but it is a more relevant and valid approach (Zweig and Campbell, 1993). In Chapter 5, we present methods for comparing the accuracy of two tests when the true diagnoses of the patients are known; in Chapter 11 we present methods for comparing two tests' accuracies when the true diagnoses are unknown.

There is no question that studies of diagnostic test accuracy are challenging to design and require specialized statistical methods for their analysis. We will present and illustrate concepts and methods for designing, analyzing, interpreting, and reporting studies of diagnostic test accuracy. In Part I (Chapters 2-7) we define various measures of diagnostic accuracy, describe strategies for designing diagnostic accuracy studies, and present the basic statistical methods for estimating and comparing test accuracy, calculating sample size, and synthesizing the literature for meta-analysis. In Part II (Chapters 8-12) we present more advanced statistical methods for describing a test's accuracy when patient characteristics affect it, for analyzing multi-reader studies, studies with verification bias or imperfect gold standards, and for performing meta-analyses.

1.2 CASE STUDIES

We introduce three diagnostic test accuracy studies to illustrate the kinds of designs, questions, and statistical issues that arise in diagnostic medicine. These case studies, along with many other examples, are used throughout the book to illustrate various statistical methods. The datasets for these case studies are given in Appendix at the end of the book.

1.2.1 Case Study 1: Parathyroid Disease

Parathyroid glands are small endocrine glands usually located in the neck or upper chest that produce a hormone that controls the body's calcium levels. Most people have four parathyroid glands. In the most common form of parathyroid disease, one of these glands grows into a benign tumor, called a parathyroid adenoma, which produces excess amounts of parathyroid hormone. In a less common condition, called parathyroid hyperplasia, all four parathyroid glands become enlarged and secrete excess parathyroid hormone. In both conditions, a patient's serum calcium levels become elevated, and the patient experiences loss of energy, depression, kidney stones, and headaches. Surgical removal of the offending parathyroid lesion is considered curative in most cases.

Single photon emission computed tomography (SPECT) using the radio-pharmaceutical Tc-99m sestamibi is a nuclear medicine imaging test used to detect and localize parathyroid lesions prior to surgical intervention. In this prospective study (Donald Neumann, MD, PhD, Cleveland Clinic, Ohio, personal communication, 2007), 61 consecutive patients with hyperparathyroidism were imaged using a hybrid SPECT/CT instrument in an attempt to localize the diseased parathyroid glands preoperatively. Each patient underwent SPECT imaging, both with and without attenuation correction, as well as SPECT combined with CT imaging. Following imaging, the patients went to surgery to remove the diseased glands. The goal of the study was to compare the accuracy of these three tests.

One expert nuclear radiologist, blinded to the surgical findings, interpreted the images. On the SPECT imaging, each gland was scored on a scale from 1-7, with 1=definitely no disease, 2=probably no disease, 3=indeterminate, 4=maybe diseased, and 5=definitely diseased. Scores of 5, 6, and 7 were all considered definitely diseased but were distinguished by the intensity of the attenuation: 5=low, 6=medium, and 7=high, respectively. The SPECT/CT images were scored using just the 1-5 part of the scale. For this study, SPECT images scored as 1-3 were considered negative and scores of 4-7 as positive. For SPECT/CT, scores of 1-3 were considered negative and scores of 4-5 were considered positive. 97 glands in 61 patients were localized by imaging prior to undergoing parathyroid surgery, the results of which were considered the gold standard.

The investigators wanted to compare the sensitivity and specificity of these three tests to determine which single test should be used for future patients. In Chapter 2, we show that one of these tests appears more sensitive than the others, while another test appears more specific. A comparison of the tests' Receiver Operating Characteristic (ROC) curves gives us a complete understanding of the strengths and weaknesses of the three tests and thus allows us to identify the most suitable test for preoperative patients.

The data from this study are complicated by the fact that many of the 61 patients had multiple glands visualized at screening, so called "clustered data." Observations from the same patient, even if from different glands, are usually correlated, at least to some small degree. If we ignore this correlation, then the resulting confidence intervals and p-values can be misleading. In Chapters 4 and 5, we describe a simple analysis method that can be used for clustered data so that confidence intervals and p-values are correct.

1.2.2 Case Study 2: Colon Cancer Detection

Polyps that form in the colon or rectum can progress to cancer without any signs or symptoms. Computed tomography colonography (CTC) is an imaging test that can detect polyps before they develop into cancer. Radiologists sometimes overlook polyps on the CTC images, however, and these missed polyps ("false negatives") can develop into cancer, which can lead to symptoms, even death. Investigators have developed a computer algorithm, called computer aided detection (CAD), to help radiologists detect polyps on the CTC. The CAD utilizes tissue intensity, volumetric and surface shape, and texture characteristics to identify suspicious areas. The CAD marks the suspicious areas for the reader to exam more closely. Often, the CAD identifies multiple suspicious areas on the same image. The radiologist must distinguish marked areas that contain a polyp ("true positive") from marked areas that do not contain a polyp, for example a folded bowel lining ("false positive").

In this study (Baker et al., 2007), the investigators wanted to compare radiologists' accuracy without CAD to their accuracy with CAD to determine if CAD improves radiologists' accuracy. Seven radiologists from two institutions participated in the study. The readers had varying levels of overall experience with abdominal imaging, as well as varying levels of training with CTC imaging technology. Overall, the 7 were considered inexperienced CTC readers.

Two hundred seventy patients from six institutions were compiled in this retrospective design. These 270 patients had undergone CTC for the following reasons: screening, follow-up exams for polyps detected in a prior exam, and failed prior colonoscopy including patients at risk for colon polyps/carcinoma but who were deemed not suitable candidates for a colonoscopy. An expert abdominal imager with extensive CTC experience and with knowledge about each patient's follow-up (clinical, imaging, pathologic, and surgical), stratified the 270-patient sample into presence versus absence of a polyp; cases with a polyp were further stratified by polyp size (less than 6 mm "small", 6-9 mm "medium", or 10 mm or larger "large"). One hundred forty-one *training cases* were randomly sampled from the different strata to improve the CAD algorithm and train the readers. From the remaining 119 *test cases*, 30 were randomly selected to be used in this reader performance study; the study sample was composed of 25 positive cases with at least one polyp of middle to large size (a total of 39 polyps) and five cases with no polyps.

The seven readers were each given a unique order for reading the 30 images. First without CAD, the reader marked all findings. The reader used a pull-down window to identify the location of each finding according to one of eight colon segments. The reader then scored each finding according to their confidence that a polyp was present: 1=definitely not a polyp; 2=probably not a polyp; 3=indeterminate; 4=maybe a polyp; and, 5=definitely a polyp. When the reader's interpretation without CAD was completed, the reader was given a list of potential polyps detected by the CAD. Any CAD marks that coincided with a lesion found by the reader without CAD were not presented to the reader and were discarded. New CAD marks were scored by the reader using the 1-5 rating scale. The investigators in this study want to know if the CAD improves inexperienced radiologists' accuracy over their accuracy without CAD ("unaided setting"). The seven-reader design helps us to get a better estimate of reader accuracy, but also complicates the analyses because the readers' findings are correlated by the fact that they all interpreted the same sample of 30 patients. Sensitivity was defined for this study as correct detection of a polyp in a patient with polyps, and, in addition, required that the reader identify the correct location of the polyp. If the wrong location was chosen, then the missed polyp was considered a false negative. In this study patients can have multiple true positives (i.e. multiple correctly located polyps in the same patient), as well as a mixture of true positive, false positive, false negative, and true negative findings. Clustered data complicates the statistical analyses, but statistical methods are presented in Chapters 4 and 5 to handle these data appropriately.

1.2.3 Case Study 3: Carotid Artery Stenosis

Excessive plaque formation, or stenosis, in the carotid (neck) artery can lead to transient ischemic attacks (TIAs) or even stroke. Conventional catheter angiography is an invasive diagnostic test used by physicians to examine the carotid arteries in patients who have suffered a TIA or stroke. Because the test is invasive, there are risks associated with the test including stroke and death. Magnetic Resonance Angiography (MRA) is a non-invasive test that may help physicians examine the carotid arteries without risk. Patients with other cardiovascular problems who are at high risk for plaque formation in the carotid arteries can also benefit from such a noninvasive screening test.

In this study, investigators (Thomas Masaryk, MD, Cleveland Clinic, Ohio, personal communication, 2007) wanted to assess the accuracy of MRA for detecting carotid artery plaque. Patients scheduled for a conventional catheter angiogram because they had suffered a recent stroke (symptomatic) or because they were at high risk for suffering a stroke in the future (asymptomatic) were asked to participate in this study. One hundred sixty-three patients were prospectively recruited for the study. These patients first underwent an MRA, then a conventional catheter angiogram.

Four radiologists from three institutions independently interpreted the conventional catheter angiograms, and the same four radiologists independently interpreted the MRA images. At least two weeks passed between the catheter angiogram and MRA interpretations; the study ID numbers were changed so that there was no obvious connection between the catheter angiogram and MRA images.

A significant stenosis requiring surgical intervention was defined as stenosis that blocked 60-99 percent of the carotid vessel. Note that arteries that are completely blocked (100 percent stenosis, or occlusions) are not considered good surgical lesions. The radiologists were asked to grade their confidence that a significant stenosis was present using a 5-point scale: 1=definitely no significant stenosis, 2=probably no significant stenosis, 3=equivocal, 4=probably significant stenosis, and 5=definitely significant stenosis. They were also asked to indicate the percent of stenosis present (a number between 0 and 100). The radiologists responded to these questions for both the left and right sides for both MRA and conventional catheter angiography.

In this study the investigators want to know the accuracy of MRA and whether or not it can replace the conventional invasive test, catheter angiography. The data are complicated by the multiple-reader design, as well as by the fact that the data are clustered (i.e. findings from both the left and right carotid arteries in the same patient). There are several patient characteristics, such as gender, age, and symptoms, which the investigators suspect may affect the accuracy of MRA. In Chapter 3, we discuss the kinds of effects that covariates can have on diagnostic test accuracy; in Chapter 8, we discuss various regression methods to handle covariate data. Finally, we note that the gold standard for this study, catheter angiography, is not a perfect test and radiologists often disagree in their interpretations of its findings. Fortunately, there are statistical methods, which we describe in Chapter 11, that deal with studies with imperfect reference standards.

1.3 SOFTWARE

A variety of software has been written to implement many of the statistical methods discussed in this book. These programs can be found in FORTRAN, SAS macros (SAS Institute, Cary, North Carolina, USA), Stata (Stata Data Analysis and Statistical Software, Stata Corp LP, College Station, Texas), and R (free software at http://www.r-project.org/). The authors have prepared a Web site (http://faculty.washington.edu/azhou/books/diagnostic.html) that contains links to some useful software. The web site will be maintained and updated periodically for at least five years after this book's publication date.

1.4 TOPICS NOT COVERED IN THIS BOOK

Although this book covers the main themes in statistical methods for diagnostic medicine, it does not cover several related topics, as follows.

Decision analysis, cost-effectiveness analysis, and cost-benefit analysis are methods commonly used to quantify the long-term, or downstream, effects of a test on the patient and society. In Chapters 2 and 4, we discuss how these methods can be applied to find the optimal cutpoint on the ROC curve. Description of how to perform these methods, however, is beyond the scope of this book. There are many excellent references on these topics, including (Gold et al., 1996), (Pauker and Kassirer, 1975), (Russell et al., 1996), (Weinstein et al., 1996), (Drummond et al., 2005), (Glick et al., 2007), and (Willan and Briggs, 2006).

Most of the methods we present for estimation and hypothesis testing are from a frequentist perspective. Bayesian methods can also be used, whereby one incorporates into the assessment of the diagnostic test some previously acquired information or expert opinion about a test's characteristics or information about the patient or population. Examples of Bayesian methods used in diagnostic testing include Gatsonis (1995); Joseph et al. (1995); Peng and Hall (1996); Hellmich et al. (1988); O'Malley and Zou (2001); Broemeling (2007).

Finally, when there are multiple diagnostic tests performed on a patient, we may want to combine the information from the tests in order to make the best possible diagnosis. See, for example, Pepe and Thompson (2000), Zhou et al. (2011), and Lin et al. (2011) for various methods for combining tests' results to optimize diagnostic accuracy.

CHAPTER 2

MEASURES OF DIAGNOSTIC ACCURACY

In this chapter we describe various measures of the accuracy of diagnostic tests. We begin by introducing measures of *intrinsic accuracy*, a test's inherent ability to correctly detect a condition when it is actually present and to correctly rule out a condition when it is truly absent. These attributes are considered fundamental to the tests themselves. They do not change for different samples of patients with different prevalence rates of disease. It is important to recognize, however, which these attributes can change somewhat over time and population as the technical specifications of the imaging machine, the clinician interpreting the test, and the characteristics of the patient (e.g. severity of disease) change.

The intrinsic accuracy of a test is measured by comparing the test results to the true condition status of the patient. We assume for most of our discussion that the true condition status is one of two mutually exclusive states: *"the condition is present"* or *"the condition is absent."* Some examples are the presence versus the absence of parathyroid disease, the presence of a malignant versus benign tumor, and the presence of one versus more than one tumor. We determine the true condition status by means of a *gold standard*. A gold standard is a source of information, completely different from the test or

Statistical Methods in Diagnostic Medicine,
Second Edition. By Xiao-Hua Zhou, Nancy A. Obuchowski, Donna K. McClish
Copyright © 2011 John Wiley & Sons, Inc.

tests under evaluation, which tells us the true condition status of the patient. Different gold standards are used for different tests and applications; some common examples are autopsy reports, surgery findings, pathology results from biopsy specimens, and the results of other diagnostic tests that have perfect or near perfect accuracy. In Chapter 3, we discuss more about the selection of a gold standard; in Chapter 11 we present statistical methods for measuring diagnostic accuracy without a gold standard.

Once a test has been shown to have some level of intrinsic accuracy, the role of the test in particular clinical situations must be evaluated. At this stage we consider not only the intrinsic accuracy of the test but also the prevalence of the disease, the consequences of the test's misdiagnoses, and the impact of the cognitive and perceptual abilities of the interpreting clinician on the diagnosis. In Sections 2.11 and 2.12, we discuss the predictive values of a test and how the order of tests can affect accuracy; in Chapters 3 and 9, we discuss the design and analysis of multi-reader studies of diagnostic accuracy.

2.1 SENSITIVITY AND SPECIFICITY

Two basic measures of diagnostic accuracy are *sensitivity* and *specificity*. Their definitions are best illustrated by a table with 2 rows and 2 columns, or *decision matrix*, where the rows summarize the data according to the true condition status of the patients and the columns summarize the test results. We denote the true condition status by the indicator variable D, where $D = 1$ if the condition is present and 0 if the condition is absent. Test results indicating the condition is present are called *positive*; those indicating the condition is absent are called *negative*. We denote positive test results as $T = 1$, negative test results as $T = 0$. Table 2.1 has such characteristics; it is called a *count table* because it indicates the numbers of patients in various categories. The total number of patients with and without the condition is, respectively, n_1 and n_0; the total number of patients with the condition who test positive and negative is, respectively, s_1 and s_0; and the total number of patients without the condition who test positive and negative, is respectively, r_1 and r_0. The total number of patients in the study group, N, is equal to $N = s_1 + s_0 + r_1 + r_0$, or $N = n_1 + n_0$.

The sensitivity (Se) of a test is its ability to detect the condition when it is present. We write sensitivity as $Se = P(T = 1 \mid D = 1)$, which is read "sensitivity (Se) is the probability (P) that the test result is positive ($T = 1$), given that the condition is present ($D = 1$)." Among the n_1 patients with the condition, s_1 test positive; thus, $Se = s_1/n_1$.

The specificity (Sp) of a test is its ability to exclude the condition in patients without the condition. We write specificity as $Sp = P(T = 0 \mid D = 0)$, which is read "specificity (Sp) is the probability (P) that the test result is negative ($T = 0$), given that the condition is absent ($D = 0$)." Among n_0 patients without the condition, r_0 test negative; thus, $Sp = r_0/n_0$.

Table 2.1 Basic 2x2 Count Table

	Test Result:		
True Condition Status:	Positive (T=1)	Negative (T=0)	total
Present (D=1)	s_1	s_0	n_1
Absent (D=0)	r_1	r_0	n_0
total	m_1	m_0	N

Count data can be summarized by probabilities as in Table 2.2. This table emphasizes that sensitivity and specificity are computed from different subsamples of patients, that is, the subsamples of patients with and without the condition. Note that the sum of the two probabilities in the top row (the $D = 1$ row) is 1.0, and similarly, the sum of the two probabilities in the bottom row (the $D = 0$ row) is one. The probability that the test will be positive in a patient with the condition (i.e., the sensitivity) is given in the $(D = 1, T = 1)$ cell of the table. Another way diagnostic accuracy is commonly

Table 2.2 2x2 Probability Table

	Test Result:		
True Condition Status:	Positive (T=1)	Negative (T=0)	total
Present (D=1)	$Se = s_1/n_1$	$FNR = s_0/n_1$	1.0
Absent (D=0)	$FPR = r_1/n_0$	$Sp = r_0/n_0$	1.0

described emphasizes the consequences associated with the test results. In this usage, sensitivity is the true-positive fraction (TPF) or rate (TPR); s_1 is the number of true positives (TPs). Specificity is the true negative fraction (TNF) or rate (TNR); r_0 is the number of true negatives (TNs). The "true" positives and negatives, are respectively, s_1 and r_0 because the diagnostic test indicated the correct diagnosis. In contrast, s_0 is the number of false negatives (FNs) and s_0/n_1 is the false negative fraction (FNF) or rate (FNR). Here, the test falsely indicates the absence of the condition in a patient who truly has the condition. False negative results cause harm by delaying treatment and providing false reassurance. Similarly, r_1 is the number of false positives (FPs), and r_1/n_0 is the false positive fraction (FPF) or rate (FPR). False detection of the condition leads to unnecessary, perhaps risky, confirmatory tests, as well as incorrect treatment and false labeling of patients.

The definition of positive and negative test results, as well as the condition of interest, must be clear because a positive finding may correspond to the presence or absence of a condition, depending upon the clinical application. For example, in a study of lung disease (Remer et al., 2000), patients with detected adrenal adenomas were labeled positive and patients with detected lung metastases were labeled negative. The fact that patients with adrenal adenomas are eligible for lung cancer surgery, whereas patients without this condition (i.e. the patients with lung metastases) are not, motivated the authors to refer to the detection of an adenoma as a positive finding.

2.1.1   Basic Measures of Test Accuracy: Case Study 2

To illustrate the foregoing calculations, consider the colon cancer case study introduced in Chapter 1. The study sample was comprised of 30 patients who had undergone computed tomography colonography (CTC) (i.e. the diagnostic test). Here, we will consider the results for Reader 1 when the reader was aided by the computer-aided detection (CAD) algorithm. Based on the compilation of results from colonoscopy (a gold standard test where a long flexible instrument connected to a camera is inserted into the rectum and moved along the colon) and surgery, an expert radiologist determined that 25 patients had 39 polyps and 5 patients had no polyps. We define a true positive, here, as a patient with one or more polyps where the reader correctly detected at least one polyp. A false negative is a patient with one or more polyps in which the reader missed all of the patient's polyps. A true negative is a patient with no polyps in which the reader did not detect any polyps. Finally, a false positive is a patient with no polyps in which the reader falsely detected one or more polyps. The data in Table 2.3 were compiled from Tables A.2 and A.3 of the Appendix (the last 5 lines of Table A.3 summarize the results for the 5 patients without polyps) of the Appendix.

Table 2.3   CAD-aided CTC Results of 25 Patients With and 5 Without Colon Polyps

	Test Result:		
Polyp Status:	*Positive*	*Negative*	*total*
Present	22	3	25
Absent	2	3	5
total	24	6	30

Of the 25 patients with polyps, 22 tested positive - that is, at least one of the patient's polyps was detected on CTC. Thus there are 22 TPs and 3 FNs; the sensitivity is 22/25 =0.88. Of 5 patients without polyps, three tested negative (TNs). The specificity is 3/5, or 0.60. The FPR was 2/5 =0.40, or 1 - the specificity.

Table 2.4 Gap Measurements of 10 Patients With and 10 Without Fractured Heart Valve

Fractured	Intact
0.58	0.13
0.41	0.13
0.18	0.07
0.15	0.05
0.15	0.03
0.10	0.03
0.07	0.03
0.07	0.00
0.05	0.00
0.03	0.00

We note that in this study, characterization of the test's rate of false detection cannot fully be understood by examining only the five cases without polyps. In this study readers were asked to find all polyps; thus, among the 25 patients with polyps there are also false positives - i.e. areas on the image where the reader falsely claimed that a polyp was present. From Table 2 of the Appendix we see that Reader 1, aided with CAD, had a total of 16 false positives in 30 patients. Researchers often report this as an average of 0.53 false positives per patient. Furthermore, we note that 12 of these false positives were reported by the reader before using CAD; only 4 of the 16 false positives were attributable to CAD.

Similarly, we could have defined sensitivity at the *polyp-level* rather than the *patient-level*. Here, a true positive is a polyp which the reader correctly detected, and a false negative is a polyp which the reader did not detect. Using this polyp-level definition for sensitivity, Reader 1's sensitivity aided by CAD is 33 TPs / 39 true polyps = 0.846.

2.1.2 Diagnostic Tests with Continuous Results: The Artificial Heart Valve Example

Many diagnostic tests yield a numeric measurement rather than a binary result (i.e. positive or negative). Consider a digital-imaging algorithm to identify patients whose implanted artificial heart valve has fractured (Powell et al., 1996). One measure used to distinguish fractured from intact valves is the width of the gap between the valve strut legs. The larger the gap, the more likely the valve has fractured. Table 2.4 lists the gap measurements of 20 patients who have undergone elective surgery for valve replacement. Figure 2.1 illustrates the data.

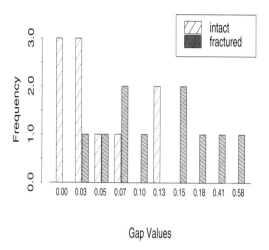

Gap Values

Figure 2.1   Histogram of Gap Measurements of Patients With and Without Fractured Heart Valves

At surgery, 10 patients were found to have fractured valves and 10 were found to have intact valves; the gap values range from 0.03 to 0.58 for patients with a fractured valve, and from 0.0 to 0.13 for patients with intact valves. To describe the sensitivity and specificity of the imaging technique, we choose a value of, say 0.05, in which case the patients with gap values greater than 0.05 are labeled positive and patients with gap values less than or equal to 0.05 are labeled negative. The corresponding sensitivity and specificity are, respectively, 0.80 and 0.70.

In this example we arbitrarily chose a gap value of 0.05 to define the test results as positive or negative. The test result of 0.05 is called a *decision threshold*, the test result used as a cutoff to define positive and negative test results, and subsequently to define sensitivity and specificity. We could have used any gap value as a decision threshold. Sensitivity and specificity would have been affected, however, by our choice.

Table 2.5 summarizes the sensitivity and specificity corresponding to several possible decision thresholds. If we choose a larger gap value of, say, 0.13, then the sensitivity decreases to 0.50 while the specificity increases to 1.0. If, however, we choose 0.03, the sensitivity increases to 0.90 while the specificity decreases to 0.60. This example illustrates that the sensitivity and specificity of a test are inherently linked - as one increases, the other decreases. Thus, in describing a diagnostic test, both sensitivity and specificity must be reported, along with the corresponding decision threshold.

Table 2.5 Estimates of Se and Sp From Heart Valve Imaging Study

Defn of + Test	Se	Sp	FNR	FPR
> 0.58	0.0	1.0	1.0	0.0
> 0.13	0.5	1.0	0.5	0.0
> 0.07	0.6	0.8	0.4	0.2
> 0.05	0.8	0.7	0.2	0.3
> 0.03	0.9	0.6	0.1	0.4
> 0.0	1.0	0.3	0.0	0.7
≥ 0.0	1.0	0.0	0.0	1.0

2.1.3 Diagnostic Tests with Ordinal Results: Case Study 1

The gap measurement is an objective test result, calculated by a computer algorithm. Other tests yield results that must be interpreted subjectively by a human reader, for example, mammographic images for the detection of breast cancer, SPECT images to detect and localize parathyroid lesions, or magnetic resonance (MR) images for the detection of multiple sclerosis. For these tests, the observer establishes a decision threshold in his/her mind and uses that threshold to label cases as positive or negative. The decision threshold that an observer adopts depends on many factors, including his or her "style," his or her estimate of the condition's likelihood in the patient before testing, and assessment of the consequences of misdiagnoses (Metz, 1978).

Consider the SPECT imaging case study introduced in chapter 1. The radiologist scored each SPECT/CT image on a 1-5 scale, with 1=definitely no parathyroid disease, 2=probably no parathyroid disease, 3=possibly parathyroid disease, 4= probably parathyroid disease, and 5=definitely parathyroid disease. Such an ordinal scale is common in diagnostic radiology studies. Another commonly used scale is the 0% to 100% scale which describes the reader's confidence in the presence of the condition: 0% is no confidence and 100% is complete confidence in the presence of the condition.

Table 2.6 summarizes the radiologist's results. If the radiologist uses a decision threshold at 4, or "probably disease," so that only cases assigned a score of 4 or 5 are called positive, then the corresponding sensitivity and specificity will be 0.70 and 0.963. Alternatively, a decision threshold at a score of 3 results in a sensitivity and specificity of 0.729 and 0.889. Here again, we see that an increase in sensitivity (from 0.70 to 0.729) is offset by a decrease in specificity (from 0.963 to 0.889).

2.1.4 Effect of Prevalence and Spectrum of Disease

Sensitivity and specificity are measures of intrinsic diagnostic accuracy; they are not affected by the prevalence of the condition. For example, compare the

Table 2.6   SPECT/CT Using 5-Category Scale from Table A.1 in Appendix

Surgery Result:	Test Result:					
	1	*2*	*3*	*4*	*5*	*Total*
Disease Present	18	1	2	9	40	70
No Disease	23	1	2	0	1	27

data in tables 2.3 and 2.7. Table 2.7 presents the test results of 5250 patients - 250 with polyps (10 times more than in Table 2.3) and 5000 without polyps (1000 times more than in Table 2.3). The prevalence rate is about 5%. The sensitivity is 0.88; specificity, 0.60. These are identical to the estimates from Table 2.3 where the prevalence was 83%. This property of sensitivity and specificity is important; in practical terms it means that the sensitivity and specificity estimated from a study sample are applicable to other populations with different prevalence rates.

Table 2.7   CTC Results of 5250 Patients

Polyp Status:	Test Result:		
	Positive	*Negative*	*Total*
Present	220	30	250
Absent	2000	3000	5000
total	2220	3030	5250

Although not affected by the prevalence of the condition, sensitivity and specificity of some diagnostic tests are affected by the *spectrum of disease*. A disease's range of clinical severity or range of anatomic extent constitutes its spectrum. For example, large polyps are easier to detect than small ones; thus CTC has greater sensitivity when it is applied to patients with more advanced disease. Similarly, patient characteristics affect sensitivity and specificity of some diagnostic tests. For example, it is well known that older women have fatty, less dense breasts than younger women; mammography is better able to detect lesions in fatty breasts. In Chapter 3, we will discuss study designs and the importance of collecting patient characteristics, or covariates, to properly measure diagnostic test accuracy.

2.1.5   Analogy to α and β Statistical Errors

There are some interesting analogies between Table 2.1 and the type I and II (or α and β) error rates used in statistical hypothesis testing. The type I (α) error rate is the probability of rejecting the null hypothesis when, in reality, the null hypothesis is true. The type II (β) error rate is the probability of failing to reject the null hypothesis when, in reality, the alternative hypothesis is true. In the diagnostic testing situation, let us define the null (H_0:) and alternative (H_1:) hypotheses as follows:

H_0: The condition is not present.

H_1: The condition is present.

Then, the type I error rate is analogous to the FPR and the type II error rate is analogous to the FNR. Statistical power, that is, 1 - type II error rate, is analogous to sensitivity. In statistical hypothesis testing it is standard to set the type I error rate at 0.05 (5%). With diagnostic tests, however, the particular clinical application dictates the allowable error rates (See Section 2.12).

2.2   COMBINED MEASURES OF SENSITIVITY AND SPECIFICITY

2.2.1   Problems Comparing Two or More Tests: Case Study 1

When comparing two or more diagnostic tests' accuracies, it is often difficult to determine which test is superior because both sensitivity and specificity must be accounted for. For example, consider the parathyroid disease study. Table 2.8 summarizes the sensitivity and specificity of the three tests using a cutpoint of three or less as "negative" and greater than three as "positive." SPECT with attenuation correction (AC SPECT) has superior sensitivity (in fact, statistically significant at the 0.05 level), while SPECT/CT has superior specificity (statistically significant at the 0.05 level). Ideally, we could find cutpoints where all the tests have the same specificities (or sensitivities) so that we could compare the tests' sensitivities (or specificities), but this is often not possible with ordinal test results or even continuous test results if the sample size is small. It would be useful, therefore, to summarize the accuracy of tests by a single number.

2.2.2   Probability of a Correct Test Result

There are several measures that incorporate sensitivity and specificity into a single index. We start with a measure seen often in the literature and often referred to simply as *accuracy*; however, we will refer to it more precisely as the *probability of a correct test result*. From Table 2.1 the probability of a correct

Table 2.8   Estimates of Accuracy for Case Study 1

	Measure of Accuracy:		
Diagnostic Test	Sensitivity	Specificity	ROC Area
No-AC SPECT	0.71	0.48	0.63
AC SPECT	0.80	0.44	0.67
SPECT/CT	0.70	0.96	0.83

test result is equal to $(s_1 + r_0)/N$ and constitutes the proportion of TPs and TNs in the entire sample. This measure is easily verified as a weighted average of sensitivity and specificity with weights equal to the sample prevalence (i.e. P(D=1)) and the complement of prevalence (i.e. P(D=0)),

$$P(TP \text{ or } TN) = (\# \text{ correct decisions})/N = Se \times P(D=1) + Sp \times P(D=0).$$

The strength of this measure of accuracy is its simple computation. However, this measure has many limitations, as will be illustrated by several examples. First, consider an 1885 editorial by Gilbert (1885) in which he writes about the extremely high "accuracy" of a fellow meteorologist in predicting tornadoes. Gilbert pointed out that because of the rarity of this meteorological event, high accuracy can be achieved simply by "calling" for "no tornado" every day.

As a second example, consider the colon polyp data in Tables 2.3 and 2.7. The sensitivity (0.88) and specificity (0.60) calculated from these two tables are the same, but note that the prevalence is different. From Table 2.3 the probability of a correct test result is (22 + 3) / 30, or 0.83. In Table 2.7, on the other hand, the probability of a correct test result is only 0.613. In Table 2.3, sensitivity is given more weight since the prevalence is 83%; in Table 2.7, specificity is given much more weight since the prevalence is very low. This example illustrates that although sensitivity and specificity *are* measures of the intrinsic accuracy of a test, the probability of a correct test result is *not* a measure of intrinsic accuracy.

Another limitation of the probability of a correct result is that it is calculated based on only one decision threshold. However, there are many potential decision thresholds, and the clinical application should determine which threshold is relevant. This is also a limitation of reporting only single pairs of sensitivity and specificity.

Still another limitation of the probability of a correct result is that it treats FP and FN results as if they were equally undesirable, but often this is not the case (Zweig and Campbell, 1993). One might be tempted to use this measure to compare two tests applied to the same population. Metz (1978) used the following example to illustrate the problem with this. Suppose test *A* has a sensitivity of 100% but specificity of 0%; test B has a specificity of 100% and sensitivity of 0%. If the prevalence of the condition is 50%, then both tests yield the same probability of a correct result, yet these two tests perform differently and patient management would be radically different.

2.2.3   Odds Ratio and Youden's Index

We mention two other measures which are often used in meta-analyses of the accuracy of diagnostic tests (See Chapter 7). One is the *odds ratio*, defined as the odds of a positive test result relative to a negative test result among patients with the condition divided by the odds of a positive test result relative to a negative test result among patients without the condition. The odds ratio can be written in terms of sensitivity and specificity:

$$ Odds\ Ratio = \frac{Se/(1-Se)}{(1-Sp)/Sp} = \frac{Se \times Sp}{FNR \times FPR}. $$

For the data in Tables 2.3 and 2.7, the odds ratio is the same, 11. An odds ratio of 1.0 indicates that the likelihood of a positive test result is the same for patients with and without the condition (i.e. Se=FPR). Odds ratios greater than 1.0 indicate that the odds of a positive test result is greater for patients with the condition; odds ratios less than one indicate that the odds of a positive test result is greater for patients without the condition.

The other index is *Youden's index*: Se+Sp-1, or written another way, Se-FPR. For the data in Tables 2.3 and 2.7, Youden's index is 0.48. It has a maximum value of 1.0 and a minimum value of 0.0; it reflects the likelihood of a positive result among patients with versus without the condition. Hilden and Glasziou (1996) showed that Youden's index can also be interpreted as a function of the expected regret achieved by the test, where regret is the difference between the action taken after performing a test and the best action that could have been taken in retrospect.

Unlike the probability of a correct test result, the odds ratio and Youden's index are not dependent on the prevalence of the condition in the sample. However, both the odds ratio and Youden's index share two limitations with the probability of a correct result. First, they are based on only one decision threshold when, in reality, many potential decision thresholds exist. To overcome this limitation, one could estimate these indices at each possible decision threshold and report the maximum value over all thresholds (Greiner et al., 2000). Second, these indices treat FP and FN results as equally undesirable. For example, suppose test A has sensitivity of 0.90 and specificity of 0.40, and test B has sensitivity of 0.40 and specificity of 0.90. The odds ratio and Youden's index of both tests are equivalent, 6.0 and 0.3, respectively, yet the two tests have very different properties.

In subsequent sections we discuss several other summary measures of accuracy which in many situations are preferable to the probability of a correct test result, the odds ratio, and Youden's index. These measures are associated with the *Receiver Operating Characteristic (ROC) curve.*

2.3   RECEIVER OPERATING CHARACTERISTIC (ROC) CURVE

In 1971 Lusted (1971) described a method, used often in psychophysics, that overcame the limitations of a single sensitivity and specificity pair by including all sensitivity and specificity pairs. A *Receiver Operating Characteristic*, or *ROC curve*, is a method of describing the intrinsic accuracy of a test apart from the decision thresholds. Since the 1970s, the ROC curve has been the most valuable tool for describing and comparing the accuracies of diagnostic tests.

An ROC curve is a plot of a test's sensitivity (plotted on the y-axis) versus its false positive rate (FPR), or (1-specificity) (plotted on the x-axis). Each point on the graph is generated by a different decision threshold. We use line segments to connect the points from the possible decision thresholds, forming an *empirical ROC curve*. We have seen that as the sensitivity of a test increases, its FPR also increases; the ROC curve shows precisely the magnitudes of the increases.

2.3.1   ROC Curves: Artificial Heart Valve and Case Study 1

Figures 2.2 and 2.3 illustrate the ROC curves for the heart valve-imaging (Table 2.4) and parathyroid gland data (Table 2.6), respectively.

In Figure 2.2 each circle on the empirical ROC curve represents a (FPR, Se) point corresponding to a different decision threshold. For example, the point at the far left (FPR=0.0, Se=0.5) corresponds to the decision threshold of > 0.13 (See Table 2.5). The point at the far right at (FPR=0.7, Se=1.0) corresponds to the decision threshold at > 0.0. Line segments connect the points generated from all possible decision thresholds. In this example data, there are nine decision thresholds that provide unique (FPR, Se) points, in addition to the two trivial points of (0,0) and (1,1). The nine thresholds were generated from the 10 different test results of the study patients (see Table 2.4).

In Table 2.6, there are k=5 categories for the test results. In the corresponding empirical ROC curve (Figure 2.3) there are k-1, or 4, nontrivial points connected with line segments. Point *A* on the curve, corresponding to the cutoff at the definitely diseased category, is a strict threshold in that only cases judged as definitely diseased are considered positive. Point *B* corresponds to the cutoff at the probably diseased category; it is a moderate threshold. Point *C* corresponds to the cutoff at the possibly diseased category and is a lax threshold.

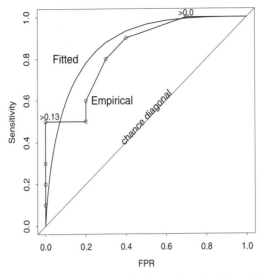

Figure 2.2   Empirical and Fitted ROC Curves for the Heart Valve-Imaging data

2.3.2   ROC Curve Assumption

An ROC curve can be constructed from objective measurements of a test (e.g. the gap value from the digitized image of a heart valve), objective evaluation of image features (e.g. attenuation coefficient of a lesion from computed tomography), or subjective diagnostic interpretations (e.g. the 5-category scale used for interpretation of SPECT images of parathyroid glands). The only requirement is that the measurements or interpretations can be meaningfully ranked in magnitude. With objective measurements the decision variable is explicit; one can choose from an infinite number of decision thresholds along the continuum of the test results. For diagnostic tests interpreted subjectively, the decision thresholds are implicit or latent, for they only exist in the mind of the observer (Hanley, 1989). An essential assumption for the ROC curve is that these decision thresholds are the same for the subsamples of patients with and without the condition. When the decision thresholds are implicit, this assumption may need to be tested (Zhou, 1995) (See Chapter 4). The concept of the ROC curve is the same whether the decision thresholds are explicit or implicit; the curve illustrates the trade-off between sensitivity and the FPR as the decision threshold changes.

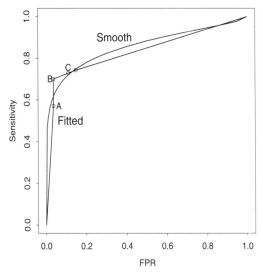

Figure 2.3 Empirical and Fitted ROC Curves of SPECT/CT in Case Study 1

2.3.3 Smooth, Fitted ROC Curves

While empirical ROC curves like the ones in Figures 2.2 and 2.3 are useful, they tend to have a jagged appearance, particularly with ordinal data and/or with small sample sizes. Alongside the empirical curve in Figures 2.2 and 2.3, we plotted an example of a *fitted ROC curve* (sometimes called a *smooth curve*). A smooth curve comes from a statistical model which one chooses to best resemble the test results from the sample of patients. In these examples we used the binormal model (i.e. two Gaussian distributions: one for the test results of patients without the condition, the other for test results of patients with the condition); it is the most commonly used model for fitting ROC curves in diagnostic medicine. When the binormal model is used, the ROC curve is completely specified by two parameters. The first parameter, denoted as a, is the standardized difference in means of the distributions of test results for patients with and without the condition. The second parameter, denoted as b, is the ratio of the standard deviations (SDs) of the distributions of test results for patients without versus with the condition. In Chapter 4, we discuss the binormal model of ROC curves in detail; in this chapter, it is important to note that the intrinsic accuracy of a test is completely defined by its ROC curve, which in many cases can be defined by the two parameters a and b.

2.3.4   Advantages of ROC Curves

The name "receiver operating characteristic" curve comes from the notion that, given the curve, we - the receivers of the information - can use (or operate at) any point on the curve by using the appropriate decision threshold. The clinical application determines which characteristics of the test are needed. Consider the heart valve data (Figure 2.2). If the imaging technique is used to screen asymptomatic people, we want good specificity to minimize the number of FPs because surgery to replace the valve is risky. We might choose a cutoff at 0.07, where the FPR is 0.20 and sensitivity is 0.60. On the other hand, if the technique is used to diagnose patients with chest pain, then a higher sensitivity is needed. In this setting, a cutoff at 0.03 is more appropriate, with sensitivity of 0.90 and FPR of 0.40. (We discuss the optimum choice of operating points for particular applications in Section 2.12.)

This example illustrates the advantages of the ROC curve over a figure such as Figure 2.1. Unlike Figure 2.1, an ROC curve is a visual representation of accuracy data: the scales of the curve (sensitivity and FPR) are the basic measures of accuracy and are easily read from the plot. Often the values of the decision variable that generated the points are labeled on the curve as well. The ROC curve does not require selection of a particular decision threshold since all possible decision thresholds are included. Because sensitivity and specificity are independent of prevalence, so, too, is the ROC curve. Like sensitivity and specificity, however, the ROC curve and associated indices may be affected by the spectrum of disease, as well as patient characteristics. We will discuss this further in Chapter 3.

Another advantage of the ROC curve is that it does not depend on the scale of the test results; that is, it is invariant to monotonic transformations of the test results, such as linear, logarithm, and square root (Campbell, 1994). In fact, the empirical curve depends only on the ranks of the observations, not on the actual magnitude of the test results.

Finally, the ROC curve provides a direct visual comparison of two or more tests on a common set of scales. As we saw in Table 2.8 with the parathyroid disease example, it is difficult to compare two tests when you only have one sensitivity, specificity pair. The performance of one test is superior to another only if the test is both more specific and more sensitive, equally specific and more sensitive, or equally sensitive and more specific. Even if one of these cases holds, however, it is difficult to determine how much better the test is when a change in the decision threshold occurs because such a change in threshold may affect the two tests differently (Turner, 1978). By constructing the ROC curve, a comparison of tests at all decision thresholds is possible.

2.4   AREA UNDER THE ROC CURVE

As noted in Section 2.2, it is often useful to summarize the accuracy of a test by a single number. Several such summary indices are associated with the ROC curve, including the most popular: the *area under the ROC curve, AUC*, or just *A*.

The ROC area is the area bounded above by the ROC curve itself, to the left and right by the parallel y-axes, and below by the x-axis. The ROC area can take on values between zero and 1.0. An ROC curve with an area of 1.0 consists of two line segments: (0,0)-(0,1) and (0,1)-(1,1). Such a test is perfectly accurate because the sensitivity is 1.0 when the FPR is 0.0. Unfortunately, such diagnostic tests are rare. In contrast, a test with an area of 0.0 is perfectly inaccurate; that is, patients with the condition are always labeled incorrectly as negative and patients without the condition are always labeled incorrectly as positive. If such a test existed, it would be trivial to convert it into one with perfect accuracy by reversing the test results. The practical lower bound for the ROC area is then 0.5. The (0,0)-(1,1) line segment has an area of 0.5; it is called the *chance diagonal*. If we relied on pure chance to distinguish patients with versus without the condition, the resulting ROC curve would fall along this diagonal line.

Diagnostic tests with ROC curves above the chance diagonal have at least some ability to discriminate between patients with and without the condition. The closer the curve gets to the (0,1) point (left upper corner), the better the test. As we will discuss in Chapter 4, it is often appropriate to test whether the ROC area is different from 0.50. Rejection of this hypothesis implies that the test has some ability to distinguish patients with versus without the condition.

2.4.1   Interpretation of the Area Under the ROC Curve

The ROC area has several interpretations: (1) the average value of sensitivity for all possible values of specificity; (2) the average value of specificity for all possible values of sensitivity (Metz, 1986) (Metz, 1989); and (3) the probability that a randomly selected patient with the condition has a test result indicating greater suspicion than a randomly chosen patient without the condition (Hanley and McNeil, 1982).

This third interpretation comes from the work of Green and Swets (1966) and Hanley and McNeil (1982). They showed that the area under the true ROC curve is linked to the *two-alternative forced choice (2-AFC) experiment* used in psychophysics. (By "true ROC curve" we mean the empirical curve if it is constructed from an infinitely large sample of patients and an infinite number of decision thresholds. Note that the fitted curve is an estimate of this true curve.) In a 2-AFC experiment two stimuli are presented to an observer, where one stimulus is *noise* and the other is *signal*. The observer identifies the signal stimulus; the area under the ROC curve is the frequency with which the observer correctly identifies the signal.

The area under the ROC curve constructed from ordinal or continuous data retains this same meaning, even though the 2-AFC experiment is not performed (Hanley and McNeil, 1982). This is easy to understand by considering how the area under the empirical ROC is estimated. Let X denote the test result for a patient with the condition and Y the test result for a patient without the condition. We have n_1 patients in the sample with the condition (i.e. we have n_1 X's) and n_0 patients in the sample without the condition (n_0 Y's). We pair up each X with each Y. For each pair, we assign a score of 1 if the patient with the condition has a more suspicious test result than the patient without the condition, we assign a score of 0 if the patient without the condition has a more suspicious test result than the patient with the condition, and we assign a score of $1/2$ if the two patients have the same test result. The sum of these scores, after all possible pairings have been evaluated, divided by the total number of these pairs, is the estimate of the area under the empirical ROC curve. We write this as

$$\hat{A} = \frac{1}{n_0 \times n_1} \sum_{all\,X's} \sum_{all\,Y's} \Psi(X,Y) \tag{2.1}$$

where $\sum_n Z$ just means to take the sum of Z over all the n's, and $\Psi(X,Y)$ is where we evaluate each X, Y pair as follows: $\Psi(X,Y) = 1$ if $X > Y$, $\Psi(X,Y) = 0$ if $X < Y$, and $\Psi(X,Y) = 1/2$ if X=Y. (See Chapter 4 for more details.)

The notion that the area under the ROC curve is the probability of correctly ordering patients, one with and one without the condition, based on their test results can be further extended to each point on the ROC curve itself. Pepe and Cai (2004) showed that the ROC curve at a certain cutpoint can be thought of as the probability that the test result of a patient with the condition is greater (more suspicious) than the test result of a patient without the condition, given that the test result of the latter is at the specified cutpoint on the ROC curve. This insight allows one to test hypotheses about the ROC curve using standard binary regression techniques (see Chapter 8).

2.4.2   Magnitudes of the Area Under the ROC Curve

Table 2.4.2 summarizes the ROC areas of several imaging and laboratory diagnostic tests. Most of these ROC areas are based on a meta-analysis of existing studies (we talk about meta-analysis more in Chapter 7 and 12). Note that there is a large range in ROC curve areas of these common diagnostic tests. It is difficult to label a certain range of ROC curve area magnitudes as "poor" and "good" because it depends on the disorder and clinical application. However, the table does allow us to put ROC areas of new tests in context with some commonly used and accepted diagnostic tests.

2.4.3   Area Under the ROC Curve: Case Study 1

In Table 2.8 we compared the sensitivity and specificity of three tests for detecting parathyroid disease and discussed the difficulty in identifying the

Table 2.9   ROC Areas for Some Diagnostic Tests

Target Disorder	Patient Population	Diagnostic Test (gold standard)	ROC Area (Ref)
Breast cancer	Women presenting for screening	film-screen mammography (biopsy or two) (years followup)	0.74 - 0.95 (Jensen et al.:2006)
Multiple Sclerosis (MS)	Patients with signs and symptoms of MS	MRI CT (expert panel)	0.82 0.52 (Mushlin et al.:1993)
Herniated nucleus pulposus-caused nerve compression	Patients with acute low back and radicular pain	MRI CT CT myelography (expert panel)	0.81-0.84 0.86 0.83 (Thornbury et al.:1993)
Fetal pulmonary maturity	Infants who were delivered within 72 hours of amniotic fluid testing	Lecithin/sphingomyelin ratio Saturated phosphatidylcholine (evaluation of newborn)	0.70-0.88 0.65-0.85 (Hunink et al.:1990)
Tumor staging in non-small cell bronchogenic carcinoma	Patients with known or suspected non-small cell bronchogenic carcinoma	CT /MRI (surgery or biopsy)	Chest Wall Invasion: 0.86 / 0.87 Bronchial Involvement: 0.83 / 0.78 Mediastinal Invasion: 0.83 / 0.92 Mediastinal Node Metastase 0.60 / 0.60 (Webb et al.:199
Obstructive airways disease	Subjects presenting to the pulmonary function test lab	Forced expiratory time (spirometry)	0.63 (Schapira et al.:1993)

best test based only on a single sensitivity, specificity pair. The last column of Table 2.8 gives the estimated areas under the empirical ROC curves. Clearly,

SPECT-CT, with an ROC area of 0.83, has superior accuracy relative to no AC-SPECT and AC-SPECT. We interpret an ROC area of 0.83 as follows: if we select, at random, two glands - one with and one without parathyroid disease - the probability is 0.83 that the diseased gland will be rated as more suspicious than the normal gland. The area under the binormal-fitted curve (see Figure 2.3) is slightly larger at 0.86. Unless the number of decision thresholds is large, the area under the empirical ROC curve is usually less than the area under the fitted curve (See Chapter 4).

In Figure 2.4 the fitted ROC curve for SPECT-CT is illustrated along with the fitted ROC curve for AC-SPECT (ROC area under this fitted curve is 0.73). Note the two labeled points on these ROC curves. These represent the sensitivity and FPR pair corresponding to a positive test criterion of "possible disease" or higher which was used in Table 2.8. Studying Figure 2.4 we see that at every FPR point, the sensitivity of SPECT-CT is superior to AC-SPECT. This example illustrates that comparison of two tests based on only a single sensitivity and FPR pair can be misleading. The ROC curves and the area under the curves nicely illustrate how the tests compare. In the next subsection we discuss situations where the area under the ROC curve can be misleading.

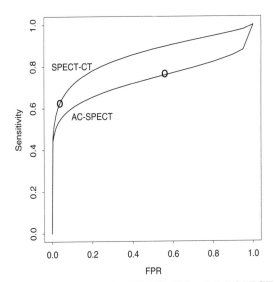

Figure 2.4 Fitted ROC Curves for SPECT-CT and AC-SPECT in Case Study 1

2.4.4 Misinterpretations of the Area Under the ROC Curve

In some situations, the ROC curve area, when used as a summary measure of diagnostic accuracy, can be misleading. Hilden (1991) offers a hypothetical example of a perfectly discriminating test with ROC curve area of only 0.5. Suppose that patients without the condition have test values between 80 and 120, while one half of patients with the condition have values less than 80 and the other half have values greater than 120. The ROC curve, shown in Figure 2.5, consists of the line segments: (0.0, 0.0)-(0.0, 0.5); (0.0, 0.5)-(1.0, 0.5); and (1.0, 0.5)-(1.0, 1.0).

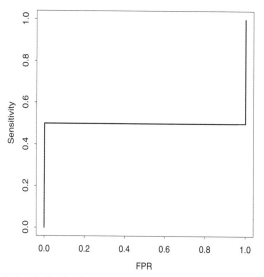

Figure 2.5   A Perfectly Discriminating Test with ROC Area of 0.5

    The ROC area is 0.5, yet the test discriminates perfectly between patients with and without the condition (i.e. there are no overlaps between patients with and without the condition). If T denotes the original test result, then constructing an ROC curve using the transformation: $T' = \mid T - 100 \mid$ leads to an ROC curve area of 1.0. For the rest of this book, we assume that, when appropriate, a test's results have been transformed so that as the value of the test result increases, the likelihood of the condition increases.

    A real example when such a transformation is necessary is a test for atherosclerosis of the carotid arteries. Ultrasound is used to measure the velocity of the blood as it passes through the vessels. The velocity increases as the extent of disease increases; however, when a vessel is completely occluded, the velocity is zero. To estimate the ROC area of the velocity measurements, Hunink et al. (1993) assigned ranks to the velocity measurements, but instead of assigning the lowest rank to the zero velocities, they assigned the highest rank so that the largest-valued test result would have the highest likelihood of atherosclerosis.

As we've learned, the ROC area describes a test's inherent ability to discriminate between patients with versus without the condition. This is because the ROC area is invariant to the prevalence of the condition and the cutoffs used to form the curve. Such a measure of diagnostic accuracy is useful in the early stages of a diagnostic test's evaluation, but once a test's ability to distinguish between patients with and without the condition is shown, its role for particular applications must be evaluated. At this stage, we may be interested only in a small portion of the ROC curve. For example, if we use the heart valve-imaging technique to screen asymptomatic patients, we are interested only in the part of the ROC curve where the specificity is high; we will adjust our decision threshold to ensure that the specificity is high. We are not interested in the average sensitivity over all specificities or the average specificity over all sensitivities. As a global measure of intrinsic accuracy, the ROC area is not always relevant.

Similarly, the ROC area may be misleading when comparing the accuracy of two tests. The ROC areas of two tests may be equal but the tests may differ in clinically important regions of the curve. Likewise, the ROC curve areas may differ but the tests may have the same area in the clinically relevant region of the curve. Figure 2.6 illustrates two ROC curves that cross at a FPR of 0.14. The area under curve A is greater than the area under curve B (i.e. 0.85 versus 0.80). If the clinically relevant region of the curve is at low FPRs, test B is preferable to test A despite the greater ROC curve area for A.

Finally, we note that while the ROC curve and its area are considered to be inherent properties of a diagnostic test, it should be recognized that the ROC curve of a diagnostic test depends on the characteristics of the patient, the clinician interpreting the test results, and the machine and technician capturing the images (Greenland, 2008). These vary across populations and time. Furthermore, while the ROC curve itself illustrates the trade-off in errors (false positives versus false negatives) at various cut-points, the ROC area does not contain this detailed information. This detail is important, however, in order to measure the utility of a diagnostic test (that is, the effect on the patient's outcome and monetary costs of incorrect and correct diagnoses) (Hilden, 2000). In fact, Hilden has shown that there exists no summary index that is both unaffected by the prevalence of the condition and able to correctly incorporate the utility of the test. Thus, in planning a diagnostic test accuracy study and reporting its result, it is important to consider how the results of the study can be generalized and how they can not.

In the next two sections we present two alternative summary measures of intrinsic accuracy which focus on only a portion of the ROC curve, thus overcoming some of the limitations of the area under the whole curve.

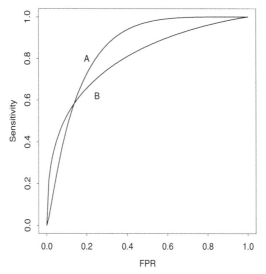

Figure 2.6   Two Tests with Crossing ROC Curves

2.5   SENSITIVITY AT FIXED FPR

An alternative summary measure of intrinsic accuracy is the *sensitivity at a fixed FPR*, or, similarly, the *FPR at a fixed sensitivity*. We write these as $Se_{(FPR=e)}$ or $FPR_{(Se=e)}$. For a predetermined FPR of e (or predetermined sensitivity of e), the sensitivity (or FPR) is estimated from the ROC curve.

This measure of accuracy allows us to focus on the particular portion of the ROC curve of clinical relevance. The characteristics of the clinical application, such as the prevalence of the condition and the consequences of misdiagnoses, determine at which FPR or sensitivity we need to operate (See Section 2.12). Consider the ROC curves of SPECT-CT and AC-SPECT illustrated in Figure 2.4. At FPR=0.05, the sensitivity of SPECT-CT is 0.65, compared to the sensitivity of AC-SPECT of 0.56. (See Chapter 4 for a description of how to estimate the sensitivity at a fixed FPR.)

The sensitivity at a fixed FPR is often preferable to the ROC curve area when evaluating a test for a particular application. This measure also has a simple and clinically useful interpretation. One disadvantage of this measure is that reported sensitivities from other studies are often at different FPRs; thus comparisons with published literature can be problematic. A second disadvantage is that published reports are not always clear regarding whether the FPR was selected before the start of the study (as it should be) or after the data were examined (a practice which can introduce bias) (Hanley, 1989).

A third disadvantage is that the statistical reliability of this measure is lower (i.e. the variance is larger) than that of the ROC curve area (Hanley, 1989; Obuchowski and McClish, 1997) (See Chapter 6).

2.6 PARTIAL AREA UNDER THE ROC CURVE

Another summary measure of a diagnostic test's intrinsic accuracy is the *partial area under the ROC curve*. As its name implies, it is the area under a portion of the ROC curve, often defined as the area between two FPRs, e_1 and e_2. We write this: $A_{(e_1 \leq FPR \leq e_2)}$. Similarly, we can define the area between two sensitivities, for which we write $A_{(e_1 \leq Se \leq e_2)}$. If $e_1 = 0$ and $e_2 = 1$, the area under the entire ROC curve is specified; if $e_1 = e_2$, then the sensitivity at a fixed FPR of e (or FPR at a fixed sensitivity of e) will be given. The partial area measure is thus a compromise between the ROC curve area and the sensitivity at a fixed FPR.

Like the sensitivity at a fixed FPR index, the partial area allows one to focus on the portion of the ROC curve relevant to a particular clinical application. In Figure 2.6, if a FPR range is restricted to 0.0-0.05, the partial area for test B will be larger than for test A. If we include larger FPRs, such as 0.0-0.30, then the partial area for test B will be similar to test A. (See Chapter 4 for a description of how to estimate the partial area under the ROC curve.)

To interpret the partial area, we must consider its maximum possible value. The maximum area is equal to the width of the interval, that is $(e_2 - e_1)$ (Mc-Clish, 1989). McClish (1989) and Jiang et al. (1996) recommend standardizing the partial area by dividing by its maximum value; Jiang et al. refer to this standardized partial area as the *partial area index*. This index is interpreted as the average sensitivity for the range of specificities examined (or average specificity for the range of sensitivities examined), an interpretation that is highly useful clinically. For example, in Figure 2.4 the partial areas under the ROC curve for SPECT-CT and SPECT in the clinically relevant range of 0.0 to 0.10 are 0.062 and 0.054. The partial area indices are 0.62 and 0.54, respectively, which we interpret as the average sensitivities of SPECT-CT and SPECT in the 0.0-0.10 FPR range.

Dwyer (1997) offers a probabilistic interpretation of the partial area index when the partial area is defined for sensitivities greater than or equal to e_1 (i.e. $A_{(e_1 \leq Se \leq 1.0)}$). The partial area index equals the probability that a randomly chosen patient without the condition will be correctly distinguished from a randomly chosen patient with the condition who tested negative for the criterion that corresponds to Se=e_1. For example, suppose we want to estimate $A_{(0.8 \leq Se \leq 1.0)}$ from the gap values in Table 2.4. From Table 2.5 we know that a cutoff of > 0.05 corresponds to an observed sensitivity of 0.80. Among the 10 patients with a fractured valve, two tested negative using this criterion (i.e. two patients had gap values ≤ 0.05). The partial area index is the probability that a randomly chosen patient with an intact valve will be correctly distinguished from a patient like one of the foregoing. An analogous interpretation for $A_{(0.0 \leq FPR \leq e_2)}$ is the probability that a randomly chosen patient with the condition will be correctly distinguished from a randomly chosen patient without the condition who tested positive for the criterion that corresponds to FPR=e_2. Note the similarities between this and the probabilistic interpretation of the ROC curve area.

A potential problem with the partial area measure is that the minimum possible value depends on the location along the ROC curve. The minimum partial area is equal to $(1/2)(e_2 - e_1)(e_2 + e_1)$ (McClish, 1989). For example, the minimum value for $A_{(0 \leq FPR \leq 0.2)}$ is 0.02 (maximum value is 0.20) and the minimum value for $A_{(0.8 \leq FPR \leq 1.0)}$ is 0.18 (maximum value is 0.20). Suppose that we estimated a partial area of 0.19 for both of these FPR ranges; the partial area index, 0.95, is the same for both ranges. However, we would probably not value these two areas the same. To remedy this problem, McClish offers a transformation of the partial area to values between 0.5 and 1.0. The formula is as follows:

$$\frac{1}{2}[1 + \frac{A_{(e_1 \leq FPR \leq e_2)} - min}{max - min}] \tag{2.2}$$

where min and max are the minimum and maximum possible values for the partial area. Continuing with this example, the partial area of 0.19 is transformed to 0.972 for the 0-0.2 FPR range and 0.75 for the 0.8-1.0 FPR range.

The partial area measure has similar limitations to the sensitivity at a fixed FPR. First, it is difficult to compare this measure with the published literature if different ranges are used. Second, the relevant range should be specified a priori; it is not always clear from published reports whether this occurs. Third, the statistical reliability of this measure is lower than that of the ROC area, but greater than that of the sensitivity at a fixed FPR (Hanley, 1989; Obuchowski and McClish, 1997) (See Chapter 6).

2.7 LIKELIHOOD RATIOS

Still another single index of diagnostic accuracy is the *likelihood ratio* (LR), the ratio of the following two probabilities: the probability of a particular test result among patients with the condition to the probability of that test result among patients without the condition. The LR can be defined as

$$LR(t) = \frac{P(T = t \mid D = 1)}{P(T = t \mid D = 0)}, \tag{2.3}$$

where t can be a single test value, an interval of test values, or one side of a decision threshold. When the test result refers to one side of a decision threshold, we have *positive and negative LRs*, where

$$LR(+) = \frac{P(T = 1 \mid D = 1)}{P(T = 1 \mid D = 0)}$$

and

$$LR(-) = \frac{P(T = 0 \mid D = 1)}{P(T = 0 \mid D = 0)}.$$

Note that the LR(+) is the ratio of sensitivity to the FPR. Likewise, LR(-) is the ratio of the FNR to specificity. The LR reflects the magnitude of evidence that a particular test result provides in favor of the presence of the condition relative to the absence of the condition. A LR of 1.0 indicates that the test result is equally likely in patients with and without the condition; a $LR > 1.0$ indicates that the test result is more likely among patients with the condition than without the condition; and a $LR < 1.0$ indicates that the test result is more likely among patients without the condition. The higher the LR, the more likely the test result is among patients with the condition relative to patients without the condition.

2.7.1   Three Examples to Illustrate Likelihood Ratios

First, consider the parathyroid example (Case Study 1) given in Table 2.6. Let's choose a decision threshold at 3, such that patients classified as 3, 4, or 5 are called positive. The LR(+) = Se/FPR = 0.729/0.111 = 6.57; LR(-) = FNR/Sp = 0.271/0.889 = 0.30. Thus, a positive test result is 6 times more likely in glands with parathyroid disease than glands without; a negative test result is 3 (i.e. 1/0.30) times more likely in glands without parathyroid disease.

Table 2.10 summarizes the probability of various gap values for patients with and without valve fractures. The last column gives the LR(t). Gap values between 0.031 and 0.050 are equally likely in patients with and without a fractured valve (i.e. probability of 0.10), whereas gap values between 0.051 and 0.070 are twice as likely in patients with a fractured valve.

Table 2.10   Estimating LR(t) from Heart Valve Imaging Study

Test Result, t	$P(T = t \mid D = 0)$	$P(T = t \mid D = 1)$	LR(t)
0.0	0.3	0.0	0.0
0.001-0.030	0.3	0.1	0.33
0.031-0.050	0.1	0.1	1.0
0.051-0.070	0.1	0.2	2.0
0.071-0.100	0.0	0.1	undefined
0.101-0.130	0.2	0.0	0.0
> 0.0	0.7	1.0	1.43
> 0.03	0.4	0.9	2.25
> 0.05	0.3	0.8	2.67
> 0.07	0.2	0.6	3.0
> 0.15	0.0	0.3	undefined

Note that the numerator of the LR(+) is the y coordinate of the ROC curve (i.e. sensitivity). The denominator of the LR(+) is the x-coordinate of the ROC curve (i.e. false positive rate). The LR for an interval of test values, t_1-t_2, corresponds to the slope of the line segment between t_1 and t_2 on the ROC curve (Choi, 1998). The ROC curve labeled 'A' in Figure 2.7 corresponds to the gap measurement of the heart valve-imaging study (see Table 2.10).

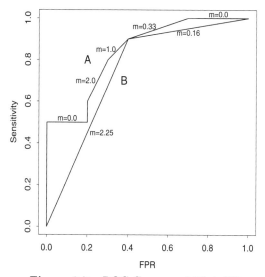

Figure 2.7   ROC Curves and Their LRs

The line connecting the (FPR,Se) coordinate for the decision threshold at 0.0 and the (FPR,Se) coordinate for the decision threshold at 0.03 has a slope of 0.33, which corresponds to the LR(0.001-0.030) from Table 2.10. One can verify this equivalence by computing the change in sensitivity divided by the change in FPR for these two points - that is, from the bottom of Table 2.10: (1.0-0.9)/(0.7-0.4) = 0.33. Similarly, the slope of the line between the (FPR,Se) coordinates corresponding to decision thresholds at 0.03 and 0.05 is 1.0, which is the LR(0.031-0.050). The ROC curve labeled B has the single point (Se=0.9, FPR=0.4) from the decision threshold > 0.03. The slope of the line from the origin to this point is 2.25 - that is, the LR(+) for the > 0.03 cutoff. For ROC curve B, the slope is the ratio of Se/FPR, or LR(+). More generally, the slope is the change in sensitivity divided by the change in FPR over the defined interval of test results as in ROC curve A (Zweig and Campbell, 1993).

As a third example, consider the study by Mushlin et al. (1993) where they used LRs to assess the accuracy of MRI in identifying multiple sclerosis (MS). Two observers assigned one of the following rating categories to each of 303 patients: "definitely not MS," "probably not MS," "possible MS," "probable MS," and "definite MS." The corresponding LRs were 0.3, 0.3, 1.3, 2.9, and 24.9. Although the accuracy of MRI was less than definitive (ROC area =0.82), the authors concluded that a "definite MS" reading essentially establishes the diagnosis of MS. However, 25% of patients with MS were classified as "probably not MS" or "definitely not MS"; thus these diagnoses are not sufficient to rule out MS.

2.7.2 Limitations of Likelihood Ratios

Zweig and Campbell (1993) note that LRs can be easily misinterpreted. Consider the CTC polyp data in Tables 2.3 and 2.7. The LR(+), 2.2, is the same in both tables; thus, it is correct to say that a positive result is 2.2 times more likely in patients with polyps as compared with patients without polyps. It is not necessarily correct to say that given a positive test result, a patient is 2.2 times more likely to have a polyp than to not have a polyp. The latter statement is a reflection of the prevalence rate in the population. For example, in Table 2.3 (prevalence of polyps is 83%), given a positive test result, the ratio of patients with polyps to without polyps is 11 (i.e. 22:2 equals 11:1). In contrast, in Table 2.7 (with a prevalence of just under 5%), the ratio is 0.11 (i.e. 220:2000), indicating that it is much more likely that a patient with a positive test result does not have polyps.

While the LR is an intrinsic measure of diagnostic accuracy because the measure itself is unaffected by the prevalence of disease (e.g. the LR(+) equals 2.2 in both Tables 2.3 and 2.7), it has some limitations when used as a single measure of accuracy. Like all ratios of two random variables, it is difficult to estimate its standard error (SE) and statistical distribution (See Chapter 4). Zweig and Campbell (1993) illustrate that a LR without an accompanying ROC curve can be misleading. They present two ROC curves with identical LRs for the line segments forming the curves, but the two curves have vastly different ROC curve areas. The two identical curves are parallel, with one located near the upper left corner and the other near the chance diagonal. Thus, we recommend that investigators using LRs also illustrate the test's ROC curve, and/or its area.

The primary role of the LR is in Bayes Theorem (see Section 2.11) and in defining the decision threshold that is optimal for particular clinical applications (Section 2.12).

2.7.3 Proper and Improper ROC Curves

Most ROC curves are concave as in Figures 2.2 and 2.3. Figure 2.8 illustrates a proper ROC curve. Occasionally, however, a diagnostic test will have a ROC curve with a "hook," defined as a portion of the ROC curve that lies below the chance diagonal (Pan and Metz, 1997). These curves are called *improper ROC curves* (Metz and Kronman, 1980). The distinction between *proper* and *improper* ROC curves is based on the LR. Figure 2.9 illustrates an improper ROC curve.

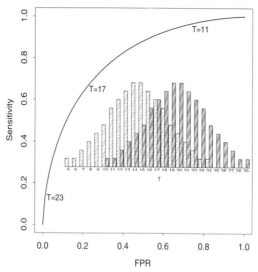

Figure 2.8 A Proper ROC Curve

The insets in both figures depict the corresponding distributions of test results for hypothetical patients: the light shading denotes the test results for patients without the condition, whereas the darker shading denotes the test results of patients with the condition. In Figure 2.8, the distributions of the test results of patients with and without the condition are identical but shifted apart. The corresponding ROC curve is a decreasing function of the LR. At the bottom left corner of the curve, corresponding to large test values, the LR is > 1.0. The LR decreases along the curve's path. At $T=17$, the LR $=1.0$. At the top right corner of the curve, corresponding to small test values, the LR is < 1.0. Proper ROC curves, such as the one depicted in Fig. 2.8, are monotonic functions of the LR (Pan and Metz, 1997).

In contrast, in Figure 2.9 there is more variability in the test results of patients without the condition. At the far bottom left corner of the ROC curve and at the far top right corner, the LR is < 1.0. The probability that $T=16$ is the same for patients with and without the condition; thus the LR $= 1.0$. Similarly, at $T=21$ the LR $= 1.0$; when T is between 16 and 21, the LR is > 1.0. This ROC curve is an improper ROC curve because it is not a monotonic function of the LR. The curve has the characteristic "hook"

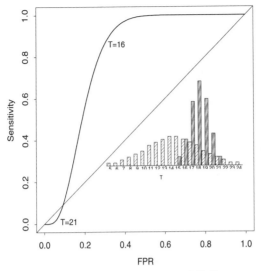

Figure 2.9   An Improper ROC Curve

(Pan and Metz, 1997) at the bottom left. Problems can occur in estimating improper ROC curves; see Chapter 4 for a discussion.

2.8   ROC ANALYSIS WHEN THE TRUE DIAGNOSIS IS NOT BINARY

In this chapter, and for most of this book, we describe methods for analyzing diagnostic test accuracy studies when the objective of the diagnostic test is to differentiate between two possible scenarios: the condition is present versus the condition is not present (binary-scale). There are many examples, however, of diagnostic tests that are performed to differentiate between more than two conditions or to measure the magnitude of a substance.

1. Computed Tomography (CT) is used to differentiate between various distinct pulmonary diseases in symptomatic patients: normal, interstitial disease, nodules, or pneumothorax (polychotomous- or nominal-scale).

2. In stroke patients, positron emission tomography (PET) classifies the regions of the heart as an ordering of a worsening condition: normal, hibernating, ischemic, or necrotic (ordinal-scale).

3. The creatinine blood test measures the amount of creatinine in the blood; creatinine is a chemical waste molecule whose concentration in the blood increases when the kidneys are not functioning correctly (continuous-scale).

The traditional ROC curve can be used to measure diagnostic test accuracy of nominal-, ordinal-, and continuous-scale tests by dichotomizing the true diagnosis. For example, we might group together the PET heart results of hibernating, ischemic, and necrotic as abnormal. Similarly, we might classify interstitial disease, nodules, and pneumothorax as abnormal lung conditions. Finally, we may define a blood creatinine of 10.0 milligrams per deciliter or greater as abnormal. This approach, however, can conceal clinically important information about the performance of the diagnostic test and can lead to biased estimates of test accuracy (Obuchowski et al., 2004).

There have been a few published papers describing measures of diagnostic accuracy for conditions that are nominal-, ordinal-, and continuous-scale. Kijewski et al. (1989) were one of the first to consider the problem of a diagnostic test for an ordinal-scale condition. They proposed an extension of the ROC curve for any number of ordinal levels, but no summary measure of accuracy was proposed. Mossman (1999) described a three-dimensional ROC curve for exactly three nominal truth states. He illustrated an ROC surface on 3D coordinates and described a summary measure of accuracy, the volume under the ROC surface (VUS), which is interpreted as the probability that test values can be used to correctly sort out a trio of patients, one patient from each of three truth states. Dreiseitl et al. (2000) later developed statistical methods for comparing competing tests' volumes. The idea was further extended to any number of truth states (Edwards et al., 2004).

An important distinction between binary-scale tests and tests with more than two truth states is the format used for assessing the reader's confidence in the presence of the condition(s). In Section 2.1.3 we talked about a five-point ordinal scale and a 0-100% confidence scale for describing a reader's confidence that a condition is present. Rockette (1994) extended this idea to the nominal scale by asking the reader to grade their confidence in the presence of each possible condition (i.e. interstitial disease, nodules, and pneumothorax) against the absence of that particular condition. He then constructed an ROC curve for each condition and took a weighted average of the curves' ROC areas as a summary measure of overall accuracy. A limitation of this approach is that the summary measure describes the test's ability to differentiate between each condition and the absence of that condition, but not between two diseased conditions (i.e. interstitial disease versus nodules). The original idea was later extended to the *differential diagnosis*, where the reader is given a list of all possible conditions and asked to assign each condition a confidence score between zero and 100, such that the sum of all of the scores for a patient is equal to 100 (Obuchowski et al., 2001). A summary measure of accuracy can be computed based on all pairwise comparisons of each condition versus all other conditions.

Obuchowski (2006) described a summary measure of test accuracy when the condition is continuous-scale. The summary measure is a simple extension of the traditional, binary-scale area under the ROC curve and can be interpreted in much the same way. Similar to the equation (2.1), the summary measure for continuous-scale tests can be written as

$$\hat{A} = \frac{1}{n \times (n-1)} \sum_{all X_1's} \sum_{all X_2's} \Psi(X_1, X_2) \qquad (2.4)$$

where X_1 and X_2 are test results from different patients, n is the total number of patients, and $\Psi(X_1, X_2)$ is where we evaluate each X_1, X_2 pair. Consider as an example a hand-held quick test to measure creatinine. The results of the quick test are compared to the gold standard blood test. To estimate the accuracy of the quick test, we evaluate each X_1, X_2 pair of patients, as follows: $\Psi(X_1, X_2) = 1$ if the quick test and blood test both measured higher creatinine for patient 1 than for patient 2, or both measure higher creatinine for patient 2 than for patient 1, $\Psi(X_1, X_2) = 0$ if the quick test measured higher creatinine for patient 2 but patient 1 had a higher blood creatinine or vice versa, and $\Psi(X, Y) = 1/2$ otherwise.

Its interpretation is similar also: given two randomly chosen patients, the summary measure is the probability that the patient with a higher gold standard outcome (e.g. higher blood creatinine) has a higher diagnostic test result (i.e. higher result on a hand-held quick test) than a randomly chosen patient with a lower gold standard outcome. This simple extension of the ROC area was extended to a family of summary measures of accuracy for tests used to interpret nominal-, ordinal-, and continuous-scale conditions (Obuchowski, 2005).

2.9 C-STATISTICS AND OTHER MEASURES TO COMPARE PREDICTION MODELS

The discussion thus far has focused on assessing the accuracy of diagnostic tests. Another application for the use of these measures, particularly the area under the ROC curve, is the assessment of prediction and prognostic models. Prediction models describe people at risk for a particular disease and give a prediction, usually a probability, for the likelihood that a patient will develop the disease. Prognostic models, on the other hand, describe people with disease and predict their prognosis (e.g. death or recovery). For example, the Framingham risk score is a model of several risk factors used to predict a person's risk of cardiovascular disease (called the "event"). When new risk factors or biomarkers are identified, physicians want to assess whether the new risk factor improves the old model's accuracy. In this section we briefly describe how measures of diagnostic accuracy are used to compare models and refer the reader to references on this topic.

One of the most common approaches to comparing prediction or prognostic models is to examine the *concordance-index*, or *c-index* of the models. The c-index is equivalent to the area under the empirical ROC curve. This metric describes how well the model discriminates between people with and without an event (Harrell et al., 1996). Another important attribute of prediction/prognostic models is their calibration (Cook, 2007). Calibration is a measure of how well the predicted probability of an event agrees with the actual frequency of the event. Discrimination, on the other hand, is a measure of how well the model separates those who will and those who will not develop the event. A model can discriminate well as long as the predicted probabilities are higher for those patients who will eventually have an event and lower for those patients who do not suffer the event; the predicted probabilities don't have to be precise for good discrimination. In the context of diagnostic tests, discrimination is important because the patient's symptoms focus attention on a particular disease and the goal is then to identify those with the disease and to send home those without it. In contrast, in prediction/prognostic models, both discrimination and calibration are important because it is important to classify patients into risk strata requiring different management strategies (Ware and Cai, 2008).

For comparing prediction/prognostic models, a global measure of model fit, such as the Bayes Information Criterion (Harrell, 2001) or metrics developed by Pencina et al. (2008) can be applied. Both calibration, using the Hosmer-Lemeshow statistic (Hosmer and Lemeshow, 1989) or the Brier score (Redelmeier et al., 1991), and discrimination, using the concordance index, can be measured separately. It is also important to determine how many subjects would be reclassified into clinical risk categories and if reclassification is more accurate with the new model (Cook, 2007; Ridker and Cook, 2004). Finally, if a new invasive or expensive biomarker is being evaluated, the costs relative to the benefit of improvement in reclassification can be measured through decision analysis (Vickers and Elkin, 2006).

2.10 DETECTION AND LOCALIZATION OF MULTIPLE LESIONS

Some diagnostic tasks are more complicated than simply detecting patients with the condition. For example, in colon cancer screening, patients can have multiple polyps; these lesions must be correctly located prior to follow-up procedures like biopsy and surgery. Another example is the detection of infarcts in a patient suspected of having a stroke. Multiple infarcts can occur and treatment depends on their location, making detection and localization of the infarcts especially critical.

For diagnostic tests designed to locate and assess lesions, estimators of sensitivity must require that the lesion be correctly located. If a lesion is found but the location does not match the gold standard's location of the lesion, then the detected lesion is a false positive and the missed true lesion is a false negative. For example, in Case Study 2, a true positive occurred when the reader correctly located a polyp and scored it as suspicious on the five-point confidence scale. If the reader did not see the true polyp but instead detected a skin fold, then the true polyp was assigned the lowest confidence score (1=definitely not a polyp), and the skin fold was a false positive.

A second important consideration in defining the accuracy of these diagnostic and screening tests is the number of true lesions among patients with the condition. If there is usually one lesion among patients with the condition, then *patient-level* estimators of diagnostic accuracy are appropriate. If diseased patients often have more than one lesion, then *lesion-level* estimators of diagnostic accuracy are needed. For example, in Case Study 2 there were 39 colon polyps in 25 patients. In Table 2.3 we summarized the patient-level data and estimated the sensitivity: 22 of 25 patients had at least one polyp detected, or 88%. At the patient-level, as long as the reader found one polyp, the patient is considered a true positive. In contrast, a lesion-level estimator of sensitivity is the proportion of true polyps that are correctly located and scored as suspicious: 33 true positive polyps among 39 true polyps, or 85%. The patient-level estimate of sensitivity can often be considerably higher than the lesion-level estimate especially when there are many lesions per diseased patient, though the bias is not serious in this example (Obuchowski et al., 2010).

To characterize the false positive rate of tests designed to detect and locate lesions, two metrics should be reported: i) the number of patients with one or more false findings among patients without the condition, and ii) the average number of false positives per patient. In Case Study 2 among the 5 patients without polyps two were falsely identified as having at least one lesion: 2 of 5 patients, or 40%. Among the 30 total patients, there were 16 total false findings: an average of 0.53 false positives per patient. Note that in some clinical applications it is important to report the average number of false positives per patient for all patients, among patients with and without the condition separately, and among patients with at least one false positive.

For diagnostic and screening tests designed to detect and locate lesions, three methods have been proposed for ROC-type analyses. We describe them briefly here and refer interested readers to Chapter 9 and to the original references for additional details.

In the *location receiver operating characteristic approach* (Starr et al., 1975, 1977; Swensson and Judy, 1981; Swensson, 1996) the reader of the image provides a rating score for the likelihood that there is at least one lesion (e.g. breast mass, lung nodule, or colon polyp) somewhere in the image; then the reader marks the single most suspicious region. In this method, the reader does not get credit for finding multiple lesions, when they exist, so this approach is appropriate when there is no more than one lesion per patient.

In the *free-response ROC curve* (FROC) method (Bunch et al., 1978; Chakraborty and Berbaum, 1989; Chakraborty, 2006), the reader is asked to locate all suspicious lesions and to score each one using a common confidence scale. The FROC curve is a plot of the proportion of lesions that were correctly located and scored as suspicious (plotted on the y-axis) versus the average number of FPs per case (x-axis). Chakraborty and Berbaum (2004) and Chakraborty (2006) developed an extension of the FROC curve called the Jackknife Free-Response (JAFROC) method which allows comparisons between modalities interpreted by a single reader or multiple readers (Penedo et al., 2005). Software for the JAFROC method is available at www.devchakraborty.com. The FROC curve for Case Study 2 is illustrated in Figure 2.10.

In the *region-of-interest* (ROI) method (Obuchowski et al., 2000), clinically relevant ROIs are defined (e.g. for detecting lung nodules, the ROIs might be the 5 lung lobes - right upper, right middle, right lower, left upper, and left lower; for colon polyp detection, the 6 colon segments - rectum, sigmoid, descending, transverse, ascending, and cecum - might be the ROIs; or for breast cancer detection, the two breasts - left and right - are the ROIs). The reader is asked to locate and score all suspicious lesions. These lesions are then mapped to an ROI. For ROIs containing a true lesion (as determined by the gold standard), the score assigned to the true lesion becomes the ROI's score; if the lesion is missed (i.e. no lesion is detected in the ROI or a lesion is found but does not match the location of the true lesion), the lowest confidence score (least suspicious) is assigned to the ROI. For ROIs not containing a true lesion, the highest score assigned to any falsely detected lesions becomes the ROI's score. An ROC curve is constructed from the scores assigned to the ROIs. Since ROIs from the same patient are not independent in a statistical sense, adjustment for the correlation between ROIs is needed (i.e. clustered data; see Chapters 4 and 5). The ROI-based ROC curve for Case Study 2 is illustrated in Figure 2.11.

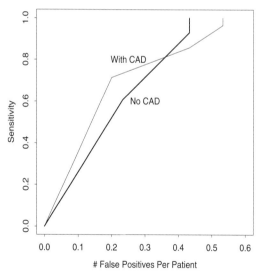

Figure 2.10   FROC Curve for Case Study 2

The two curves in Figures 2.10 and 2.11 represent Reader 1's performance without and with CAD. In the FROC curve the reader's sensitivity with CAD is higher up to about 0.35 false positives per patient; here, the curves cross, and the reader's sensitivity without CAD is higher. In the ROI-based method the two ROC curves are similar with slightly greater overall area under the curve with CAD. Because there are so few points on both sets of curves, it is difficult to compare the two methods with this example.

2.11 POSITIVE AND NEGATIVE PREDICTIVE VALUES, BAYES THEOREM, AND CASE STUDY 2

In this section we address a question important to clinicians: What does a positive (or negative) test result mean? For a patient with a positive test result, we want to know the probability that the patient has the condition; for a patient with a negative test result, we want to know the probability that the patient does not have the condition. We can write this as $P(D = 1 \mid T = 1)$ and $P(D = 0 \mid T = 0)$, respectively. The key concept to answering these questions is recognizing that these probabilities depend not only on the sensitivity and specificity estimates of the test but also on the probability of the condition before the test is performed.

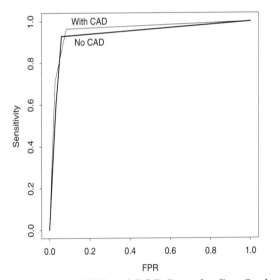

Figure 2.11   ROI-based ROC Curve for Case Study 2

Consider as an example a 45-year old patient who has undergone a screening CT colonoscopy, the result of which is positive. What is the probability that this patient has a colon polyp? Suppose Table 2.7 describes the results of a prospective study of 5250 45-year old patients who underwent screening with CT colonoscopy. We can compute the probability of a polyp after a positive

CT directly from these data. The number of patients who tested positive is 2220, and of these patients, 220 actually had a polyp; thus, $P(D = 1 \mid T = 1) = 220/2220$, or 0.10. The probability of the condition, given a positive test result, is the *positive predictive value*, or *PPV*. Similarly, the probability that the patient does not have a polyp following a positive CT colonoscopy, $P(D = 0 \mid T = 1)$, is $2000/2220 = 0.90$, or simply 1-PPV.

Now suppose this patient had a negative CT. The probability the patient does not have polyps following a negative test result, $P(D = 0 \mid T = 0)$ is the *negative predictive value* (*NPV*). Here NPV=3000/3030, or 0.99. Similarly, the probability of a polyp after a negative test result is 1-NPV, 0.01.

Recall that sensitivity and specificity calculated from Tables 2.3 and 2.7 were identical: 0.88 and 0.60. However, the PPV and NPV calculated from these two tables are not identical; from Table 2.3, PPV=0.92 and NPV=0.50 (compared with 0.10 and 0.99 from Table 2.7). The discrepancy is due to the different prevalence rates. PPV and NPV are *not* measures of the intrinsic accuracy of a test; they are functions of both the intrinsic accuracy and the prevalence of the condition. Both the study design and sampling scheme will affect the prevalence rate in a study sample (See Chapter 3). These factors must be taken into account when estimating PPV and NPV.

Continuing with this example, consider a 70-year old patient with a history of polyps. Since PPV and NPV are functions of the prevalence of the condition, we cannot compute PPV and NPV directly from Table 2.7. However, we can still use the intrinsic accuracy estimates from Table 2.7 (or Table 2.3) to compute the PPV and NPV using *Bayes Theorem.*

2.11.1   Bayes Theorem

Bayes' theorem, named after the reverend and mathematician who developed it (Bayes, 1763), is a method of determining the PPV and NPV, given both the intrinsic accuracy of a test and the probability of the condition before the test is applied. The latter probability is the *pre-test probability* and is based on the patient's history, signs and symptoms, and the results of any diagnostic tests performed earlier. The PPV and NPV are the *post-test probabilities* of the condition (also called *revised* or *posterior probabilities*) because they represent the probability of the condition after the test result is known. Bayes' theorem, then, gives us the post-test probability of the condition as a function of the pre-test probability of the condition and the sensitivity and specificity of the test. Bayes theorem is expressed as:

$$P(D = d \mid T = t) = \frac{P(T = t \mid D = d)P(D = d)}{P(T = t \mid D = 0)P(D = 0) + P(T = t \mid D = 1)P(D = 1)}. \tag{2.5}$$

For example, to compute the PPV and NPV,

$$PPV = P(D = 1 \mid T = 1) = \frac{Se \times P(D = 1)}{Se \times P(D = 1) + (1 - Sp) \times P(D = 0)} \tag{2.6}$$

and

$$NPV = P(D = 0 \mid T = 0) = \frac{Sp \times P(D = 0)}{Sp \times P(D = 0) + (1 - Se) \times P(D = 1)}. \quad (2.7)$$

Figure 2.12 illustrates the relationship between the pre- and post-test probabilities after a positive test result. Here, the sensitivity is constant at 0.95 and the FPR is 0.01, 0.10, or 0.25. When the pre-test probability is very low, a positive test greatly increases the probability of the condition. In contrast, if the pre-test probability is very high, a positive test has little effect on the probability of the condition. A positive test has greatest impact when the FPR is low. In contrast, sensitivity has a large impact when a test result is negative - the greater the sensitivity, the larger the impact.

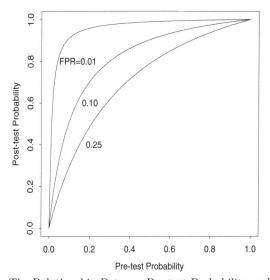

Figure 2.12   The Relationship Between Pre-test Probability and the PPV

An alternative form of Bayes theorem uses odds ratios and LRs (Sox et al., 1989):

$$post-test\,odds = pre-test\,odds \times LR. \quad (2.8)$$

The odds are formed by dividing a probability by its complement: odds = P/(1-P). For example, if we divide the equation (2.6) by $P(D = 0 \mid T = 1)$ then:

$$\frac{PPV}{(1 - PPV)} = \frac{P(D = 1)}{P(D = 0)} \times \frac{Se}{(1 - Sp)}.$$

Similarly, $NPV/(1 - NPV) = P(D = 0)/P(D = 1) \times Sp/(1 - Se)$. The odds is then converted to a probability by: probability = odds/(odds+1).

Suppose the pre-test probability of colon polyps is 10% for a 65-year old patient with a family history of polyps. The pre-test odds are 0.10/0.90 to 1, or 0.1111 to 1. From Table 2.7 (or Table 2.3) the LR(+) is 2.2, in which case the post-test odds is 0.1111 x 2.2 = 0.244, which is equivalent to a probability (i.e. PPV) of 0.196. Note that in the equation (2.7) a LR of 1.0 does not alter the odds, large LRs increase the odds, and small LRs decrease the odds.

Radack et al. (1986) give a nice illustration of the use of LRs and their effect on the post-test odds for a continuous-scale laboratory test, creatine kinase concentration. They show that patients with acute myocardial infarction (AMI) are more likely to have higher creatine kinase values; in other words, higher creatine kinase values have higher LRs. They reported the LRs for different ranges of creatine kinase values. They show that patients with similar pre-test odds can have very different post-test odds depending on their creatine kinase value.

Several assumptions are made when applying Bayes' theorem (Sox et al., 1989). One is that sensitivity and specificity are constant, regardless of the pre-test probability. This assumption is violated if, for example, a test is less sensitive in detecting a condition in its early stages when its pre-test probability is low. For example, CT colonoscopy is less sensitive when polyps are small, as occurs before the patient develops symptoms (low pre-test probability). Later, when the polyp is larger and easier to detect, the test's sensitivity increases, and at the same time, the patient's symptoms may develop (higher pre-test probability). The post-test probability calculated from Bayes' theorem could be misleading if based on data from a study of a mixture of patients having both early and late stages of colon cancer.

A second assumption is important when calculating the probability of a condition after a sequence of tests (Sox et al., 1989). To use Bayes' theorem, the sensitivity and specificity of a test must be independent of the results of other tests - meaning that if two tests are to be performed in sequence, the sensitivity of the second test must be equivalent for patients who test positive and for patients who test negative on the first test. We can write this assumption as

$$P(T_2 = 1|T_1 = 1, D = 1) = P(T_2 = 1|T_1 = 0, D = 1),$$

where T_1 and T_2 denote results of the first and second test, respectively. The foregoing assumption also applies to specificity, as follows:

$$P(T_2 = 0|T_1 = 1, D = 0) = P(T_2 = 0|T_1 = 0, D = 0).$$

If this assumption is met, then the post-test probability of the first test in the sequence is the pre-test probability of the second test (and so forth). If the equation (2.8) is used, the LRs of multiple tests can be multiplied.

The use of Bayes' theorem to interpret diagnostic tests has an interesting analogy in the interpretation of statistical tests in clinical research (Browner and Newman, 1987). As with diagnostic testing, errors occur in statistical hypothesis testing. The results of statistical tests, like diagnostic tests, cannot be interpreted properly without knowledge of the prior probability of the research hypothesis. Although difficult to quantify, the prior probability of the research hypothesis can be used in Bayes' theorem to calculate the probability that the research hypothesis is true.

2.12 OPTIMAL DECISION THRESHOLD ON THE ROC CURVE

In some clinical situations, it may be desirable to find a test result value for a diagnostic test that is optimal in some sense. For example, Somoza and Mossman (1991) wanted to determine the optimal operating point of a diagnostic test for depression, such that patients with a test value greater than the cutpoint would be treated for depression and patients with test values less than the cutpoint would be monitored but not treated.

In this section we present three approaches to determining the *optimal decision threshold* on the ROC curve of a diagnostic test. The first two criteria identify the decision threshold that maximizes the overall rate of correct classification (i.e. maximize the sensitivity and specificity). The last criterion takes into account the particular clinical circumstances of the application, including the financial and/or health effects (i.e., the "costs"), to identify the decision threshold that minimizes the average overall costs.

2.12.1 Optimal Thresholds for Maximizing Classification

We begin with two basic assumptions for the optimal threshold (Dwyer, 1997). First, we assume that two options exist for managing the patient: give treatment when the condition is believed to be present or withhold treatment when the condition is believed not to be present. Second, we assume the decision to give or withhold treatment is based on the results of the test; positive results imply treatment should be given and negative results imply treatment should be withheld.

Two methods commonly used for establishing the optimal threshold to maximize classification are the point on the ROC curve closest to the $(0,1)$ point and the point on the ROC curve farthest from the chance diagonal. The cutpoint on the ROC curve closest to the $(0,1)$ point is defined as the point c that satisfies (Coffin and Sukhatme, 1997):

$$min[((1 - Se(c))^2 + (1 - Sp(c))^2)^{1/2}] \qquad (2.9)$$

$$\text{or}$$
$$min[(1 - Se(c))^2 + (1 - Sp(c))^2],$$

where min means "the minimum of".

The second index is based on Youden's index and is defined as the point c^* that satisfies (Schisterman et al., 2005):

$$max[Se(c*) + Sp(c*) - 1] \tag{2.10}$$

where max means "the maximum of".

Perkins and Schisterman (2006) have shown that c in the equation (2.9) equals c^* in the equation (2.10) when the sensitivity at c equals the specificity at c and the sensitivity at c^* equals the specificity at c^*; otherwise, the criteria do not agree. When the criteria do not agree, Perkins et al. show that c^* is preferable because it maximizes the overall rate of correct classification.

2.12.2   Optimal Threshold for Minimizing Cost

In many applications it is important to minimize the average loss in classifying patients. To minimize the average loss we take into account the patient's pre-test probability of the condition and the different costs of misclassification errors. Depending on the relative costs of errors, the optimal threshold for minimizing cost may not maximize the overall classification.

The cost of performing the test is denoted by C_o. Here, C_o may include the technical and professional costs of performing the test, as well as any health costs caused by test complications. The costs of each diagnostic decision's consequences are denoted by C_{TP}, C_{FP}, C_{TN}, and C_{FN}, where, for example, C_{TP} denotes the cost of a true positive result. We weigh each of these costs by the probability of its occurrence. The average overall cost of performing a test, C, is then (Metz, 1978):

$$C = C_o + P(TP) \times C_{TP} + P(FP) \times C_{FP} + P(TN) \times C_{TN} + P(FN) \times C_{FN} \tag{2.11}$$

where P(TP) denotes the probability of a true positive result and is equal to $Se \times P(D = 1)$. Thus, the cost of performing a test depends on the sensitivity and specificity of the test, the pre-test probability of the condition, and the consequences of the test decisions.

The point on the ROC curve where the average overall cost is at a minimum for a particular application has a slope, m, equal to (Metz, 1978):

$$m = \frac{P(D=0)}{P(D=1)} \times \frac{C_{FP} - C_{TN}}{C_{FN} - C_{TP}} \tag{2.12}$$

If the ROC curve is smooth, the optimal operating point is where a line with this slope is tangent to the curve. When the empirical ROC curve is used, the optimal operating point is where a line - with the slope calculated from the equation (2.12) - moves down from above and to the left to intersect the ROC curve plot (Zweig and Campbell, 1993). Another way to find the optimal operating point is to find the sensitivity and specificity pair that maximizes the function [sensitivity - m(1-specificity)], where m is from Equation(2.12) (Zweig and Campbell, 1993).

Note that the best operating point on the ROC curve does not depend on C_o. Instead, it depends on the consequences of the test's results only in terms of the difference in costs between FPs and TNs relative to the difference in costs between FNs and TPs.

The slope of the ROC curve is steep in the lower left where both the TP and FP rates are low, and flat near the upper right where the TP and FP rates are high. The best operating point is near the lower left if the condition is rare and/or treatment for the condition is harmful to healthy patients and of little benefit to patients with the condition (Metz, 1978). In contrast, when the condition is common and/or treatment is highly beneficial and poses little harm to healthy patients, the best operating point is toward the upper right where the FNR is low.

The financial and health costs used in determining the optimal threshold must be calculated with great care. Estimation of these costs is a specialized field in medicine. A few relevant references are Gold et al. (1996), Pauker and Kassirer (1975), Russell et al. (1996), Weinstein et al. (1996), Drummond et al. (2005), Glick et al. (2007), and Willan and Briggs (2006).

2.12.3   Optimal Decision Threshold: Rapid Eye Movement as a Marker for Depression Example

Somoza and Mossman (1991) used the equation (2.12) to determine the optimal operating point for a biological marker used to detect depression. The biological marker is rapid eye movement (REM) latency, the time between sleep onset and the start of the first rapid eye movement period. REM latency is shorter in patients with depression. Somoza and Mossman fit ROC curves to the data of four studies of REM latency in patients suspicious for depression. They use patient "utility" values to describe the relative costs of the test's decision, with values ranging from 0.0 (the lowest health value) to 1.0 (the highest health value). Somoza and Mossman assigned a utility value of 1.0 to patients in whom depression was correctly diagnosed and for whom treatment could be offered (TPs); 0.9 to patients in whom depression was correctly ruled out but for whom no treatment could be offered (TNs); 0.7 to patients for whom an incorrect diagnosis of depression was made and, consequently, an unnecessary treatment regimen was given (with needless exposure to treatment side effects) (FPs); and 0.0 to depressed patients in whom depression went undetected and for whom an effective treatment was not given (FNs). If the prevalence of depression in the presenting population is 0.10, then the slope of the ROC curve at the optimal operating point is 1.8. The optimal decision threshold is between 47 and 60 minutes, depending on which ROC curve of the four studies is used. Patients with a REM latency of less than this decision threshold are diagnosed with depression and are treated; otherwise, the patient is considered negative for depression and is not treated.

2.13   INTERPRETING THE RESULTS OF MULTIPLE TESTS

Few diagnostic tests are both highly sensitive and specific. To diagnose patients, clinicians often order two or more tests, which can be performed *in parallel* (i.e. at the same time and interpreted in combination) or *serially* (i.e. the results of the first test determine whether the second test is performed). The advantage of serial testing is its cost-effectiveness, because some patients receive only one test. The potential disadvantage is the delay in treatment while one awaits the results of the second test (Hershey et al., 1986). We talk briefly about these two scenarios, beginning with parallel testing.

2.13.1   Parallel Testing

Griner et al. (1981) give hypothetical data for two tests, A and B, for diagnosing pancreatic cancer. We assume that the sensitivity and specificity of each test are independent of the results of the other test (See Section 2.12). Individually, test A has sensitivity and specificity of 0.8 and 0.6, respectively; test B 0.9 and 0.9, respectively. There are several ways in which the tests can be interpreted in parallel:

The OR rule (sometimes called "believe the positive"), in which the diagnosis is positive if either A or B is positive. Both must be negative for the diagnosis to be negative.

The AND rule (sometimes called "believe the negative"), in which the diagnosis is positive only if both A and B are positive. Either A or B can be negative for the diagnosis to be negative.

Using the OR rule, the sensitivity of the combined result is: $Se_A + Se_B - (Se_A \times Se_B) = 0.8 + 0.9 - (0.8 \times 0.9) = 0.98$. The specificity is $(Sp_A \times Sp_B) = 0.54$. With the OR rule the sensitivity of the combined result is higher than either test individually, but the specificity is lower than either test individually. Using the AND rule the combined sensitivity is $(Se_A \times Se_B) = 0.72$, whereas the specificity is $Sp_A + Sp_B - (Sp_A \times Sp_B) = 0.96$. Thus with the AND rule, specificity is higher than either test individually, but the sensitivity is lower than either test individually.

An example of parallel testing is given by Beam et al. (1996) in a study of the effect of double reading mammograms. Here, two readers interpreted each mammogram, and their results were combined using the OR rule. The result was generally an increase in sensitivity offset by an increase in the FPR.

An alternative approach to assessing the accuracy of parallel tests is identifying the optimal linear combination of the tests and/or biomarkers to maximize the area under the empirical ROC (Pepe and Thompson, 2000; Pepe et al., 2006).

2.13.2   Serial, or Sequential, Testing

The basic decision rules in serial testing are as follows:

For the OR Rule ("believe the positive"), if the first test is positive, then the diagnosis is positive; otherwise, perform the second test. If the second test is positive, the diagnosis is positive; otherwise the diagnosis is negative.

For the AND Rule ("believe the negative"), if the first test is positive, apply the second test. If the second test is also positive, the diagnosis is positive; otherwise the diagnosis is negative.

Again using the hypothetical data from Griner et al. (1981), suppose test A is the first test applied. Using the AND rule, the sensitivity is $Se_A \times Se_B = 0.72$ and the specificity is $Sp_A + (1 - Sp_A) \times Sp_B = 0.96$; the accuracy is the same as for the AND rule for parallel testing. Using the OR rule, the sensitivity is $Se_A + (1 - Se_A) \times Se_B = 0.98$. The specificity is $Sp_A \times Sp_B = 0.54$; the accuracy is the same as for the OR rule for parallel testing.

Case Study 2 is an example of serial testing using the OR rule. If the radiologist detects a polyp while reading the image unaided, then the radiologist recommends follow-up. If no polyps are detected initially, then the radiologist applies the CAD algorithm. All CAD marks are assessed and, if the radiologist determines that a polyp exists, then the patient is recommended for follow-up.

Serial testing is particularly common in repeated screening of asymptomatic people, for example screening for breast or colon cancer or diabetes. In this book, we defined accuracy for the simplest situation of two tests with binary results. Polistser (1982) presented the accuracy results of multiple binary tests; Kraemer (1992) considered multiple tests with continuous results; Thompson (2003) described the accuracy of multiple tests with binary and/or continuous results, and when the decision thresholds for defining positive vary over repeated screenings or vary based on the subject's characteristics.

CHAPTER 3

DESIGN OF DIAGNOSTIC ACCURACY STUDIES

Diagnostic accuracy studies are challenging to design, often more so than a study of the efficacy of a new treatment. There are many issues to consider, including identifying the relevant patient population (and sometimes, reader/interpreter/rater population), determining the gold standard, choosing an appropriate measure of accuracy, and accounting for the effects of covariates on the measured accuracy. We must be aware of and carefully avoid bias, and there are many potential sources of bias: in the selection of the patient sample (i.e. spectrum bias); in the accessibility and validity of the gold standard (i.e. verification bias, disease progression bias, imperfect gold standard bias); in the setting for the interpretation of the tests (i.e. review bias, context bias); and in the analysis of the results (i.e. bias from indeterminate test results, failing to adjust for important covariates).

We stress at the onset that sophisticated statistical analyses and large sample sizes can never compensate for a poor study design. Large samples may produce precise estimates of test accuracy, but if they are strongly biased, then they are meaningless. (By "precise" we mean that the estimates of accuracy have small variances; "bias" refers to the situation where the estimates of accuracy do not match the test's true accuracy.) Designing sound diag-

Statistical Methods in Diagnostic Medicine,
Second Edition. By Xiao-Hua Zhou, Nancy A. Obuchowski, Donna K. McClish
Copyright © 2011 John Wiley & Sons, Inc.

nostic accuracy studies is a crucial first step in the assessment of diagnostic technology.

This chapter is organized according to the steps involved in planning a diagnostic accuracy study. The ten steps are outlined in Table 3.1. These steps are not truly sequential. For example, the sampling plan for the patients (step 3) and the gold standard used for evaluation of accuracy (step 4) are often considered simultaneously. Also, the sample size determination (step 10) often influences the sampling plan for the patients (step 3) and readers (step 7). In order to organize these materials, however, we have separated these into distinct steps.

We begin with a discussion of the objective of the study.

3.1   ESTABLISH THE OBJECTIVE OF THE STUDY

The first step in designing a diagnostic accuracy study is to determine the objective of the study. The objective must be clearly stated to prevent overzealous conclusions and to help in selecting the appropriate patients (and readers, when appropriate) for the study. Some important questions to ask are: What modality will be evaluated? What is the condition which the modality will attempt to detect? What is the clinical application of interest in the study? Is this a new modality being evaluated, a mature modality in a new application, or a mature modality in an established application? Is there an existing or competing modality? And, since the characteristics of a test often change dramatically over time due to improvements and innovations in the technology, how might the modality and/or application change during the course of the study?

For some studies the condition to be detected by the test(s) is easily defined (e.g. pregnancy, bone fracture); however, sometimes the condition is difficult to define (e.g. atherosclerosis, colon cancer, congestive heart disease). The thresholds for detection of these conditions continue to be lowered by advances in imaging (Black and Welch, 1993), making it difficult to define what "disease" is and when it begins. For these studies, it's critical that we define the condition in a clinically meaningful way. For a study of atherosclerosis, our operational definition of disease might be one or more stenotic vessels reducing the lumen by more than 70%, corresponding to an increased risk of stroke and cardiac events. For a study of colon cancer, our operational definition of disease might be based on the size and/or invasive characteristics of the lesion (e.g. colon polyps ≥ 2 cm, recognizing that about 50% of these lead to invasive cancer).

The objective of the study is guided by the published literature on similar studies and by the investigator's own previous work. From the literature we can determine the setting in which the modality has already been evaluated, if at all. We need to consider the i) internal validity (i.e. whether previous studies were designed in such a way that their results would be repeatable at

Table 3.1 Steps in Designing Diagnostic Accuracy Studies

Step	Brief Description
(1) Establish objective of study	Identify modality and clinical application; determine role of the study and phase of assessment.
(2) Identify target patient population	Specify characteristics of target patients, including signs, symptoms, extent, severity, pathology, and co-morbidity.
(3) Select sampling plan for patients	Consider possible sampling plans appropriate for phase of study; select one and recognize limitations.
(4) Select the gold standard	Assess if the gold standard is "gold" and feasible for all patients. If not, consider options.
(5) Choose a measure of accuracy	Match measure of accuracy to goals of study and particular clinical application.
(6) Identify target reader population	Specify characteristics of target readers, including training, experience, employment.
(7) Select sampling plan for readers	Consider possible sampling plans; select one and recognize limitations.
(8) Plan data collection	Determine the format for the test results; plan reading sessions; train the readers.
(9) Plan data analyses	Specify statistical hypotheses; plan analyses and reporting of results.
(10) Determine sample size	Determine range of input parameters; calculate sample size.

the same institution with similar patients), ii) external validity (i.e. whether previous studies were designed so that their results would be repeatable at a different but similar institution with similar patients), and iii) generalizability (i.e. whether previous studies were designed so that their results would be repeatable at different institutions and/or with different patient populations). We may choose to repeat a published study, paying more attention to avoiding bias or including a more representative sample of patients (or readers). We may want to measure accuracy in a different clinical setting than previously published, or compare the test's accuracy to a competing test. We may also decide to estimate accuracy for important patient subgroups, overlooked or pooled together in previous studies. Thus, in determining the objective of the study, it is important to recognize the possible contribution of the planned study to the existing literature.

There are different kinds of diagnostic accuracy studies, each with specific roles in the complete assessment of diagnostic test accuracy. It is helpful to recognize the different kinds of studies and classify previous studies and the planned study accordingly. Several authors have proposed phases for the assessment of diagnostic accuracy (Nierenberg and Feinstein, 1988; Zweig and Robertson, 1982; Robertson et al., 1983). We have synthesized and modified these, and propose our own three phases, summarized in Table 3.2. The three phases in Table 3.2 involve testing with human patients. Animal and phantom studies often precede the exploratory phase in the development of a new test; we do not discuss these studies here.

In the **Exploratory Phase** we get our first approximation of a new technology's diagnostic ability. The objective of these studies is to determine if a new test has *any* diagnostic value. Usually, we want to answer this basic question in as short a period of time as possible. In a typical exploratory study, we compare cases of confirmed disease with normal volunteers (controls). Often these studies are methodologically weak and tend to overestimate accuracy.

In the second phase (**Challenge Phase**) we want to challenge the test's accuracy by applying the test to potentially difficult subgroups of patients with and without the condition. As we discussed in Chapter 2, the accuracy of a diagnostic test is often affected by patient characteristics. The same patient characteristics may affect two tests differently. This is the stage where these relationships are revealed. For these studies we need to speculate on the conditions that might affect the absolute accuracy of the test and the comparative accuracies of competing tests. Ransohoff and Feinstein (1978) recommend that we consider the pathologic, clinical, and co-morbid conditions of the patients with the disease and similarly the conditions that might mimic the disease among patients without the disease. Statistical methods for covariate adjustment, such as the covariate-adjusted ROC curve (Janes and Pepe, 2008a), are often used in these studies.

In phase II studies where the test must be interpreted by trained readers (e.g. imaging tests such as MRA), multiple-reader multiple-case ("MRMC") studies are used. The study readers interpret the test results retrospectively,

Table 3.2 Phases in Assessment of a Test's Diagnostic Accuracy

Phase	Typical Design	Typical Patient Sampling Plan	Accuracy Measure
I. "Exploratory" (Early)	Retrospective (10-50 pts)	Typical cases of disease vs. normals (healthy volunteers).	crude estimates of ROC curve area, TPR, FPR
II. "Challenge" (Intermediate)	Retrospective (10-100 pts)	Cases of disease from spectrum of pathologic, clinical, co-morbid conditions vs. patients with pathologic, clinical, co-morbid conditions mimicking disease.	ROC curve area with adjustment for covariates; For comparative studies, the clinically relevant FPR and FNR range.
III. "Clinical" (Advanced)	Prospective (100s of pts)	Representative sample from target population.	application-dependent

knowing that their interpretations will not affect the clinical management of the patient. Thus, the reader is taking part in a kind of experiment, which often does not represent the readers' accuracy in a clinical setting.

From the challenge phase we determine the *existence* of differences in test accuracy for different patient subpopulations (and the *existence* of differences between two tests for some patient subpopulations). It is not straight-forward, however, to estimate the test's accuracy (or the size of the difference in accuracy between two tests) from a phase II study because the study sample does not reflect the relative prevalences of subpopulations from the target population (Metz, 1989; Begg, 1989). Thus, in the third phase of assessment (**Clinical Phase**) we want to measure the accuracy of the test(s) when applied to a representative sample of patients from a well-defined clinical population. In these phase III studies, it is important to avoid bias.

For example, for diagnostic tests that require interpretation by a trained reader, we want to avoid bias associated with a simulated reading setting. Thus, readers in a Phase III study would typically interpret the test results as part of their usual clinical workload. While demonstrating internal validity is sufficient for phase I and II studies, for phase III studies we want to demonstrate external validity. This is established by performing studies that repeat other phase III studies at a different institution with a patient population with the same characteristics as the original study (Van den Bruel et al., 2006).

Since phase III studies tend to be expensive and of long duration, some (Phelps and Mushlin, 1988; Mooney et al., 1990) recommend and provide methodology to determine if these clinical studies are justified.

Each of the three phases plays a distinct role in the evaluation of a diagnostic test's accuracy. Thus, it's important that studies be performed in each phase. Dexamethasone suppression test (DST) for diagnosing depression is an example of a test which was not properly assessed before it became widely used (Nierenberg and Feinstein, 1988). At the time it was recommended for clinical use it had not undergone any clinical evaluations (phase III studies) and the few intermediate studies did not include some key patient groups (e.g. patients with dementia of the Alzheimer's type, obsessive-compulsive disorders, and normal patients with sleep deprivation). Subsequent studies revealed the test's high FPR among these key patient subgroups, but by then the test was in widespread use.

We now illustrate this first step in designing diagnostic accuracy studies with our three case studies.

In Case Study 1, the test combination of SPECT and CT has not been evaluated in a clinical setting. Our objective is to determine if SPECT/CT has any incremental ability over SPECT alone to localize diseased parathyroid glands. SPECT/CT, if found to have incremental ability, would be used before surgery to guide surgeons to the diseased glands. The competing modality is SPECT alone. The study will be part of a Phase I (exploratory) assessment of SPECT/CT.

In Case Study 2, the diagnostic accuracy of computed tomography colonography (CTC) has been studied extensively in the literature, while the added value of this particular computer aided detection (CAD) algorithm has been investigated in a few small Phase I studies. The objective of the study is to compare the diagnostic accuracy of readers without and with CAD for patients with various sized polyps. If found to increase readers' accuracy, CAD will be used to help readers screen for colon polyps. The competing modality is CTC without CAD. The study will be part of a Phase II (challenge) MRMC assessment of CTC with CAD.

Case Study 3 is an example of a Phase III study. There are several published studies looking at the accuracy of MRA for detecting carotid artery plaque. This study will look at MRA's accuracy in two well-defined patient populations - symptomatic and asymptomatic patients at risk for stroke. No competing test will be evaluated.

3.2 IDENTIFY THE TARGET PATIENT POPULATION

The second step in designing a diagnostic accuracy study is to identify the target patient population. This is the patient population to whom you intend to offer the test if it is determined to be accurate enough.

We need to answer two questions: What are the characteristics of these patients (e.g. demographics; signs and symptoms; comorbidities; stage, extent, location, and severity of the condition)? And, are there any characteristics which would exclude patients from undergoing the test (e.g. patients with a pacemaker for studies of MRI)? For Phase III studies especially, it is important to look beyond the patient population at a single institution or single geographic location. Patients at different clinical and geographic sites can have different signs and symptoms before presenting for medical treatment, as well as different comorbidities.

Diagnostic test accuracy and/or cut-points for defining test results may vary, sometimes dramatically, with patients' demographics, disease severity, and clinical site. Age, gender, and clinical setting can also influence test accuracy if they correlate with disease severity or comorbidities. For example, in studying the accuracy of oligoclonal bands in the cerebrospinal fluid of MS patients, the specificity is much lower among controls who present with symptoms similar to MS (e.g. systemic lupus) than among healthy controls (West et al., 1995). Thus, it is critical that the target population represent the complete spectra of patients who would be considered for the test.

The study of the accuracy of MRI to diagnose Multiple Sclerosis (MS) (Mushlin et al., 1993) illustrates the process of selecting the target patient population. These authors did not consider patients with previously diagnosed MS. Rather, their target population was patients suspected of having MS in whom the diagnosis of MS was uncertain. This characterizes the population of patients who might undergo MRI in a clinical setting.

In Case Study 1 the target population would be adult patients with hyperparathyroidism who plan to undergo surgery for removal of diseased glands. The target population would include a wide spectra of symptom severity and duration. The normal glands in patients with hyperparathyroidism will serve as the controls. The exclusion criteria might include patients with contra-indications to the contrast agents used.

In Case Study 2 the target population would be adult patients undergoing CTC for screening, as well as patients recalled following polyp detection in a prior exam, or as a follow-up for a failed prior colonoscopy. These patients should represent a wide range of patient demographics, as well as a wide spectra of disease characteristics.

In the carotid artery stenosis study (Case Study 3), the target population is patients at high risk for stroke who are surgical candidates for carotid endarterectomy. This population would include both symptomatic and asymptomatic patients, an age range appropriate for this kind of surgery (e.g. 50-80 years), a complete spectrum of risk factors (e.g. bruit, previous TIAs, etc), and a broad spectrum of symptoms. The exclusion criteria might include contra-indications to MRI, as well as patients who are too ill for surgery.

3.3 SELECT A SAMPLING PLAN FOR PATIENTS

In this step we consider the various options for obtaining patients for the study in order to meet the study's objective. The three phases in the assessment of test accuracy require different sampling strategies, so we divide this section accordingly.

3.3.1 Phase I: Exploratory Studies

Exploratory studies often use a **retrospective** sampling plan for patients, which means that the true disease status of the patients is already known at the time the patient is selected for the study. The usual sources of patients for a retrospective design are test records and disease-specific registries. In contrast, in **prospective** designs the true disease status is unknown when the patient is recruited for the study. The usual sources of patients for prospective designs are clinical settings where patients present with signs or symptoms (e.g. primary care, emergency department) and where patients are referred for testing (e.g. radiology department, laboratory medicine department).

In a typical exploratory study, we select from the target patient population both subjects known to have the condition and subjects known not to have the condition. Note that the prevalence of the condition in the sample does not need to correspond to the prevalence in the population. In fact, most diagnostic accuracy study samples have a much higher prevalence rate than in the population so that the study will have sufficient numbers to evaluate the test's sensitivity. Usually the subjects with the condition represent typical cases of disease (in contrast to difficult to diagnose cases). The subjects without the condition are often normal volunteers. Sox et al. (1989) refer to the patients in these early studies as "the sickest of the sick" and the "wellest of the well." The rationale for this patient sample is that if the new test cannot distinguish the sickest from the wellest patients, then there is no need to continue with the test's assessment. A natural consequence of using such a patient sample is that the estimates of accuracy are often overly optimistic (i.e. estimates of sensitivity, specificity, and ROC indices are higher than they would be for the target patient population as a whole). It is important that investigators recognize this. Findings from exploratory studies are useful for weeding out the useless tests and for refining tests which show some diagnostic value; they are not useful for estimating the accuracy of the test for a clinical population.

SPECT/CT (Case Study 1) is an example of a test in the exploratory phase. One possible sampling plan is to recruit patients with hyperparathyroidism and some healthy volunteers. Healthy volunteers would not normally have a SPECT study, however, and we would not want to subject healthy volunteers to such a test. Furthermore, the objective of this study is to locate the diseased glands, not to differentiate patients with and without hyperparathyroidism. Since hyperparathyroidism patients have both diseased and normal glands, both sensitivity and specificity can be estimated; the correlation between glands from the same patient, however, must be accounted for (see Chapters 4 and 5). Patients must be recruited prospectively in this study because the test (SPECT and SPECT/CT) cannot be performed after the gold standard (surgery) is performed. Thus, the sampling plan for the SPECT/CT is atypical of most Phase I studies.

3.3.2 Phase II: Challenge Studies

The first step in choosing a sampling plan for a Phase II study is careful consideration of the spectrum of characteristics of the target patient population. Ransohoff and Feinstein (1978) recommend that we focus on the pathologic, clinical, and co-morbid components of the target patients' characteristics.

The pathologic component refers to the extent, location, and cell type (Ransohoff and Feinstein, 1978). For example, for a diagnostic test for colon cancer, we should not just include cases with large polyps (i.e. > 10 mm), but also patients with moderate and small sized polyps, various types of polyps (e.g. adenomatous versus nonadenomatous), polyps of different morphologies (e.g. sessile, flat, pedunculated), and polyps in various locations (e.g. rectum, sigmoid, descending segment, transverse segment, etc). For patients without the condition (i.e. without colon cancer), we need to consider patients with a different process but in the same anatomic location (e.g. severe colitis).

The clinical component refers to the chronicity and severity of symptoms (Ransohoff and Feinstein, 1978), as well as patient variables like age, gender, and body habitus (Black, 1990). For example, body fat may affect the accuracy of tests, generally increasing accuracy for CT and decreasing the accuracy of ultrasound (US). Thus, for comparing CT and US we need to consider a range of body habitus for both patients and controls.

The co-morbid component refers to co-existing ailments (Ransohoff and Feinstein, 1978). For example, for a test to detect pneumothorax we should include patients with pneumothorax and other pulmonary diseases (e.g. cystic fibrosis, interstitial lung disease) and patients without pneumothorax but with these other pulmonary diseases.

Phase II studies usually use a retrospective sampling plan so that challenging cases with and without the condition can be selected. **Matching** is a strategy commonly used in retrospective studies to minimize differences in patients with and without the condition. For example, one might randomly sample patients from a list of patients with a known condition (e.g. colon cancer), and then identify one or more patients without the condition that match each diseased patient with respect to variables that could affect diagnostic test accuracy (e.g. age, gender, disease risk factors, and co-morbidities). Matching is an effective way to ensure that patients with and without the condition are similar with respect to covariates that might affect diagnostic accuracy. Statistical adjustment for the matching covariates, however, is required; in other words, matching is not an alternative to statistical adjustment (Janes and Pepe, 2008a).

If the goal of the study is to measure the incremental improvement in accuracy of a diagnostic test over the accuracy achieved with just the covariates, then matching should not be used (Janes and Pepe, 2008a). For example, in a study to assess the incremental accuracy of prostate-specific antigen (PSA) for diagnosing prostate cancer over the accuracy achieved with just patient age, matching on age should not be performed. The reason is that the distribution of the covariates (i.e. age) in the controls is artificial, i.e. it is not a natural distribution because controls were sampled based on the value of the covariate. Thus, in a study with age-matched controls we cannot accurately measure the diagnostic performance of age. Investigators need to think carefully about whether matching is appropriate for their study.

Phase II (and III) studies often involve a comparison of two (or more) tests' accuracies. In these comparison studies, we need to decide whether to use a **paired** or **unpaired** design. In a paired design, the same patients undergo all of the tests being evaluated in the study. In Case Study 2, for example, all images were interpreted without CAD and with CAD. In an unpaired design, different patients undergo the different tests. For example, some patients' CTC images would be interpreted without CAD and others patients' images would be interpreted with CAD. The paired design requires fewer patients than the unpaired design (often, substantially fewer patients). In some circumstances, however, a paired design is not possible; e.g. the tests are mutually exclusive because of their invasiveness, it's unethical to expose patients to both tests' risk of complications and/or discomfort, or there are time constraints on treatment that do not allow more than one test to be performed.

In both types of comparative designs (i.e. paired and unpaired), it is important to recognize that one test may be superior to the other for one subgroup of patients and inferior for another. We must never assume that because a test is superior for one subgroup that it will be superior to, or at least as good as, the competing test for all patients (Swets et al., 1991). Rather, each subgroup must be studied; this is the role of Phase II studies.

The lower test accuracy observed in Phase II studies can be beneficial when planning sample size for comparative studies. For easy-to-diagnose patients, both tests will tend to have high accuracies (e.g. ROC areas near 1.0), and a large sample size will be needed to detect a small difference between the tests. In Phase II studies, the tests are challenged with difficult cases; the difference in the tests' accuracies is likely to be largest for these difficult cases. Rockette et al. (1995) determined that sample size can be reduced by as much as 45-90% by sampling only difficult cases for a study. They warn, however, that for unpaired study designs the ratio of easy to difficult cases for the two samples must be the same for both tests.

A study by Slasky et al. (1990) provides a nice example of a Phase II study. The goal of the study was to compare the accuracies of three radiographic display modes for detecting three chest abnormalities: interstitial disease, nodules, and pneumothorax. The authors selected patients for the study based on their known disease status (retrospective design) and difficulty for detection. A paired study design was used. The final study sample consisted of 62 patients with interstitial disease only, 44 with nodules only, 34 with pneumothorax only, 19 with interstitial disease and nodules, 2 with nodules and pneumothorax, 16 with interstitial disease and pneumothorax, and 10 with all three abnormalities; in addition, there were 113 patients with none of these abnormalities. Each case was classified a priori as subtle, typical, or gross (very easy to detect). All easily detected cases were omitted from the final sample, and the ratio of subtle to typical in the final sample was about 1:1.

3.3.3   Phase III: Clinical Studies

The goal of Phase III studies is to measure, without bias, the accuracy of a test and the difference in accuracy of two or more tests. This is in contrast to Phase II studies where the goal is to determine if a test has any diagnostic value for discriminating difficult cases and to simply rank multiple tests according to their accuracies. Thus, Phase III studies are much more demanding than Phase II studies. The sample of patients (and readers, when appropriate) must closely represent the target population(s), and biases which commonly occur in patient selection and in determining the true diagnosis must be avoided (Metz, 1989). For Phase II studies, issues of sampling and bias are important, but the only requirement is that these factors not affect the overall conclusions about the usefulness of the test nor the relative rankings of multiple competing tests.

Bias in diagnostic accuracy studies can lead to over- or under-estimation of diagnostic test accuracy. Lijmer et al. (1999) and Rutjes et al. (2006) investigated study design characteristics to see which ones led to over- or under-estimation of test accuracy. These studies found that nonconsecutive sampling of patients for a study leads to overestimation of test accuracy (i.e. the estimates of sensitivity and specificity are often artificially high). Studies that selected patients based on whether they had been referred to the diagnostic test (i.e. **referral bias**), as opposed to sampling from patients with a common set of symptoms, tended to under-estimate diagnostic accuracy.

We begin with a discussion of Case Study 3 to illustrate some of the issues involved in sampling patients for Phase III studies. Table 3.3 summarizes three possible sampling plans for Case Study 3.

Table 3.3 Possible Sampling Plans for Case Study 3 (Phase III)

Sampling Plan	Example
1. Retrospective sample of patients having undergone a particular test(s)	Review registries to identify all patients who have undergone both MRA and catheter angiography
2. Prospective sample of patients referred for a particular test	Recruit people who are referred to MRA by their primary care doctor
3. Prospective sample of patients with particular characteristics	Recruit patients at high-risk for stroke from a CVD prevention clinic

One possible study design is a retrospective design (plan 1 in Table 3.3), where the patient sample consists of those who have already undergone a particular test(s) (e.g. MRA and catheter angiography, the gold standard procedure). The patients are identified by reviewing a registry of all exams performed during a certain time period. The results of the tests are available from patient records or registry. Often, however, the tests must be re-interpreted for the study to control for review bias (See Section 3.8). In this design it is relatively easy and inexpensive to accumulate patients, and the study can be carried out quickly; however, there are some serious problems with this design. First, since the test has already been performed, there is no way to standardize the administration of the test for the study patients (e.g. same dose of contrast agent, same imaging parameters). Second, we cannot be sure that the test was performed independently of other tests (e.g. catheter angiogram performed without knowledge of the MRA findings). Third, we must rely on the medical records for information on the patients' signs and symptoms and pertinent histories; often this information is collected and recorded in an inconsistent fashion, or not at all. Fourth, patients who have undergone the test(s) may not be representative of patients from the target population. Rather, these patients have been selected to undergo the test; other patients from the target population may not have been referred for the test or may have been referred at a different rate (e.g. patients with bruits may get referred for MRA at a higher rate than patients with other risk factors). It is usually impossible to determine the factors which influenced the evaluating physicians' referral patterns. When there are two tests involved, other problems can occur. For example, patients may be referred for the more expensive test only after the less expensive test is performed and determined to be equivocal or suspicious. Any sort of comparison between these two tests will lead to biased estimates of accuracy because the patients are only those with particular findings on the first test. In this situation, the more expensive test's estimated accuracy may be misleadingly higher than the first test.

When the composition of a sample has been influenced by external factors so that it is not representative of the target population, we have **selection bias**. The term covers a wide variety of situations which lead to a skewed sample of patients. **Spectrum bias** often is a consequence of selection bias. Spectrum bias occurs when the composition of the patient sample is missing important patient subgroups (Ransohoff and Feinstein, 1978). Table 3.4 summarizes the common biases that we will be covering in this chapter.

A classic example of selection bias is found in the mammography literature, where full-field digital mammography (FFDM) is compared to conventional film-screen. To perform a prospective comparison of these two modalities requires a very large sample size because the prevalence of breast cancer in the screening population is only 0.5% (i.e. 5000 women must be recruited in order to find 25 cases of cancer). One strategy to reduce the sample size is to consider only women who test positive on standard film screen. These women return for follow-up tests and some undergo biopsy. Prior to biopsy, the FFDM is performed. The advantages to this design are that the prevalence of cancer in this subgroup is much higher than 0.5%, and all patients in this subgroup have a gold standard, i.e. biopsy. This strategy has a serious problem, however: in comparing film to FFDM the study sample includes only the film-positive patients, i.e. TPs and FPs. The sensitivity of film will be greatly overestimated (making FFDM look artificially inferior) and the specificity of film will be greatly underestimated (making FFDM look artificially superior). Thus, even though the patient sample includes diseased and nondiseased patients from the target population, the strong selection bias leads to biased estimates of accuracy.

Probably the most popular approach for recruiting patients for a phase III study is the second design in Table 3.3. It is a prospective design where patients who are referred for testing by their doctor are recruited for the study. The advantages of this study over the first design are that we can (1) standardize the administration of the test for all study patients, (2) blind the person performing the test to information we do not want them to have (e.g.

Table 3.4   Common Biases in Studies of Diagnostic Test Accuracy

Bias	Description
Selection Bias	The composition of the sample is influenced by external factors, so that the study sample is not representative of the target population
Spectrum Bias	The study sample does not include the complete spectrum of patient and disease characteristics
Imperfect Gold Standard Bias	The reference procedure is not 100% accurate
Work-up Bias	The results from the diagnostic test influence the subsequent clinical work-up needed to establish the patient's diagnosis
Incorporation Bias	The results from the diagnostic test under evaluation are incorporated, in full or part, into the evidence used to establish the gold standard diagnosis
Verification Bias	Patients with positive (or negative) test results are preferentially referred for the gold standard procedure; the bias occurs when estimates of accuracy are based only on the verified patients
Disease Progression Bias	The disease progresses (or regresses) between when the test and gold standard are performed
Treatment Paradox Bias	Treatment is administered between when the test and gold standard are performed; treatment alters the disease
Test Review Bias	The diagnostic test is evaluated without proper blinding of the results from the gold standard or competing test
Diagnostic Review Bias	The gold standard is evaluated without proper blinding of the results from the test(s) under study
Reading-Order Bias	When comparing two or more tests, the reader's interpretation is affected by his memory of the results from the competing test
Context Bias	When the sample prevalence differs greatly from the population prevalence, readers' interpretations may be affected, resulting in biased estimates of test accuracy
Location Bias	A positive finding in a diseased patient is considered a true positive whether the true lesion or a false finding is located by the reader

the results of the competing test and gold standard), and (3) collect information (signs, symptoms, history) in a standardized fashion without reliance on the patient's medical record. However, this design still relies on patients from the target population who have been *referred* for the test; thus, selection bias still exists. Using such a "convenience sample," it is difficult to know to whom the test results and study findings apply.

Thornbury et al. (1991) suggest one way to get a broader spectrum of patients for a study is to include patients referred from a variety of sources (e.g. neurosurgery, primary care, outpatient clinics, ED). This approach is likely to provide a broader spectrum of patients, i.e. low, moderate, and high-risk patients. Recruiting patients from multiple institutions across a variety of geographic locations can also help provide a broader spectrum of patients.

The ideal approach, however, is to prospectively recruit patients directly from the target population. For Case Study 3 we might identify high risk patients from a cardiovascular disease prevention center (design 3 in Table 3.3) and determine their willingness to participate in the study. This design provides all of the advantages of design 2, yet avoids referral bias.

For prospective studies comparing two tests, we can randomize patients to one of the two tests (for an unpaired design) or randomize the order in which the two tests are administered (for a paired design). In the unpaired design, the purpose of randomization is to ensure that the patients who undergo the two tests are similar. Note that it is not appropriate to allow the patient or ordering physician to decide which test the patient should receive; this can lead to serious bias. In the paired design the purpose of randomizing the order of the tests is to (1) avoid more drop-outs occurring from one test because it is always performed last, and (2) reduce the risk of systematic differences in the two tests because of changes in the disease (for rapidly progressing conditions) (Freedman, 1987). While randomization is absolutely critical for the unpaired design, for paired designs there are situations where randomization is impractical or impossible (e.g. one test is invasive so must be performed second).

Instead of using random sampling, where all patients in the population have an equal chance of being selected for the study, we could use stratified sampling. One usually stratifies on factors that are expected to be related to the prevalence of the condition and/or to the accuracy of the test. For example, patients at high risk for stroke could be stratified on age, which is correlated to the prevalence of stenosis. Then, within each stratum (e.g. within each age decile group) we would randomly sample patients. We may decide to sample all high-risk patients in the 60-70 year old age group, but only a small portion of patients in the youngest age group. For unpaired designs we need to randomize patients within each stratum; this ensures a balance of the two tests for each stratum. Unbiased estimates of accuracy are obtained from a stratified sample by appropriately weighting the estimates of accuracy from each stratum (Rockette et al., 1991; Sukhatme and Beam, 1994).

An example where stratification was used successfully is a study comparing three psychiatric screening tests (Weinstein et al., 1989). Members of an HMO were mailed a 30-item General Health Questionnaire (GHQ). The authors created 5 strata corresponding to the results of the GHQ: stratum 1 respondents had GHQ scores between 0 and 4, stratum 2 respondents had scores between 5 and 7, etc. The investigators sampled respondents from each stratum to participate in their research study. The sampling rates were higher for strata with higher GHQ scores because they expected increasing prevalence rates of depression and anxiety as the scores increased. For example, although 74% of respondents were in stratum 1, only 2.2% were sampled; in contrast, 11.9% of stratum 5 subjects were sampled even though only 5% of respondents fell into this stratum. ROC curves were constructed by weighting subjects in proportion to the prevalence in the parent population of respondents.

Another nice example of stratified sampling is the mammography study by Beam et al. (1996). Their sampling frame consisted of all women who were screened at their institution during a 4-year period and who had a biopsy or follow-up mammogram at least two years later. They stratified the sampling frame by age (40-49, 50-59, and 60-69) and breast disease status (normal, benign, and cancer). Then, from each age and breast disease combination, they randomly sampled patients.

3.4 SELECT THE GOLD STANDARD

Selecting the gold standard for a study is often the most difficult part of planning a study. We must first consider whether or not a reasonable gold standard exists. If one does exist, we must determine whether all patients have or will undergo the gold standard, or only a subset of the patients. We begin with a discussion of the types of problems that can occur when there is no reasonable gold standard.

Some would argue that there is no such thing as a true gold standard, in the sense that no test or procedure is 100% accurate at determining the presence/absence of disease. Even surgery and pathology, which are often considered true gold standards, are not always perfect. Pathology is an interpretative discipline, like radiology. Pathologists often do not agree with each other when examining the same slide. Also, pathologists and radiologists may be looking at different locations, or the abnormalities observed by the pathologist may not have been present when the test was performed. Furthermore, the pathologist's language for describing disease may differ from the clinician interpreting the test (Swets, 1988). Thus, for all studies of diagnostic test accuracy, it is important that we establish operational standards for diagnostic truth. These operational standards should take into account the phase of the study, the specific goals of the study, and the potential effects of bias on estimates of test accuracy and comparisons of test accuracy. A good dose of common sense is also needed (Metz, 1978).

Consider Case Study 1. Surgical findings will be the gold standard for this Phase I study. The surgeon will look for the glands and determine whether each gland is diseased or not. There is the possibility that one or more glands examined at surgery will be mismatched to the glands seen at imaging. However, for this Phase I study, examination of the glands at surgery is a reasonable gold standard.

Now consider Case Study 3. The gold standard is catheter angiography (CA). CA has sensitivity and specificity probably exceeding 0.90 and has been shown to correlate well with clinical outcome. For a Phase I or II study, this gold standard is reasonable. For a Phase III study with a goal of estimating without bias the accuracy of MRA, CA is probably not adequate because the accuracy of CA is not nearly 100%. In this study there is no true gold standard.

Imperfect gold standards, such as CA, are used in many diagnostic accuracy studies. If an imperfect reference test is used as a gold standard, then the estimates of test accuracy will usually be biased. This is called **Imperfect Gold Standard Bias** (see Table 3.4). If the test and imperfect gold standard are independent (no tendency to make the same errors), then sensitivity and specificity of the test will be underestimated. In fact, in most situations an imperfect gold standard will lead to underestimation of the test's accuracy (Valenstein, 1990). The exception occurs when the test and imperfect gold standard are highly correlated. Here, the test is credited for misclassifying the same patients as the imperfect gold standard, so its accuracy is overestimated.

Consider the following example which illustrates the typical effect of imperfect gold standards. Suppose 100 patients with disease and 400 patients without disease undergo the test and imperfect gold standard. Furthermore, suppose that the test and imperfect gold standard are independent. Let the gold standard and test both have Se and Sp of 0.95. When comparing the test to this imperfect gold standard, the estimated Se of the test is only 0.79 and Sp is 0.94 (see Table 3.5).

There are several approaches to minimizing the bias from imperfect gold standards. One approach is to frame the problem in terms of the clinical outcome, instead of test accuracy (Valenstein, 1990). For example, for a test to detect the location in the brain responsible for triggering epilepsy seizures, one could compare the test results to the patients' seizure status after nerve stimulation at various locations and report the strength of this relationship. This can provide useful clinical information, even when the test's accuracy cannot be adequately evaluated. A similar approach is used in "diagnostic randomized clinical trials (D-RCT)" (de Graaff et al., 2004). In this type of study, patients are randomized either to the conventional diagnostic work-up strategy or to the new diagnostic work-up strategy under investigation. Patients in the two study arms are followed and their outcomes (e.g. morbidity, mortality, health care utilization, quality-of-life) are compared. Although diagnostic accuracy cannot be estimated from such a study, this design allows one to evaluate the effect of the diagnostic test on the diagnostic process, the

Table 3.5   Example Illustrating the Typical Effect of an Imperfect Gold
Standard on the Estimates of Accuracy

	True Disease Status		Imperfect Standard	
Test Result	+	-	+	-
+	95	20	91	24
-	5	380	24	361
	Se=0.95	Sp=0.95	Se=0.79	Sp=0.94

The true Se and Sp of the test are both 0.95,
yet compared against the imperfect gold standard,
the estimated Se is only 0.79 and Sp is 0.94.

therapeutic process, as well as patient outcomes. Other limitations of this
design are that it is not well suited to early phase studies because of their
large sample size and study duration. Second, it cannot be used when it is
unethical to withhold the conventional diagnostic test. Lastly, since the study
outcomes are not measured until after treatment, the effect of treatment may
confound (enhancing or mitigating) the effects of the new diagnostic test.

Another solution is to use an expert review panel to arrive at a less error-
prone diagnosis. In a study by Thornbury et al. (1993) an expert gold standard panel was established to determine the diagnosis of patients receiving
MRI and CT for acute low back pain. The panel was comprised of an expert
neurosurgeon and neurologist; the process was moderated by a physician experienced in technology assessment. For each case the initial history, physical
exam, and laboratory findings were first presented to the panel. Then the
panel considered the treatment results and follow-up information (through 6
months) and decided whether or not a herniated disc (HNP) was present. The
diagnosis of the expert panel, based on all clinical and surgical (if available)
information, excluding the MRI and CT results, was used as the gold standard
against which the MRI and CT results were compared.

When using such a review panel to determine "truth," it is important to
avoid **incorporation bias**. This bias occurs when the results of the test(s) are
incorporated into the evidence used to establish the true diagnosis (Ransohoff
and Feinstein, 1978). The usual effect of this bias is overestimation of test
accuracy. This overestimation occurs because cases of FPs are wrongfully
arbitrated as TPs and cases of FNs are wrongfully arbitrated as TNs. This
bias can be eliminated by establishing the diagnosis independently of the
diagnostic test(s) under study, as was done in the low back pain study by
Thornbury et al. (1993).

Incorporation bias is particularly common in studies assessing the effect of computer-aided detection (CAD) on readers' accuracy. CAD has been used extensively to improve readers' accuracy to find colon polyps and lung nodules. A colon polyp, however, is not synonymous with colon cancer, and a lung nodule is not synonymous with lung cancer. The role of screening tests, such as CTC, is to detect these suspicious lesions that need further follow-up, not to differentiate benign from malignant (which can only be done with biopsy). In studies comparing readers' accuracy for detecting suspicious lesions without and with CAD, an expert panel often reviews the screening test and determines whether or not a suspicious lesion is present. An example is Case Study 2 where an expert abdominal imager, not otherwise involved in the study, reviewed the clinical and imaging results, including CTC results, of each patient; any available optical colonoscopy and surgical data were also reviewed. The expert radiologist made a determination about the presence or absence of colon polyps. Here, the test under evaluation, i.e. CTC, was incorporated into the gold standard evaluation. For studies measuring the effect of CAD, there are several ways to minimize the effects of incorporation bias: 1) include multiple expert readers in the expert panel and use the majority opinion as the gold standard diagnosis, 2) provide the expert readers only the images without the CAD marks for determining the gold standard diagnosis, and 3) for very large studies and/or when image interpretation is very time consuming, show the expert readers the compilation of findings found by the study readers and/or by CAD - ask them to make a determination about the presence or absence of a suspicious lesion, and do not tell the experts which lesions were identified by CAD and which were identified without CAD.

A third option for avoiding imperfect gold standard bias is to use a mathematical correction. There exists several such mathematical corrections; these methods are the subject of Chapter 11. A mathematical correction would probably be the best approach for case study 3.

Two biases caused by delays between when the diagnostic test and gold standard are performed are **treatment paradox bias** and **disease progression bias** (Scott et al., 2008). In treatment paradox bias an effective treatment is started following the results of the diagnostic test and the gold standard is performed sometime thereafter; the disease may be less severe and/or more difficult to identify after treatment so the gold standard results do not reflect the disease status at the time the diagnostic test was performed. In disease progression bias the gold standard is again performed sometime after the diagnostic test, but the disease may have progressed or regressed since the diagnostic test and thus the gold standard may identify more or less disease than was present at the time the diagnostic test was performed. For chronic conditions, a few days between diagnostic test and gold standard is unlikely to be a problem, whereas a few days could introduce bias for an infectious disease.

Another concern when choosing a gold standard is **work-up bias** (Ransohoff and Feinstein, 1978). Work-up bias occurs when the results of the test influence the subsequent clinical work-up needed to establish the diagnosis of the patient. Consider as an example a study assessing the accuracy of a new digital enhancement algorithm for distinguishing benign and malignant breast lesions. When a suspicious lesion is detected on mammography, the patient usually undergoes needle biopsy. If the biopsy is positive, then a core biopsy and/or surgery is performed. Core biopsy and surgery have much higher accuracy than needle biopsy. If we used the results of the needle biopsy as the gold standard for confirming lesions that are classified as benign, and if we used core biopsy and surgery for confirming lesions which are classified as malignant, then our estimates of accuracy will be biased. Whiting et al. (2003) refers to this type of work-up bias as **differential verification bias**. Lijmer et al. (1999) and Rutjes et al. (2006) found that studies with differential verification bias tend to overestimate test accuracy (i.e. the estimates of sensitivity and specificity are artificially high).

We now consider the most common type of work-up bias: **verification bias**. Consider the following example. Eighty-seven patients who recently underwent aortic graft surgery presented to their cardiologist with fever and chest pain. The cardiologist ordered a MRI to check for infection of the graft. The MRI was positive in 30 and negative in 57 cases. Of the 30 MR-positive cases, 24 (80%) went to surgery, which is considered the gold standard for assessing the presence/absence of graft infection. In contrast, only 15 of the 57 MR-negative cases (26%) went to surgery. The data are displayed in Table 3.6. There is a statistically significant association between the MR result and whether the patient went to surgery (p=0.001, chi-square test), indicating that the MR results indeed influenced the decision to perform surgery. Suppose we estimate sensitivity and specificity based on only those 39 patients who underwent surgery (see Table 3.7). The estimated sensitivity is 20/25, or 0.80, and the specificity is 10/14, or 0.71. As we will see shortly, these estimates of sensitivity and specificity are biased because they are calculated on a highly selected sample of patients, i.e. patients who underwent surgery.

Table 3.6   Verification Status of 87 Patients with Suspected Graft Infection

	MRI Result:		
Surgery?	Positive (T=1)	Negative (T=0)	total
Yes	24	15	39
No	6	42	48

Verification bias is probably the most common type of work-up bias. It occurs when patients with positive (or negative) test results are preferentially referred for the gold standard procedure, and then we calculate sensitivity and specificity based only on those cases who underwent the gold standard procedure (Begg, 1987). This bias is counterintuitive in that investigators

Table 3.7   Accuracy Data for 39 Surgical Patients. Estimated Se=0.80, Sp=0.71

	MRI Result:		
Surgery Result:	Positive (T=1)	Negative (T=0)	total
Infection	20	5	25
No Infection	4	10	14

usually believe that by including only cases with rigorous verification of the presence or absence of the condition, their study design will be ideal (Begg and McNeil, 1988). In fact, those studies requiring the most stringent verification of disease status, and discarding those cases with less definitive confirmation, often report the most biased estimates of accuracy (Begg, 1987; Black, 1990).

There are a number of solutions to the problem of verification bias. The first solution is simply to verify all test results. Depending on the gold standard, however, this may be unrealistic (e.g. when the gold standard exposes the patient to risk of serious complications). In these situations, we can minimize bias by allowing patients to be verified with different gold standards. For example, in evaluating the accuracy of mammography for screening for breast cancer, some patients, particularly those with positive results, will undergo core biopsy and surgery; those with negative test results can be followed clinically and radiographically for a specified period of time (maybe two years for breast cancer) to detect misclassifications. Note that we never assume that patients with negative test results are disease-free; this can lead to serious overestimation of test specificity (Begg, 1987). In avoiding verification bias, however, it is important to avoid other biases that we have talked about, including differential verification bias, disease progression bias, and treatment paradox bias.

Consider another example. The PIOPED (PIOPED Investigators, 1990) study was performed to measure the accuracy of ventilation/perfusion (V/Q) scans for detecting pulmonary embolism. Of the 1493 patients who consented to the study protocol, a random sample of 931 were selected for mandatory angiography (considered the gold standard) if the V/Q scan was positive. All patients were contacted by phone at 1, 3, 6, and 12 months after their exam to assess relevant events (i.e. death, major bleeding complications, etc.). An Outcomes Classification Committee was established to review all the available information for each patient to establish the final (definitive) diagnosis. Of the 931 patients selected, 176 did not undergo angiography: 69 had negative V/Q scans and 107 were protocol violations. The data show a clear relationship between less suspicious findings on the V/Q scan and absence of angiography. However, using the clinical follow-up information, the committee was able to arbitrate a final diagnosis for 901 patients (97%), including 4 cases where the Committee overturned the angiography diagnosis on the basis of other available information.

In the graft infection study described earlier, the verification bias was avoided by following patients who did not undergo surgery. All of the 48 patients who didn't undergo surgery were followed clinically for at least three months during which time no antibiotics were administered. During this three-month period, two patients' symptoms worsened and required hospitalization and antibiotic treatment. These two patients were classified as disease positive; the remaining 46 patients were classified as disease negative. The accuracy data for all 87 suspected graft infection patients are illustrated in Table 3.8. From these data, the estimated sensitivity is 20/27 or 0.74, and the specificity is 50/60 or 0.83. We now see that our original estimates of accuracy (Table 3.7) were biased: sensitivity was overestimated and specificity was underestimated.

Table 3.8   Accuracy Data for 87 Patients

	MR Result:		
Surgery Result:	Positive (T=1)	Negative (T=0)	total
Infection	20	5	25
No Infection	4	10	14
Follow-Up Result:			
Infection	0	2	2
No Infection	6	40	46

Estimated Se=0.74, Sp=0.83.

A second approach to avoiding verification bias is to avoid the situation where the diagnostic test determines which patients undergo verification.

In other words, the study patients are selected for undergoing the gold standard based on their signs and symptoms, but not the test(s) evaluated in the study. One example of this is the study of ultrasound (US) for diagnosing leaks in silicone gel breast implants (Chilcote et al., 1994). Twenty-five women with signs or symptoms of implant failure presented to a plastic surgeon for removal or replacement of their implant(s). US was performed prior to surgery but had no bearing on the women's decisions to undergo surgery. A second example is the study of prostate cancer by Rifkin et al. (1990). The goal of the study was to compare the accuracy of magnetic resonance (MR) and US for staging prostate cancer. Any patient who, based on clinical evaluation and non-imaging tests, was thought to have prostate cancer and was scheduled for surgery was enrolled into the study. After signing informed consent, patients were scheduled for both MR and US prior to surgery.

A third approach to avoiding verification bias is to apply a mathematical correction to the estimates of accuracy. A number of correction methods have been proposed. Most of them are based on the assumption that the decision to verify a patient is a conscious one and must be based on visible factors, such as the test result and possibly other clinical information such as signs and symptoms. Thus, conditional on these factors, the true disease status is independent of the selection mechanism; this is referred to as the conditional independence assumption (Begg, 1987). Regardless of the assumptions and methods used, it is important that we record the test results of *all* patients who undergo the test, not just those who undergo the test and gold standard. In Chapter 10 we describe in detail various correction methods for verification bias.

3.5 CHOOSE A MEASURE OF ACCURACY

In this section we discuss the choice of an appropriate measure of test accuracy for the study. Depending on how the data are collected, several different measures of test accuracy can be estimated from a single study. Here, we will focus on which measure should be the primary focus of the study; sample size calculations are usually based on this primary measure.

The measure of accuracy chosen for a study should depend on the phase of the study, the objective of the study, and the particular clinical application. In Phase I (exploratory) studies, the ROC area is often used because it directly addresses the fundamental question asked in exploratory studies: can the test distinguish patients with and without the condition?

In Phase II (challenge) studies the ROC area is again very relevant for assessing a test's ability to discriminate various subgroups within the target patient population. When comparing tests, however, the ROC area can cover up important differences between the tests or can favor one test when, in fact, the tests are identical for the clinically relevant region of the ROC curve (see Chapter 2). Thus, for Phase II comparative studies the portion of the ROC curves in the clinically relevant region should at least be examined. An example is the Phase II study of film-screen vs. digital mammography (Powell et al., 1999). The authors used the ROC area as their primary measure of accuracy; however, they also report the estimated FPR at a fixed sensitivity of 0.90. The partial area under the ROC curve and sensitivity (or specificity) at a fixed FPR (FNR) are not usually used as the primary measure of accuracy in Phase II studies because the sample size required for a study using these measures is considerably greater than for a study using the area under the entire ROC curve (see Chapter 6).

In studies assessing the accuracy of tests to find lesions (e.g. diseased glands, colon polyps), correctly locating the lesion is an important part of the overall diagnostic process and thus needs to be accounted for in the measure of test accuracy (Obuchowski et al., 2010). **Location bias** occurs when readers of a test (e.g. radiologist interpreting a CT image of the colon) are credited with a true positive finding for detecting *any* lesion in a patient who has one or more true lesions. For example, a radiologist might find a false lesion in the transverse segment of the colon, while missing the true polyp in the cecum. Location bias occurs when this case is considered a true positive result in estimating sensitivity. In Chapter 2 we discussed measures of test accuracy that account for both correct detection and localization of lesions, thereby avoiding location bias. To appropriately measure test accuracy in these studies, each detected lesion needs to be scored with respect to the suspicion level. For example, in Case Study 1, the location of each gland was recorded and the gland was scored according to the reader's suspicion that it was diseased. In Case Study 2, each reader recorded the coordinates of each detected polyp and then scored each polyp. Sensitivity and ROC type measures of accuracy (e.g. FROC and the ROI-based ROC) can then be estimated.

In Phase III (clinical) studies it's critical that the measure of accuracy be highly relevant to the clinical application and have a clinically useful interpretation. For these studies we do not recommend the ROC curve area as the primary measure of accuracy because it is too global. The appropriate measure of accuracy will depend on the particulars of the study; we illustrate this with several examples.

The American College of Radiology (ACR) recommends that screening mammograms be scored using the BIRADS (Breast Imaging and Reporting Data System) (American College of Radiology, 1995). The BIRADS consists of 6 ratings describing the reader's degree of suspicion and a recommended action step: category 0 indicates that the mammogram contained insufficient information to make a diagnosis and follow-up imaging is necessary, category 1 indicates that the image is negative and routine screening is recommended, 2 indicates a definite benign finding and routine follow-up is recommended, 3 indicates that the findings are probably benign and a six-month follow-up is recommended, 4 indicates that a suspicious lesion was found with reasonable probability of being malignant and biopsy should be considered, and 5 indicates that a highly suspicious lesion was found with a high probability for malignancy with appropriate action recommended. After follow-up imaging, the category 0 images are reclassified as 1-5. A common definition of a positive screening mammogram is a score of 4 or higher since this is when there is an immediate step taken in the management of the patient. In Phase III studies of mammography it makes good sense to use this well-established cutoff and estimate the sensitivity and specificity at this cutoff. In their Phase III study Beam et al. (1996) estimated sensitivity and specificity at this cutoff to characterize the variability between U.S. mammographers. Similarly, Pepe et al. (1997) describe their plan to estimate sensitivity and specificity at this cutoff when comparing accuracy pre- and post-intervention. Pepe et al. present a bivariate statistical method to deal with the difficulty of comparing two tests' accuracies based on only a single point on the ROC curve.

Consider as a second example the study by Baul et al. (1995) of the accuracy of Magnetic Resonance Angiography (MRA) in the presurgical evaluation of patients with severe lower limb atherosclerosis. The critical issues for these presurgical patients are to (1) locate the occlusion causing the disease and (2) identify normal segments which can be used as the distal terminus of the graft. The readers graded each vessel as "no disease," "minimally diseased (one area of less than 50% stenosis)," "stenotic (a single lesion of more than 50% and less than 100% stenosis)," "diffusely diseased (multiple lesions with greater than 50% stenosis)," and "fully occluded." The authors estimated the sensitivity and specificity of MRA for distinguishing vessels with any flow (no disease, minimally diseased, stenotic, or diffusely diseased) from fully occluded vessels, and the sensitivity and specificity of MRA for distinguishing normal vessels (no disease or minimally diseased) from vessels with any disease. Thus, like the mammography studies, there was clear rationale for the cutoffs used, so simply estimating sensitivity and specificity at these cutoffs was a reasonable approach for this study.

In contrast, in the study by Mushlin et al. (1993) to assess the accuracy of MRI for diagnosing MS, there was no standardized way to interpret the MRI results. Thus, the authors estimated the ROC curve and constructed simultaneous confidence bands for the curve (see Chapter 4). From the curve and using their knowledge about the disease and the consequences of incorrect diagnoses, the authors identified a cutoff that essentially confirms the diagnosis of MS, but they could not identify a cutoff to exclude the diagnosis of MS.

Measures of test accuracy that adjust for covariates are often needed in Phase II and III studies. Consider a study looking at the accuracy of a diagnostic test to detect lesions. Readers' confidence in the presence of a lesion probably depends, in part, on the size of the lesion, and the size of the lesion will likely correlate with the patient's status of asymptomatic or symptomatic. Thus, some adjustment for the patients' symptom status is needed in order to properly describe the accuracy of the test. A second example is a study of the diagnostic accuracy of PSA for diagnosing prostate cancer. PSA values increase naturally with a patient's age, thus age-adjustment is needed to properly describe the diagnostic accuracy of PSA. There are several methods of adjusting the ROC curve for covariates. The simplest option is covariate-specific ROC curves, where a separate ROC curve is constructed for each level of the covariate. This works well for studies with large sample sizes and with one covariate with just a few levels. For studies with small Ns or lots of levels of the covariate, a covariate-adjusted ROC curve, written AROC, can be used (Janes and Pepe, 2008a). The AROC is a weighted average of the covariate-specific ROC curves and is estimated by standardizing the diseased patients' test results with respect to the test results of patients without the disease but with the same value of the covariate. It provides a single ROC curve that can be used to compare two diagnostic tests in paired studies. Chapter 8 describes various methods of adjusting for covariates in measures of test accuracy.

In Case Studies 1 and 2 the ROC curve area is the primary measure of test accuracy. An AROC curve may be appropriate in Case Study 2 to adjust for

CTC's and CAD's accuracies for detecting lesions of different sizes. In Case Study 3 (Phase 3 study) there is no standardized way to interpret the MRA results and there are likely to be differences in test accuracy for symptomatic and asymptomatic patients. Thus, we might construct covariate-specific ROC curves and find the optimal cutpoint based on the relative consequences of FPs and FNs. The clinical situation may demand different cutpoints depending on whether the patient is symptomatic or asymptomatic. For symptomatic patients, a low FNR (i.e. high sensitivity) may be needed because the risk of mortality or serious morbidity from stroke is high in this population. For asymptomatic patients, the risk of stroke is lower, and the risks from unnecessary follow-up tests and procedures need to be considered; thus a cutpoint with a low FPR may be needed.

3.6 IDENTIFY TARGET READER POPULATION

Some diagnostic tests require a trained reader to interpret the test. This is particularly common for diagnostic imaging tests, such as chest x-rays, CT, MRA, and mammography. The diagnostic accuracy of these tests is a function of both the machine and the reader who utilizes the machine (Beam, 1992). Since readers differ in their cognitive and perceptual abilities, it is important to include multiple readers in such studies. The goal of multi-reader studies is then to estimate the accuracy of the machine and reader combination. Note that this goal cannot be achieved when readers interpret cases by consensus or majority rule (Obuchowski and Zepp, 1996). Rather, the accuracy of each reader should be estimated separately (see Section 3.9.3).

The target reader population is the population of readers who will be interpreting the test(s) if the test(s) is shown to be accurate enough. Most of the published research studies on diagnostic tests have a very narrow target reader population. For example, a mammography study comparing standard film and digitized images (Powell et al., 1999) included seven board-certified mammographers all from the same institution. Thus, the effective target reader population for this Phase II study was the mammographers at that single institution.

There are several important questions about test accuracy that can be addressed properly only with a broad target reader population. Some of these questions are (Beam et al., 1992): How much variability is there between radiologists in the general population of radiologists? How is accuracy related to the readers' personal characteristics (experience, training, etc.)? How much disagreement in diagnosing a case is normal/natural/typical between and within radiologists? These questions are very pertinent to Phase III studies.

In Phase II studies it is important to begin to get a handle on the diversity of readers' diagnostic performance. For these studies a narrower target reader population, such as the readers at a single institution, may suffice, but even in Phase II studies investigators are becoming increasingly aware of the need for better reader representation.

A nice example of a study using a broad target reader population is the mammography study by Beam et al. (1996). The target reader population was all mammographers working in ACR-accredited mammography centers in the U.S.

In Case Study 3 the ideal target reader population is all neuroradiologists in the U.S. Various radiology societies could be contacted to obtain a membership list by specialty. A registry of neuroradiologists practicing in the U.S. could be created from these lists and serve as the target reader population for the study.

3.7   SELECT SAMPLING PLAN FOR READERS

For Phase II studies with a narrowly defined target reader population (e.g. readers from a single institution), readers are usually selected based on their expertise and availability to participate in the study. Selection of readers in this fashion could lead to a biased sample (e.g. readers familiar with digital display might be more willing to participate in a study of digital mammography than readers unfamiliar with this format). However, this sampling approach is inexpensive and convenient and, thus, for Phase II studies it has become the norm.

For Phase III studies, where it is important to have as unbiased a reader sample as possible, random sampling or stratified random sampling should be used to select readers. In the mammography study by Beam et al. (1996) a random sample was used. They identified all of the ACR-accredited mammography centers in the U.S. There were 4611 such centers in the U.S. at the time of the study. Then they randomly sampled 125 centers from the 4611 and mailed letters to these centers to assess their willingness to participate. Fifty centers (40%) agreed to take part in the study. 108 radiologists from these 50 centers actually interpreted images for the study.

In Case Study 3, we could mail an invitation to neuroradiologists belonging to one of the imaging professional societies. Of the radiologists responding with interest in the study, we might stratify them according to 3 or 4 levels of experience (because we expect reader accuracy to vary by experience level). We could then take a random sample of readers from each stratum as our sample for the study. We note again that this reader sample may be biased because selection for the study depends on the reader's motivation to participate, which, in turn, may be associated with his skill and experience level. Instead of this sampling plan, however, Case Study 3 used a more convenient sample. Four neuroradiologists from three institutions who were friends of the study's principal investigator composed the reader sample. These four neuroradiologists were all highly experienced and research-oriented. This sampling strategy limits the generalizability of the study results.

3.8 PLAN DATA COLLECTION

In this section, we discuss the data that needs to be collected for a diagnostic accuracy study, the process of collecting data when there are one or more readers in the study, and training of readers. We begin with a discussion of the data that needs to be collected.

3.8.1 Format for Test Results

The primary piece of data to collect is, of course, the results of the test(s). For quantitative tests the results can be easily expressed. For example, in a study of the accuracy of PSA in screening for prostate cancer, we can simply record the numerical PSA values. For tests requiring interpretation by trained readers, there are a number of possible ways to express the reader's confidence in the presence of the condition. Some commonly used options are (1) a binary result indicating whether the test is positive or negative for the condition, (2) an ordinal score (e.g. the ACR's BIRADS score (American College of Radiology, 1995)), and (3) a percent confidence score. If the intent is to construct a ROC curve, the first approach is not adequate; however, the two latter approaches are appropriate for constructing a ROC curve.

Rockette et al. (1992) performed an empirical study to assess if the estimates of accuracy are affected by whether a percent confidence or ordinal scale is used. On two different occasions, they asked five readers to evaluate a sample of 95 CT abdominal images to determine the presence/absence of masses; a different scale was used on each occasion. The authors reported nearly identical results for the two scales for all five readers. The authors note, however, several disadvantages with the ordinal scale: (1) more likely to produce degenerate datasets (See Chapter 4), (2) more reader training required to ensure that readers spread results out across the categories, and (3) more artificial, thus less able to reflect clinical thinking and reporting. Readers, however, also need training to ensure that they spread out their percent confidence scores rather than binning their scores at either end. Furthermore, some readers find a five-choice ordinal scale easier to use than a 100-point percent scale. Finally, with the ordinal scale we can easily attach follow-up action steps to each category, as with the BIRADS score. These action steps are particularly important in Phase III studies. Clearly, both the ordinal and percent confidence scales have their advantages and disadvantages. For some studies, a reasonable compromise between the two scales is the percent confidence scale broken up by deciles (e.g. 0%, 10%, 20%, etc). This option reduces the number of possible responses to a more reasonable number (11 choices), yet maintains the probability-based interpretation.

Depending on the clinical application, we may need to collect other diagnostic information about the condition. These might include the size and type of the lesion, and the severity, intensity, or stage of the condition. In Case Study 2 the readers should record the size and type (i.e. flat, sessile, pedunculated) of polyps. In Case Study 3 the readers should record the percent of the artery lumen blocked by the stenosis (i.e. the readers not only record their confidence that there is a significant lesion that needs surgical intervention, but also the severity of the blockage).

In addition to recording the test results, it is important to record available clinical data (e.g. demographics, signs and symptoms, and relevant history) for two reasons. First, the diagnostic accuracy or comparative accuracies of tests may vary with these clinical factors. For Case Study 3 we suspect that the accuracy of MRA may be higher for symptomatic patients, so we record the symptom status of patients for later analyses. Second, given these clinical data, the results of the test may not have any incremental diagnostic value (Begg, 1989). For example, age is a strong predictor of prostate cancer, so it is important to assess the incremental value of PSA over age alone.

Thornbury et al. (1991) recommend that for advanced studies (i.e. stage III) we collect data for cost-effectiveness studies. These data might include costs of tests and procedures performed as a consequence of the test results (e.g. biopsy, surgery, radiation, medicine prescribed), costs of complications attributable to the tests and to the subsequent patient management, costs of hospitalizations, length of hospital stay, and absentee days.

3.8.2 Data Collection for Reader Studies

We now discuss the process of collecting the accuracy data when the test(s) are interpreted by readers. There are three relevant issues: reader masking, randomization of the reading order, and the setting/environment for the readers' interpretations.

The test(s) must be interpreted without knowledge of the final (gold standard) diagnosis. If the reader is not "masked" (or "blinded"), his interpretation of the test(s) may be affected (Black, 1990). This is called **test review bias** (Ransohoff and Feinstein, 1978). The usual effect of this bias is overestimation of test accuracy. The best way to avoid this bias is to have the gold standard procedure interpreted after the diagnostic test is interpreted or by different people. Similarly, two tests being compared must be interpreted independently of one another, and both must be independent of the gold standard.

Diagnostic review bias occurs when the gold standard procedure is performed and/or interpreted with knowledge of the test results. This bias occurs often in retrospective studies because clinicians are not masked to the results of other tests in routine practice. Lijmer et al. (1999) and Rutjes et al. (2006) found that studies where the interpretation of the gold standard was not masked to the results of the test(s) under study often leads to overestimation of test accuracy (i.e. the estimates of sensitivity and specificity are artificially high). In these studies it is sometimes possible to avoid bias by re-interpreting the gold standard, masked to the test results. In some cases, however, the manner in which the gold standard was performed or administered was influenced by the results of the test (e.g. multiple, nonstandard views of a certain location where a lesion was detected by the test). In these situations there is no way to avoid the bias in a retrospective study. In a prospective study, however, we can standardize the imaging protocols to avoid this type of bias.

When two images (e.g. MRI and CT) from the same patient are read by the same reader, the image read last will tend to be interpreted more accurately than the image read first if any relevant information is retained by the observer (Metz, 1989). If all images using test A are interpreted first, followed by all images from test B, the results of the study are potentially biased in favor of test B. This is called **reading-order bias**. It can have the effect of (1) negating a real difference (i.e. if A is really superior to B), (2) inflating the true difference (i.e. if B is really superior to A), or (3) creating a difference when no true difference exists.

The simplest way to reduce or eliminate reading order bias is to vary the order in which the tests are interpreted and to include a wash-out period. For example, suppose we have 100 patients who underwent both test A and B. We decide that 25 cases per reading session is appropriate. We randomly assign patients to one of four sets (denoted 1, 2, 3, and 4). Then, the reading sessions might be organized as: patient set 1 using test A (denoted 1A), 2B, 3A, 4B, 1B, 2A, 3B, 4A. If there are multiple readers, it is best if each observer interprets the cases in a different sequence, for example, (1B, 2A, 3B, 4A, 1A, 2B, 3A, 4B), (4A, 3B, 2A, 1B, 4B, 3A, 2B, 1A), and (4B, 3A, 2B, 1A, 4A, 3B, 2A, 1B). With such a design each reader interprets half the cases in test A first and the other half in test B first, and there is at least one reading session between the interpretations of the same case (Metz, 1989). Ideally, a wash-out period is included after the readers have interpreted the test results of each patient for the first time and before the second interpretation with the competing test (i.e. 1A, 2B, 3A, 4B, wash-out period, 1B, 2A, 3B, 4A). The duration of the wash-out period depends on several factors, including the complexity of the interpretations and the volume of study cases and clinical cases the reader is interpreting. A typical wash-out period is 4-6 weeks.

A nice example of a study avoiding reading-order bias is the study of ovarian cancer by Fultz et al. (1999). The goal of the study was to compare the accuracy of four methods of interpreting CT scans: method A = paired simultaneous reading by two observers, B = reading with a checklist, C = standard single-observer interpretation, and D = combination of two independent readings (the results for method D were derived from method C). The patients were randomly assigned to three groups; there were four readers. There were four reading sessions, each separated by at least two months. In the first reading session each reader used three interpretation methods, one for each of the patient groups. For example, in reader one's first reading session he used method A for group 2 patients, B for group 3 patients, and C for group 1 patients. In the second reading session Reader 1 used method C for group 3 patients, A for group 1 patients, and B for group 2 patients. In the third session Reader 1 used method B for group 1 patients, C for group 2 patients, and A for group 3 patients. Each of the four readers followed a different schedule. In the fourth reading session the readers reread a sample of cases so that intraobserver agreement could be estimated. Thus, all the readers interpreted all of the cases using all four methods.

In designing the setting/environment for the reader interpretations it is important to determine whether the study should assess the value of the test(s) "in the field" (i.e. typical clinical setting) or assess the value of the "test per se" (i.e. experimental setting) (Begg and McNeil, 1988). For field studies readers have access to whatever information is customarily provided, *except results of competing tests and the gold standard procedure*, and the interpretations are performed in as nearly a clinical set-up as possible. The additional information provided to readers might include the patient's signs and symptoms, age, and results of previous tests. For the "test per se" style no additional information is provided to the readers. In addition, sometimes restrictions are put on the readers, such as limits on the time the reader is allowed to view each image, specifications on the ambient light, access to various image enhancement features, and control of possible distractions (i.e. beepers and phone access). There are no strict criteria for when the interpretations should be performed in the field or when more experimental conditions are appropriate. It is important to note, though, that the estimates of test accuracy from the more experimental type settings may have limited generalizability (Gur, 2007; Rutter and Taplin, 2000). In other words, readers' performance in these experimental settings often does not mimic their performance in a clinical setting. In general, then, in Phase II studies readers are often blinded to clinical history and asked to perform the readings under more experimental conditions so that two or more tests can be compared on their own merits. In Phase III studies it is sometimes appropriate to provide readers with customary information in order to estimate the accuracy of the test(s) in a clinical setting. For each study the appropriate setting for the reader interpretations should be decided through discussions between the clinical and methodologic investigators and with some common sense.

There are a variety of designs for collecting the interpretations in multiple reader studies. We start with some broad definitions. When comparing two or more tests, we need to decide whether a paired-reader or unpaired-reader design will be used. In a **paired-reader design** each reader interprets the results of all tests being studied. The paired-reader design can be used with either the **unpaired-patient design** (i.e. different patients undergo the tests) or the **paired-patient design** (the same patients undergo all of the tests being studied). In Case Study 2 each reader interpreted the CTC results both without and with CAD; the same patients' CTC images were interpreted without and with CAD. Thus, Case Study 2 is an example of a paired-reader, paired-patient design, also referred to as the "traditional" design (Obuchowski, 1995).

In an **unpaired-reader design** different readers interpret the results of the different tests (e.g. some readers interpret the CTC results without CAD while different readers interpret the CTC results with CAD). The paired-reader design is usually preferred over the unpaired-reader design because it requires fewer patients and readers. For the same reason, the paired-patient design is usually preferred over the unpaired-patient design. There are situations, however, that do not permit a paired design. For example, sometimes different expertise is required to interpret the two tests and readers do not have equivalent expertise in both tests. Another situation is when readers have a vested interest in one test, so either consciously or subconsciously, they might perform their interpretations more carefully on the preferred test. Gelfand and Ott (1985) describe this latter situation and the resulting bias as it relates to the comparison of colonoscopy and barium enema. For these situations an unpaired-reader design is appropriate. Similarly, when patients cannot undergo both tests because it is unethical, the tests are contraindicated, or for monetary reasons, an unpaired-patient design must be used. Pepe et al. (1997) describe a mammography study that used an unpaired-reader, unpaired-patient design. The goal of the study was to assess the impact of an intervention (i.e. an educational program for mammographers) on reader accuracy. The mammographers were randomized to either the intervention or control group. The study cases were randomly assigned to two sets, A and B. One half of the mammographers in the intervention group read the A set prior to the intervention and B after the intervention; the other half read B first, then A. The mammographers in the control group were similarly split so that half of them read A first, then B, and the other half read B first, then A. A paired-reader design could not be used because readers have a natural tendency to improve over time and the order of the two readings cannot be randomized (i.e. the intervention must be second). The authors chose not to use a paired-patient design because they were concerned that readers might recall cases which they had seen prior to the intervention. Since they wanted to avoid any bias that favored the intervention, they used an unpaired-patient design.

The paired-reader, paired-patient set-up is illustrated in Table 3.9. Here, T_{kj1} and T_{kj2} denote the test results for the k-th patient, interpreted by the j-th reader, using test 1 and 2, respectively. There are a total of N patients and J readers. This conventional design is popular because it requires the smallest number of patients (Obuchowski, 1995). Furthermore, compared with other designs, it demands one of the smaller reader samples and one of the fewer number of interpretations per reader. In contrast, the unpaired-reader unpaired-patient design (See Table 3.10) is the most inefficient design in that it requires the largest reader and patient sample sizes.

The unpaired-patient, paired-reader design (see Table 3.11) and the paired-patient, unpaired-reader designs (Table 3.12) are improvements over the unpaired-patient, unpaired-reader design but are inferior to the traditional design. Still, these designs may be necessary when the tests are mutually exclusive or when the readers of the tests require different expertise, respectively.

Table 3.9   Data Set-Up for Traditional MRMC Design

	Reader 1		Reader j		Reader J	
Patient	Test 1	Test 2	Test 1	Test 2	Test 1	Test 2
1	T_{111}	T_{112}	T_{1j1}	T_{1j2}	T_{1J1}	T_{1J2}
2	T_{211}	T_{212}	T_{2j1}	T_{2j2}	T_{2J1}	T_{2J2}
k	T_{k11}	T_{k12}	T_{kj1}	T_{kj2}	T_{kJ1}	T_{kJ2}
N	T_{N11}	T_{N12}	T_{Nj1}	T_{Nj2}	T_{NJ1}	T_{NJ2}

This design requires N total patients and J total readers.

Table 3.10   Data Set-Up for Unpaired-Patient, Unpaired-Reader MRMC Design

	Test 1			Test 2		
Patient	Reader 1	Reader j	Reader J	Reader 1$'$	Reader j'	Reader J'
1	T_{111}	T_{1j1}	T_{1J1}			
2	T_{211}	T_{2j1}	T_{2J1}			
k	T_{k11}	T_{kj1}	T_{kJ1}			
N	T_{N11}	T_{Nj1}	T_{NJ1}			
1$'$				$T_{1'1'2}$	$T_{1'j'2}$	$T_{1'J'2}$
2$'$				$T_{2'1'2}$	$T_{2'j'2}$	$T_{2'J'2}$
k$'$				$T_{k'1'2}$	$T_{k'j'2}$	$T_{k'J'2}$
N$'$				$T_{N'1'2}$	$T_{N'j'2}$	$T_{N'J'2}$

The balanced version of this design requires $I \times N$ total patients and $I \times J$ total readers,
where I is the number of diagnostic tests under study.
There are N interpretations per reader. (Note that I=2 in the table.)
In the unbalanced version of this design,
the number of patients and/or number of readers is different for
the I diagnostic tests.

Table 3.11   Data Set-Up for Unpaired-Patient, Paired-Reader MRMC Design

	Test 1			Test 2		
Patient	Reader 1	Reader j	Reader J	Reader 1	Reader j	Reader J
1	T_{111}	T_{1j1}	T_{1J1}			
2	T_{211}	T_{2j1}	T_{2J1}			
k	T_{k11}	T_{kj1}	T_{kJ1}			
N	T_{N11}	T_{Nj1}	T_{NJ1}			
$1'$				$T_{1'12}$	$T_{1'j2}$	$T_{1'J2}$
$2'$				$T_{2'12}$	$T_{2'j2}$	$T_{2'J2}$
k'				$T_{k'12}$	$T_{k'j2}$	$T_{k'J2}$
N'				$T_{N'12}$	$T_{N'j2}$	$T_{N'J2}$

The balanced version of this design requires $N \times I$ total patients and J total readers, where I is the number of diagnostic tests under study.
There are $N \times I$ interpretations per reader. (Note that I=2 in the table.)
In the unbalanced version of this design,
the number of patients is different for the I diagnostic tests.

Table 3.12   Data Set-Up for Paired-Patient, Unpaired-Reader MRMC Design

	Test 1			Test 2		
Patient	Reader 1	Reader j	Reader J	Reader $1'$	Reader j'	Reader J'
1	T_{111}	T_{1j1}	T_{1J1}	$T_{11'2}$	$T_{1j'2}$	$T_{1J'2}$
2	T_{211}	T_{2j1}	T_{2J1}	$T_{21'2}$	$T_{2j'2}$	$T_{2J'2}$
k	T_{k11}	T_{kj1}	T_{kJ1}	$T_{k1'2}$	$T_{kj'2}$	$T_{kJ'2}$
N	T_{N11}	T_{Nj1}	T_{NJ1}	$T_{N1'2}$	$T_{Nj'2}$	$T_{NJ'2}$

The balanced version of this design requires N total patients and $J \times I$ total readers, where I is the number of diagnostic tests under study.
There are N interpretations per reader. (Note that I=2 in the table.)
In the unbalanced version of this design,
the number of readers is different for the I diagnostic tests.

There are several variations on these designs. In the "hybrid" design (Obu-chowski, 1995) each reader interprets the test results of a different sample of patients. Each patient undergoes all I tests being studied. The reader interpreting a patient's test results interprets the results of all I tests for that patient. Thus, this "hybrid" design is a paired-patient-per-reader, paired-reader design. There are J total readers and $J \times N$ total patients undergoing all I tests. This design requires the fewest number of readers, but requires many more patients than the traditional design. It can be an efficient design when patients can be accrued into the study quickly and inexpensively.

A variation of this hybrid design was developed to take advantage of the savings in the number of readers required with the hybrid design but also reduce the number of patients required with the hybrid design. In the "mixed" design (Obuchowski, 2009), readers are randomized to several groups (usually 2 or 3 groups). Each group of readers interprets a different sample of patients. As in the hybrid design, each patient undergoes all I tests, and the readers interpret all I test results for a patient. This design is ideal for large MRMC studies where it can reduce the number of interpretations that readers must perform for a study. There are many other variations to these designs.

The choice of study design for MRMC studies depends on (1) the nature of the diagnostic tests, i.e. are they mutually exclusive? Do they require specialized training/expertise to interpret? (2) the available resources, i.e. are patients, readers, and/or reader-time limiting resources? and (3) prior information about the patterns of correlations between the tests due to the paired-patient and/or paired-reader design (see chapter 6).

Computer-aided detection (CAD) studies, such as Case Study 2, pose unique challenges to the MRMC study design (Dodd et al., 2004; Wagner et al., 2007). These studies are often performed using the traditional MRMC design, though the hybrid and mixed designs are also viable options. In these studies the readers' interpretations with CAD can be collected in two ways: **sequential read** (the reader first interprets the image without CAD, then immediately is given the CAD marks and asked to re-interpret the image) or **concurrent read** (the reader is given the CAD marks at the start of the interpretation). The readers' unaided interpretation (i.e. without CAD) can be collected in one of three ways: i) historically (i.e. document readers' performance before CAD was available), ii) in a separate reading session where CAD is not used, or iii) in the first part of the sequential reading format (i.e. the readers' unaided interpretations prior to seeing the CAD marks can be recorded and saved). While readers' performance with historical controls offers some information about the effect of CAD, there are many other factors (in addition to CAD) that can cause changes in readers' performance over time; thus, these studies do not permit precise estimation of the effect of CAD.

Two common CAD study designs, along with their advantages and disadvantages, are summarized in Table 3.13. In design 1 the sequential reading format is used, with the unaided interpretation occurring prior to displaying the CAD marks. Design 2 is a fully crossed design with separate reading sessions with and without CAD; in the CAD sessions either the sequential or concurrent reading formats can be used. Design 1 is a more efficient design in terms of reducing readers' time, but there is the potential for readers to perform differently when they know they will soon see the CAD marks. Also, a randomized reading order is not possible because all of the patients' images are first interpreted without CAD. Design 2 requires a longer study because readers must interpret each image at two different reading sessions (i.e. once unaided, and once aided with CAD). Also, in design 2, when comparing readers' interpretations with and without CAD, there is more total variability in the difference in accuracy with vs. without CAD because the readers are interpreting the image with and without CAD on different days (i.e. there is **intra-reader variability**, the variability in a reader's interpretation when reading the same image or test result on different occasions).

A randomized reading order can and should be implemented with design 2. The patients can be randomized to two groups: the first group's images are first interpreted in reading sessions without CAD. The second group's images are first interpreted in reading sessions with CAD (either sequential or concurrent reading formats). After a wash-out period, the first group's images are interpreted in reading sessions with CAD, and the second group's images are interpreted in reading sessions without CAD.

Table 3.13   Two Common Study Designs for Computer-Aided Detection (CAD) Studies

Design	Description	Advantages	Disadvantages
1 Sequential	An image is interpreted without CAD and saved as "unaided;" then the CAD marks are displayed and the image is re-interpreted with CAD. This process is repeated for all images.	No wash-out period needed; Less variability in interpretations between unaided and aided readings; Shorter study duration.	Potential reading order bias; Readers may pay less or more attention to the unaided image, knowing they will get the CAD marks soon.
2 Crossed	Separate reading sessions are used for "unaided" readings and for CAD readings. Either the sequential or concurrent CAD reading format can be used.	Reading order bias can be negated; Readers in the "unaided" session do not anticipate the CAD marks.	Wash-out period needed; Longer study duration; More variability in interpretations.

Another issue to consider in planning reader studies, particularly in Phase III studies, is the prevalence of patients with the condition in the study sample. Readers in diagnostic accuracy studies are often asked to review samples with an augmented prevalence rate. Egglin and Feinstein (1996) performed a study to assess the impact of prevalence of disease on test interpretation. They assembled a test set of pulmonary arteriograms with a prevalence of 33% and embedded it into two larger groups of films such that Group A had an overall prevalence rate of 60% and Group B had an overall prevalence rate of 20%. After blinded randomized reviews by six readers, they found that reviewers' accuracies of the embedded set differed, depending on the context (i.e. Group A or B). The mean sensitivity for diagnosing pulmonary emboli was significantly higher in group A (0.75 versus 0.60). Mean specificity was lower in group A but the change was not statistically significant (0.64 versus 0.68). Egglin and Feinstein defined **context bias** as the bias in estimates of accuracy which can occur when the sample prevalence differs greatly from the population prevalence. Gur et al. (2003) performed a comprehensive evaluation of context bias. Their study included 14 readers, 1632 patients (including a nested test set of 179), and five conditions (lung nodules, pneumothorax, interstitial disease, alveolar disease, and rib fracture). They found no change in observer performance as the prevalence rate varied from 2% to 28%. The absence of bias was consistent over readers and conditions. Most studies of diagnostic test accuracy include a sample with a prevalence rate much higher than occurs in a clinical population. This strategy reduces the overall sample size required of these studies and saves reader time and study expense. Given the findings of Gur et al, this strategy seems appropriate.

3.8.3 Reader Training

The last topic we discuss in this section is reader training. The goal of most training is to familiarize the reader with the interpretation setting and format to be used in the study. Straub et al. (1990) looked at the effect of three types of training: (1) a general instructional session describing the study protocol, (2) practice with a teaching file that allowed readers to get accustomed to the modalities being evaluated and gave them feedback on the accuracy of their results for the teaching cases, and (3) a training session to encourage readers to distribute their ratings over the five-point confidence scale to produce more visually-appealing and hopefully more reliable ROC curves. After the first training session the readers asked significantly fewer questions about the type of abnormalities being investigated, and the session was judged useful by the authors. After the second training session the readers usually improved their accuracy once they became accustomed to the modalities and display modes. This type of training was also viewed as essential to the success of the study. For the third type of training they found that for some readers there was a significant reduction in accuracy post-training (Gur et al., 1990). Their findings suggest that this type of training can alter reader performance and possibly affect the conclusions of studies.

We recommend that investigators provide readers with general instructions about the study (e.g. purpose of study, definition of terms, general description of sample population, diagnostic tests, availability of any diagnostic tools (e.g. image optimization tools such as window/leveling), and any standard criteria for interpreting cases) and also perform training using non-study patients. This will allow readers to become familiar with the types of patients used, the approximate sample prevalence rate, the study forms, the imaging software, and the setting for the interpretations. When selecting cases for training, we need to be careful not to bias the readers; this could happen, for example, if the cases were all more easily diagnosed on one modality than the other.

In our experience some discussion with the readers about the confidence scale to be used in the study is necessary. Readers can be shown cases of different complexity and subtleness, and the investigators can suggest how the confidence scale might be distributed across these cases. We should avoid prescribing what scores should be used on various types of cases, as differences in how readers apply the scale is natural and should not be standardized.

3.9   PLAN DATA ANALYSES

In this section we talk about the statistical hypotheses commonly used in diagnostic accuracy studies, adjustment for covariates, and how the test results should be reported. We begin with a discussion of the statistical hypotheses.

3.9.1   Statistical Hypotheses

Most diagnostic accuracy studies have one (or more) of the following goals: (1) measure the accuracy of a single diagnostic test, (2) compare a test's accuracy to a prespecified value, (3) determine whether the accuracies of two or more diagnostic tests are different, (4) assess whether two diagnostic tests have equivalent accuracies, (5) assess whether a new test's accuracy is non-inferior to a standard test, (6) measure the added diagnostic value of a new test to existing tests or (7) identify a suitable cutoff value for the test result.

For the first goal we need to construct a confidence interval for the diagnostic accuracy of the test (see Chapter 4 for details about constructing and interpreting confidence intervals). In Case Study 3 we want to construct a confidence interval for the accuracy of MRA. We might also want to test whether or not MRA's accuracy is sufficient to replace Catheter Angiography. The appropriate null, H_0, and alternative, H_1, hypotheses are

$$H_0: \theta_{MRA} \leq \theta_o$$

$$H_1: \theta_{MRA} > \theta_o,$$

where θ_{MRA} is the diagnostic accuracy for MRA (which could be measured in terms of sensitivity, specificity, ROC area, or the partial area under the ROC curve) and θ_o is a prespecified value such that values less than or equal to it are evidence that MRA cannot replace CA, and values greater than it are evidence that MRA can replace CA. In order to establish the appropriate value for θ_o, we would need to consider the risks and costs of false positives and false negatives with both MRA and CA, probably using decision analysis to appropriately weigh the risks.

In phase I studies we often want to know if the new test has any diagnostic value. Specifically, we want to know if the ROC area of the new test exceeds 0.5. We would use a similar set of hypotheses:

$$H_0: \theta_{newtest} \leq \theta_o$$

$$H_1: \theta_{newtest} > \theta_o,$$

where $\theta_{newtest}$ is the ROC area of the new test and θ_o is 0.5.

In Case Study 2 we want to compare the accuracy of readers without versus with CAD to determine which reading format is better. The null hypothesis is that the two tests are equal in accuracy. The alternative hypothesis is that the tests' accuracies are different.

$$H_0: \theta_{withoutCAD} = \theta_{CAD}$$

$$H_1: \theta_{withoutCAD} \neq \theta_{CAD}.$$

The alternative hypothesis is two-tailed because we are interested in both situations, i.e. without CAD is better than with CAD, and CAD is better than without CAD. Depending on how CAD is scored, however, a one-tailed alternative may be appropriate. For example, in some studies using a sequential design readers are allowed only to add lesions to the list of lesions seen unaided. If θ denotes test sensitivity, then θ_{CAD} can only be equal to or greater than $\theta_{withoutCAD}$. More recently, investigators have avoided this bias by requiring readers to re-evaluate, or even re-record, any suspicious findings seen prior to the CAD marks. For these studies, a two-tailed alternative is appropriate.

As an example of testing for equivalence, suppose we are comparing digitized film (new test) to plain film screen mammography (standard test). We want to test whether the accuracy of the digitized image is the same as plain film. We must first specify the smallest difference between the two tests which would not be considered equivalent. For example, suppose that if the two tests' ROC areas differ by 0.05 or more, then they would not be considered equivalent; if they differ by less than 0.05, then they are considered equivalent. The appropriate hypotheses are

$$H_0: \theta_{film} \geq \theta_{digital} + \Delta_M$$

$$H_1: \theta_{film} < \theta_{digital} + \Delta_M,$$

where Δ_M is the smallest difference that is unacceptable. Here, $\Delta_M = 0.05$. Note that the alternative hypothesis is one-tailed.

In the sixth goal, we want to measure the incremental value of a new test. For example, in Case Study 1 we want to test whether the addition of CT images to SPECT improves readers' diagnostic accuracy over SPECT alone. The incremental value is quantified by comparing the ROC curve for the combination of the existing and new tests with the ROC curve for the existing test alone. In our example, the reader looks at both the CT and SPECT images, weighs the information from the two in his mind, and then assigns a single confidence score. In other studies, a statistical model is needed to optimally combine the results of two or more tests. For example, in detecting prostate cancer we might want to test whether PSA adds value over just using the patient's age to predict prostate cancer. The ROC area with just patient age would be compared to the ROC area with age and PSA; logistic regression could be used to optimally weigh age and PSA to create a single test result incorporating both variables. The set of hypotheses are

$$H_0: \theta_{age+PSA} \leq \theta_{age}$$

$$H_1: \theta_{age+PSA} > \theta_{age}$$

.

3.9.2   Planning for Covariate Adjustment

In designing a study, it's important to plan not only for the collection of possible covariates, but also how their relationship to test accuracy will be evaluated and handled. The importance of covariate adjustment cannot be overstated. Test accuracy can be over-estimated or under-estimated by failing to adjust for important covariates. Furthermore, the generalizability of the study results are in jeopardy. Test accuracy must be evaluated and reported for patient groups with different symptoms and clinical characteristics in order for study results to be transferable to populations at other institutions (Scott et al., 2008).

Covariates can impact diagnostic accuracy in two ways (Janes and Pepe, 2008a,b) (see Table 3.14):

Covariates may influence the test results of patients while not altering the ROC curve. This happens when the inherent ROC curve is the same at each level of the covariate, but the cutpoints that generate the curves differ depending on the level of the covariate. Without adjustment, the pooled, or unadjusted, ROC curve (and summary measures of accuracy estimated from the ROC curve) will under-estimate the accuracy of the diagnostic test. If matching is used in the study so that controls are matched to cases on the covariate, the unadjusted ROC curve is still biased. In other words, matching does not eliminate confounding. Covariate-adjusted ROC curves are needed to

Table 3.14   Steps in Determining When Covariate Adjustment is Needed

Step	Description
1	Test for association between each covariate and the test results of patients without the condition. For disease-specific covariates, test for association with the test results of patients with the condition.
2	If no associations, no covariate-adjustment is needed (skip step 3). If associations are evident, determine their effect on test accuracy in step 3.
3	If covariates affect cutpoints but not the ROC curve, covariate-adjusted ROC curves are needed. If covariates change the ROC curve, covariate-specific ROC curves are needed.

appropriately characterize the diagnostic accuracy of the test; the adjustment is needed in both unmatched and matched studies.

The second way that covariates can impact diagnostic accuracy is by altering the inherent accuracy of the test, i.e. the separation between the patients without and with the condition differs depending on the value of the covariate. In this situation, there is effect modification (Janes and Pepe, 2008a). The pooled or unadjusted ROC curve may over- or under-estimate the true accuracy. An example of a covariate that causes effect modification is severity of disease; test accuracy is often higher for more severe disease and lower for more subtle, less severe disease. Covariate-specific ROC curves should be used to describe the test's accuracy for each level of the covariate. However, if the sample size is small or it is desirable to have a single summary curve to compare against a competitor diagnostic test, then a covariate-adjusted (AROC) curve can be used. Covariate-specific ROC curves and covariate-adjusted ROC curves (which are simply a weighted average of the covariate-specific ROC curves) are discussed further in Chapter 8.

In Case Study 3 we suspect that symptom status could affect MRA's accuracy. We could look at the distribution of MRA scores for asymptomatic patients without stenosis and the distribution of MRA scores for symptomatic patients without stenosis. We might compare the two distributions using a Mann-Whitney U test. If there is evidence of an association (i.e. the distributions differ), then two ROC curves - one for symptomatic patients and one for asymptomatic patients - could be constructed and compared. If the ROC curves differ, then there is evidence of effect modification. If the curves do not differ, then a single covariate-adjusted curve can be estimated. Another potential confounder is the percent of stenosis. It is a measure of the severity of disease and may be an effect modifier. The distribution of MRA scores for patients with mild, moderate, and severe stenosis could be compared using a Kruskal-Wallis test. If there is evidence of association, then covariate-specific ROC curves may be needed.

3.9.3   Reporting Test Results

In reporting the results of a diagnostic accuracy study, there are several characteristics of the study design that should be described so that readers will be able to determine if the results of the study (i.e. the measured accuracy of a diagnostic test) are transferable (generalizable) to another setting (Irwig et al., 2002). For transferability of test results to be possible, the definition of the disease must be constant, the same diagnostic test must be used, and the definitions of test results (e.g. positive and negative results) must be the same. In addition to study design characteristics, there are several questions about the reported test accuracy: (1) What is the estimated accuracy and how is it interpreted for the study? (2) With what precision was the accuracy estimated? (3) How does the accuracy vary across patient subgroups? and (4) To whom do the results apply?

In addressing the first question, what is the estimated accuracy and how is it interpreted for the study, it is important to first clearly define "the condition" being studied (e.g. "detection of colon polyps ≥ 2.0 cm"). We need to specify how the results of the test were quantified and then report the estimated accuracy and its interpretation relevant to the study. When reporting sensitivity and specificity, we need to indicate the cutoff value used because without the cutoff value the estimates of sensitivity and specificity are meaningless. When reporting positive and negative predictive values we must specify the prevalence of the condition in the study sample. Some (Eisenberg, 1995) have even suggested reporting PPVs and NPVs at standardized prevalence rates. For multi-reader studies the accuracy of each reader should be estimated (i.e. no "pooled" or consensus accuracy estimates). When there are fewer than about 10 readers, often the accuracy of each reader is reported, along with the average reader accuracy. For larger studies we should report the average reader accuracy, the minimum and maximum estimates, and the variability between the readers. The study by Beam et al. (1996) is an excellent illustration of reporting accuracy from multi-reader studies. From a sample of 108 ACR-accredited mammographers interpreting 79 screening films (paired-patient, paired-reader design), the authors estimated and reported the readers' sensitivities which varied by 53% (47% to 100%, average of 79%), specificities which varied by 63% (36% to 99%, average of 89%), and ROC areas which varied by 21% (74% to 95%, average of 85%).

For tests that can produce uninterpretable results, it's important to specify the frequency and cause of uninterpretable results, how these results were accounted for in the statistical analysis, and the rationale for their handling. Here, **uninterpretable** means technically unacceptable; these are not the same as equivocal, intermediate, or indeterminate test results (Begg et al.,

1986). Examples of uninterpretable test results are insufficient cell specimens when performing needle biopsy, abdominal gas interfering with pelvic US studies, and too dense breast tissue for mammography screening. When comparing two tests, the frequency of uninterpretable results may differ; this may be very important in ranking the performance of the tests (Begg et al., 1986). Although the indeterminate results may be excluded from calculation of diagnostic test accuracy, a test with more indeterminate results has less diagnostic accuracy (Scott et al., 2008). For example, Poynard et al. (1982) describe the assessment of three tests for diagnosing extrahepatic cholestasis. They show that the usefulness of the three tests is strongly influenced by the different frequencies of uninterpretable results.

There are two important considerations in dealing with uninterpretable test results (Begg et al., 1986): (1) the potential repeatability of the test and (2) the possible association between the uninterpretable test result and both the true disease status and unobserved test result (if the test is repeatable). Repeatable, here, means that the cause of the uninterpretability is transient (in which case it is possible to repeat the test and observe the test result) and not an inherent property of the subject (e.g. obesity interfering with the US exam, in which case the test result will never be interpretable).

If the test is not repeatable, then Begg et al. (1986) recommend that the uninterpretable result be considered as another possible outcome of the test. For constructing an ROC curve, they suggest that the likelihood ratio (See Chapter 2) be computed for all the possible outcomes of the test; then the uninterpretable result can be ranked with the other test outcomes according to the value of its LR.

If the test is repeatable and the uninterpretable test results occur randomly (i.e. are not related to either the unobserved/underlying test result or the true disease status), then unbiased estimates of accuracy can be obtained by simply ignoring (discarding) the uninterpretable cases (Begg et al., 1986).

Another situation occurs when the test is repeatable and the uninterpretable test results are correlated to the true disease status. For example, Poynard et al. (1982) report uninterpretable test results in 36% of patients with versus 7% without extrahepatic cholestasis for one of the three tests under study (percutaneous transhepatic cholangiography). These uninterpretable test results provide relevant information about the unknown status of the condition. This information should not be overlooked, but rather used in a decision rule for diagnosing the patient.

Finally, when the test is repeatable and the test is correlated to the underlying test result, then the uninterpretable results again cannot be ignored. Begg et al. (1986) recommend that the test be repeated for those cases whose initial test was uninterpretable. Then, the second (or third, if necessary) test result for these patients should be used for estimation of diagnostic accuracy. This assumes, of course, that the disease process hasn't changed during the time between the first and subsequent test(s).

In addressing the second question regarding the precision of the accuracy estimates, it is critical that we report the standard errors and confidence intervals (CI) for accuracy. There are several potential sources of variability in diagnostic accuracy studies: variability between and within patients, variability between and within readers interpreting the tests, and variability between and within the diagnostic device/modality. It's important to state which sources of variability are included in standard errors and CIs. Estimation of standard errors and construction of CIs for single-modality, single-reader studies are discussed in Chapter 4; for studies comparing two tests, see Chapter 5; and for multi-reader studies, see Chapter 9.

In addressing the third question, i.e. accuracy for various patient subgroups, we need to assess and report how test accuracy is affected by 1. patient covariates (e.g. demographics, signs and symptoms, comorbidities, and clinical site (if applicable)), 2. factors associated with the condition (e.g. size, severity, location), 3. factors associated with the device/modality (i.e. particularly for retrospective studies and/or studies of long duration because the imaging parameters and machines themselves may have changed), and 4. reader covariates (if applicable) (e.g. experience, training). Chapters 8 and 9 discuss various statistical methods for adjusting for covariates.

Finally, when reporting test accuracy, we need to be clear about the generalizability of the test results. The generalizability of a study depends on the study's target populations (patients and readers) and how well the samples represent these populations. As we discussed throughout this chapter, Phase I and II studies usually have narrowly defined populations. In contrast, it is the role of Phase III studies to estimate, without bias, the accuracy of tests for a specific clinical application. For these studies, if we have been able to properly sample patients (and readers) from the target populations, then the study results are generalizable to our target populations.

The **STARD committee** (Bossuyt et al., 2003) created a 25-item checklist, along with a flow diagram of the study execution, for study investigators to use in preparing their manuscripts; the checklist and flow diagram also allow readers to assess the potential for bias and to evaluate the generalizability of a study. The checklist identifies items that a diagnostic accuracy study should include in each section of the manuscript, from Title to Discussion. Briefly, the 25 items are as follows: In the title/abstract/keywords, the study should be identified as a study of diagnostic accuracy. In the Introduction, the research questions should be clearly stated. In the Methods section, the type of study (prospective or retrospective), the study population, method of patient recruitment, and the sampling method should be described. The gold standard and technical description of the test and by how and whom they were interpreted should be clearly described. The methods used to estimate and compare diagnostic accuracy should be reported. The Results section should include when the study was performed, basic characteristics of the study population, the number of eligible patients that did and did not undergo the diagnostic test(s) and gold standard, the time interval between diagnostic test and gold standard, the distribution of disease severity and comorbidities in the study sample, a table or plot comparing test and gold standard results, any adverse events of the test or gold standard, estimates of test accuracy with 95% CIs, the number and handling of indeterminate test results, variability in test results for subgroups of patients, and estimates of test reproducibility. Finally, in the Discussion the authors should discuss the clinical applicability of the study results.

3.10   DETERMINE SAMPLE SIZE

Often the last step in designing a diagnostic accuracy study is determining the number of patients, and readers when appropriate, needed for the study. The information needed for sample size determination, the various issues to consider, the formulae for calculating sample size, and examples are given in Chapter 6.

CHAPTER 4

ESTIMATION AND HYPOTHESIS TESTING IN A SINGLE SAMPLE

In Chapter 2, we introduced several measures of the accuracy of diagnostic tests. The choice of appropriate methods to estimate these accuracy measures and their variability is a function of the type of data and the assumptions we are willing to make concerning the distribution of the data.

Some tests produce only two results: positive or negative for the condition. This type of data is called binary data. Accuracy for binary data can be assessed by measures such as sensitivity, specificity, odds ratio, and likelihood ratio (LR).

Other tests produce results that can take on more than two values. Data that take on only a few ordered values, such as the breast imaging and reporting system (BIRADs) scale used in mammography, are called ordinal data. Test results can also be continuous (numeric, quantitative), taking on an unlimited number of values; these results include objective measures such as laboratory values (e.g., creatine phosphokinase (CPK) enzymes), objective assessments of images (e.g., attenuation values), and subjective assessments (e.g., ratings of confidence, ranging from 0% to 100%, that a malignancy is present).

Statistical Methods in Diagnostic Medicine,
Second Edition. By Xiao-Hua Zhou, Nancy A. Obuchowski, Donna K. McClish
Copyright © 2011 John Wiley & Sons, Inc.

Accuracy for ordinal or continuous scale tests can be assessed by measures such as the receiver operating characteristic (ROC) curve, the area and partial area under the curve, and the sensitivity at a specific false positive rate (FPR). The most appropriate method of estimating these accuracy measures depends on whether the data are ordinal or continuous, as well as the assumptions we wish to make about the distribution of the test results. If the distribution of test results is assumed to follow a particular probability distribution, the methods used will be called parametric. Methods not relying on any distributional assumptions, known as nonparametric methods, will also be used. Methods that make some distributional assumptions, but leave others unspecified fall in between parametric and non-parametric and are often referred to as semi-parametric methods. In addition, design considerations, such as whether all tested units are independent, will be a factor.

In this chapter, we discuss how to estimate these accuracy measures and estimate the variances and confidence intervals for them. The results are presented separately for binary (Section 4.1), ordinal (Section 4.2) and continuous (Section 4.3) data. We also discuss both parametric and nonparametric methods and consider some basic hypothesis testing in a single sample situation (Section 4.4).

We assume that the true condition status of each individual is known - and known without error (i.e., there is no verification bias or imperfect standard bias). Methods dealing with these issues are discussed in Chapters 10 and 11.

For sake of simplicity (unless otherwise specified), for all ordinal- and continuous-scale test, we assume that larger values of the test result imply a higher likelihood of the condition of interest. For example, if an image is rated on a 1-5 scale, we assume that a value of 5 is more likely to be associated with the condition than a value of 3 or 1.

4.1 BINARY-SCALE DATA

4.1.1 Sensitivity and Specificity

Suppose we want to assess the accuracy of computer-aided detection (CAD) for enhancing the detection of polyps when using computed tomography colonography (CTC). As described in detail in Chapter 1 (Case Study 2), 30 patients were part of a reader performance study designed to compare the accuracy of CTC in detecting polyps 6mm or larger with and without the use of CAD. We would like to estimate the sensitivity of CAD for detection of these polyps.

We introduced estimates for sensitivity and specificity of test results in Chapter 2, but we repeat the topic here for completeness. Suppose we have a study with a single diagnostic test applied to each patient. The sensitivity of the diagnostic test is simply the proportion of patients with the condition that have a positive test. The specificity of the diagnostic test is the proportion of patients without the condition that have a negative test. As we saw in

Chapter 2, the data for binary test results can be displayed as in Table 4.1. Estimates of sensitivity and specificity are then:

Table 4.1   Display of Binary Data

True Condition Status	Test Result Positive ($T = 1$)	Negative($T = 0$)	Total
Present ($D = 1$)	s_1	s_0	n_1
Absent ($D = 0$)	r_1	r_0	n_0
Total	m_1	m_0	N

$$\widehat{Se} = \frac{s_1}{n_1}, \widehat{Sp} = \frac{r_0}{n_0}. \tag{4.1}$$

The variances of these estimators follow from the variance of a sample proportion and are estimated by

$$\widehat{Var}(\widehat{Se}) = \frac{\widehat{Se}(1 - \widehat{Se})}{n_1} = \frac{s_1 s_0}{n_1^3}, \widehat{Var}(\widehat{Sp}) = \frac{r_1 r_0}{n_0^3}. \tag{4.2}$$

The usual approach to constructing a confidence interval for a measure of diagnostic accuracy assumes a large sample size, so that it is reasonable for the estimated measure to follow a normal distribution. The confidence interval, usually referred to as an asymptotic interval, generally has the following form with upper (UL) and lower (LL) limits:

$$(LL, UL) = \left(\widehat{\theta} - z_{1-\alpha/2}\sqrt{\widehat{Var}(\widehat{\theta})}, \widehat{\theta} + z_{1-\alpha/2}\sqrt{\widehat{Var}(\widehat{\theta})}\right), \tag{4.3}$$

where $\widehat{\theta}$ is the estimate of the accuracy measure, θ; $z_{1-\alpha/2}$ is the $1 - \alpha/2$ percentile of the standard normal distribution; and $100(1 - \alpha)\%$ is the confidence level. Since sensitivity and specificity are proportions, we can construct an asymptotic $100(1 - \alpha)\%$ confidence interval based on the equation (4.3), often referred to as the Wald's interval. For example, for the sensitivity, $Se = \theta$ and the confidence interval is:

$$\left(\widehat{Se} - z_{1-\alpha/2}\sqrt{\widehat{Se}(1 - \widehat{Se})/n_1}, \widehat{Se} + z_{1-\alpha/2}\sqrt{\widehat{Se}(1 - \widehat{Se})/n_1}\right) \tag{4.4}$$

Unfortunately, this formula has two major drawbacks. First, the percentage of time that the confidence interval actually includes the true value of the accuracy parameter (i.e., the coverage) is often much smaller than desired. This situation is particularly true for small sample size, and for accuracy values close to 0 or 1. Second, when the accuracy is close to 1, the upper limit of the confidence interval often exceeds 1.0 (a value that we know is impossible). Many alternative confidence intervals have been suggested. Based on a recent article by Zhou et al. (2008) we suggest two alternatives as the best. The confidence interval by Agresti and Coull (1998) is recommended as being simple computationally and having good coverage as long as the proportion is not near 0 or 1. (Even near 0, according to Brown et al. (2001), the Agresti-Coull (AC) interval is conservative with greater than $100(1-\alpha)\%$ coverage). The estimate of the proportion (here, the sensitivity) is modified by adding $z^2_{1-\alpha/2}/2$ to the numerator and $z^2_{1-\alpha/2}$ to the denominator of the usual sensitivity estimator, so that

$$\widehat{Se}_{AC} = \frac{s_1 + z^2_{1-\alpha/2}/2}{n_1 + z^2_{1-\alpha/2}}, \widehat{Var}\left(\widehat{Se}_{AC}\right) = \frac{\widehat{Se}_{AC}(1-\widehat{Se}_{AC})}{n_1 + z^2_{1-\alpha/2}}. \tag{4.5}$$

This is substituted into the equation (4.3). (Note that often the AC interval is approximated by adding two positive results and two negative results.) The other interval, referred to as the ZL interval, and particularly recommended when the sensitivity is near 0 or 1, is

$$\left(\frac{e^{LL}}{1+e^{LL}}, \frac{e^{UL}}{1+e^{UL}}\right), \tag{4.6}$$

where the limits (LL, UL) are

$$LL = \ln[\widehat{Se}/(1-\widehat{Se})] - n^{-1/2}[\widehat{Se}(1-\widehat{Se})]^{-1/2}g^{-1}(z_{1-\alpha/2}) \tag{4.7}$$

$$UL = \ln[\widehat{Se}/(1-\widehat{Se})] - n^{-1/2}[\widehat{Se}(1-\widehat{Se})]^{-1/2}g^{-1}(z_{\alpha/2}). \tag{4.8}$$

Here

$$g^{-1}(x) = -n^{1/2}(\hat{\gamma}/6)^{-1}[(1-(\hat{\gamma}/2)(n^{-1/2}x - n^{-1}\hat{\gamma}/6))^{1/3} - 1], \tag{4.9}$$

and

$$\hat{\gamma} = (1 - 2\widehat{Se})/\sqrt{\widehat{Se}(1-\widehat{Se})}. \tag{4.10}$$

Both the AC and ZL confidence intervals have coverage usually greater than the nominal level, but the expected width of the ZL interval is shorter than that of the AC interval, particularly for values of sensitivity near 0 or 1. Also, the limits of the ZL confidence interval will never be less than 0 or greater than 1. The confidence interval for the specificity, since it is a proportion, can be estimated the same way.

4.1.1.1 Sensitivity: Case Study 2

In our example of assessing the accuracy of CAD-enhanced CTC to detect polyps, there were 30 patients, 25 of whom had at least one polyp diagnosed ($n_1 = 25$). While there were seven readers, we focus here on the accuracy of a single reader (the first). For the initial analysis, we say that the reader was correct if she or he detected at least one polyp. This occurred for 22 of the 25 subjects. We call these true positives ($s_1 = 22$). The estimate of sensitivity is $\widehat{Se} = 22/25 = 0.88$, with a variance of $(0.88 \times 0.12)/25 = 0.00422$. Using the equation (4.4), (setting $\alpha = 0.05$; $z_{1-\alpha/2} = 1.96$) we estimate the limits of the 95% confidence interval as

$$0.88 \pm 1.96\sqrt{0.00422},$$

which gives the confidence interval of (0.753, 1.007). Note that the estimated upper limit is greater than 1. If we estimate the confidence interval, instead, using the AC method, the 95% CI is (0.690, 0.965), while the 95% CI is (0.710, 0.967) using the ZL method. As expected, the ZL interval has shorter width than the AC interval.

4.1.2 Predictive Value of a Positive or Negative

When accuracy data are collected from a cohort or cross-sectional study, the predictive value of a positive (PPV) or negative test (NPV) can be estimated as

$$\widehat{PPV} = \frac{s_1}{m_1} \text{ and } \widehat{NPV} = \frac{r_0}{m_0} \tag{4.11}$$

with variance

$$\widehat{Var}(\widehat{PPV}) = \frac{s_1 r_1}{m_1^3}, \text{ and } \widehat{Var}(\widehat{NPV}) = \frac{r_0 s_0}{m_0^3}. \tag{4.12}$$

As PPV and NPV are proportions, confidence intervals can be constructed in the same way as described in Section 4.1.1.

Direct estimates of PPV and NPV as proportions are not appropriate if accuracy of a test is assessed using data from a case-control study. In addition, as discussed in Chapter 2, direct estimates of PPV and NPV from a sample may not be relevant to the clinical question, if the prevalence of the patient population of interest is different from that of the population represented by the sample estimates. Bayes theorem can be used to estimate predictive values for any set of values for sensitivity, specificity and prevalence, even if derived from different populations.

A paper by Mercaldo et al. (2007) recommended confidence intervals for the PPV based on the logit transformation of the Bayes formula:

$$logit(PPV) = ln\left[\frac{p \times Se}{(1 - Sp)(1 - p)}\right]; logit(NPV) = ln\left[\frac{(1 - p)Sp}{(1 - Se)p}\right], \tag{4.13}$$

$$Var(logit(PPV)) = \left[\frac{1 - Se}{Se}\right]\frac{1}{n_1} + \left[\frac{Sp}{1 - Sp}\right]\frac{1}{n_0}, \tag{4.14}$$

$$\text{and } Var(logit(NPV)) = \left[\frac{Se}{1 - Se}\right]\frac{1}{n_1} + \left[\frac{1 - Sp}{Sp}\right]\frac{1}{n_0}. \tag{4.15}$$

The equation (4.3) can be used to construct a confidence interval for $logit(PPV)$ or $logit(NPV)$. The $100(1-\alpha)\%$ confidence limits for the PPV, for example, would look like

$$\frac{e^{logit(\widehat{PPV}) \pm z_{1-\alpha/2}\sqrt{\widehat{Var}(logit(\widehat{PPV}))}}}{1 + e^{logit(\widehat{PPV}) \pm z_{1-\alpha/2}\sqrt{\widehat{Var}(logit(\widehat{PPV}))}}}. \qquad (4.16)$$

Mercaldo et al. (2007) found this confidence interval to have good coverage except when PPV or NPV were estimated as 1.0. In that case, they suggested adding a continuity correction, $k^2/2$, $k = z_{1-\alpha/2}$ to each cell prior to estimating Se and Sp. It is important to note that they assumed a known value of prevalence, and thus did not take into account the additional variability introduced in the PPV estimate when prevalence is estimated.

Mossman (2001) compared five methods for constructing confidence intervals which took into account the variability of estimated prevalence: an objective Bayesian method, two log-odds methods, a likelihood ratio method and a delta method. He concluded that the objective Bayesian method performed best, with the delta method the best of the three methods with explicit formulae. We describe these two methods here.

The objective Bayesian Method for the confidence interval of PPV involves drawing repeated random samples of prevalence, sensitivity and specificity from prior distributions for these parameters, estimating the PPV (similar to Bootstrap percentile confidence intervals described in Appendix B4.3) and choosing appropriate quantiles from these values. More specifically, a $100(1-\alpha)\%$ confidence interval for the PPV using the objective Bayesian method can be constructed as follows:

(1) Draw B random samples from the Beta distribution $\beta(x; s_i + 1/2, m_1 - s_i + 1/2)$, $\beta(x; r_i + 1/2, m_0 - r_i + 1/2)$, and $\beta(x; n_1 + 1/2, N - n_1 + 1/2)$ to get values for sensitivity $(Se^{(i)})$, specificity $(Sp^{(i)})$ and prevalence $(p^{(i)})$, respectively, $i = 1, 2, \ldots, B$ where

$$\beta(x; a, b) = [\Gamma(a+b)/\Gamma(a)\Gamma(b)]x^{a-1}(1-x)^{b-1}.$$

(2) For the i-th draw, substitute into the formula for the PPV

$$PPV^{(i)} = \frac{p^{(i)}Se^{(i)}}{p^{(i)}Se^{(i)} + (1-p^{(i)})(1-Sp^{(i)})}.$$

(3) The $B(\alpha/2)$ and $B(1-\alpha/2)$ ordered values of these B estimates provide lower and upper limits of a $100(1-\alpha)\%$ confidence interval for the PPV. Mossman (2001) suggested that B be large, perhaps 10,000.

The less computationally intense delta method uses the equation (4.3), along with a variance estimate using the delta method. This variance is as follows:

$$Var(\widehat{PPV}) = \left(\frac{\partial PPV}{\partial p}\right)^2 Var(\widehat{p}) + \left(\frac{\partial PPV}{\partial Se}\right)^2 Var(\widehat{Se})$$

$$+ \left(\frac{\partial PPV}{\partial Sp}\right)^2 Var(\widehat{Sp}). \tag{4.17}$$

Estimates of the partial derivatives are as follows:

$$\frac{\partial PPV}{\partial p} = \frac{\widehat{Se}(1 - \widehat{Sp})}{[\widehat{p}\widehat{Se} + (1 - \widehat{p})(1 - \widehat{Sp})]^2}, \tag{4.18}$$

$$\frac{\partial PPV}{\partial Se} = \frac{(1 - \widehat{p})\widehat{p}(1 - \widehat{Sp})}{[\widehat{p}\widehat{Se} + (1 - \widehat{p})(1 - \widehat{Sp})]^2}, \tag{4.19}$$

and

$$\frac{\partial PPV}{\partial Sp} = \frac{-(1 - \widehat{p})\widehat{p}\widehat{Se}}{[\widehat{p}\widehat{Se} + (1 - \widehat{p})(1 - \widehat{Sp})]^2}. \tag{4.20}$$

The variance of the NPV can be derived similarly. See Mossman (2001) for more details of all methods and their comparison.

4.1.2.1 Predictive values: Case Study 3   Case Study 3 looked at the use of MRA for detection of significant carotid stenosis in patients who had suffered TIA or stroke. Four different radiologists scored the MRAs of the left and right carotid arteries from 1 to 5, with increasing values indicating more likelihood of stenosis. Here we convert the data to binary, considering a positive test result for a score of 4 or 5. Looking only at Radiologist 4 (see Table 4.6), left carotid, 56 of 62 subjects with significant carotid stenosis were called positive by MRA and 23 of 101 subjects without significant carotid stenosis were called positive by MRA. A direct estimate of PPV would be $56/79 = 0.709$. Note that this estimate of PPV is meaningful for a clinician if the prevalence of significant carotid stenosis for the population she or he treats is similar to that of this study, $\widehat{p} = 62/163 = 0.38$. A study in Japan (Tanimoto et al., 2005) found carotid stenosis in 124 of 632 (0.196) consecutive patients scheduled to undergo coronary angiography due to suspected CAD. The predictive value of a positive for MRA estimated above (0.709) would not apply to this Japanese population. Assuming the same sensitivity and specificity of MRA as in Case Study 3 ($\widehat{Se} = 56/62 = 0.903; \widehat{Sp} = 78/101 = 0.772$) and using Bayes Theorem, we can estimate PPV for this Japanese population as

$$\widehat{PPV} = \frac{0.903 \times 0.196}{0.903 \times 0.196 + (1 - 0.772) \times (1 - 0.196)} = 0.491.$$

As expected, the PPV is lower in the Japanese population. Estimate of 95% confidence intervals based on the work of Mercaldo et al. (2007) yields (0.401, 0.583). Using the delta method (Mossman, 2001), the confidence interval is estimated as (0.388, 0.596). As expected, the Mossman confidence interval is wider, since the standard error of PPV accounts for the variability in the estimate of prevalence.

4.1.3   Sensitivity, Specificity and Predictive Values with Clustered Binary-Scale Data

In the previous section, we introduced a reader accuracy study to estimate the sensitivity of CAD-enhanced CTC for the detection of polyps (Case Study 2). In that study, there were actually multiple polyps found in some patients - 39 polyps in these 25 patients. Each patient had from 1 to 3 polyps. These data are displayed in Table 4.2. Previously, we summarized the results for each patient, so that we had a single data point for each patient (any patient with at least one polyp detected was called positive for CAD-enhanced CTC). This summarization is unlikely to be optimal. We should, instead, use the results of each of the 39 polyps to estimate sensitivity. We realize, though, that the detection capabilities for each patient may be correlated (i.e., in simplistic terms, the ability to detect multiple polyps in the same patient may be expected to be more similar than for different patients). Thus we need some different methods specific to this kind of data, called clustered data.

In general, clustered data occur when the units being tested for the condition are not all independent of each other. Beam (1998) referred to the diagnostic unit of study (DUOS) as the smallest "unit" that is tested. For the CTC study described, the polyp is the smallest unit that is tested; the patients constitute the cluster and the polyps are the DUOS within the cluster. Other examples of clustered data include multiple lymph nodes from the same patient evaluated for evidence of cancer and several aortoiliac segments in a patient scanned for evidence of peripheral arterial disease. In studies of this design, the patients constitute the clusters and the lymph nodes and aortoiliac segments constitute the units within the cluster. Note that the units within a cluster do not necessarily all have the same gold standard diagnosis (i.e., some units may have the condition while others may not).

Assume there are I clusters. Let N_i be the number of elements in the i-th cluster that were found positive on the gold standard and $\widehat{Se}_i$ the sensitivity estimated from data using those elements from the i-th cluster only. Sensitivity can be estimated as

$$\widehat{Se} = \sum_{i=1}^{I} N_i \widehat{Se}_i \bigg/ \sum_{i=1}^{I} N_i. \tag{4.21}$$

This estimate of sensitivity is actually equivalent to the proportion of all units in the sample found positive for the condition by the test, where the denominator is the total number of truly positive units, taken over all clusters (Equation 4.1). In contrast, the variance of the sensitivity estimated from a clustered design is larger than that from an independent design (assuming that the correlation between units is positive, which is the most likely scenario). A ratio estimator for the variance has been derived (Cochran, 1977; Rao and

Scott, 1992), as

$$\widehat{Var}(\widehat{Se}) = \frac{1}{I(I-1)} \sum_{i=1}^{I} \left(\frac{N_i}{\bar{N}}\right)^2 (\widehat{Se}_i - \widehat{Se})^2, \tag{4.22}$$

where $\bar{N} = \sum_i N_i/I$ is the mean cluster size. The estimate of specificity, and direct estimates of predictive value of a positive or predictive value of a negative test result and appropriate variances can be derived similarly. With this appropriate estimate of the variance, confidence intervals can be estimated using the equation (4.4) or equations (4.5)-(4.10). Alternatively, Rutter (2000) suggested using bootstrapping to estimate the variance. This would be implemented by stratifying clusters according to whether or not any of the units within the cluster have the condition, and then drawing patients with replacement from each stratum. Resampling at the cluster level simultaneously incorporates all sources of within-cluster variability.

4.1.3.1 Sensitivity of Clustered Data: Case Study 2 We can now appropriately estimate the sensitivity, variance and confidence interval of CAD-enhanced CTC for detecting polyps, using all available information for Reader 1. Recall that there were $\sum_i N_i = 39$ polyps (units) in $I = 25$ patients (clusters). Table 4.2 has the data along with some calculations needed to use equations (4.21)-(4.22). Column 1 of the table has the ID, column 2 has the number of polyps detected by Reader 1 using CAD-enhanced CTC, and column 3 has the total number of polyps that could have been detected. The mean number of polyps per patient is $\bar{N} = 1.56$ (mean of column 3). There were 33 polyps found by Reader 1, out of the possible 39, giving an overall estimate of sensitivity of $\widehat{Se} = 33/39 = 0.8462$. In order to calculate an estimate for the variance which takes into account the clustering, we need to estimate a sensitivity for each patient, as well as the weighting factor $N_i/\bar{N}$. Columns 4 and 5 have these values. For each patient, if we multiply the values in column 5 by $(\widehat{Se}_i - \widehat{Se}) = (\widehat{Se}_i - 0.8462)$ and square the product, we get the results in column 6. The sum of column 6, divided by $I(I-1) = 25 \times 24$ yields the final variance estimate of $2.5676/(25 \times 24) = 0.00428$. For comparison, ignoring the clustering and analyzing the data as if it were from 39 patients would yield a variance of $(0.8462 \times 0.1538)/39 = 0.0033$. This value is inappropriately small, because it ignores the correlation amongst polyps. Even if the amount of correlation amongst units within a cluster is small, the estimate of variance will be biased if it is ignored. The asymptotic 95% confidence interval, using the equation (4.5) is (0.718, 0.974).

4.1.4 Likelihood Ratio (LR)

A study was conducted to determine the usefulness of serum creatine kinase (CK) for diagnosing acute myocardial infarction (AMI) (Radack et al., 1986). A positive (i.e., abnormal) CK test was defined as a serum CK value of over

Table 4.2   CAD Enhanced Computed Tomography Colonography Results for Detection of Colon Polyps (Reader 1)

ID	No. TN	No. Polyps	$\widehat{Se}_i$	N_i/N	$(N_i/N)^2 \times (\widehat{Se}_i - \widehat{Se})^2$
1	1	1	1.000	0.641	0.0097
2	2	2	1.000	1.282	0.0389
3	2	2	1.000	1.282	0.0389
4	1	1	1.000	0.641	0.0097
5	2	2	1.000	1.282	0.0389
6	2	2	1.000	1.282	0.0389
7	1	1	1.000	0.641	0.0097
8	1	1	1.000	0.641	0.0097
9	1	1	1.000	0.641	0.0097
10	1	1	1.000	0.641	0.0097
11	2	2	1.000	1.282	0.0389
12	0	1	0.000	0.641	0.2842
13	2	3	0.667	1.923	0.1191
14	2	2	1.000	1.282	0.0389
15	1	1	1.000	0.641	0.0097
16	1	1	1.000	0.641	0.0097
17	1	1	1.000	0.641	0.0097
18	2	1	1.000	1.282	0.0389
19	1	2	0.500	1.282	0.1970
20	0	2	0.000	1.282	1.1768
21	1	1	1.000	0.641	0.0097
22	2	2	1.000	1.282	0.0389
23	2	2	1.000	1.282	0.0389
24	2	2	1.000	1.282	0.0389
25	0	1	0.000	0.641	0.2942

120, while a negative (normal) test result was 120 or less. Investigators wanted to know how much more likely it was for a positive CK result to occur in someone with AMI as compared to someone without AMI.

In Chapter 2, the LR was defined as

$$LR(t) = \frac{P(T = t|D = 1)}{P(T = t|D = 0)}, \tag{4.23}$$

where t is a single test value, an interval of test values, or one side of a decision threshold. For binary variables we have

$$LR(+) = \frac{P(T = 1|D = 1)}{P(T = 1|D = 0)} = \frac{Se}{1 - Sp}, \tag{4.24}$$

and the estimate of the LR is obtained by substituting estimates of sensitivity and specificity into the equation. The distribution of the LR is skewed (i.e., non-symmetric), but the (natural) logarithm of the LR has better properties, and more closely follows a normal distribution. The estimate of the variance of the logarithm of the positive LR is (Simel et al., 1991)

$$\widehat{Var}(\ln(\widehat{LR}(+))) = \frac{1 - \widehat{Se}}{s_1} + \frac{\widehat{Sp}}{r_1}. \tag{4.25}$$

A confidence interval can be fashioned first for the logarithm of the LR. The confidence interval for the LR itself can then be obtained by exponentiating the confidence limits of the $\ln(\widehat{LR}(+))$. Assuming asymptotic normality, the $100(1 - \alpha)\%$ confidence limits for the positive LR are

$$\frac{\widehat{Se}}{1 - \widehat{Sp}} \exp\left(\pm z_{1-\alpha/2} \sqrt{\frac{1 - \widehat{Se}}{s_1} + \frac{\widehat{Sp}}{r_1}} \; Bigr). \tag{4.26}$$

Estimates of the negative LR and its confidence interval can be estimated similarly, noting that

$$\widehat{LR}(-) = \frac{1 - \widehat{Se}}{\widehat{Sp}}, \widehat{Var}(\ln(\widehat{LR}(-))) = \sqrt{\frac{\widehat{Se}}{s_0} + \frac{1 - \widehat{Sp}}{r_0}}. \tag{4.27}$$

Although the confidence interval based on this log transformation is relatively easy to compute, Gart and Nam (1988) showed that a better method is an iterative procedure based on likelihood scores. The score method, as it is referred to, provided better coverage (i.e., it is more likely to include or "cover" the true LR $100(1 - \alpha)\%$ of the time). Software to estimate LRs and their confidence intervals includes STATA.

4.1.4.1 Likelihood Ratio: CK to Diagnose AMI The 2×2 table containing the CK data for our example is in Table 4.3. Based on this table, the sensitivity of the serum CK test is $28/51=0.55$, and the specificity of the test is $471/722 = 0.65$. An estimate of the positive $LR(+)$ can be computed as

$$\widehat{LR}(+) = \frac{\widehat{Se}}{1 - \widehat{Sp}} = \frac{0.55}{0.35} = 1.58.$$

Using the log transformation, the 95% confidence interval is $(1.21, 2.06)$. The 95% confidence interval using the score method is $(1.17, 2.00)$. Since the LR is greater than one, the investigator can conclude that it is more likely for a positive serum CK result to occur in someone with an AMI, although the results are not strong.

Table 4.3   Display of CK Results (2 categories) for Diagnosis of AMI

AMI	Serum CK Result		
	CK> 120	CK≤ 120	Total
Present $(D = 1)$	28	23	51
Absent $(D = 0)$	251	471	772
Total	279	494	773

The serum CK results were also presented in five categories, as displayed in Table 4.4. If we think of each category, in turn, as defining a positive result (with the remaining category defining negative results) then we can calculate five LRs - one for each category. Table 4.5 shows these LRs and confidence intervals. Both the log transformation and score methods were used to compute confidence intervals. Two of these LRs are less than one: for CK≤ 120 and for CK between 121 and 240. Point estimates for the LRs for values greater than 240 range from 4.13 to 9.10. These values show a much stronger relationship of CK to diagnosis of AMI than the simple binary results. Although the point estimates show an increasing trend with increasing values of serum CK, the confidence intervals are wide enough that we really cannot say with certainty that these values have different LRs. The lack of certainty is probably caused by the small number of people in the study with these CK values.

4.1.5   Odds Ratio

In the CK example discussed in the previous section regarding the usefulness of serum CK to diagnose AMI, we could have used the odds ratio as an alternative method of assessment. The odds ratio will tell investigators whether the odds of a positive test are greater for those with AMI than without AMI.

Table 4.4 Display of CK Results (5 categories) for Diagnosis of AMI

AMI	Serum CK Result					Total
	>480	381-480	241-380	121-240	1-120	
Present ($D = 1$)	9	6	7	6	23	51
Absent ($D = 0$)	14	12	24	201	471	772
Total	23	18	31	207	494	773

Table 4.5 Likelihood Ratio Results for AMI

CK Results	LR	95% Confidence Intervals	
		log transform	Score
1-120	0.69	(0.51, 9.94)	(0.49, 0.90)
121-240	0.42	(0.20, 0.90)	(0.20, 0.85)
241-360	4.13	(1.87, 9.12)	(1.87, 8.70)
361-480	7.08	(2.77,18.08)	(2.81,17.17)
>480	9.10	(4.14,20.01)	(4.15,19.30)

The odds ratio, introduced in Chapter 2, can be estimated as

$$\widehat{OR} = \frac{\widehat{Se}/(1 - \widehat{Se})}{(1 - \widehat{Sp})/\widehat{Sp}} = \frac{s_1 r_0}{s_0 r_1}. \tag{4.28}$$

As for the LR, the distribution of the estimated odds ratio is skewed, but the distribution of the logarithm of the estimated odds ratio is approximately normally distributed. Thus, confidence intervals are usually derived through the log of the odds ratio. The variance of the log of the estimated odds ratio can be estimated as

$$\widehat{Var}(ln(\widehat{OR})) = [\frac{1}{s_1} + \frac{1}{s_0} + \frac{1}{r_1} + \frac{1}{r_0}]. \tag{4.29}$$

The $100(1 - \alpha)\%$ confidence limits for the odds ratio

$$\frac{s_1 r_0}{s_0 r_1} \exp\left(\pm z_{1-\alpha/2}\sqrt{1/s_1 + 1/s_0 + 1/r_1 + 1/r_0}\right). \tag{4.30}$$

If the confidence interval excludes 1, then the odds of a disease is different depending on the results of the medical test (i.e., the test discriminates between those with and without disease).

If one of the cells in the table is zero (i.e., if s_1, s_0, r_1 or r_0 is zero), a reasonable estimate of the odds ratio is not possible. Cox (1970) suggested that 0.5 be added to each cell entry before computing the estimates of the odds ratio and the variance of the odds ratio or log odds ratio. The resulting values have smaller asymptotic bias and mean square error.

Odds ratios of 2 or 3 are often considered important in epidemiologic research. In contrast, a variable with an associated odds ratio of 3 is a very poor discriminator of disease from non-disease (Pepe, 2000). In fact, odds ratios need to be more in the range of 30 and above to represent both good sensitivity and specificity (for example, a sensitivity of 0.9 and odds ratio of 3 would imply specificity of only 0.25, but an odds ratio of 30 would imply specificity of 0.77 and odds ratio of 40 would be associated with specificity of 0.82).

In Chapters 7 and 12, the odds ratio will be used to facilitate the summary of sensitivity and specificity across studies, in meta-analysis. In the meta-analysis literature, the odds ratio is often referred to as the diagnostic odds ratio.

4.1.5.1 Odds Ratio: CK to Diagnose AMI   The odds ratio for the AMI data is computed as $\hat{o} = (28 \times 471)/(251 \times 23) = 2.28$. The 95% confidence interval based on the log transformation is $(1.29, 4.05)$. Thus we estimate the odds of a positive serum CK test result is 2.28 times greater for someone with AMI than without, with a confidence interval of $(1.29, 4.05)$. Note that the sensitivity here is 0.55 and the specificity is 0.65.

4.2   ORDINAL-SCALE DATA

In Case Study 3, described in Chapter 1, investigators were interested in determining whether MRA could be used as a non-invasive test to detect significant carotid stenosis. Recall that radiologists used an ordinal scale to rate the carotid as 1=definitely no significant stenosis, 2=probably no significant stenosis, 3=equivocal, 4=probably significant stenosis, 5=definite significant stenosis. While there were four radiologists assessing MRA for both the left and right carotid, in this section we focus on the accuracy for the left carotid, for Radiologist 4 only. We take as the gold standard, the majority diagnosis for the catheter angiogram results of the four radiologists, where percent stenosis between 60% and 99% was taken as indication of significant stenosis requiring surgery (in the seven instances where there was no majority, a positive diagnosis was assigned if the mean estimated stenosis was at least 60%). Table 4.6 has the results. We are interested in using these data to assess the accuracy of MRA through use of the ROC curve and its associated summary measures.

Table 4.6   Results of Magnetic Resonance Angiography (MRA) to Detect Significant Carotid Stenosis, Radiologist 4

| Disease Status | MRA Results | | | | | |
	1	2	3	4	5	Total
Significant Stenosis	1	2	3	14	42	62
No Significant Stenosis	38	25	15	19	4	101
Total	39	27	18	33	46	163

As mentioned in Chapter 2, an ROC curve can be estimated from ordinal data, such as the 5-category scale to interpret MRA data mentioned above. Suppose we represent our K ordered categories numerically as 1 through K, where 1 represents a patient who is most likely to not have the condition, and K represents a patient who is most likely to have the condition. The ordinal test data can be displayed in a $2 \times K$ table that looks like Table 4.7.

4.2.1   Empirical ROC Curve

If the diagnostic test produces only ordinal results, with K categories, then K values of sensitivity and false positive rate can be determined, with one set corresponding to each of the K categories. For each value of T, we estimate the sensitivity and FPR by assuming that values equal to, or to the right of T (i.e., equal to or larger) are positive, and those to the left of T (i.e., smaller)

Table 4.7   Display of Ordinal Data

| | Test Results | | | | |
Disease Status (D)	1	2	...	K	Total
$D = 1$	s_1	s_2	...	s_K	n_1
$D = 0$	r_1	r_2	...	s_K	n_0
Total	m_1	m_2	...	m_K	N

are negative. Then

$$\widehat{Se}(i) = \widehat{TPR}(i) = P(T \geq i | D = 1) = \frac{1}{n_1} \sum_{j=i}^{K} s_j, \qquad (4.31)$$

and

$$\widehat{FPR}(i) = 1 - \widehat{Sp}(i) = P(T \geq i | D = 0) = \frac{1}{n_0} \sum_{j=i}^{K} r_j. \qquad (4.32)$$

The plot of the pairs $(\widehat{FPR}(i), \widehat{Se}(i))$ over all values i of the ordinal rating scale constitutes the empirical ROC curve for ordinal data.

4.2.2   Fitting a Smooth Curve

The empirical ROC curve estimated from the $2 \times K$ table of ordinal data is jagged, because the curve drawn by connecting the few observed points is crudely fit. To better characterize the relationship between the test and the condition of interest, it would be desirable to fit a smooth curve to the data. One way to accomplish this task is to hypothesize an explicit functional form for the ROC curve itself. While such models have been suggested in the past (Egan, 1975), new methods suggested by Pepe (2003) have helped popularize this approach. Estimation of the curve involves the methods of generalized estimating equations and generalized linear models and can incorporate covariate information (This subject is discussed in Chapter 8).

The most popular way of fitting a model to the data is to hypothesize ordinal-scale test results, T_1 and T_0, of patients with and without the condition as a categorization of two unobserved or latent continuous-scale random variables, T_1^* and T_0^*, respectively. We generally assume that distributions of the latent variables are overlapping (see Figure 4.1). To be more specific, we assume that T_1^* is the underlying random variable for the latent result of a diagnostic test for a patient with the condition and has distribution F_1 and that T_0^* is the underlying random variable for the latent result of a patient without the condition and has a distribution F_0. Let c be a cutoff or decision threshold. Then the FPR and sensitivity associated with c, where $-\infty < c < \infty$, are:

$$FPR(c) = P(T_0^* > c|D = 0) = 1 - F_0(c), \tag{4.33}$$

$$TPR(c) = P(T_1^* > c|D = 1) = 1 - F_1(c). \tag{4.34}$$

For an ordinal-scale test result T_i which can take on one of the K ordered values, we assume that there are $K - 1$ unknown decision thresholds $\tilde{c}_1$, $\tilde{c}_2$, ..., $\tilde{c}_{K-1}$, so that

$$\text{if } T_i^* \le \tilde{c}_1, \text{ then } T_i = 1, \tag{4.35}$$

$$\text{if } \tilde{c}_{j-1} < T_i^* \le \tilde{c}_j, \text{ then } T_i = j \text{ for } j = 2, 3, \cdots, K - 1. \tag{4.36}$$

$$\text{if } T_i^* > \tilde{c}_{K-1}, \text{ then } T_i = K. \tag{4.37}$$

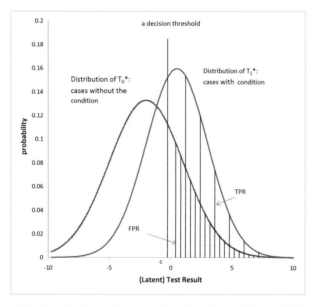

Figure 4.1 The Distribution of Latent Test Variables of Those With and Without the Condition

Often it is assumed that F_1 and F_0 are both normal distribution functions, in which case, we refer to T_1^* and T_0^* as following the binormal distribution. More exactly, the binormal assumption refers to the assumption that there exists a (usually unknown) monotonic transformation such that the transformation yields normal distributions. We assume that T_1^* and T_0^* have been suitably transformed. Then

$$T_1^* \sim N(\mu_1, \sigma_1^2); T_0^* \sim N(\mu_0, \sigma_0^2), \tag{4.38}$$

where μ_1, μ_0 are the means and σ_1^2, σ_0^2 are the variances of the normal distributions of the underlying latent test responses for those with and without the condition. We can then determine the probability of the observed test results based on the distribution of these latent responses:

$$\widehat{P}_{0j} = P(T_0 = j|D = 0) = \Phi(c_j) - \Phi(c_{j-1}) \tag{4.39}$$

$$\widehat{P}_{1j} = P(T_1 = j|D = 1) = \Phi(bc_j - a) - \Phi(bc_{j-1} - a), \tag{4.40}$$

where $c_j = (\tilde{c}_j - \mu_0)/\sigma_0$, $b = \sigma_0/\sigma_1$ and $a = (\mu_1 - \mu_0)/\sigma_1$; $c_0 = -\infty$, $c_K = +\infty$ and Φ is the cumulative normal distribution. Maximum likelihood (ML) methods are used to estimate the parameters a and b, as well as the $K-1$ nuisance parameters $c_1, \cdots, c_{K-1}$. These methods can also provide estimates of the variances of the estimated parameters as well as the correlation among estimated parameters.

Algorithms have been described in Dorfman and Alf (1968). Metz et al. (1998) developed software, which has implemented these techniques, dubbed "ROCKIT". The "ROCKIT" contained an algorithm to estimate the parameters a and b and standard errors for the binormal models, the unknown decision thresholds $\tilde{c}_j$, as well as the total ROC curve area, the variances, and a test for equality of the area under the ROC curves. The algorithms in ROCKIT are appropriate for ordinal- and continuous-scale data, for independent, completely dependent and partially paired designs. Because the completely independent and the completely paired design are special instances of the partially paired designs, ROCKIT has now subsumed much of their previously used software (ROCFIT, INDROC, CORROC, LABROC and CLABROC). This software is available from the Kurt Rossman Laboratories (`http://xray.bsd.uchicago.edu/kr/roc_soft.htm`). Some other standard statistical software packages, such as STATA, can also estimate these parameters.

Once estimates of the parameters a and b have been obtained, the ROC curve can be plotted as the collection of points $(1 - \Phi(c), 1 - \Phi(\widehat{bc} - \widehat{a}))$, where $-\infty < c < \infty$ ranges over the possible threshold values of the latent variable. Note, this could also be written as the points $(FPR, \Phi(\widehat{a} + \widehat{b}\Phi^{-1}(FPR))$ for $0 \leq FPR \leq 1$ or can be written $(FPR, 1 - \Phi(\widehat{b}Z_{FPR} - \widehat{a}))$ where, Z_{FPR} is the upper FPR percentage point of the standard normal distribution; i.e., $\Phi(Z_{FPR}) = 1 - FPR$.

Some may question the almost universal use of the binormal assumption. Rating scales such as the one used to evaluate MRA for carotid stenosis do not represent a specific numerical scale. Simple changes in scale of the decision variable can make the distributions of those with and without the condition look like almost any pair of distributions. Similarly, a transformation could easily change almost any pair of distributions to look like a pair of normal curves. Thus, when we speak of a binormal ROC curve, we are speaking of the functional form of the ROC curve, and not the form of the underlying distributions of the test results for people with and without the condition of interest. As Hanley (1988) pointed out, most diagnostic tests that produce ordinal results have only a few values or categories so that many different distributions could fit the tables.

Swets (1986a), examining data from psychology, determined that the binormal model is reasonable. Through simulation, Hanley (1988) examined a variety of ROC forms and underlying distributions including power law, binomial, Poisson, chi-square and gamma distributions, and found that the ROC curve was well approximated by a curve based on a binormal model. Walsh (1997), though, showed that the use of the binormal model with non-normal data, if the set of decision thresholds is too narrow, may result in biased ROC curve area estimates, as well as increased variance and decreased size and power of tests comparing areas.

Until recently, the only other distribution that had received much attention was the logistic distribution (Ogilvie and Creelman, 1968; Grey, 1972), which is almost indistinguishable from the normal distribution. Although the logistic distribution may in fact be easier to work with, the computer techniques and software that were first popularized − RSCORE II (Dorfman and Alf) and LABROC (Metz) − were based on the binormal assumption and most likely influenced the choice of other researchers. More recently, some additional distributions have been considered that created "proper" ROC curves and are used primarily to avoid the problems of degenerate data sets (See Section 4.2.7).

As alluded to above, it may not be necessary to make assumptions regarding the specific underlying distributions of the test results to model the ROC curve. Directly modeling the ROC curve as

$$ROC(t) = \Phi(a + b\Phi^{-1}(t)) \tag{4.41}$$

allows various semi-parametric methods to be used to estimate the parameters a and b. While some semi-parametric methods may only apply to continuous data, others have been shown to apply to ordinal data (Pepe, 2000; Alonzo and Pepe, 2002). Semi-parametric methods are discussed a bit more in Section 4.3.2 and in Chapter 8, the latter in the context of regression and covariates.

We might like to formally test whether the binormal assumption seems reasonable for a particular data set. To do that, we compare the observed probability of a particular test result, with the expected result when binormality is assumed. Dorfman and Alf (1968) suggested such a test, called a goodness of fit test:

$$\chi^2 = \sum_{i=0}^{1} \sum_{k=1}^{K} n_i \frac{[\widehat{P}(T_i = k|D = i) - P(T_i = k|D = i)]^2}{\widehat{P}(T_i = k|D = i)}, \tag{4.42}$$

where $P(T = k|D = 1) = s_K/n_1$, and $P(T = k|D = 0) = r_K/n_0$ are the observed probabilities of results and $\widehat{P}(T = k|D = i)$ is the expected probability as estimated under the binormal assumption, using equations (4.39) and (4.40) . This test statistic is distributed approximately as χ^2 with $K-3$ degrees of freedom.

An important assumption for the binormal model to hold is that the decision thresholds are the same regardless of the condition of the subject (i.e., no interaction between decision threshold and condition). Zhou (1995) questioned this assumption, suggesting that this goodness of fit test actually assesses not only the binormal assumption but also whether the decision points are the same. Still assuming binormality, Zhou (1995) proposed a separate test of this assumption of interaction between decision thresholds and condition. This test statistic is proportional to the difference of the log-likelihood under the interaction assumption ($\ln L_1$) and the log-likelihood under the assumption of no interaction ($\ln L_0$). The test statistic,

$$2(\ln L_1 - \ln L_0)), \tag{4.43}$$

has a Chi-square distribution with $K-2$ degrees of freedom. Estimates of the log-likelihoods can be obtained as follows. Under the interaction assumption (that there are different decision threshold for those with and without the condition), $\ln L_1$ can be estimated (Zhou, 1995) as

$$\ln L_1 = \sum_{k=1}^{K} [s_k \ln(s_k/n_1) + r_k \ln(r_k/n_0)]. \tag{4.44}$$

Under the assumption of no interaction, the log likelihood is

$$\ln L_0 = \sum_{k=1}^{K} [s_k \ln(\widehat{P}_{1k}) + r_k \ln(\widehat{P}_{0k})], \tag{4.45}$$

where $\widehat{P}_{ik}$, $i = 0, 1$; $k = 1, 2, \cdots, K$, are as in equations (4.39) and (4.40) with estimates of a and b substituted into the equations. Note that in (4.44), if there are zero cells, some accommodation needs to be made. Since the term $s_i ln(s_i/n)$ comes from the likelihood function term $(s_i/n_1)^{s_i}$, and by convention $0^0 = 1$, and $ln(1) = 0$, we will set such terms equal to zero.

Zhou (1995) provided a method for testing this assumption that can be used with other distributional forms for the latent variable (see Zhou (1995) for details). In a more recent work, Walsh (1999) provided a different interpretation of Zhou's results, asserting other explanations for lack of fit in Equation (4.43). Currently this issue is unresolved.

4.2.2.1 Estimating the ROC Curve: Case Study 3   We can construct an empirical ROC curve for the use of MRA to detect significant carotid stenosis. For this example, $K = 5$, with test results numbered from 1=definitely no significant stenosis to 5=definitely significant stenosis. Figure 4.2 plots the pairs of $(\widehat{FPR}, \widehat{Se})$ for the ROC graph. The points are (0.0,0.0); (0.04,0.68); (0.23,0.90); (0.38,0.95); (0.62,0.98); and (1.0,1.0).

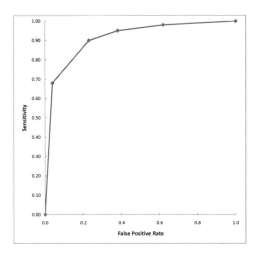

Figure 4.2   Empirical ROC Curve for the Use of MRA to Detect Significant Carotid Stenosis

As an alternative to the jagged, empirical plot of the ROC curve, we can instead plot a smooth curve based on the binormal assumption. We estimate the binormal parameters using ROCKIT to obtain $\hat{a} = 1.9070$, $\hat{b} = 0.8217$, with $\widehat{Var}(\hat{a}) = 0.0880$, $\widehat{Var}(\hat{b}) = 0.0398$ and $\widehat{Cov}(\hat{a}, \hat{b}) = 0.0432$. Estimates of the four threshold values are -0.314, 0.313, 0.745, 1.759. To plot the ROC curve we use the fact that the points of interest are

$$(FPR, \Phi(\hat{a} + \hat{b}\Phi^{-1}(FPR)) = (FPR, \Phi(1.9070 + 0.8217 \times \Phi^{-1}(FPR)).$$

For example, for $FPR = 0.1$, we have $\Phi^{-1}(0.1) = -1.282$ and

$$\widehat{Se} = \widehat{TPR} = \Phi(1.9070 + 0.8217 \times (-1.282)) = \Phi(0.8536) = 0.803.$$

Table 4.8 is a worksheet for determining points on the ROC curve. Column 2 has values of $\Phi^{-1}(FPR)$ for $FPR = 0.10$ to 0.90. Column 3 has values $\hat{a} + \hat{b} \ \Phi^{-1}(FPR)$ which are needed to determine the TPR (column 4). We plot these points to draw a smooth ROC curve (see Figure 4.3)

The validity of the estimates of the binormal ROC curve is based on the binormal model being a reasonable fit to the data. We can assess the goodness of fit of the binormal model to the data with the Dorfman-Alf test statistic, the equation (4.42), which we find to be 3.285. Since this value is less than $\chi^2_{5-3,0.05} = 5.99$, we do not reject the null hypothesis.

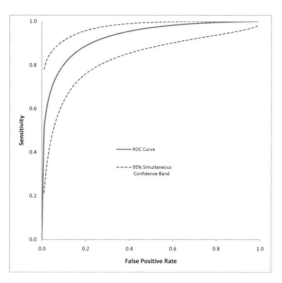

Figure 4.3   Smooth ROC Curve for Use of MRA to Detect Significant Carotid Stenosis

We can also compute Zhou's test statistic to determine whether the assumption of no interaction of condition and decision points is reasonable for these data. The value of $\ln L_0$ is computed to be $\ln L_0 = -202.595$. The value of $\ln L_1$ can be easily calculated to be $\ln L_1 = -203.041$. The test statistic is $2 \times (-202.595 - (-203.041)) = 0.893$, which is not statistically significant since it is less than $\chi^2_{5-2, 0.05} = 7.81$. For these data, the assumption that the decision thresholds are independent of condition is reasonable.

4.2.3   Estimation of Sensitivity at a Particular False Positive Rate

Continuing with our MRA example, suppose the investigators wish to determine the sensitivity of MRA to detect significant carotid stenosis when the specificity is 0.90. They would like both a point estimate and an interval estimate.

Using parametric methods as described in the previous section, we can easily determine the sensitivity corresponding to any fixed value of specificity. We saw that the ROC curve is plotted as the points $(FPR, TPR) = (FPR, \Phi(a + b\Phi^{-1}(FPR)))$. That is, for a fixed false positive rate e, and estimates of $\widehat{a}$ and $\widehat{b}$, the sensitivity, or true positive rate (TPR), can be estimated as

$$\widehat{TPR}_e = \widehat{Se}_{(FPR=e)} = \Phi(\widehat{a} + \widehat{b}\Phi^{-1}(e)). \qquad (4.46)$$

In other words, the quantile associated with the TPR can be written as

$$\Phi^{-1}(\widehat{TPR}_e) = \widehat{a} + \widehat{b}\Phi^{-1}(e). \qquad (4.47)$$

Table 4.8 Estimation of ROC Curve Points for Smooth ROC Curve

| FPR | $\Phi^{-1}(TPR)$ | $\widehat{b}\Phi^{-1}(TPR) + \widehat{a}$ | TPR | $V(\Phi^{-1}(TPR))$ | 95% Confidence Interval | |
					Pointwise	Simultaneous
0.10	-1.282	0.854	0.803	0.043	(0.674, 0.896)	(0.636, 0.913)
0.20	-0.842	1.215	0.888	0.043	(0.790, 0.948)	(0.760, 0.958)
0.30	-0.524	1.476	0.930	0.054	(0.847, 0.973)	(0.818, 0.979)
0.40	-0.253	1.699	0.955	0.069	(0.882, 0.987)	(0.855, 0.990)
0.50	0.000	1.907	0.972	0.088	(0.908, 0.994)	(0.881, 0.996)
0.60	0.253	2.115	0.983	0.112	(0.928, 0.997)	(0.902, 0.998)
0.70	0.524	2.338	0.990	0.144	(0.944, 0.999)	(0.920, 0.999)
0.80	0.842	2.599	0.995	0.189	(0.960, 1.000)	(0.938, 1.000)
0.90	1.282	2.960	0.998	0.264	(0.975, 1.000)	(0.956, 1.000)

If such points were plotted in normal deviate space, they would all lie on the straight line with slope $\hat{b}$ and intercept $\hat{a}$.

The variance can easily be determined in normal deviate space, since we know $Var(\Phi^{-1}(\widehat{TPR}_e)) = Var(\hat{a} + \hat{b}\Phi^{-1}(e)$ when $FPR = e$. Then

$$Var(\Phi^{-1}(\widehat{TPR}_e)) = Var(\hat{a}) + [\Phi^{-1}(e)]^2 Var(\hat{b}) + 2\Phi^{-1}(e)\ Cov(\hat{a}, \hat{b}). \quad (4.48)$$

As mentioned previously, estimates of the variances and the covariances are available from programs such as ROCKIT. An alternative approach to estimating the variance of $\Phi^{-1}(\widehat{TPR})$ is to use the jackknife, as was done in McNeil and Hanley (1984), or to use bootstrap methods (see also Appendices B4.1−B4.5).

Once estimates of the parameters' variances and covariances are obtained, they can be used to estimate the confidence limits of the sensitivity corresponding to a particular $FPR = e$. Assuming asymptotic normality, the $100(1 − \alpha)\%$ confidence interval for the sensitivity, in normal deviate space, is easily determined from the confidence limits (LL, UL):

$$\Phi^{-1}(\widehat{TPR}_e) \pm z_{1-\alpha/2}\sqrt{Var(\Phi^{-1}(\widehat{TPR}_e))}. \quad (4.49)$$

The confidence limits for sensitivity, in the usual space, are $(\Phi(LL), \Phi(UL))$. Research into the adequacy of coverage of the asymptotic confidence limits for various sample sizes is needed.

Confidence intervals constructed in this way are called pointwise confidence intervals. The confidence level, α, applies to a probability statement around the sensitivity corresponding to a single, specific FPR. We can also construct simultaneous confidence bands around the ROC curve. A simultaneous confidence band has a confidence level that applies to the entire, or possibly a portion of, the ROC curve. Statements made regarding the simultaneous confidence bands refer to every possible value along the ROC curve, not just to individual points along the curve, for which reason these simultaneous bands are by necessity wider than pointwise bands.

Ma and Hall (1993) specified simultaneous confidence bands based on the Working-Hotelling model in the form of

$$\left(FPR, \Phi(\hat{a} + \hat{b}\Phi^{-1}(FPR) \pm k\sqrt{Var(\Phi^{-1}(\widehat{TPR}))}\right), \quad (4.50)$$

where $Var(\Phi^{-1}(\widehat{TPR}))$ is as in (4.48) above. The constant k takes on the value 2.448 for a two-sided 95% simultaneous confidence band and $k = 2.146$ for a two-sided 90% simultaneous confidence band. Note that this is virtually identical to pointwise confidence intervals, except that the constant is different (we would have used a constant 1.96 for 95% pointwise confidence and 1.645 for 90% pointwise confidence intervals). The simultaneous confidence band is a vertical band, in that it is a band around the $\widehat{Se}$ for each corresponding value of FPR. For details regarding one-sided confidence bands, or bands about only a portion of the ROC curve, see Ma and Hall (1993).

4.2.3.1 Sensitivity at a Particular Specificity Value: Case Study 3 We can now answer the investigator's questions and determine the sensitivity of MRA when the specificity is 0.90. We have already gone through the steps to estimate the sensitivity at a particular FPR, e, when we estimated points on the smooth ROC curve. Table 4.8 has the values of sensitivity (TPR) for various values of FPR. In particular, for $FPR = 0.10$, $\Phi^{-1}(0.1) = -1.282$ and the point estimate for sensitivity is 0.8034. Confidence intervals for individual points can be determined easily once the variance at each point is estimated. For $FPR = 0.10$ we calculate the variance as

$$
\begin{aligned}
Var(\Phi^{-1}(\widehat{TPR}_{0.10})) &= 0.0880 + (-1.282)^2 \times 0.0398 \\
&\quad + 2 \times (-1.282) \times 0.0432 \\
&= 0.04264.
\end{aligned}
$$

The bounds at that point would be

$$
\left(\Phi(0.85395 - 1.96\sqrt{0.04264}), \Phi(0.85395 + 1.96\sqrt{0.04264}) \right) = (0.674, 0.896).
$$

Column 6 in Table 4.8 has 95% confidence intervals for sensitivities corresponding to FPRs from 0.1 to 0.9.

We can also plot the 95% simultaneous confidence band about our ROC curve. The calculations are exactly as we did for the pointwise interval except for the constant. For example, at $FPR = 0.1$, the bounds at that point would be

$$
\left(\Phi(0.85395 - 2.448\sqrt{0.04264}), \Phi(0.85395 + 2.448\sqrt{0.04264}) \right) = (0.636, 0.913).
$$

The limits of the simultaneous confidence band for false positive rates from 0.1 to 0.9 are in the last column of Table 4.8, and the simultaneous confidence bands are drawn in Figure 4.3. We can say, roughly, that with 95% confidence (all) the points of the true ROC curve fall within these two bands. This should be contrasted to the situation where we are only interested in a particular sensitivity along the curve, rather than with the entire curve. In that case we would say that we have 95% confidence that the true sensitivity corresponding to one particular false positive rate lies within the pointwise confidence interval (such as saying that we are 95% confident that the true sensitivity corresponding to a false positive rate of 0.1 is between 0.674 and 0.896).

Note that these simultaneous confidence intervals in this last column of the table are wider than the pointwise estimate we would have for a specific sensitivity. For example, for $FPR = 0.1$, the 95% pointwise confidence limits would be (0.674, 0.896) vs. the 95% simultaneous confidence limits of (0.636, 0.913). That is the "cost" of being able to make a statement that applies, simultaneously, to all points along the ROC curve.

4.2.4   Area and Partial Area under the ROC Curve (Parametric Methods)

A general form for the area under the ROC curve allows us to look at the area between two false positive rates $FPR_1 = e_1$ and $FPR_2 = e_2$:

$$A_{(e_1 \leq FPR \leq e_2)} = \int_{e_1}^{e_2} ROC(c)dc. \tag{4.51}$$

When we assume binormality, this integral can be written as

$$A_{(e_1 \leq FPR \leq e_2)} = \int_{e_1}^{e_2} \Phi[a + b\Phi^{-1}(v)]dv. \tag{4.52}$$

At times, for brevity, we will write $A_{(e_1 \leq FPR \leq e_2)} = A_{e_1, e_2}$. This partial area as it is known, is evaluated by numerical integration (McClish, 1989). When we are interested in the area under the entire curve, then $e_1 = 0$, and $e_2 = 1$. In that case, the area under the entire curve can be written in simpler, closed form, as

$$A = \Phi\left(\frac{a}{\sqrt{1 + b^2}}\right). \tag{4.53}$$

The variance of the estimated partial area can be derived (McClish, 1989; Obuchowski and McClish, 1997) as

$$Var(\widehat{A}_{(e_1 \leq FPR \leq e_2)}) = f^2 Var(\widehat{a}) + g^2 Var(\widehat{b}) + 2fg\ Cov(\widehat{a}, \widehat{b})), \tag{4.54}$$

where

$$f = \frac{e^{-a^2/2(1+b^2)}}{\sqrt{2\pi(1 + b^2)}}[\Phi(h_2) - \Phi(h_1)], \tag{4.55}$$

$$g = \frac{e^{-a^2/2(1+b^2)}}{2\pi(1 + b^2)}[e^{-h_1^2/2} - e^{-h_2^2/2}] - \frac{abe^{-a^2/2(1+b^2)}}{\sqrt{2\pi(1 + b^2)^3}}[\Phi(h_2) - \Phi(h_1)], \tag{4.56}$$

and

$$h_i = [\Phi^{-1}(e_i) + ab/(1 + b^2)]\sqrt{1 + b^2}. \tag{4.57}$$

The variance formula simplifies when applied to the area under the entire ROC curve. In that case we have that

$$f = \frac{e^{-a^2/2(1+b^2)}}{\sqrt{2\pi(1 + b^2)}}, g = -\frac{abe^{-a^2/2(1+b^2)}}{\sqrt{2\pi(1 + b^2)^3}}. \tag{4.58}$$

The area and variances can be estimated by substituting estimates of the parameters a and b into equations (4.52)–(4.58). Estimates of a, b and their variances may be obtained as described in section 4.2.2 with parametric, or semi-parametric methods, usually a result of modeling the full ROC curve. Alonzo and Pepe (2002) also suggested using the binary regression approach to model the ROC curve over a restricted range directly.

Note that if the role of positive and negative test results are reversed, then the ROC curve can be used directly to determine the area for a range of true positive rates. For other early work on partial areas, see Jiang et al. (1996), Thompson and Zucchini (1989), and Wieand et al. (1989).

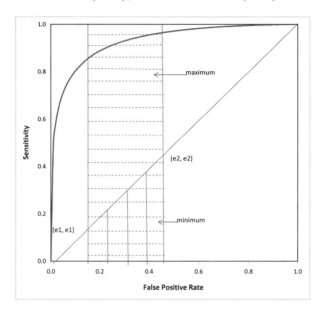

Figure 4.4   The Partial ROC Curve Area Minimum and Maximum Values

As discussed in Chapter 2, the area under the entire ROC curve takes on values between 0.5 and 1.0 and bounds can also be determined for the area under a portion of the ROC curve. The partial area of an ROC curve between false positive rates e_1 and e_2 is bounded above by the area of the rectangle that encloses it, i.e. the rectangle with corners $(e_1, 0.0)$, $(e_1, 1.0)$, $(e_2, 0.0)$, $(e_2, 1.0)$. This rectangle has sides of length 1.0 and $e_2 - e_1$ (see Figure 4.4). Thus the maximum area would be

$$A_{mx(e_1,e_2)} = e_2 - e_1. \tag{4.59}$$

The lower bound for the partial area can be found by looking at the trapezoid with corners $(e_1, 0.0)$, (e_1, e_1), (e_2, e_2), $(e_2, 0.0)$. This is the trapezoid bounded above by the line $y = x$ and below by the horizontal axis. This trapezoid has area

$$A_{mn(e_1,e_2)} = \frac{1}{2}(e_2 - e_1)(e_2 + e_1), \tag{4.60}$$

which is the minimum value that the partial area could take.

The partial area under the ROC curve between two false positive rates e_1 and e_2 can be difficult to interpret. McClish (1989) and Jiang et al. (1996)

suggested dividing the partial area by its maximum $(e_2 - e_1)$. This so called partial area index (Jiang et al., 1996) can be interpreted as the average sensitivity between those false positive values. Yet this transformation may still not be helpful if we want to compare areas under different portions of the ROC curve. Suppose, hypothetically, the partial area under the ROC curve between false positive rates 0.7 and 0.9 is $A_{(0.7 \leq FPR \leq 0.9)} = 0.18$. The maximum value this area could attain is 0.2, while the minimum is 0.16. Looking at a different part of the ROC curve, we could also have $A_{(0.3 \leq FPR \leq 0.5)} = 0.18$. In this case, the maximum would still be 0.2, but the minimum value would be 0.08. Although the partial area index would be the same for both partial areas (0.90), we might not want to value the partial areas the same. A transformation suggested by McClish (1989) would help solve this.

$$A^*_{(e_1 \leq FPR \leq e_2)} = \frac{1}{2}\left[1 + \frac{A_{e_1,e_2} - A_{mn}}{A_{mx} - A_{mn}}\right], \qquad (4.61)$$

where for brevity we use $A_{mx} = A_{mx(e_1,e_2)} = e_2 - e_1$ and $A_{mn} = A_{mn(e_1,e_2)} = (e_2 - e_1)(e_2 + e_1)/2$. This transformation yields values between 0.5 (no discrimination) and 1.0 (perfect discrimination), so it is possible to view the partial area on the same scale as the total area. The variance of the estimated transformation is

$$Var(\widehat{A}^*_{(e_1 \leq FPR \leq e_2)}) = \frac{Var(\widehat{A}_{e_1,e_2})}{4(A_{mx} - A_{mn})^2}. \qquad (4.62)$$

In the above hypothetical example, $A^*_{(0.7 \leq FPR \leq 0.9)} = 0.75$ and $A^*_{(0.3 \leq FPR \leq 0.5)} = 0.92$. The partial area in the lower part of the curve appears to reflect better accuracy than the partial area in the upper portion of the curve.

4.2.5   Confidence Interval Estimation

Confidence intervals for the area and partial area estimates when test results are ordinal scale generally are based on the assumption of asymptotic normality of the estimates of these quantities, using the equation (4.3). If the area or partial area is large, adequate coverage with the confidence interval may require a transformation. One such transformation is based on the logit

$$\text{logit}(\widehat{A}) = \ln(\widehat{A}/(1 - \widehat{A})). \qquad (4.63)$$

This transformation tends to have a more symmetric distribution. The $100(1-\alpha)\%$ confidence interval around the (untransformed) area is

$$\left(\frac{e^{LL}}{1 + e^{LL}}, \frac{e^{UL}}{1 + e^{UL}}\right), \qquad (4.64)$$

where the lower and upper limits (LL, UL) are

$$\text{logit}(\widehat{A}) \pm z_{1-\alpha/2}\sqrt{\widehat{Var}(\text{logit}(\widehat{A}))}, \qquad (4.65)$$

and

$$\widehat{Var}(\text{logit}(\widehat{A})) = \frac{Var(\widehat{A})}{[\widehat{A}(1 - \widehat{A})]^2}. \tag{4.66}$$

For the partial area, the logit transformation is best used with the partial area index, which we will write $A_{e_1,e_2}/A_{mx}$. The confidence interval for the partial area in this case would be

$$\left(\frac{e^{LL}}{1 + e^{LL}}, \frac{e^{UL}}{1 + e^{UL}} \right), \tag{4.67}$$

where the limits (LL, UL) are

$$\text{logit}\left(\frac{\widehat{A}_{e_1,e_2}}{A_{mx}} \right) \pm z_{1-\alpha/2} \sqrt{\widehat{Var}\left[\text{logit}\left(\frac{\widehat{A}_{e_1,e_2}}{A_{mx}} \right) \right]}, \tag{4.68}$$

$$\text{and } \widehat{Var}\left[\text{logit}\left(\frac{\widehat{A}_{e_1,e_2}}{A_{mx}} \right) \right] = \frac{A_{mx}^2 Var(\widehat{A}_{e_1,e_2})}{[\widehat{A}_{e_1,e_2}(A_{mx} - \widehat{A}_{e_1,e_2})]^2}. \tag{4.69}$$

Another, related transformation, suggested by McClish (1987) is

$$\ln\left(\frac{A_{mx} + \widehat{A}_{e_1,e_2}}{A_{mx} - \widehat{A}_{e_1,e_2}} \right) = \ln\left(\frac{1 + \widehat{A}_{e_1,e_2}/A_{mx}}{1 - \widehat{A}_{e_1,e_2}/A_{mx}} \right). \tag{4.70}$$

Based on this transformation, the $100(1 - \alpha)\%$ confidence interval is

$$\left(A_{mx} \frac{1 - e^{LL}}{1 + e^{LL}}, A_{mx} \frac{1 - e^{UL}}{1 + e^{UL}} \right), \tag{4.71}$$

where the limits (LL, UL) are

$$\ln\left(\frac{A_{mx} + \widehat{A}_{e_1,e_2}}{A_{mx} - \widehat{A}_{e_1,e_2}} \right) \pm z_{1-\alpha/2} \sqrt{Var\left[\ln\left(\frac{A_{mx} + \widehat{A}_{e_1,e_2}}{A_{mx} - \widehat{A}_{e_1,e_2}} \right) \right]}, \tag{4.72}$$

with

$$\widehat{Var}\left[\ln\left(\frac{A_{mx} + \widehat{A}_{e_1,e_2}}{A_{mx} - \widehat{A}_{e_1,e_2}} \right) \right] = \frac{4A_{mx}^2 Var(\widehat{A}_{e_1,e_2})}{(A_{mx}^2 - \widehat{A}_{e_1,e_2}^2)^2}. \tag{4.73}$$

Other potential methods to construct confidence intervals include the jack-knife and various bootstrap methods (bootstrap percentile, bias-corrected and accelerated bootstrap, bootstrap-t). These methods are described in the Appendix B.

Obuchowski and Lieber (1998) performed a study to determine how large the sample size needed to be in order for the asymptotic confidence interval of the total area to be appropriate. They also examined alternative bootstrap confidence intervals to determine the best approach when asymptotic methods were not appropriate. When the ROC area was moderate (around 0.80), and sample sizes of subjects with and without the condition were less than 50, they did not recommend the asymptotic methods. The best alternative was determined to be the bootstrap percentile method, which was found to provide good coverage as long as the sample size of subjects with and without the condition did not differ substantially (in which case the bootstrap t was preferred). If the area of the ROC curve was high (around 0.95), the data sets were often degenerate, particularly if the samples were small. For non-degenerate data sets, if the number of subjects without the condition was at least 30, the authors determined asymptotic methods to be adequate; however with smaller samples, the authors could not find any methods (including asymptotic and various bootstrap methods) that appeared to work well.

When the estimate of the area under the ROC curve is 1.0, confidence intervals cannot be estimated by any of the methods described. But it is important not to assume that the diagnostic test is perfectly accurate, based on this estimate. Obuchowski and Lieber (2002), using simulation, provided tables with suggested lower bounds for confidence intervals. Results varied depending on whether the test results were ordinal- or continuous- scale, the sample size, and the ratio of standard deviations of the test results. We are unaware of studies that have been published that evaluate coverage of confidence intervals for non-parametric estimates of partial areas when test results are ordinal-scale.

4.2.5.1   Area and Partial Area Under the ROC Curve: Case Study 3   We can estimate the area under the entire ROC curve for the MRA data in Table 4.6. Using the equation (4.53) the area is estimated as

$$\Phi(1.9070/\sqrt{1 + 0.8217^2}) = \Phi(1.4734) = 0.9297,$$

which agrees with ROCKIT. ROCKIT gives the standard deviation of the estimated area as 0.0213. With a sample size of 62 for those with, and 101 without significant stenosis, the asymptotic confidence interval may supply adequate coverage:

$$(0.9297 - 1.96 \times 0.0213, 0.9297 + 1.96 \times 0.0213) = (0.8880, 0.9714).$$

Suppose we are not interested in the accuracy of MRA for the entire curve, but rather only when the FPR is low. The area under the curve for $FPR \leq 0.10$ will be $A_{(0 \leq FPR \leq 0.1)} = 0.06721$ with a SE of 0.008392 (using equations (4.52), (4.54)). An asymptotic 95% confidence interval for the partial area will be

$$(0.06721 - 1.96 \times 0.008392, 0.06721 + 1.96 \times 0.008392) = (0.0508, 0.0837).$$

The partial area index is $0.06721/0.1 = 0.6721$. As suggested in the previous section, we might prefer to estimate the confidence interval using the logit transformation and Eqs (4.67)-(4.69). The logit of the partial area index is

0.7717; the standard error of the logit of the partial area index is

$$\frac{0.1 \times 0.008392}{0.06721 \times (0.1 - 0.06721)} = 0.38079.$$

Limits of the logit transformation (LL, UL) are:

$$(0.7717 - 1.96 \times 0.38079, 0.7717 + 1.96 \times 0.38079) = (0.02535, 1.51805).$$

Finally, the 95% confidence interval for this would be

$$\left(\frac{e^{0.02535}}{1 + e^{0.02535}}, \frac{e^{1.51805}}{1 + e^{1.51805}} \right) = (0.50534, 0.82025).$$

The maximum this partial area could attain will be $e_2 - e_1 = 0.1 - 0.0 = 0.10$; the minimum will be $(e_2 - e_1)(e_2 + e_1)/2 = (0.1 - 0.0)(0.1 + 0.0)/2 = 0.005$. For interpretative purposes, the transformation of this area will be

$$A_t = \frac{1}{2} \left\{ 1 + \frac{0.06721 - 0.005}{0.1 - 0.005} \right\} = 0.827.$$

Thus the average sensitivity of MRA for detecting significant carotid stenosis can be thought of as equivalent to a moderate area under an entire ROC curve (when $FPRs$ are no greater than 0.1).

4.2.6 Area and Partial Area Under the ROC Curve (Nonparametric Methods)

The area under an ROC curve can be estimated directly without making distributional assumptions (i.e., nonparametrically) by summing the area of trapezoids formed by connecting the points of the ROC curve (see Figure 4.5.) This is equivalent to the Mann-Whitney version of the statistic for the rank sum test, and we will refer to it as the MW area estimate. The trapezoidal method provides a systematic underestimate of the area under the true, unknown ROC curve (Bamber, 1975; Hanley and McNeil, 1982). This bias is greater when the medical test results take on only a few categories, and can be small if the test results take on many categories.

Let T_{0i} represent the observed test result for the i-th subject without the condition and T_{1i} the observed test result for the i-th subject with the condition. A formula for the nonparametric estimate of the entire area, denoted as A_{MW}, useful for both ordinal and continuous data, is

$$\widehat{A}_{MW} = \frac{1}{n_0 n_1} \sum_{i=1}^{n_1} \sum_{j=1}^{n_0} \Psi(T_{1i}, T_{0j}), \tag{4.74}$$

where Ψ is a function of two variables: $\Psi(X, Y) = 0$ if $Y > X$, $\Psi = 1/2$ if $Y = X$ and $\Psi = 1$ if $Y < X$. Here we have $X = T_{1i}$ and $Y = T_{0j}$.

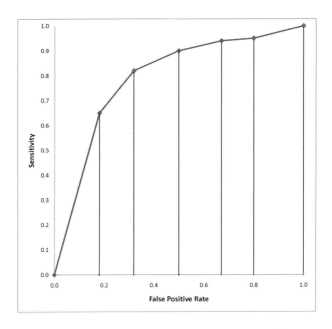

Figure 4.5   The Nonparametric Area under the ROC Curve (Trapezoidal Rule)

The expected value of $\widehat{A}_{MW}$ is equal to $P(T_0 < T_1) + 1/2 \times P(T_0 = T_1)$. With ordinal data, there will be many ties (i.e., test results with the same value) so that the second term, $P(T_0 = T_1)$, will be greater than zero. That is, with ordinal data, we will have that the expected value of the area estimate, $\widehat{A}_{MW}$, is greater than $P(T_0 < T_1)$. Thus we see that with ordinal data, the nonparametric estimate of the area is an underestimate of the true area.

A number of different methods to estimate the variance of the nonparametric area have been suggested. One uses the relationship of the nonparametric (trapezoidal) area under the curve to the Mann-Whitney version of the rank sum test to provide the estimate of the asymptotic variance $Var(\widehat{A}_{MW})$ as:

$$\frac{A_{MW}(1 - A_{MW}) + (n_1 - 1)(Q_1 - A_{MW}^2) + (n_0 - 1)(Q_2 - A_{MW}^2)}{n_0 n_1}, \quad (4.75)$$

where Q_1 is the probability that two randomly chosen subjects with the condition will be ranked above (i.e., have higher test scores than) one randomly chosen subject without the condition, and Q_2 is the probability that one randomly chosen subject with the condition will be ranked above two randomly chosen subjects without the condition (Bamber, 1975; Hanley and McNeil, 1982). Because the probabilities Q_1 and Q_2 can be difficult to estimate, Hanley and McNeil (1982) suggested using an approximation based on the exponential distribution

$$\widehat{Q}_1 = \frac{\widehat{A}_{MW}}{2 - \widehat{A}_{MW}} \text{ and } \widehat{Q}_2 = \frac{2\widehat{A}_{MW}^2}{1 + \widehat{A}_{MW}}. \tag{4.76}$$

This approximation can produce an underestimate when the area is close to 0.5 (Hanley and McNeil, 1982; Hanley and Hajian-Tilaki, 1997) or the ratio of SDs of patients with and without the condition is different from one (Obuchowski, 1994), and an overestimate when the area is close to 1 (Hanley and McNeil, 1982; Hanley and Hajian-Tilaki, 1997). These estimates are most useful in sample size estimation (see Chapter 6).

An estimate of the variance that is free of such assumptions, was provided by DeLong et al. (1988). Their method is useful in other contexts, for which reason we describe it here. Define the T_1 component for the i-th subject, $V_{10}(T_{1i})$, as

$$V_{10}(T_{1i}) = \frac{1}{n_0} \sum_{j=1}^{n_0} \Psi\left(T_{1i}, T_{0j}\right), \tag{4.77}$$

and the T_0 component for the j-th subject, $V_{01}(T_{0j})$, as

$$V_{01}(T_{0j}) = \frac{1}{n_1} \sum_{i=1}^{n_1} \Psi\left(T_{1i}, T_{0j}\right). \tag{4.78}$$

The (total) area under the curve can be estimated using either the T_1 components or the T_0 components as

$$\widehat{A}_{DL} = \sum_{i=1}^{n_1} V_{10}(T_{1i})/n_1 = \sum_{j=1}^{n_0} V_{01}(T_{0j})/n_0, \tag{4.79}$$

which provides the same area estimate as $\widehat{A}_{MW}$ in (4.74). The variance of the area under the curve is estimated by

$$\widehat{Var}(\widehat{A}_{DL}) = \frac{1}{n_1} S_{10} + \frac{1}{n_0} S_{01}, \tag{4.80}$$

where S_{10} and S_{01} are variance estimates for the T_1 and T_0 components, given as

$$S_{10} = \frac{1}{n_1 - 1} \sum_{i=1}^{n_1} [V_{10}(T_{1i}) - \widehat{A}_{DL}]^2 \tag{4.81}$$

and

$$S_{01} = \frac{1}{n_0 - 1} \sum_{j=1}^{n_0} [V_{01}(T_{0j}) - \widehat{A}_{DL}]^2. \tag{4.82}$$

DeLong et al. (1988) have made available a SAS macro which calculates the area and variance. This macro is now included as part of the SAS statistical software. Other software programs such as STATA also can be used to estimate the area under the ROC curve and its variance in this way.

Another method of estimating the variance of the area under the curve is to use either the jackknife or the bootstrap (see Appendix B). Hanley and Hajian-Tilaki (1997) showed that the jackknife and the method of DeLong et al. (1988) produced essentially equivalent results for the area under the curve and its variance.

A nonparametric estimate of the partial area under the curve for ordinal data can be found by summing the area of the trapezoids restricted to the partial area of interest (Zhang et al., 2002; He and Escobar, 2008). Suppose we are interested in the partial area between the FPRs e_1 and e_2, which correspond to the p-th and $(p + s)$-th ordinal test results, T_{0p} and $T_{0(p+s)}$. The area would be estimated as

$$\widehat{A}_{N(e_1<FPR<e_2)} = \frac{1}{n_0 n_1} \sum_{i=1}^{m} \sum_{j=1}^{n} \Psi_{p,s}(T_{1i}, T_{0j}), \qquad (4.83)$$

where $\Psi_{p,s}(T_1, T_0) = 1$ if $T_1 > T_0$ and $T_0 \in [T_{0p}, T_{0(p+s)}]$, $\Psi_{p,s}(T_1, T_0) = 1/2$ if $T_1 = T_0$ and $T_0 \in [T_{0p}, T_{0p+s}]$, and $\Psi_{p,s}(T_1, T_0) = 0$ otherwise (i.e., similar to $\Psi(X, Y)$ as defined above but restricted to false positive values in the range of interest).

The variance presented by Zhang et al. (2002) has been shown to be wrong (He and Escobar, 2008). The correct variance is presented in the context of continuous test results in section 4.3.4, equations (4.106). Confidence intervals for the area and partial area can be constructed using the asymptotic formula the equation (4.3) with any of the variance formulae. Transformations described for use with parametric estimates (equations (4.63)-(4.73)) can also be used. Bootstrap methods also apply.

Obuchowski and Lieber (1998) considered the adequacy of using asymptotic confidence intervals with the nonparametric estimate of the total area, when sample sizes were small, and made recommendations. They found that there must be at least 30 subjects with and without the condition for the asymptotic confidence interval, using standard errors of DeLong et al. (1988), to provide adequate coverage. This minimum is increased to 150 for large areas (0.95). The bias-corrected and accelerated bootstrap confidence interval appeared to be the best alternatives in most circumstances (see article for details).

4.2.6.1   Nonparametric Estimate of the Area and Partial Area Under the ROC Curve: Case Study 3   In Sections 4.2.1–4.2.5, we analyzed data assessing the accuracy of MRA to detect coronary stenosis, assuming the ROC curve follows a binormal form. We could easily estimate the area under the ROC curve nonparametrically as described above. Using SAS, PROC LOGISTIC, we find that the nonparametric estimate is 0.913, with variance 0.000514. Note that the nonparametric estimate of the area is slightly smaller than the parametric estimate of 0.930, as expected, since the nonparametric estimate is biased. As a comparison, using equations (4.75)-(4.76), we can estimate the variance, using the approximations for Q_1 and Q_2, where $\widehat{Q}_1 =$

$(0.913)/(2-0.913) = 0.8399$ and $\widehat{Q}_2 = 2(0.913)^2/(1+0.913) = 0.87148$ to get $\widehat{Var}(\widehat{A}_{MW}) = 0.00068$. This estimate is larger than the DeLong et al. (1988) estimate, which is expected, since the area is close to 1.0.

If we only wanted to assess accuracy of MRA to detect significant carotid stenosis when $FPRs$ are small, we can estimate the partial area. There are only a few points on the curve, so we are limited in what we can consider. In particular, we consider the area under the curve from $FPR = 0.0$ to $FPR = 0.23$. Analysis with the equation (4.83) will have $p = 4$, $s = 2$.

$$\widehat{A}_{N(0 \leq FPR \leq 0.23)} = \frac{19 \times (14 \times 0.5 + 42 \times 1) + 4 \times (42 \times 0.5)}{62 \times 101} = 0.162.$$

An estimate of the area under the same portion of the curve, using parametric methods, has a similar, but slightly larger value of $\widehat{A}_{(0 \leq FPR \leq 0.23)} = 0.177$.

4.2.7 Nonparametric Analysis of Clustered Data.

The issue of clustered data was raised in section 4.1.2 with regards to binary data and estimation of sensitivity and specificity. If the clustered data are ordinal or continuous (quantitative), then appropriate analysis of the ROC curve area also requires that the clustering be taken into account. The methods are described in detail in Obuchowski (1997a), following the general method of DeLong et al. (1988).

We let T_{1ij} denote the test result of the j-th unit affected by the condition in the i-th cluster $j = 1, 2, \cdots, n_{1i}$; $i = 1, 2, \cdots, I$, and similarly, T_{0ik} denote the test results of the kth unit not affected by the condition in the i-th cluster ($k = 1, 2, \cdots, n_{0i}$) where n_{1i} and n_{0i} are the number of units affected and unaffected by the condition in the i-th cluster. Let $N_i = n_{1i} + n_{0i}$ be the total number of units in the i-th cluster. One can envision tables like Table 4.7 created for each cluster. The total number of units with the condition is $n_1 = \sum n_{1i}$ and the total number of units without the condition is $n_0 = \sum n_{0i}$. The total number of clusters with at least one affected unit is denoted by I_{10} and the total number of clusters with at least one unaffected unit is denoted by I_{01}. The estimate of the area is then

$$A_C = \frac{1}{n_0 n_1} \sum_{i=1}^{I} \sum_{i'=1}^{I} \sum_{j=1}^{n_{1i}} \sum_{k=1}^{n_{0i'}} \Psi(T_{1ij}, T_{0i'k}). \tag{4.84}$$

Note that this estimate gives equal weight to all pairwise rankings within and between clusters. Similar to before, we define the components

$$V_{10}(T_{1ij}) = \frac{1}{n_0} \sum_{i'=1}^{I_{01}} \sum_{k=1}^{n_{0i'}} \Psi(T_{1ij}, T_{0i'k}), \tag{4.85}$$

and

$$V_{01}(T_{0i'k}) = \frac{1}{n_1} \sum_{i=1}^{I_{10}} \sum_{j=1}^{n_{1i}} \Psi(T_{1ij}, T_{0i'k}). \tag{4.86}$$

As we saw in the previous section with unclustered data, an alternate form for the area estimate is

$$\widehat{A}_C = \sum_{i=1}^{I}\sum_{j=1}^{n_{1i}} V_{10}(T_{1ij})/n_1 = \sum_{i=1}^{I}\sum_{j=1}^{n_{0i}} V_{01}(T_{0ij})/n_0.$$

Let $V_{10}(T_{1i.})$ and $V_{01}(T_{0i.})$ denote the sums of the T_1 and T_0 components of the i-th cluster. The sum of squares of the components is

$$S_{10} = \frac{I_{10}}{(I_{10}-1)n_1} \sum_{i=1}^{I_{10}}[V_{10}(T_{1i.}) - n_{1i}\widehat{A}_C]^2, \tag{4.87}$$

$$S_{01} = \frac{I_{01}}{(I_{01}-1)n_0} \sum_{i=1}^{I_{01}}[V_{01}(T_{0i.}) - n_{0i}\widehat{A}_C]^2, \tag{4.88}$$

and

$$S_{11} = \frac{I}{(I-1)} \sum_{i=1}^{I}[V_{10}(T_{1i.}) - n_{1i}\widehat{A}_C][V_{01}(T_{0i.}) - n_{0i}\widehat{A}_C]. \tag{4.89}$$

The estimator of the variance of $\widehat{A}_C$ is then

$$\widehat{Var}(\widehat{A}_C) = \frac{1}{n_1}S_{10} + \frac{1}{n_0}S_{01} + \frac{2}{n_0 n_1}S_{11}. \tag{4.90}$$

Rutter (2000) suggested using the bootstrap to construct confidence intervals for clustered data. She found that for the area under the ROC curve, both Obuchowski's method and the bootstrap percentile method provided reasonable coverage.

4.2.7.1 Nonparametric Estimate of the Area for Clustered Data: Case Study 3

The MRA study presented at the beginning of Section 4.2 was more complex than we dealt with. In the study, both the left and right carotids were assessed for stenosis (see Chapter 1). This is an example of clustered data. Each person is a cluster, and the units of the cluster are the left and right carotids. Previously we assessed the accuracy for the left carotid, for Radiologist 4 only. It would be better, though, to assess the accuracy of MRA by using the assessment of both carotids in a single analysis. The details of the calculations for the area are similar to that of the previous section, except more involved and we don't do the calculations here. The area, calculated to take into account the clustering, is 0.914. Components of the variance are $S_{10} = 0.016625$, $S_{01} = 0.026185$, $S_{11} = 0.40843$, with variance 0.000293539 (standard error: 0.01713). If we ignore clustering, then the area estimate is 0.914 with a standard error of 0.0156, which is somewhat smaller (and incorrect). Ignoring clustering will result in somewhat inflated test statistics and thus levels of significance that are too small.

4.2.8   Degenerate Data

Occasionally when diagnostic accuracy is estimated from data under the binormal assumption, there may be problems in estimating the binormal parameters. Estimation programs such as RSCORE and ROCKIT may not converge, or they may estimate either the parameter b, or some of the decision thresholds as infinite. Metz calls these data sets degenerate (Metz, 1989). Degenerate data sets generally occur when the sample size is small, and when the test results are not well distributed across the possible response categories. Often times a test result category will be zero.

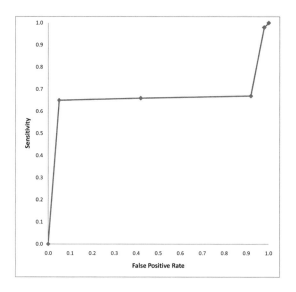

Figure 4.6   Example of an ROC Curve for Degenerate Data

A plot of the points on the ROC curve when the data are degenerate often will reveal a problem. An ROC curve derived from binormal data that are not degenerate will have a particular shape. The curve starts at (0,0), rises relatively rapidly and then bends smoothly as it turns toward (1,1). In contrast, for degenerate data, a plot of the points on the ROC curve may show sensitivities on or near the vertical axis (i.e., sensitivities near zero). A binormal curve that would be an exact fit to the data might consist of a vertical line from (0,0) to some point on the vertical axis, then a horizontal line across the unit square through a single interior point (FPR^*, TPR^*), and then finally a vertical segment at $FPR = 1$ up to the point (1,1). Figure 4.6 is an example of the ROC curve from such a (hypothetical) degenerate data set. Dorfman and Berbaum (1995) illustrated a number of possible degenerate data sets, which they attributed to Metz (1989).

There are a number of possible solutions. Rockette et al. (1990) suggested estimating the area under the curve nonparametrically. Doing so would be a simple solution, but unfortunately, the bias in the area estimate is considerable for ordinal data (Dorfman and Berbaum, 1995). Dorfman and Berbaum (1995) have developed new computer software, RSCORE4, that is more successful at estimation of the binormal parameters. The program gives identical results to RSCORE and ROCKIT when the data are not degenerate. If the data are grouped in only two categories, it is assumed that the parameter b has value 1 ($b = 1$) and standard methods are used to estimate the parameter a. If more categories are used, but there are some test response categories with no observations, then a small value is added to each test result (value 10^{-k}, where k is between 1 and 7) and standard methods used for estimation. In the unusual circumstances that the parameters still cannot be estimated (i.e., the algorithm does not converge, and/or some estimates are infinite), then a pattern-search algorithm is used.

Metz (1989) suggested a solution to the problem of degeneracy that assumed that the ROC curve belonged to a family of curves with monotonically decreasing LRs. A couple of such "proper" ROC curves have been suggested. Pan and Metz (1997) proposed the proper binormal model, in which the decision threshold is a monotonic transformation of the LR of the underlying pair of normal distributions. They developed the method, identified the likelihood equations (which are difficult to maximize) and developed software, called PROPROC, to estimate ROC curve parameters, as well as the area and partial area under the curve and the corresponding SEs. An updated curve fitting algorithm, along with software implemented on the website provides superior numerical stability (`http://xray.bsd/uchicago.edu/krl/`; Pesce and Metz (2007)).

Another model for a proper ROC curve is the bigamma model. Dorfman et al. (1997) proposed a model in which the distribution of test results for those with the condition followed a gamma distribution with shape parameter r and scale parameter λ. The bigamma model has two parameters, r and λ, similar to the binormal model. The gamma distribution approaches the normal distribution as the shape parameter enlarges. Thus, the bigamma distribution should be similarly flexible and able to accommodate most diagnostic testing data. Simulations showed that the binormal model is not robust when sample sizes are small and that the bigamma model has a smaller bias for estimating total or partial area under the ROC curve (Dorfman et al., 1997). In a series of articles, Dorfman and Berbaum (2000a,b) presented a contaminated binormal model that could handle degenerate data as well as or better than the standard binormal or bigamma models and also worked with data that are not degenerate.

Of course, it would be better if degenerate data sets were avoided in the first place. This can be achieved in the study design stage by having larger samples, and by training observers to distribute their responses more evenly across the response categories (See Chapter 3).

4.2.9   Choosing Between Parametric, Semi-parametric and Nonparametric Methods

The choice between parametric, semi-parametric and nonparametric methods with ordinal data depends in part on the comfort level with the binormal assumptions and the distribution of the data. In addition, one has to take into consideration the ROC curve measures that are of interest, as well as the resources available for computation.

Parametric and semi-parametric methods have an advantage with ordinal test results, as they allow an estimate of the smooth ROC curve. The area estimate is generally unbiased. The binormal assumption and maximum likelihood estimates of the binormal parameters allow estimation of the total area, as well as the partial area and the sensitivity at a specified FPR. Computer programs implementing the maximum likelihood algorithms are available, particularly ROCKIT and STATA. But if the sample size is small, data sets will often be degenerate, some of the maximum likelihood estimates of the parameters will be infinite and the computer algorithms will not converge. No ROC curve measures will be estimable.

The nonparametric approach to ROC curve analysis for ordinal test results does not require distributional assumptions for the test results or the ROC curve. While the binormal assumption has been shown repeatedly to provide good approximations to ROC curves arising from many different forms, some do not feel comfortable with the assumption. This discomfort is relieved when using nonparametric methods. The nonparametric estimate of the ROC curve is very rough. The area estimate is easy to calculate, even by hand, and can be determined for any data-set, even if small, without regard to the distribution of the operational points (i.e. degeneracy is not a problem). While degeneracy may not make estimation impossible, when the operating points are maldistributed, the nonparametric (trapezoidal) estimate of the area will greatly underestimate the true area under the ROC curve. The variance calculation can be time consuming, but computer programs for estimation are readily available.

4.3   CONTINUOUS-SCALE DATA

In addition to their use to assess the accuracy of diagnostic medical tests, ROC curves are also useful as a means of assessing the accuracy of variables to predict prognosis. As an example of such a use, as well as an example of using continuous or quantitative data, we consider the use of cerebrospinal fluid CK-BB isoenzyme measured within 24 hours of injury as a means of predicting the outcome of severe head trauma. We are interested in determining which patients will have a poor outcome (death, vegetative state or severe disability) after suffering a severe head trauma. A sample of 60 subjects admitted to a hospital with severe head trauma are considered with 19 eventually having moderate to full recovery, with the remaining 41 poor or no recovery (Hans et al., 1985). The data are in Table 4.9. We know that the area under an ROC curve is a measure of discrimination between those with and without disease. In this circumstance, we will use the ROC curve to assess the discrimination between those with and without a poor outcome. We would like to know if CK-BB isoenzyme is a good predictor of the outcome.

Table 4.9   Data for 60 Patients with Severe Head Trauma

Poor Outcome				Good Outcome	
Age	CK-BB	Age	CK-BB	Age	CK-BB
4	140	21	463	6	136
7	1087	22	60	6	286
8	230	23	509	7	281
11	183	23	576	8	23
15	1256	24	671	8	200
16	700	29	80	10	146
16	16	29	490	11	220
16	800	29	156	12	96
17	253	30	356	12	100
18	740	40	350	16	60
18	126	41	323	17	17
18	153	45	1560	18	27
19	283	45	120	18	126
19	90	50	216	19	100
19	303	51	443	24	253
19	193	56	523	28	70
20	76	59	76	35	40
20	1370	61	303	38	6
20	543	61	353	46	46
20	913	62	206		
20	230				

Some diagnostic tests, as well as predictive measures such as the above prognostic variable for head trauma outcome, produce continuous or quantitative, numerical test results. Examples include biochemical tests such as CPKs or glucose levels. Confidence ratings given on a 0-100% scale may also be considered quantitative if the readers provide a reasonable spread of answers. Some of the methods to deal with these data are similar to that of ordinal data, yet some provide opportunities for different methods. We discuss both below.

4.3.1   Empirical ROC Curve

The theoretical ROC curve is a plot of the points $(FPR(c), TPR(c))$ for each value of c with $-\infty < c < \infty$. For continuous data, Campbell (1994) suggested plotting the estimated cumulative distribution functions. As in Section 4.2, let T_0 be a random variable representing the continuous test result of someone without the condition, with the distribution function F_0. Let T_1 be the random variable representing the continuous test result of someone with the condition, with the distribution function F_1. The theoretical ROC curve is a plot of $(\bar{F}_0(c), \bar{F}_1(c))$, for all possible values of c, where $\bar{F}_i(c) = 1 - F_i(c)$ are the survivor functions, as described earlier. For a random sample of size n_0 without the condition and n_1 with the condition, the empirical ROC curve would be the plot of the pairs $(\bar{F}_{n_0}(c_i), \bar{F}_{n_1}(c_i))$, where c_i ranges over the observed values of the test. $\bar{F}_{n_0}(c_i)$ and $\bar{F}_{n_1}(c_i)$, of course, are one minus the sample cumulative distribution functions

$$\bar{F}_{n_0}(c_i) = \frac{1}{n_0} \sum_{j=1}^{n_0} I_{[T_{0j} > c_i]}, \bar{F}_{n_1}(c_i) = \frac{1}{n_1} \sum_{j=1}^{n_1} I_{[T_{1j} > c_i]}, \qquad (4.91)$$

where $I_{[T_{0j} > c_i]}$ is equal to 1 if $T_{0j} > c_i$; otherwise it is 0 (similarly for $I_{[T_{1j} > c_i]}$). The plot of $(\bar{F}_{n_0}(c), \bar{F}_{n_1}(c))$ will consist of at most $n_0 + n_1 + 1$ points (depending on "ties"). Since the data are continuous, adjacent points can be connected by vertical lines of length $1/n_0$ and horizontal lines of length $1/n_1$, to form a step function that runs from $(0, 0)$ to $(1, 1)$.

4.3.2   Fitting a Smooth ROC Curve - Parametric, Semi-parametric and Nonparametric Methods

As with ordinal scale test results, the usual distributional assumption made to fit a smooth ROC curve is that the test results are binormal or that there exists a (perhaps unknown) monotone transformation of the original data which follows a binormal distribution. When the test results are actually normally distributed, the parameters a and b can be estimated directly from the means and variances of the test results of those with and without the condition of interest. Thus we would have

$$\widehat{b} = \widehat{\sigma}_0/\widehat{\sigma}_1 \text{ and } \widehat{a} = (\bar{T}_1 - \bar{T}_0)/\widehat{\sigma}_1, \qquad (4.92)$$

where $\widehat{\sigma}_i$ is the estimated standard deviation and $\bar{T}_i$ is the estimated mean of the continuous test results, $i = 0, 1$. Variance-covariance estimates of $\widehat{a}$ and $\widehat{b}$ are

$$\widehat{Var}(\widehat{a}) = \frac{n_0(\widehat{a}^2 + 2) + 2n_1\widehat{b}^2}{2n_0n_1}, \qquad (4.93)$$

$$\widehat{Var}(\widehat{b}) = \frac{(n_1 + n_0)\widehat{b}^2}{2n_0n_1}, \qquad (4.94)$$

$$\widehat{Cov}(\widehat{a}, \widehat{b}) = \frac{\widehat{a}\widehat{b}}{2n_1}. \tag{4.95}$$

In most instances, continuous test results are not binormal. A Box-Cox transformation can be used to transform the data to binormality (Box and Cox, 1964; Zou et al., 1998; Zou and Hall, 2000b). The Box-Cox transformation is

$$\psi_\lambda(T_{kj}) = \frac{(T_{kj})^\lambda - 1}{\lambda} \text{ for } \lambda \neq 0; \ k = 0, 1; \ j = 1, \cdots, n_k, \tag{4.96}$$

$$\psi_\lambda(T_{kj}) = \ln(T_{kj}) \text{ for } \lambda = 0; \ k = 0, 1; \ j = 1, \cdots, n_k. \tag{4.97}$$

where T_{kj} is the continuous observed result of the test for the j-th subject with ($k = 1$) or without ($k = 0$) the condition. The parameter λ can be estimated via maximum likelihood. The TRANSREG procedure in SAS is one program that will estimate λ. Once the parameter λ is estimated, the original test data can be transformed. These transformed data can be used to directly estimate the binormal parameters and their variances, as in equations (4.92)-(4.95). Note that the same transformation, ψ_λ, must be applied to patients both with and without the condition of interest. Faraggi and Reiser (2002) show that this method often gives good results.

Goddard and Hinberg (1990) showed that when the binormal assumption was violated, directly estimating the parameters gave seriously biased estimates of the area. Thus, we do not recommend casual use of the estimator in (4.92) unless the data or their transformation have been shown to satisfy the normality assumption. Goodness-of-fit tests, such as those in Bozdogan and Ramirez (1986) and Lin and Mudholkar (1980), can be used to assess the normality assumptions.

Zou et al. (1997) described a nonparametric (kernel) method to estimate a smooth ROC curve from continuous data. They suggested estimating the points on the ROC curve, $(\bar{F}_0(c), \bar{F}_1(c))$, through the integral of the density function, where the density function f was estimated as

$$\widehat{f}_i(x) = \frac{1}{n_i h_i} \sum_{j=1}^{n_i} k\left(\frac{x - T_{ij}}{h_i}\right), i = 0, 1. \tag{4.98}$$

The function k is called the kernel and h_i is the bandwidth. Thus we can write that

$$\bar{F}_i(c) = \sum_{j=1}^{n_i} \int_c^\infty \frac{1}{n_i h_i} k\left(\frac{x - T_{ij}}{h_i}\right) dx, i = 0, 1. \tag{4.99}$$

These integrals can be evaluated with numerical integration. Zou et al. (1997) and Zou et al. (1998) suggested a bandwidth

$$h_i = 0.9 min(SD, IQR/1.34)/\sqrt[5]{n_i}, \tag{4.100}$$

where SD is the standard deviation and IQR is the interquartile range (i.e., 75th percentile minus 25th percentile) for the observations of those with (T_{1j})

and without(T_{0j}) the condition. This bandwidth is optimized if the distribution of the data are approximately bell-shaped.

Zou et al. (1997) initially suggested using the biweight kernel

$$k\left(\frac{x - T_{ij}}{h_i}\right) = \frac{15}{16}\left[1 - \left(\frac{x - T_{ij}}{h_i}\right)^2\right]^2 \text{ for } x \in (T_{ij} - h_i, T_{ij} + h_i). \quad (4.101)$$

In subsequent work, Zou et al. (1998) suggested the Gaussian kernel $\phi(x)$, that is, the density of the standard normal distribution

$$\phi(x) = \frac{1}{\sqrt{2\pi}}e^{-x^2/2},$$

so that the integral above can be written as

$$\bar{F}_i(c) = \frac{1}{n_i}\sum_{j=1}^{n_i}\Phi\left(\frac{T_{ij} - c}{h_i}\right).$$

It is worth noting that the bandwidth choice proposed by Zou et al. (1997) is not optimal for ROC curve estimation, because the true ROC curve is a plot of $\bar{F}_1(c)$ versus $\bar{F}_0(c)$ for $-\infty < c < +\infty$ and the optimality in density estimation does not carry over to distribution estimation. Lloyd (1998), Lloyd and Yong (1999), and Zhou and Harezlak (2002) have improved on the above estimator by choosing asymptotically optimal bandwidths that are for the estimation of distribution functions.

Semi-parametric methods are also available to estimate the ROC curve. In general, these methods do not assume a distribution for the test results, but rather assume a parametric form for the ROC curve itself. In particular, the ROC curve can be written as

$$ROC(t) = F_1(\alpha_0 + \alpha_1 F_0(t)).$$

Most semi-parametric methods assume $F_1(x) = F_0(x) = \Phi(x)$, the standard normal distribution and

$$ROC(t) = \Phi(a + b\Phi^{-1}(t)). \quad (4.102)$$

This assumes a binormal form for the ROC curve itself, but not for the underlying diagnostic test results. Various methods have been proposed to estimate α_0 and α_1 or, equivalently, a and b in (4.102). We briefly describe some below. More detail on some of these methods can be found in Chapter 8, in the context of regression analysis.

Metz et al. (1998) suggested categorizing or binning continuous test results, so they resemble ordinal-scale data. The binormal parameters can then be estimated with the Dorfman-Alf method, as implemented in the LABROC family of programs, now subsumed in ROCKIT. Concerns with the original LABROC algorithm involved the possibility that the results were dependent on the categorization scheme. Later work by Metz et al. (1998) showed that a new algorithm, revolving around "truth-state runs" (transformation of the ordered test results into sequences of positive and negative outcomes), produced reliable MLEs of the binormal ROC curve parameters. Their algorithms, LABROC4 (a true maximum likelihood algorithm) and LABROC5 (a less computationally intense quasi-maximum likelihood algorithm), are also available as part of ROCKIT.

Zou et al. (1998) and Zou and Hall (2000b) presented a semiparametric method that assumed there existed a monotone function that transformed the data to follow a binormal distribution, but that function was left unspecified. A likelihood equation was developed, based on the ranks of test results in the combined sample. The likelihood equation that they found required, in part, Monte Carlo methods to evaluate. Zou et al. (1998) recommended the parametric transformation method over the kernel and semiparametric methods, which are computer intensive.

A number of methods have been developed around the placement value

$$U = 1 - F_0(T).$$

Alonzo and Pepe (2002) suggested a procedure that involved fitting a binary generalized linear model to placement values U_{it} which was defined as

$$U_{it} = I(T_{1i} > \widehat{F}_0^{-1}(t)).$$

for a fixed, finite set of values t, $0 < t < 1$, where $I(.)$ was an indicator function taking the value of 1 if $T_{1i} > \widehat{F}_0^{-1}(t)$ and 0 otherwise. $\widehat{F}_0$ was estimated from the test results of those without the condition. Pepe and Cai (2004) proposed an approach where estimated placement values would be substituted into a log-likelihood to form a pseudo log-likelihood approach to estimating a and b. Cai and Moskowitz (2004) proposed both a pseudo maximum likelihood and a profile maximum likelihood estimation method to estimate a and b. Zhou and Lin (2008) extended their work, with a new profile maximum likelihood approach that had computational advantages over the method of Cai and Moskowitz (2004).

In simulations, Pepe and Cai (2004) found their pseudo likelihood approach to be more efficient than Pepe's original binary glm approach (Pepe, 2000) when test results were normally distributed. Cai and Moskowitz (2004) also compared estimates of parameters a and b from their pseudo and profile maximum likelihood estimates with that of Alonzo and Pepe (2002) and Metz et al. (1998). Simulations based on binormal data found little bias with any of the 4 methods. The pseudo and profile maximum likelihood estimates had slightly more bias, yet were more efficient than estimates using methods of Alonzo and Pepe (2002) and the binning method of Metz et al. (1998). Zhou and Lin (2008) compared estimates of parameters a and b from their new profile likelihood approach with estimators calculated using the methods of Metz et al. (1998), Alonzo and Pepe (2002), Pepe and Cai (2004), and Cai and

Moskowitz (2004). In a simulation study, they found that all estimators had similar efficiency and robustness, except those estimated using the method of Pepe and Cai (2004), which tended to have more bias than the other estimators. The estimators of Zhou and Lin (2008) were slightly more efficient and robust than the others. While the semi-parametric method of Zou and Hall (2000a) was not evaluated in the simulation, in examples this method was found to produce similar ROC curve estimates.

4.3.2.1 ROC Curve Estimation: Head Trauma Data We consider the head trauma example, and examine the discriminatory ability of CK-BB isoenzymes to predict poor outcome in this patient sample. Figure 4.7 has a plot of the empirical ROC curve.

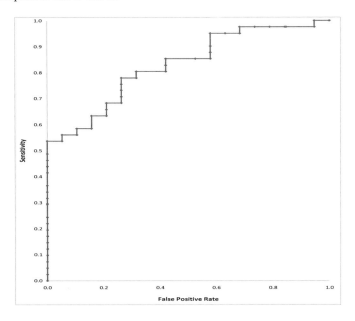

Figure 4.7   Empirical ROC Curve for the Head Trauma Data

A smooth ROC curve can be drawn if we assume binormality and estimate the parameters a and b. Direct calculation of the parameters a and b from the means and standard deviations (Table 4.10) gives us

$$\widehat{a} = \frac{427.3 - 117.5}{372.6} = 0.83, \ \widehat{b} = \frac{91.1}{372.6} = 0.24.$$

The area estimate would then be $\Phi(0.83/\sqrt{1 + 0.24^2}) = 0.790$. Estimation of the parameters via ROCKIT gives $\widehat{a} = 1.1451$, $\widehat{b} = 0.6514$, and an area estimate of $\widehat{A} = 0.831$ which are quite different than the direct estimates. One reason for these differences is that the data are not normally distributed.

Table 4.10   Descriptive Data for CK-BB Measurements in 60 Severe Head Trauma Patients with Good or Poor Outcome

	Mean	SD	25th percentile	75th percentile
Untransformed				
Good Outcome	117.5	91.1	40.0	200.0
Poor Outcome	427.3	372.6	156.0	543.0
Box-Cox Transformation				
Good Outcome	8.29	2.96	6.06	11.04
Poor Outcome	12.97	3.89	10.14	15.31

Table 4.11   Estimation of Parameters and the Total Area under the ROC Curve for the CK-BB Test to Predict Poor Outcome of Severe Head Trauma

Method	$\widehat{a}$	$\widehat{b}$	area
Direct-untransformed	0.83	0.24	0.790
Direct-transformed	1.20	0.76	0.831
ROCKIT	1.14	0.65	0.831
SAS NLMIXED-untransformed	0.84	0.24	0.793
SAS NLMIXED - transformed	1.22	0.75	0.835

The Box-Cox transformation (using SAS PROC TRANSREG) on these data suggest $\widehat{\lambda} = 0.25$ would be appropriate. After transformation, statistical tests do not reject the null hypothesis of normally distributed data. Means and standard deviations of the transformed data are also in Table 4.10. Direct estimates are now

$$\widehat{a} = \frac{12.97 - 8.29}{3.89} = 1.20, \ \widehat{b} = \frac{2.96}{3.89} = 0.76, \ \Phi\left(\frac{1.20}{\sqrt{1 + 0.76^2}}\right) = 0.830.$$

The direct estimates of $\widehat{a}$ and $\widehat{b}$ from the transformed data are closer to the values estimated via ROCKIT, and the area estimates agree (see Table 4.11). These same values can be found using PROC NLMIXED in SAS, with the added benefit that the standard error of the area estimate will also be provided (in this case, the standard error for the transformed data, as estimated by NLMIXED is 0.5114). We use the maximum likelihood estimates to draw a smooth ROC curve (Figure 4.8).

Alternatively, we can use the nonparametric kernel method to plot a smooth ROC curve for the head trauma data. As suggested by Zou et al. (1997), we first transform the data, as described above, so that its distribution is approx-

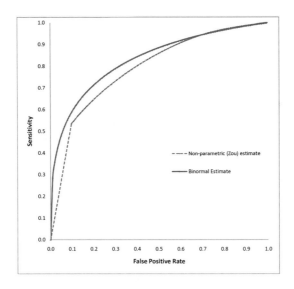

Figure 4.8 Smooth ROC Curve for Head Trauma Data

imately bell-shaped. The necessary information to estimate the bandwidth is in Table 4.10.

The bandwidth for head trauma patients with a poor outcome is

$$
\begin{aligned}
h_1 &= 0.9 \times \min[3.89, (15.31 - 10.14)/1.34]/\sqrt[5]{41} \\
&= 0.9 \times \min(3.89, 5.17)/2.10 = 1.67,
\end{aligned}
$$

and for those with good outcome is

$$
\begin{aligned}
h_0 &= 0.9 \times \min[2.96, (11.04 - 6.06)/1.34]/\sqrt[5]{19} \\
&= 0.9 \times \min(2.96, 4.98)/1.80 = 1.48.
\end{aligned}
$$

The smooth, nonparametric estimate of the ROC curve, using the Gaussian kernel, also appears in Figure 4.8, along with the smooth curve based on the binormal assumption.

4.3.3 Confidence Bands Around the Estimated ROC Curve

Assuming binormality, pointwise and simultaneous confidence intervals can be constructed around the estimated ROC curve using methods described in Section 4.2.3 for ordinal-scale data. Non-parametric and semi-parametric alternatives have been suggested specifically for quantitative, continuous-scale data. Corresponding to their non-parametric kernel estimated smooth ROC curve, Zou et al. (1997) proposed using a logit transformation to find pointwise confidence intervals, or a similar probit transformation (Zou et al., 1998). Lloyd

(1998) used percentiles of a nonparametric bootstrap and Schafer (1994) based pointwise estimates on a statistical test of Greenhouse and Mantel (1950). The method that Hilgers (1991) proposed was related to distribution-free tolerance limits. These methods have not been directly compared.

A number of methods have been suggested for simultaneous confidence intervals. Campbell proposed 3 different non-parametric methods. Two were based on (1- and 2-sided) Kolmogorov-Smirnov sample statistics, and another on bootstrap resampling. Li et al. (1996) also suggested simultaneous confidence intervals using quantiles, based on bootstrap Kolmogorov-type test. Claeskens et al. (2003) used bootstrap smoothed empirical likelihood methods to construct both pointwise and simultaneous confidence bands. They found in a simulation study that their pointwise intervals had better coverage than confidence intervals based on both normal approximation estimators as well as bootstrap percentile methods.

Jensen et al. (2000) introduced the idea of regional confidence bands. Regional confidence bands simultaneously cover the ROC curve corresponding to a subset of false positive rates that constitute a "region of interest," rather than the entire ROC curve (which they termed global confidence bands). They postulated that confidence bands constructed specifically for a region of interest would be narrower than considering global confidence intervals restricted to the area of interest. Their method was based on Monte Carlo simulation, and thus was computer intensive. Simulations verified that, indeed, regional confidence intervals are narrower than "global" ones in the area of interest. In addition, considered as a global CI, they found that their Monte Carlo method was superior to Campbell's 2-sample KS and bootstrap methods when data were normal, but inferior for skewed distributions.

4.3.4   Area and Partial Area Under the ROC Curve - Parametric, Nonparametric and Semi-parametric Methods

Parametric and semi-parametric estimation of the full and partial area under the ROC curve, for continuous data, can be done essentially the same way as for ordinal data. In general, this involves estimating the binormal parameters a and b in Equation (4.41). There are many options, though, for estimating these parameters, as described in Section 4.3.2. If the test results are truly binormal, then the parameters a and b can be estimated directly using the equation (4.92). A Box-Cox transformation to normality may also allow direct estimates on the transformed values. Since Goddard and Hinberg (1990) have shown that direct estimation of the binormal parameters can give seriously biased estimates of the area when the binormal assumption is violated, we do not recommend casual use of the direct estimates of these parameters. Alternatives to assumptions of binormality include semi-parametric methods which can be used to estimate the parameters a and b. Nonparametric estimation of the full area under the ROC curve and its variance can be accomplished as with ordinal data, using equations (4.74)−(4.82). The nonparametric estimate, in this case, though, is unbiased for the true area. This is true because continuous data have few ties (theoretically, if level of measurement permits, there are no ties), so that essentially $P(T_1 = T_0) = 0$. Clustering methods described in Section 4.2.6 can be applied to continuous data in the same way as was done for ordinal data.

The kernel method provides another non-parametric approach to estimating the area under the ROC curve. Lloyd (1998) showed that the area under the entire ROC curve, using the Gaussian kernel, was

$$\frac{1}{n_0 n_1} \sum_{i=1}^{n_i} \sum_{j=1}^{n_0} \Phi\left(\frac{T_{1i} - T_{0j}}{\sqrt{h_1^2 + h_0^2}}\right). \tag{4.103}$$

Faraggi and Reiser (2002) compared parametric and non-parametric area estimates in terms of bias and mean square error when sample sizes were small ($n_i = 20, 50, 100$). They considered direct estimation under the assumption of binormality, the Box-Cox transformation to transform to binormality, followed by direct estimation of the area, the Mann-Whitney non-parametric area estimate, the binning method of Metz et al. (1998), and kernel smoothing with area estimation under the ROC curve by numerical integration. They found that for normal data, all methods produced good estimates of the area. For non-normal, skewed data, the transformation and binning methods were preferred unless the data for those diseased or non-diseased follow a strongly bimodal distribution. In the latter case, for high area (0.9) the normal transformation method was superior, but for moderate area (0.7, 0.8) the choice of method was not clear.

If a full ROC curve has been estimated using any of the parametric or semi-parametric methods, the partial area estimates can be obtained by integrating numerically over the region of interest. This is also true of curves estimated using kernel non-parametric methods described in Section 4.3.2. See, for example, Zou et al. (1997) and Pepe and Cai (2004). Some semi-parametric methods can also be used to directly model only the portion of the curve of interest, rather than the full curve. This has the potential to give a better partial area estimate.

A non-parametric estimator for the partial area, analogous to the Mann-Whitney approach (Equation 4.74) was suggested by Dodd and Pepe (2003) for continuous data as

$$A_{N(e_1 < FPR < e_2)} = \frac{1}{n_0 n_1} \sum_{j=1}^{n_0} \sum_{i=1}^{n_1} I_{[T_{1i} > T_{0j}, \, T_{0j} \in (c_1, c_2)]}, \tag{4.104}$$

where $c_1 = \bar{F}_0^{-1}(e_1)$ and $c_2 = \bar{F}_0^{-1}(e_2)$ are threshold values of the observations associated with the false positive rates of interest and I is the indicator function. If empirical quantiles must be used, yet don't coincide exactly with the values desired, then Dodd and Pepe (2003) suggested using linear interpolation. For the variance of the partial area estimate, they suggested using a bootstrap method.

Alternatively, He and Escobar (2008) presented a very similar estimator, with a specific equation for the variances:

$$\widehat{A}_{N(e_1<FPR<e_2)} = \frac{1}{n_0 n_1} \sum_{j=1}^{n_0} \sum_{i=1}^{n_1} \Psi_{e_1,e_2}(T_{1i}, T_{0j}), \tag{4.105}$$

where $\Psi_{e_1,e_2}(T_0, T_1) = 1$ if $T_1 > T_0$ and $T_0 \in (c_1, c_0)$, $\Psi_{e_1,e_2}(T_0, T_1) = 1/2$ if $T_1 = T_0$ and $\Psi_{e_1,e_2}(T_0, T_1) = 0$ otherwise, where c_1 and c_2 are as defined above. The only difference between this estimator and that of Dodd and Pepe (2003) occurs when the value of those with and without disease are the same (which theoretically doesn't occur with continuous data). He and Escobar (2008) provided the following explicit estimator of the variance for this partial area:

$$\begin{aligned} Var(\widehat{A}_{N(e_1<FPR<e_2)}) &= \left(\frac{n_p}{n}\right)^2 \left[\frac{1}{n_P} \frac{1}{n_P - 1} \sum_{T_{0i} \in (c_1, c_2)} \{V_{10}(T_{0i}) - \widehat{\tau}\}^2 \right. \\ &\left. + \frac{1}{n_1} \frac{1}{n_1 - 1} \sum_{j=1}^{n_1} \{V_{01}(T_{1j}) - \widehat{\tau}\}^2\right], \end{aligned} \tag{4.106}$$

where

$$V_{10}(T_{0i}) = \frac{1}{n_0} \sum_{j=1}^{n_1} \Psi_{e_1,e_2}(T_{1j}, T_{0i}), \ (T_{0i} \in [c_1, c_2]), \tag{4.107}$$

$$V_{01}(T_{1j}) = \frac{1}{n_p} \sum_{T_{0i} \in [c_1, c_2]} \Psi_{e_1,e_2}(T_{1j}, T_{0i}), \ j = 1, 2, \ldots n_1, \tag{4.108}$$

$\widehat{\tau} = (n_p/n_0) A_{N(e_1<FPR<e_2)}$, and n_p is the number of test results of those without disease (T_0) that lie between c_1 and c_2. This variance estimator corrected a similar variance formula presented in Zhang et al. (2002).

Wieand et al. (1989) provided a framework for non-parametric estimation of the full area, partial area and sensitivity at a fixed false positive rate, which is based on a weighted average of sensitivities. Results for the full and partial area and sensitivity concur with the work of others.

4.3.5   Confidence Intervals for the Area Under the ROC Curve

As we saw with ordinal-scale test results, there are a number of possible methods that can be used to construct confidence intervals for the area and partial area estimates. Many methods are based on the assumption of asymptotic normality of the area and partial area, using the equation (4.3). The area and variance may be estimated parametrically, semi-parametrically or non-parametrically. Bootstrapping may also be used to estimate the variance of the area. Transformations of area estimates, as described in Section 4.2.5

may be a good alternative. The transformed area estimates tend to conform better to the normal distribution and are particularly useful when the area or partial area estimates are near 1.0. Methods not relying on the equation (4.3) include various bootstrap methods (see Appendix B) and an empirical likelihood method of Qin and Zhou (2006) based on placement values which involves iterative methods (R program available from authors). Qin and Hotiloac (2008) presented a nice summary of many of these methods as it pertains to the full area under the curve.

Obuchowski and Lieber (1998) assessed the adequacy of confidence intervals for the total area under the ROC, when the data are continuous and sample sizes are small. The results differ somewhat from that of ordinal data. If the area under the ROC curve is moderate (around 0.80), asymptotic methods should be adequate as long as the number of subjects with and without the condition is at least 50. This is true for both parametric and nonparametric estimates. For smaller samples, the bootstrap t method is preferred with parametric estimates, and the bias-corrected and accelerated (BCa) bootstrap method is generally preferred with nonparametric estimation. For ROC curve areas near 1.0, the number of subjects with and without the condition needs to be at least 150 each for the asymptotic methods to provide good coverage. While no methods appear adequate for parametric estimation with smaller samples, the BCa method can be used for nonparametric area estimates.

Qin and Zhou (2006) compared coverage of confidence intervals using their empirical likelihood approach with a couple of methods based on asymptotic normality (Equation 4.3) - the Mann-Whitney non-parametric estimator as well as a logit transformation of the Mann-Whitney estimator. They also looked at two bootstrap methods. They found that their empirical likelihood method had better coverage than Mann-Whitney estimator, particularly when the area was high. The logit transformation also had good coverage, but longer width. They also found that the empirical likelihood method produced confidence intervals with better coverage than the bootstrap percentile method, and that the bootstrap t confidence intervals over-covered the area.

Qin and Hotiloac (2008) compared finite sample performance of asymptotic confidence intervals including non-parametric (Mann-Whitney and De-Long), logit transformation of Mann-Whitney estimator, the empirical likelihood method of Qin and Zhou (2006) as well as 5 different bootstrap methods. They found that all methods had good coverage when the area was low-moderate (0.7), but coverage fell below the nominal value as the area increased for most methods. The logit transformation of the Mann-Whitney estimator, and the empirical likelihood based method provided the best coverage, except when the area was near 1 (area$\geq$ 0.95). In the latter case, as with Obuchowski and Lieber (1998), they recommended the bootstrap t.

As with ordinal test results, when the estimate of the area under the curve is 1.0, confidence intervals cannot be estimated by any of the methods described. Obuchowski and Lieber (2002), using simulation, provided tables with suggested lower bounds for confidence intervals. Results varied depending on the sample size, and the ratio of standard deviations of the test results.

Little has been published regarding adequacy of confidence intervals for partial area. McClish (1987), in a small simulation study, found that confidence intervals for the partial area based on the transformation the equation (4.70) gave superior coverage to the usual asymptotic confidence intervals (without transformations), even with moderate sized areas. In unpublished work, she also found that the logit transformation based on the partial area index was also appropriate, particularly for partial areas close to maximum value.

Dodd and Pepe (2003) evaluated the small sample performance of parametric and non-parametric estimators of the partial area and confidence intervals. They compared estimators which integrate under the appropriate portion of the curve, where the ROC curve was generated assuming binormality (McClish, 1989), using the method of Metz et al. (1998) and Pepe (2003) with their non-parametric estimator (both with quantiles estimated and assumed known). They found that when the test results were far from normally distributed, only the non-parametric results were without unacceptably large bias, and that confidence intervals had good coverage. They attributed this to the idea that methods which directly model the portion of ROC curve of interest could be more appropriate than integrating portions of ROC curves which were estimated for the entire curve. They noted that bias in area estimates decreased as a larger portion of the curve was integrated. This would coincide with the often found result that the estimates of the area under the curve are reasonably robust to departures from binormality (see Section 4.2.2). When test-results were normally distributed, the non-parametric results were unbiased but not robust.

4.3.6   Fixed False Positive Rate - Sensitivity and the Decision Threshold

Investigators want the specificity of CK-BB to predict poor recovery or death from severe head injury to be at least 0.90. They want to know what the corresponding sensitivity of CK-BB is, and also would like to find the threshold that will produce a value of specificity at least that high.

Under the binormal model assumptions, the sensitivity at a fixed false positive rate can be estimated for continuous data the same way as for ordinal data. These methods were described in Section 4.2.3. Estimates for the binormal parameters a and b and their variance covariance matrix can be derived using a program such as ROCKIT, and substituted into equations (4.46)-(4.48). Similarly, either pointwise confidence intervals (4.49) or simultaneous confidence intervals can be determined such as in (4.50). This method, while relying on the parametric nature of the binormal curve, does not provide an estimate of the decision threshold corresponding to this sensitivity and specificity. When a threshold value is needed, other methods need to be used.

When a threshold value is used with a quantitative test, that means that clinically the quantitative variable is being used in a binary fashion. In particular, the results of the quantitative test are compared to a predetermined decision threshold. If the value is greater than the threshold, the patient is said to have the condition, else the patient is said to be free of the condition of interest. We consider the situation where there is a minimum value of specificity we must exceed, say SP, and we wish to choose a decision threshold to achieve this, along with the corresponding estimate of sensitivity.

Two approaches that have been proposed (Greenhouse and Mantel, 1950; Linnet, 1987) to choose the decision threshold corresponding to the target specificity, SP, are 1) use of the corresponding SP-quantile of the sample of test results from those without disease, or 2) the upper confidence limit for the unknown true SP-fractile of the distribution.

We begin with the former approach. The threshold of a continuous diagnostic test corresponding to a specificity SP is the SP-th quantile of the distribution of test results for people without the condition. We denote this by T_{SP}. That is, it is the test result T_{0i} such that there are no more than $n_0 SP$ test results smaller, and no more than $n_0(1 - SP)$ test results larger than T_{SP}. This threshold is estimated nonparametrically as $\widehat{T}_{SP}$ = the $n_0 SP$ ranked value from the sample of test results of those without the condition. The corresponding sensitivity can be estimated straightforwardly as the proportion of the test results from the sample of patients with the condition that exceed the estimated decision threshold $\widehat{T}_{SP}$. We write this formally as

$$\widehat{Se}(\widehat{T}_{SP}) = \frac{1}{n_1} \sum_{i=1}^{n_1} I_{[T_{1i} > \widehat{T}_{SP}]}, \tag{4.109}$$

where $I_{[T_{1i} > \widehat{T}_{SP}]}$ equals 1 if $T_{1i} > \widehat{T}_{SP}$ and is zero otherwise. The notation $\widehat{Se}(\widehat{T}_{SP})$ indicates that this sensitivity is associated with the estimated decision threshold $\widehat{T}_{SP}$. When it is understood, we may drop the parenthetic notation for simplicity.

In estimating the variance of this sensitivity, we might mistakenly treat the sensitivity as if it arose from truly binary data. In that case, the variance of the sensitivity would be estimated as $\widehat{Se}(1 - \widehat{Se})/n_1$. This would be true if the threshold, T_{SP}, were known without error. With quantitative rather than truly binary data, though, T_{SP} is unknown and must be estimated from the sample. This variance estimate based on binary data ignores the contribution of the estimated threshold to the variation of the sensitivity and thus is an underestimate.

An appropriate estimate of the variance must incorporate both sources of variability (Linnet, 1987). This estimate is

$$\widehat{Var}(\widehat{Se}) = \frac{\widehat{Se}(1 - \widehat{Se})}{n_1} + \widehat{\sigma}^2_{T_{SP}} \, \widehat{f}^2_1(\widehat{T}_{Sp}), \tag{4.110}$$

where f_1 is the density of the distribution of test results of those with disease and $\widehat{\sigma}^2_{T_{SP}}$ is the estimated asymptotic variance of the estimated quantile. This latter variance estimate is

$$\widehat{\sigma}^2_{T_{SP}} = \frac{SP\,(1 - SP)}{\widehat{f}_0^2(\widehat{T}_{SP})n_0}, \tag{4.111}$$

and $\widehat{f}_0$ and $\widehat{f}_1$ can be estimated as shown previously in (4.101)-(4.102), or more simply as

$$\widehat{f}_i(\widehat{T}_{SP}) = \frac{\#\text{ sample points in interval from } \widehat{T}_{SP} - r \text{ to } \widehat{T}_{SP} + r}{2rn_i} \tag{4.112}$$

for some value of r.

If both test distributions (or their transforms) are actually Gaussian, the quantile would actually be estimated as $\widehat{T}_{SP} = \bar{T}_0 + \widehat{\sigma}_0 z_{SP}$, where z_{SP} is the ordinate of the tail probability such that $\Phi(z_{SP}) = 1 - SP$, as defined in Section 4.2.2, $f_1 = \phi$, the normal density evaluated at the value, and the estimated variance of the quantile would be

$$\widehat{\sigma}^2_{T_{SP}} = \frac{\widehat{\sigma}_0^2}{n_0}\left(1 + \frac{z_{SP}^2}{2}\right). \tag{4.113}$$

Confidence intervals for the estimated sensitivity, based on asymptotic theory, can be constructed as in the equation (4.3), substituting the equation (4.111) or the equation (4.113) for the variance. Other methods provide intervals with better coverage. One alternative that has been suggested is a BCa bootstrap confidence interval presented by Platt et al. (2000). Zhou and Qin (2005) showed that this interval did not have coverage or length as good as a new bootstrap interval they suggested. Briefly, the confidence interval with the best performance was

$$\left(\bar{R}^*(SP) - z_{1-\alpha/2}\sqrt{V^*(SP)},\ \bar{R}^*(SP) + z_{1-\alpha/2}\sqrt{V^*(SP)}\right), \tag{4.114}$$

The variance was estimated by drawing bootstrap samples of the n_1 test results T_{1i}^* and n_0 test results T_{0i}^*, calculating

$$\tilde{R}^*(SP) = \frac{\sum_{i=1}^{n_1} I_{[T_{1i}^* \geq \widehat{F}_0^{-1*}(SP)]} + z_{1-\alpha/2}^2/2}{n_1 + z_{1-\alpha/2}^2}, \tag{4.115}$$

where $\widehat{F}_0^{-1*}(SP) = \widehat{T}_{SP}^*$ is the SP-th sample quantile based on bootstrap re-samples of T_{0j}. After B bootstrap replications ($B \geq 500$), the bootstrap variance estimate, $V^*(SP)$ is

$$V^*(SP) = \frac{1}{B-1}\sum_{b=1}^{B}(\tilde{R}^{*b}(SP) - \bar{R}^*(SP))^2, \tag{4.116}$$

where

$$\bar{R}^*(SP) = (1/B) \sum_{b=1}^{B} \tilde{R}^{*b}(SP). \tag{4.117}$$

Another approach to the problem of finding a threshold insures that the specificity is at least SP with a certain a priori probability. That is, we will choose a decision threshold that corresponds to the upper confidence limit of the true (but unknown) SP-th quantile of the distribution of test results for patients without the condition. We can then determine a lower confidence bound for the corresponding sensitivity. If we choose $\sqrt{1-\alpha}$ as the confidence level for each confidence limit, then we have a simultaneous probability of $1-\alpha$ that the true value of specificity at this cutoff value is at least the desired SP, and that true value of sensitivity is at least greater than the lower confidence bound for the estimated sensitivity.

The decision threshold is estimated as the upper one-sided confidence limit for T_{SP} (with confidence probability $\sqrt{1-\alpha}$)

$$c = \widehat{T}_{SP} + z_{\sqrt{1-\alpha}}\, \widehat{\sigma}_{T_{SP}}, \tag{4.118}$$

where $\widehat{\sigma}_{T_{SP}}$ is the square root of the variance as given in the equation (4.111) or Equation (4.113) above, depending on whether you take a nonparametric or parametric approach. For the sensitivity, we determine the lower $\sqrt{1-\alpha}$ confidence bound

$$Se_l(c) = Se(c) - z_{\sqrt{1-\alpha}}\sqrt{Se(c) \times (1 - Se(c))}/n_1. \tag{4.119}$$

Again, in the normal case, the upper confidence limit of the SP-th quantile, is

$$T_{SP} = \bar{T}_0 + \widehat{\sigma}_0 z_{SP} + z_{\sqrt{1-\alpha}}\, \widehat{\sigma}_{T_{SP}}, \tag{4.120}$$

and the estimate of the lower confidence bound of sensitivity is approximately

$$\Phi(Z - z_{\sqrt{1-\alpha}} s_Z), \tag{4.121}$$

where

$$Z = \frac{\bar{T}_1 - T_{Sp}}{\widehat{\sigma}_1} \quad \text{and} \quad s_Z = \sqrt{\frac{(1 + Z^2/2)\widehat{\sigma}_1^2}{n_1}}. \tag{4.122}$$

4.3.6.1 Sensitivity at a Particular FPR Value: Head Trauma Data

Referring to the head trauma example, we can determine the sensitivity corresponding to a specificity of 0.90 from the smooth binormal ROC curve. We have that

$$Se_{(FPR=0.1)} = \Phi(1.145 + 0.65\Phi^{-1}(0.1)) = \Phi(0.31) = 0.62.$$

But this estimate does not provide a threshold value. If we look at the CK-BB data for the 19 people with a good recovery, we see that 10.5% of the patients had a value greater than 253, and 5.2% had a value greater than 281.

Our threshold value is $T_{0.9} = 281$. Looking in turn at the patients with poor outcome of the head trauma, we have 23 of 41 or 56.1% have values greater than 281. Thus, our estimate of sensitivity corresponding to this threshold is 56.1%. To estimate the variance of this sensitivity estimate we need to estimate the variance of the decision threshold:

$$\widehat{\sigma}^2_{T_{SP}} = \frac{0.90 \times 0.10}{19 \times f_0^2(T_{SP})} = \frac{0.09}{19 \times 0.00263^2} = 684.8,$$

$$f_0(\widehat{T}_{SP}) = \frac{4}{2 \times 40 \times 19} = 0.00263, \text{ with } r = 40.$$

Then an estimate of the variance of estimated sensitivity is

$$\widehat{Var}(\widehat{Se}) = \frac{0.900 \times 0.10}{41} + 684.8 \times 0.00125^2 = 0.00220 + 0.00107 = 0.0032,$$

and

$$f_1(\widehat{T}_{SP}) = \frac{4}{2 \times 40 \times 41} = 0.00125, \text{ with } r = 40.$$

We can also determine a decision threshold such that we have a simultaneous probability of 95% that the true value of specificity at this cutoff value is at least the desired 0.90, and that the true value of sensitivity is at least greater than the lower confidence bound for the estimated sensitivity. The decision threshold in this case is approximated by

$$c = 281 + 1.954 \times s_{T_{SP}} = 281 + 1.954 \times 26.17 = 332.1.$$

The estimate of sensitivity at this decision threshold is $19/41 = 0.463$. Finally, the lower confidence bound for sensitivity is

$$0.464 - 1.954\sqrt{0.464 \times 0.536/41} = 0.312.$$

We can say with 95% confidence that the specificity is at least 0.90 and sensitivity is at least 0.312 for predicting poor outcome of head trauma using CK-BB when using the decision threshold 332.

4.3.7 Choosing the Optimal Operating Point and Decision Threshold

Investigators have examined the ROC curve and its summary parameters in order to assess the accuracy of CK-BB for predicting outcome of severe head trauma. They now would like to address the more practical issue of determining the threshold value of CK-BB to use in decision making. They don't have a particular specificity they are trying to achieve (as in the previous section), but rather want this threshold to give them the "best" set of sensitivity and specificity, realizing, of course, that there is a tradeoff between the two accuracy measures.

In Chapter 2 we considered the issue of choosing the "optimal" point on the ROC curve. One way of defining "optimal" is to minimize the "cost" of a decision. A decision can be thought of as a function of the (relative) costs of correct and incorrect decisions based on the threshold. We saw that the total cost of a decision (C) could be written as

$$
\begin{aligned}
C \;=\; & C_0 + P(T) \times C_{TP} + P(FP) \times C_{FP} \\
& + P(TN) \times C_{TN} + P(FN) \times C_F,
\end{aligned}
\tag{4.123}
$$

where C_0 is the cost of performing the test, C_{TP} is the cost of a true positive, C_{FP} is the cost of a false positive, C_{TN} is the cost of a true negative and C_{FN} is the cost of a false negative. This is sometimes referred to as Bayes cost. It is this total cost that we want to minimize when we choose a threshold.

It may not be obvious that the total cost is a function of the prevalence, as well as the costs of individual decisions. The equation (4.123) can be written to show explicitly the relationship of cost and prevalence, since $P(TP) = TPR \times p$, $P(FP) = FPR \times (1 - p)$, etc., where p is the prevalence of the condition of interest. We can rewrite

$$
\begin{aligned}
C \;=\; & C_0 + TPF \times p \times C_{TP} + FPR \times (1 - p) \times C_{FP} \\
& + (1 - FPR) \times (1 - p) \times C_{TN} + (1 - TPR) \times p \times C_{FN},
\end{aligned}
$$

or more succinctly as

$$
\begin{aligned}
C \;=\; & TPR \times p \times [C_{TP} - C_{FN}] + FPR \times (1 - p) \times [C_{FP} - C_{TN}] \\
& + C_0 + pC_{FN} + (1 - p)C_{TN}.
\end{aligned}
\tag{4.124}
$$

To find the minimum cost, we would differentiate C with respect to FPR and set the derivative equal to zero. When we do this, and then solve for the derivative of TPR with respect to FPR (which is the slope of the ROC curve), we find that the optimal point on the ROC curve is that point for which the slope (m) is

$$
m = \frac{(1 - p)}{p} \frac{(C_{FP} - C_{TN})}{(C_{FN} - C_{TP})} = \frac{1 - p}{p} R,
\tag{4.125}
$$

where $R = (C_{FP} - C_{TN})/(C_{FN} - C_{TP})$ is the ratio of the costs.

We can find this point on the ROC curve in a few different ways. If we have a smooth plot of the ROC curve, then the point at which a line with this slope just touches the curve (i.e., is tangent to the curve) is the optimal operating point. However, if we are using the empirical plot then the plot is actually a step function, and won't have a tangent, per se. The operating point can be found by taking a line with slope m through the point $(0,1)$ (i.e. the upper left hand corner of the unit square), and moving it toward the ROC curve until it first intersects the curve. The point at which this happens is the optimal operating point, and the threshold that generates that point is the optimal threshold (Zweig and Campbell, 1993).

If we assume binormality, then the optimal operating point can be determined by the following (Somoza and Mossman, 1991): for $b = 1$

$$FPR_{opt} = \Phi[-a/2 - ln(m)/a], \tag{4.126}$$

$$TPR_{opt} = \Phi[1/2 - ln(m)/a], \tag{4.127}$$

and for $b \neq 1$

$$FPR_{opt} = \Phi\{[ab - \sqrt{a^2 + 2(1 - b^2)ln(m/b)}\,]/(1 - b^2)\}, \tag{4.128}$$

$$TPR_{opt} = \Phi\{[a - b\sqrt{a^2 + (1 - b^2)ln(m/b)}]/(1 - b^2)\}. \tag{4.129}$$

We substitute estimates of a and b into the equations (4.126, 4.127) or (4.128,4.129). To relate the optimal (FPR, TPR) pair to the actual threshold, Somoza and Mossman (1991) suggested fitting a polynomial. An alternative, more in keeping with the binormality assumption is to recognize that since

$$FPR(c) = \Phi\left(\frac{\mu_0 - c}{\sigma_0}\right),$$

the optimal point can be written as

$$c_{opt} = \mu_0 - \sigma_0\Phi^{-1}(FPR_{opt}). \tag{4.130}$$

If the data are not binormal, a power transformation of the Box-Cox type ψ_λ can be used to transform the data to be binormal (as described in section 4.3.2). Using the means and variances of the transformed data, a threshold can be determined. The threshold in original units would be $\psi_\lambda^{-1}(c^*)$.

In current literature, the optimal decision threshold tends to appear in conjunction with the Youden index. Recall from Chapter 2 that the point that minimizes the overall rate of misclassification is the point c^* that maximizes the Youden Index:

$$J = max_c\{TPR(c) - FPR(c)\} = max_c\{F_0(c) - F_1(c)\}.$$

While the classic Youden Index does not take costs or prevalence into account, the Generalized Youden Index does:

$$J_G = max_c\{TPR(c) - mFPR(c))\}, \tag{4.131}$$

where m is as above.

Formulae for the optimal operating point and decision threshold corresponding to the Youden and Generalized Youden Index give results identical to that above (Halpern et al., 1996; Fluss et al., 2005; Skaltsa et al., 2010). Fluss et al. (2005) compared various estimation methods for the optimal decision threshold in terms of bias and root mean squared error. Methods compared included using the Box-Cox transformation to obtain binormality and then substituting into the above formulae, as well as a couple of non-parametric methods: estimating TPR and FPR with the empirical cumulative distribution functions and then finding the maximum over the observations, and a Kernel method which smooths the CDF estimates using the Gaussian kernel as suggested by Zou et al. (1998). Fluss et al. (2005) found that the Box-Cox transformation method was best with most distributions of the data; the kernel method also gave reasonable results. Schisterman and Perkins (2007) used the delta method to derive the variance and confidence interval for the optimal decision threshold under the binormality assumption when costs and prevalence were ignored (m=1). Jund et al. (2005) and Skaltsa et al. (2010) extended these results to include costs and prevalence.

We note again, as we did in Chapter 2, that a critical step in this process is to determine the costs, or at least the ratio of these costs. This is a very difficult task, and, as mentioned previously, a specialized field of study in medicine has grown up around this.

4.3.7.1 Optimal Point on the ROC Curve: Head Trauma Data

If we want to find the optimal point on the ROC curve of CK-BB for predicting poor outcome of severe head trauma, using the method of Somoza and Mossman (1991) we need to determine the inputs to the equation (4.123). In Section 4.3.2.1 we found that a Box-Cox transformation with $\widehat{\lambda} = 0.25$ made the CK-BB data seem to follow a normal distribution. Estimated binormal parameters were $\widehat{a} = 1.20$ and $\widehat{b} = 0.76$. Since it is so difficult to assess the costs of false positives and false negatives related to CK-BB, we might choose to look at the optimal point on the ROC curve for a range of possible values of R. This is sometimes referred to as a "sensitivity analysis," as it determines how sensitive the optimal point is to the choice of costs. The prevalence of bad outcomes in our study was 0.67. For such a prevalence, we find that the optimal point (FPR, TPR) ranges from $(0.19, 0.70)$ when the ratio of costs is $R = 2$ to $(0.38, 0.84)$ when the costs are equal, to $(0.69, 0.94)$ when $R = 0.5$. For smaller prevalence, the operating points occur on the lower part of the curve (See Table 4.12).

Table 4.12   Optimal Operating Points: Using the CK-BB Test to Predict Poor Outcomes of Severe Head Trauma as a Function of the Prevalence and Relative Costs

	Relative Costs (R)		
Prevalence (p)	0.5	1.0	2.0
0.20	(0.08, 0.55)	(0.03, 0.42)	(0.01, 0.31)
0.50	(0.38, 0.83)	(0.18, 0.70)	(0.08, 0.55)
0.67	(0.69, 0.94)	(0.38, 0.84)	(0.19, 0.70)

To find the value of CK-BB which correspond to an optimal point, we note that

$$c_{opt} = \mu_N - \sigma_N \Phi^{-1}(FPR_{opt}) = 8.28 - 2.96\Phi^{-1}(FPR_{opt}).$$

Then, for example, when prevalence is 0.67, $R = 2$ and the optimal point is (0.19, 0.70) we have that $c_{opt} = 10.93$. Since we transformed the data, this threshold is in transformed units. The threshold in original units would be calculated as

$$c_{opt-original} = (0.25 \times c_{opt-transf} + 1)^4 = (0.25 \times 10.93 + 1)^4 = 193.6.$$

If the prevalence of poor outcome for severe head trauma is as in our study example, and the ratio of costs is 2, then the optimal decision threshold for CK-BB is around 194, resulting in a FPR of 0.19 and a TPR of 0.70. In our sample of subjects with severe head trauma, 28 of the 41 subjects with poor outcome had CK-BB$\geq$194 ($\widehat{TPR} = 0.68$) and 5 of the 19 subjects with good outcome had similar high CK-BB values ($\widehat{FPR} = 0.26$).

4.3.8   Choosing between Parametric, Semi-parametric and Nonparametric Methods

Hajian-Tilaki et al. (1997) found that parametric and nonparametric methods produced very similar results for both the ROC curve area estimate and its variance, even when the data were not binormal. Faraggi and Reiser (2002) further compared a wider range of parametric and nonparametric methods to estimate the area under the ROC curve and found that, for non-normal data, the transformation and binning methods (Metz et al., 1998) were preferred unless the test results followed a strongly bimodal distribution. Qin and Hotiloac (2008) found that confidence interval coverage was adequate for the semi-parametric empirical likelihood method, as well as the non-parametric Mann-Whitney estimator as long as the logit transformation was used. Bootstrapping area estimates were shown to provide reasonable coverage in many instances, and could be applied to parametric, non-parametric and semi-parametric estimates of the ROC curve and the area. The implication of this research is that we can choose a method without being very concerned about binormality. Other issues including ease of use and practicality can then be used in choosing.

Parametric modeling, including the possibility of a Box-Cox transformation to normality may be the simplest method to use. It has the advantage of allowing smooth ROC curves to be constructed, area to be estimated and confidence intervals to be constructed. Semi-parametric methods may be the more difficult as far as computation is concerned. Once software becomes more available, this may be a more reasonable option. Parametric and semi-parametric methods also have an advantage over non-parametric methods when the addition of covariates is of interest (see Chapter 8).

Nonparametric estimates of the area do not require assumptions concerning the distribution of the data, which some people feel uncomfortable with, regardless of the current research to the contrary. Even most semi-parametric estimation methods make assumptions regarding the functional form of the ROC curve (the equation (4.102)) The area estimate is easy to calculate, and, in fact can be determined for any sample size without regard to the distribution of the operational points (i.e., degeneracy is not a problem when data are continuous). Estimation of the variance can be time consuming to do by hand, but software such as to implement the methods of DeLong et al. (1988) is becoming readily available. Issues with ordinal data regarding lack of smoothness of the ROC curve with parametric methods do not necessarily carry over to continuous data, since kernel methods are available.

These results, and hence suggestions above may not apply to partial areas. Dodd and Pepe (2003), comparing parametric and non-parametric methods when data do not follow a binormal model, found that the parametric models produced biased results, particularly when the range of false positives covered was very small. As the portion of the ROC curve increased the bias decreased, which is consistent with the findings of Hanley (1988) and Swets (1986b,a) that the binormal model is relatively robust for the full area under the ROC curve. Parametric methods provide estimates of smooth ROC curves. Software is widely available to estimate the parameters of the binormal curve and their variance-covariance matrix. With this, smooth ROC curves and summary measures can readily be estimated. The efficiency and robustness of semi-parametric methods for partial areas have not been evaluated and compared to parametric or non-parametric methods, although the comment above regarding lack of software still holds.

4.4   TESTING THE HYPOTHESIS THAT THE ROC CURVE AREA OR PARTIAL AREA IS A SPECIFIC VALUE

In some studies we are interested in testing whether or not the diagnostic test has any ability to discriminate between those with and without the condition of interest. A useless test that had no discrimination ability would have sensitivity=1-specificity. The ROC curve for such a test would be the $y = x$ line and would have area $A = 0.50$. The null and alternative hypotheses would be

$$H_0 : A = 0.50, \ H_1 : A \neq 0.50.$$

A test statistic would be

$$z = \frac{\widehat{A} - 0.5}{\sqrt{\widehat{Var}(\widehat{A})}}. \tag{4.132}$$

This would have approximately a standard normal distribution. If we are assuming binormality, then the estimate of the area and its variance would be substituted based on that assumption. Similarly, if the area is estimated nonparametrically, that estimate along with the appropriate standard error would be substituted into the equation.

In a similar manner, it could be determined whether a medical test has the ability to discriminate under a more limited range of false positive values. For any particular values of e_1 and e_2 the null and alternative hypotheses would be written as

$$H_0 : A_{(e_1 \leq FPR \leq e_2)} = A_{mn(e_1, e_2)},$$

$$H_1 : A_{(e_1 \leq FPR \leq e_2)} \neq A_{mn(e_1, e_2)}.$$

where $A_{mn(e_1, e_2)}$ is as given in the equation (4.60). A test statistic would be

$$Z = \frac{\widehat{A}_{(e_1 \leq FPR \leq e_2)} - A_{mn(e_1, e_2)}}{\sqrt{\widehat{Var}(\widehat{A}_{(e_1 \leq FPR \leq e_2)})}}. \tag{4.133}$$

which would have approximately a standard normal distribution.

More generally, we could test whether the total area or partial area had any specific hypothesized value A_0 using the test statistic

$$Z = \frac{\widehat{A}_{(e_1 \leq FPR \leq e_2)} - A_0}{\sqrt{\widehat{Var}(\widehat{A}_{(e_1 \leq FPR \leq e_2)})}}. \tag{4.134}$$

where $e_1 = 0$, $e_2 = 1$ if we are referring to the total area.

4.4.1   Testing Whether MRA has Any Ability to Detect Significant Carotid Stenosis

Referring back to the MRA example, we could test whether the MRA has any ability to distinguish between arteries with significant stenosis and those without. The test statistic is

$$Z = \frac{0.9297 - 0.50}{0.0213} = 20.2, \text{ with } p < 0.0001$$

which is highly statistically significant. Not surprisingly, since the ROC curve area is close to 1.0, we conclude that MRA has some discriminating ability. If we wish to determine whether the MRA has any discriminating ability in the more limited area where the false positive rates are less than 0.1, we can use equation (4.134)

$$Z = \frac{0.0672 - 0.005}{0.008392} = 7.41, \text{ with } p < 0.0001$$

which is also highly significant.

CHAPTER 5

COMPARING THE ACCURACY OF TWO DIAGNOSTIC TESTS

When we wish to compare the accuracy of two diagnostic tests, we often compare their summary measures of accuracy. The usual null hypothesis is that the summary measure of accuracy for the two diagnostic tests is the same. The alternative is that they are different. These hypotheses can be expressed formally as

$$H_0 : \theta_1 = \theta_2 \text{ vs } H_1 : \theta_1 \neq \theta_2,$$

where θ_i is the true summary measure of the ith diagnostic test and can represent sensitivity, specificity, area or partial area under the curve and so on. Note that these hypotheses as written are for a 2-sided test; a 1-sided test and alternative can also be expressed.

Hypotheses of this nature are usually assessed with the general test statistic:

$$Z = \frac{\widehat{\theta}_1 - \widehat{\theta}_2}{\sqrt{Var(\widehat{\theta}_1 - \widehat{\theta}_2)}}, \tag{5.1}$$

where the variance of the difference is

$$Var(\widehat{\theta}_1 - \widehat{\theta}_2) = Var(\widehat{\theta}_1) + Var(\widehat{\theta}_2) - 2Cov(\widehat{\theta}_1, \widehat{\theta}_2), \tag{5.2}$$

Statistical Methods in Diagnostic Medicine,
Second Edition. By Xiao-Hua Zhou, Nancy A. Obuchowski, Donna K. McClish
Copyright © 2011 John Wiley & Sons, Inc.

and $Cov(\widehat{\theta}_1, \widehat{\theta}_2)$ is the covariance between $\widehat{\theta}_1$ and $\widehat{\theta}_2$. This test statistic usually follows a normal distribution asymptotically (i.e., for large samples).

In Chapter 3 we learned that a study design can be paired or unpaired. Recall that in a paired design, all diagnostic tests are applied to the same set of patients. In an unpaired design, independent groups of patients each undergo a different test. The statistical analysis to compare two diagnostic tests must consider the design. In particular, if a paired design is used, then the accuracy measures for any tests will be correlated, resulting in a nonzero value for $Cov(\widehat{\theta}_1, \widehat{\theta}_2)$ in the equation (5.2). On the other hand, if an unpaired design is used (independent samples of patients), the covariance term will be zero. Failure to recognize the paired design (and to incorporate the covariance) will generally result in a variance estimate that is too large, making it less likely to reject the null hypothesis.

This chapter is devoted to methods for comparing the accuracy of diagnostic tests in two samples. These methods can be used to compare two different tests (with a single reader, if applicable), a single test with two readers, a single test with two patient subgroups, and so forth. Methods to compare the accuracy of more than two samples are discussed in Chapters 8 and 9. As in Chapter 4, results for binary-scale data (Section 5.1) are presented separately from ordinal- and continuous- scale data (Section 5.2). Parametric and nonparametric methods are presented for both paired and unpaired designs. Finally, even though the emphasis of the chapter is on how to test for accuracy differences, we briefly consider methods of judging the equivalence between two tests (Section 5.3).

5.1 BINARY-SCALE DATA

5.1.1 Sensitivity and Specificity

In Chapter 4 we analyzed rating data from Case Study 3 which looked at the use of MRA for detection of significant stenosis requiring surgery. Four different radiologists scored the MRAs of the left and right carotid arteries. We are interested in determining whether the sensitivity of MRA is consistent across radiologists.

Comparison of the sensitivity or specificity of two binary diagnostic tests estimated on independent (unpaired) samples is simply the comparison of two independent proportions. We test the null hypothesis that the two diagnostic tests are equal on this measure versus the alternative hypothesis that they are not. For example, for sensitivity the hypotheses are stated

$$H_0 : Se_1 = Se_2 \text{ vs } H_1 : Se_1 \neq Se_2$$

The data to estimate the sensitivity of two tests can be displayed as in Table 5.1. The notation is the same as in Chapter 4 except that the first

Table 5.1 Display of Unpaired Binary-Scale Data to Compare Sensitivity of Two Medical Tests (Subjects with the Condition)

	Positive Results	Negative Results	Total
Test 1	s_{11}	s_{10}	n_{11}
Test 2	s_{21}	s_{20}	n_{21}.

subscript indexes the medical test. For example s_{11} is the number of true positive (TP) test results for diagnostic test 1 in the first sample. The test statistic is

$$Z = \frac{\widehat{Se}_1 - \widehat{Se}_2}{\sqrt{Var(\widehat{Se}_1 - \widehat{Se}_2)}} \tag{5.3}$$

$$= \frac{\widehat{Se}_1 - \widehat{Se}_2}{\sqrt{\widehat{Se}_1(1 - \widehat{Se}_1)/n_{11} + \widehat{Se}_2(1 - \widehat{Se}_2)/n_{21}}}, \tag{5.4}$$

where n_{i1} is the number of subjects with the condition in the ith sample, $i = 1, 2$. This test statistic is normally distributed asymptotically. Comparing the specificity of two diagnostic tests is done in the same manner. For small sample sizes, the data in Table 5.1 should be compared using Fisher's exact test (Bradley, 1968), the calculation of which is rather labor-intensive. Most statistical packages include the test with their contingency-table analysis.

If the study design is paired, with the two diagnostic tests evaluated on the same set of patients, different methods will be needed. Instead, we use a test, known as McNemar's test, for dependent proportions. Suppose that we are interested in comparing the sensitivity of two tests. We look only at those who have the condition according to the gold standard, displaying data as in Table 5.2, on the right. Here m_{111} is the number of patients with the condition for whom both tests are positive, m_{100} is the number of patients for whom both tests are negative, m_{110} is the number of patients for whom test 2 is positive but test 1 is negative, and m_{101} is the number of patients for whom test 1 is positive but test 2 is negative. (A similar table to compare specificities would have entries m_{0ij}, marginal totals r_{ij} and total n_0). The estimate of sensitivity for each of the two diagnostic tests is $s_{i1}/n_1, i = 1, 2$. To test the hypothesis that the two sensitivities are equal, the test statistic is usually written in the following form:

$$X^2 = \frac{(m_{110} - m_{101})^2}{m_{110} + m_{101}}. \tag{5.5}$$

It has a chi-square distribution with one degree of freedom (asymptotically).

If the number of patients with differing test results is small ($m_{110} + m_{101} < 20$), using an exact test will be better. Such a test might be referred to as the sign test or binomial test, with a probability of $1/2$. Tables exist with p values for this test; otherwise p values can be computed as follows: Let $m = m_{110} + m_{101}$ (the number of test results that differ) and $k = \min(m_{110}, m_{101})$. For a 2-sided test, the p value can be calculated as

$$p = 2 \times \sum_{j=1}^{k} \binom{m}{j} \left(\frac{1}{2}\right)^m, \tag{5.6}$$

where

$$\binom{m}{j} = \frac{m!}{j!(m-j)!},$$

and

$$m! = m \times (m-1) \times \cdots \times 1.$$

Comparison of specificities in the paired sample design would proceed in a similar manner.

Table 5.2   Display of Paired Binary Data to Compare Sensitivity, Specificity and Predictive Values of Two Medical Tests

		NO DISEASE					DISEASE		
		Test 1					Test 1		
		$+$	$-$	Total			$+$	$-$	Total
Test 2	$+$	m_{011}	m_{010}	r_{21}	Test 2	$+$	m_{111}	m_{110}	s_{21}
	$-$	m_{001}	m_{000}	r_{20}		$-$	m_{101}	m_{100}	s_{20}
	Total	r_{11}	r_{10}	n_0		Total	s_{11}	s_{10}	n_1

5.1.1.1 Comparing Sensitivities: Case Study 3   In Chapter 4 we analyzed rating data from Case Study 3 which looked at the use of MRA for detection of significant stenosis requiring surgery. Four different radiologists scored the MRAs of the left and right carotid arteries from 1 (definitely no significant stenosis) to 5 (definite significant stenosis). For purposes of this example we will convert the data to binary, considering a positive diagnosis a score of 4 or 5. Looking at the data displayed in Table 4.6, $56(= 14 + 42)$ of the patients that were positive according to the gold standard were diagnosed as positive with MRA by radiologist 4. This is a sensitivity of 0.903. We can also consider the scores of radiologist 3. This radiologist diagnosed 50 of 62 as positive, for a sensitivity of 0.806. In order to determine if the sensitivity of the two radiologists is truly different, or the values just reflect chance variation, we create a table comparing results for all 62 patients that have significant carotid stenosis according to the gold standard (see Table 5.3, right). With $m_{101} = 7$ and $m_{110} = 1$, McNemar's test gives $X^2 = (7-1)^2/(7+1) = 4.5$. This exceeds the value of a Chi-Square with 1 degree of freedom (3.84), so we would conclude that the sensitivity of MRA interpreted by Radiologist 4 is significantly different (in fact higher) than that of Radiologist 3. But McNemar's test is not the most appropriate to use in this situation, as $m_{110} + m_{101} = 8 < 20$. Instead, the exact test should be used. Using the equation (5.6) above, with $m = m_{110} + m_{101} = 8$ and $k = min(m_{110}, m_{101}) = 1$ we have

$$p = 2 \times \sum_{j=1}^{1} \binom{8}{j}\left(\frac{1}{2}\right)^8 = 2 \times \binom{8}{1}\left(\frac{1}{2}\right)^8 = 0.0625.$$

If we are using a significance level of $\alpha = 0.05$, then we do not have quite enough evidence to conclude. Based on the exact test, that the sensitivities are different.

Table 5.3   Paired Test Results of Radiologists 3 and 4 for Using MRA to Detect Significant Carotid Stenosis

		No Significant Carotid Stenosis				Significant Carotid Stenosis		
		Rad4					Rad4		
		+	−	Total			+	−	Total
Rad3	+	12	7	19	Rad3	+	49	1	50
	−	11	71	82		−	7	5	12
	Total	23	78	101		Total	56	6	62

5.1.2 Sensitivity and Specificity of Clustered Binary Data

The concept of clustered data was introduced in Chapter 4. There we saw that when our data are clustered, both the variance and covariance of sensitivity and specificity differs from that of a simple proportion. However, with the correct estimates of variance and covariance, we can use equations (5.1) and (5.2) to test whether two sensitivities or two specificities are the same. For example, we can adapt the equation (4.22) to estimate the variance of the estimated sensitivity for each of the two diagnostic tests:

$$\widehat{Var}(\widehat{Se}_i) = \frac{1}{I_i(I_i - 1)} \sum_{j=1}^{I_i} \left(\frac{N_{ij}}{\bar{N}_i}\right)^2 (\widehat{Se}_{ij} - \widehat{Se}_i)^2, i = 1, 2, \qquad (5.7)$$

where $\widehat{Se}_{ij}$ is the estimate of the sensitivity for the ith diagnostic test in the jth cluster, N_{ij} is the number of elements in the jth cluster for the ith diagnostic test, and I_i and $\bar{N}_i$ are the numbers of clusters and mean cluster size for the ith diagnostic test.

Under the null hypothesis that the two sensitivities are equal, the covariance of the two estimated sensitivities can be estimated as

$$\widehat{Cov}\left(\widehat{Se}_1, \widehat{Se}_2\right) = \frac{1}{I(I-1)} \sum_{j=1}^{I} \left(\frac{N_j}{\bar{N}}\right)^2 (\widehat{Se}_{1j} - \overline{Se})(\widehat{Se}_{2j} - \overline{Se}), \qquad (5.8)$$

where $\overline{Se} = (\widehat{Se}_1 + \widehat{Se}_2)/2$ is the pooled estimate of sensitivity. For an unpaired design, the covariance is assumed to be zero, whereas for a paired design, the covariance term must be included in the equation (5.2) to properly estimate the variance of the difference of the two proportions estimated from clustered binary data. Note that for a paired design, the number of clusters, the cluster size and so forth, will be the same for both samples. Hence we have dropped the subscript for test in the equation (5.8). As mentioned in Chapter 4, another method to deal with clustered data would be to use a bootstrap method Rutter (2000). Bootstrapping would involve drawing subjects (clusters) with replacement. In a paired design, re-sampling at the cluster level would allow for simultaneous incorporation of within-cluster variability both within and between tests.

5.1.2.1 Comparing Sensitivities of Clustered Data: Case Study 2   In Chapter 4, Section 4.1.2.1 we estimated the sensitivity of CAD-enhanced computed tomography colonography (CTC) for detecting polyps in 39 polyps of 25 patients. Looking at Reader 1, we saw that the sensitivity was 0.8462 with variance 0.00428. We now wish to compare this sensitivity to that of CTC that has not been enhanced, for the same 25 patients (see Table 5.4).

The estimated sensitivity of CTC is $27/39 = 0.6923$, with variance 0.00658. The sensitivity of CAD-enhanced CTC appears to be superior, but we need to determine whether this difference is statistically significant. To do so, we need to determine the variance of the difference of these two sensitivities. As we already have the variance of each, we need only an estimate of the covariance. Using the equation (5.8) and the pooled sensitivity of $(0.6923 + 0.8462)/2 = 0.7693$, we calculate the estimate as $Cov(\widehat{Se}_1, \widehat{Se}_2) = 0.00387$. Then, using the equation (5.2), we estimate the variance of the difference as

$$Var(\widehat{Se}_1 - \widehat{Se}_2) = 0.00428 + 0.00658 - 2 \times 0.00387 = 0.00312.$$

Using the equation (5.2) our test statistic is

$$Z = \frac{0.8462 - 0.6923}{\sqrt{0.00312}} = 2.76.$$

The associated 2-sided p-value is 0.006. Because this value is less than $\alpha = 0.05$, we reject the null hypothesis and conclude that CAD-enhanced CTC has higher sensitivity to detect colon polyps.

Table 5.4 Computed Tomography Colonography (CTC) Without CAD Enhancement, for Detection of Colon Polyps with Reader 1

ID	No. of TN	No. of Glands	ID	No. of TN	No. of Glands
1	0	1	2	2	2
3	2	2	4	0	2
5	2	2	6	2	2
7	1	1	8	1	1
9	0	1	10	1	1
11	2	2	12	0	1
13	1	3	14	2	2
15	1	1	16	1	1
17	1	1	18	1	2
19	1	2	20	0	2
21	1	1	22	2	2
23	1	2	24	2	2
25	0	1			

5.1.3 Predictive Probability of a Positive or Negative

Since estimates of predictive values are a function of the prevalence of the condition in the sample, comparison of predictive values of two tests are best done when both tests are assessed on the same sample of subjects. Data from such a study would consist of two tables such as Table 5.2, one for those with the condition, and one for those without. It is interesting to note that while estimates of sensitivity and specificity require data from a single table, the predictive values, being dependent on the test result, rather than the condition, uses data from both tables. Subjects provide 0, 1 or 2 observations depending on whether they had (for estimate of PPV) a positive test on one, both or neither test. This complicates matters.

Leisenring et al. (2000) presented a score test to compare predictive values of diagnostic tests. In terms of the data in Table 5.2, the test statistic T_{PPV} can be written as the ratio of the following numerator and denominator:

$$\text{Numerator} = \{m_{111}(1 - 2\bar{Z}) + m_{110}(1 - \bar{Z}) + m_{101}(0 - \bar{Z})\}^2 \qquad (5.9)$$

$$\text{Denominator} = (1 - \bar{D})^2\{m_{111}(1 - 2\bar{Z})^2 + m_{110}(1 - \bar{Z})^2 + m_{101}(0 - \bar{Z})^2\}$$
$$+(0 - \bar{D})^2\{m_{011}(1 - 2\bar{Z})^2 + m_{010}(1 - \bar{Z})^2 + m_{001}(0 - \bar{Z})^2\},$$

where

$$\bar{Z} = \frac{m_{111} + m_{110} + m_{011} + m_{010}}{2m_{111} + m_{110} + m_{101} + 2m_{011} + m_{010} + m_{001}} \qquad (5.10)$$

is the proportion of all positive tests that were from Test 2, and

$$\bar{D} = \frac{2m_{111} + m_{110} + m_{101}}{2m_{111} + m_{110} + m_{101} + 2m_{011} + m_{010} + m_{001}} \qquad (5.11)$$

is the proportion of all positive tests that are from subjects with disease. This test statistic (T_{PPV}) follows a Chi-square distribution with 1 degree of freedom. A similar score test could be developed for NPV. Leisenring et al. (2000) also presented a more complicated test statistic that allowed for analysis of a clustered study design.

Moskowitz and Pepe (2006) offered an alternative test, considering the comparison of predictive values of paired data in terms of their ratio,

$$PPV_{X_1}/PPV_{X_2} \text{ or } NPV_{X_1}/NPV_{X_2},$$

which they referred to as relative predictive probabilities $(rPPV, rNPV)$. If these ratios are significantly different from 1 (or the logarithm of the ratio different from zero), then the predictive values of the two tests are significantly different. They found that the natural logarithm of the predictive value is asymptotically normally distributed. As with the odds ratio, this fact can be used to construct a test statistic to test whether $ln(rPPV)$ is significantly different from 0. The variance estimate for $ln(rPPV)$ is $\hat{\sigma}_P^2/(n_0 + n_1)$, where

$$
\begin{aligned}
\hat{\sigma}_P^2 &= \frac{n_1^2}{(m_{111} + m_{110})(m_{111} + m_{101})} \left\{ \frac{m_{101}}{n_1}(1 - \widehat{PPV}_2) \right. \quad (5.12) \\
&+ \frac{m_{111}}{n_1}(\widehat{PPV}_2 - \widehat{PPV}_1) + 2(\frac{m_{110}}{n_1} + \frac{m_{010}}{n_0})\widehat{PPV}_1 \times \widehat{PPV}_2 \\
&+ \left. \frac{m_{110}}{n_1}(1 - 3\widehat{PPV}_1) \right\}.
\end{aligned}
$$

The relative negative predictive probability $(rNPV)$ was defined similarly, and the variance estimate for $ln(rNPV)$ is $\hat{\sigma}_N^2/(n_0 + n_1)$, where

$$
\begin{aligned}
\hat{\sigma}_N^2 &= \frac{n_0^2}{(m_{001} + m_{000})(m_{010} + m_{000})} \left\{ \widehat{PPV}_2(-\frac{m_{010}}{n_0} + \frac{m_{000}}{n_0} - \right. \\
&\quad 2(\frac{m_{000}}{n_0} + \frac{m_{100}}{n_1})\widehat{NPV}_1) + (\frac{m_{001}}{n_0} + \frac{m_{010}}{n_0}) \\
&- \left. \widehat{NPV}_1(\frac{m_{001}}{n_0} - \frac{m_{000}}{n_0}) \right\}. \quad (5.13)
\end{aligned}
$$

Finally, both Moskowitz and Pepe (2006), and Leisenring et al. (2000) indicated that generalized estimating equations methods could be used to compare predictive values of diagnostic tests, using the following models:

$$g[P(D = 1|Z, X = 1)] = \alpha_P + \beta_P Z \quad (5.14)$$

$$g[P(D = 1|Z, X = 0)] = \alpha_N + \beta_N Z, \quad (5.15)$$

where g is the link function. For this analysis, data would be arrayed separately for each test result, and the added variable Z an indicator of the corresponding test type (where $Z = 1$ for test 1 and 0 for test 2 and X represents the test result). Analysis for (5.14) uses only observations with test positive test results while (5.15) uses observations with negative test results. The null hypothesis $H_0 : \beta_P = 0$ tests for differences between diagnostic tests. Leisenring et al. (2000) used a logit link, while Moskowitz and Pepe (2006) pointed out that if the natural log link is used instead, $e^{\hat{\beta}_P}$ estimates the relative positive predictive value.

5.1.3.1 Comparing PPV's: Case Study 3

We continue the analysis of Case Study 3 started in Section 5.1.1.1, looking at the use of MRA to diagnose significant carotid stenosis. Table 5.3 has data necessary to estimate predictive values of a positive for both radiologist 3 and 4. In particular, $PPV_3 = 50/69 = 0.7246$ and $PPV_4 = 56/79 = 0.7089$. While it is unlikely that these two are significantly different (and clinically, such a difference would not be important), we will compare them to illustrate the methods above. Using Leisenring et al. (2000) methods, we first calculate $\bar{Z}$ and $\bar{D}$ as $\bar{Z} = (49 + 1 + 12 + 7)/(24 + 7 + 11 + 98 + 1 + 7) = 69/148 = 0.4662$ and $\bar{D} = (98 + 1 + 7)/(24 + 7 + 11 + 98 + 1 + 7) = 106/148 = 0.7162$. Then

$$\text{Numerator} = [49 \times (1 - 2\bar{Z}) + 1 \times (1 - \bar{Z}) + 7 \times (0 - \bar{Z})]^2 = [0.5828]^2 = 0.3397,$$

and

$$\text{Denominator} = (1 - \bar{D})^2 \{49 * (1 - 2\bar{Z})^2 + 1 \times (1 - \bar{Z})^2 + 7 \times (0 - \bar{Z})^2\}$$

$$+ (0 - \bar{D})^2 \{12 * (1 - 2\bar{Z})^2 + 7 \times (1 - \bar{Z})^2 + 11 \times (0 - \bar{Z})^2\} = 2.4411.$$

The test statistic is $T_{PPV} = 0.3397/2.4411 = 0.139$. T_{PPV} is distributed as a Chi Square with 1 degree of freedom. The p-value associated with the test statistic is 0.71, which confirms that we do not have evidence that the predictive values are different.

We can also approach the question of the equality of the predictive values by looking at their ratio, $r\widehat{PPV} = PPV_3/PPV_4 = 1.02215$. We can calculate the variance of the natural logarithm of the ratio as

$$\hat{\sigma}_P^2 = \frac{62^2}{(49 + 1)(49 + 7)} \left\{ \frac{7}{62}(1 - \widehat{PPV}_3) + \frac{49}{62}(\widehat{PPV}_4 - \widehat{PPV}_3) \right.$$

$$\left. + 2(\frac{1}{62} + \frac{7}{101})\widehat{PPV}_3 \times \widehat{PPV}_4 + \frac{1}{62(1 - 3\widehat{PPV}_3)} \right\} = 384.45.$$

Then the test statistic is

$$\frac{\ln(1.02215)}{\sqrt{384.45/(101 + 62)}} = 0.014.$$

The p-value is 0.99. The conclusion agrees with that of Leisenring et al. (2000).

5.2   ORDINAL- AND CONTINUOUS-SCALE DATA

In Chapter 4, we examined the usefulness of CK-BB enzyme, a continuous variable, to predict the prognosis of patients with severe head trauma. We now want to know whether the predictive ability varies according to patient age. In particular, we suspect that CK-BB may be a better predictor in patients 20 years of age or older.

Also, in Chapter 4, we examined data from Case Study 3, regarding the usefulness of MRA to detect significant carotid stenosis. Our dataset had scores from 4 different radiologists whose performance could be compared. In fact, in Section 5.1.1.2 we considered the data as binary. More appropriately, we can evaluate and compare the accuracy using the full ordinal scores.

We saw from Chapter 4 that with ordinal- and continuous-scale data, the accuracy measures of interest are based on the ROC curve. The following are three primary approaches to comparing two ROC curves:

1. Determine whether two ROC curves are exactly the same. In doing so, we are interested in knowing whether the true-positive rates ($TPRs$) are the same for every false-positive rate (FPR). In terms of the binormal model, this is a test of whether the binormal parameters a_i and b_i are equal for the two ROC curves. In other words, we want to test the hypotheses:

$$H_0 : a_1 = a_2 \text{ and } b_1 = b_2 \text{ vs } H_1 : a_1 \neq a_2 \text{ or } b_1 \neq b_2.$$

2. Determine whether the two ROC curves agree at a particular $FPR = e$; that is

$$H_0 : Se_1(e) = Se_2(e) \text{ vs } H_1 : Se_1(e) \neq Se_2(e), 0 < e < 1.$$

3. Determine whether the areas (or partial areas) under the two ROC curves are the same:

$$H_0 : A_{(e_1 \leq FPR_1 \leq e_2)} = A_{(e_1 \leq FPR_2 \leq e_2)} \text{ vs } H_1 : A_{(e_1 \leq FPR_1 \leq e_2)} \neq A_{(e_1 \leq FPR_2 \leq e_2)}.$$

Note that approaches 1 and 3 do not test the same null hypothesis. Of course, if the two ROC curves are exactly the same, then the areas and partial areas will also be the same. On the other hand, two ROC curves may have different shapes but the same area (or partial area) under the curve. For example, suppose that $a_1 = 1.9101, b_1 = 1.0$ and $a_2 = 0.941, b_2 = 0.5$. Then

$$A_1 = \Phi(1.1901/\sqrt{1+1}) = \Phi(0.8417) = 0.80,$$

and

$$A_2 = \Phi(0.941/\sqrt{1+0.5^2}) = \Phi(0.8417) = 0.80.$$

In fact, if two ROC curves cross, one diagnostic test may be superior for some sets of $FPRs$, and inferior for others, even though the full areas may be similar. Note also that when we compare ROC curves in terms of total areas of the entire curve, we make global assessments, considering curves over the entire range of FPRs and TPRs, whereas when we compare the curve at a specific FPR, we focus on the opposite extreme: only one point on the curve. Comparing partial areas provides a middle ground.

5.2.1   Testing the Equality of Two ROC Curves

Because the binormal ROC curve can be described by parameters a and b, a test for the equality of the two curves under the binormal assumption is a test of the equality of the two sets of parameters. Thus, we have a statistical test of the composite hypothesis:

$$H_0 : a_1 = a_2 \text{ and } b_1 = b_2 \text{ vs } H_1 : a_1 \neq a_2 \text{ or } b_1 \neq b_2.$$

As described in Chapter 4, the binormal parameters a and b are usually estimated via parametric or semi-parametric methods related to maximum likelihood (sometimes pseudo- profile or quasi-likelihood methods are used). The estimates of the two parameters are asymptotically normally distributed, and the pair, which are generally correlated, follow a bivariate-normal distribution. To determine whether two binormal ROC curves are identical, we compare the two pairs of parameter estimates $(\widehat{a}_1, \widehat{b}_1)$ and $(\widehat{a}_2, \widehat{b}_2)$, using the test statistic presented by Metz and Kronman (1980) and Metz et al. (1984):

$$X^2 = \frac{\widehat{a}_{12}^2 Var(\widehat{b}_{12}) + \widehat{b}_{12}^2 Var(\widehat{a}_{12}) - 2\widehat{a}_{12}\widehat{b}_{12}Cov(\widehat{a}_{12}, \widehat{b}_{12})}{Var(\widehat{a}_{12})Var(\widehat{b}_{12}) - [Cov(\widehat{a}_{12}, \widehat{b}_{12})]^2}, \tag{5.16}$$

where we write $a_{12} = a_1 - a_2$ and $b_{12} = b_1 - b_2$ for the differences between the parameters. If the diagnostic tests are assessed on independent samples of patients, the foregoing variances and covariance may be estimated as

$$\widehat{Var}(\widehat{a}_{12}) = \widehat{\sigma}_{a_1}^2 + \widehat{\sigma}_{a_2}^2, \tag{5.17}$$

$$\widehat{Var}(\widehat{b}_{12}) = \widehat{\sigma}_{b_1}^2 + \widehat{\sigma}_{b_2}^2, \tag{5.18}$$

$$\text{and } \widehat{Cov}(\widehat{a}_{12}, \widehat{b}_{12}) = \widehat{\sigma}_{a_1 b_1} + \widehat{\sigma}_{a_2 b_2}, \tag{5.19}$$

respectively, where $\widehat{\sigma}_{a_i}^2$ is the estimated variance of $\widehat{a}_i$, $\widehat{\sigma}_{b_i}^2$ is the estimated variance of $\widehat{b}_i$, and $\widehat{\sigma}_{a_i b_i}$ is the estimated covariance of $\widehat{a}_i$ and $\widehat{b}_i$.

If the design of the study is paired, the dependence of the samples will be incorporated into the variances of the estimated differences $\widehat{a}_{12}$ and $\widehat{b}_{12}$. Each variance includes a covariance component:

$$\widehat{Var}(\widehat{a}_{12}) = \widehat{\sigma}_{a_1}^2 + \widehat{\sigma}_{a_2}^2 - 2\widehat{\sigma}_{a_1 a_2}, \tag{5.20}$$

$$\widehat{Var}(\widehat{b}_{12}) = \widehat{\sigma}_{b_1}^2 + \widehat{\sigma}_{b_2}^2 - 2\widehat{\sigma}_{b_1 b_2}, \tag{5.21}$$

and

$$\widehat{Cov}(\widehat{a}_{12}, \widehat{b}_{12}) = \widehat{\sigma}_{a_1 b_1} + \widehat{\sigma}_{a_2 b_2} - \widehat{\sigma}_{a_1 b_2} - \widehat{\sigma}_{a_2 b_1}. \tag{5.22}$$

Under the null hypothesis of equality of the binormal parameters, the test statistic asymptotically follows a chi-square distribution with two degrees of freedom for both paired and unpaired designs. Estimates of parameters, variances and covariances obtained from parametric or semi-parametric methods described in Chapter 4, Subsection 4.3.2 can be used in equations (5.16) - (5.22). Metz et al. (1984) performed a simulation to assess the performance of the statistical test in small samples. A brief summary is that for Type I error α in the range $0 < \alpha < 0.1$ and $m = 50$ pairs of cases, the test was conservative (i.e., the actual Type I error was less than α), although not greatly so. In the worst case considered, the actually Type I error was 0.03 when the target was 0.05. For larger m the Type I error was at the nominal level.

Venkatraman and Begg (1996) and Venkatraman (2000) proposed alternative methods to assess the equality of two ROC curves that do not require the binormality assumption. The methods, both based on permutation tests, varied slightly, depending on whether the samples were independent or dependent (paired). In general, however, the methods were based on a test statistic that was proportional to the unsigned area or difference between the two ROC curves. A permutation-reference distribution was generated to test that the difference was zero; that is, that the two curves were the same at all operating points.

Regression methods, as discussed in detail in Chapters 8 (independent samples) and 9 (dependent samples) can be used to compare ROC curves by including a covariate that is an indicator of test modality.

5.2.1.1 Comparing ROC Curves: Head Trauma Data   We are interested in determining whether the ROC curves are identical for the CK-BB test used for predicting a poor outcome of head trauma in younger and older patients. (The data are displayed in Chapter 4, Table 4.9). Using ROCKIT, we estimate the parameters as displayed in Table 5.5. We need to estimate a_{12} and b_{12} as well as their variances and covariances. We have $\hat{a}_{12} = 2.7378 - 0.8443 = 1.8935$ and $\hat{b}_{12} = 1.6307 - 0.6275 = 1.0032$. Since we are comparing independent samples (younger and older patients) we use equations (5.17)-(5.19) to estimate the variances and covariances; then $\widehat{Var}(\hat{a}_{12}) = 1.7061 + 0.1340 = 1.8401$, $\widehat{Var}(\hat{b}_{12}) = 1.5863 + 0.0624 = 1.6487$; $\widehat{Cov}(\hat{a}_{12}, \hat{b}_{12}) = 1.1290 + 0.0375 = 1.1665$. The test statistic can be calculated as

$$X^2 = \frac{1.8935^2 \times 1.6487 + 1.0032^2 \times 1.8401 - 2 \times 1.8935 \times 1.0032 \times 1.1665}{1.8401 \times 1.6487 - 1.1665^2}$$

$$= 1.99.$$

The critical value for a Chi-square distribution with 2 degrees of freedom and a Type I error of $\alpha = 0.05$ is 5.99. Thus we do not reject the null hypothesis. There is insufficient evidence to conclude that the ROC curves differ for the older and younger head trauma patients. To some, this results may seem surprising; the small sample size may be responsible for the lack of sufficient evidence.

Table 5.5   Parameter Estimates, Variances and Covariances for CK-BB Enzyme Data for Younger and Older Head Trauma Patients

	Younger	Older
$\widehat{a}_i$	2.7378	0.8443
$\widehat{b}_i$	1.6307	0.6275
$\widehat{Var}(\widehat{a}_i)$	1.7061	0.1340
$\widehat{Var}(\widehat{b}_i)$	1.5863	0.0624
$\widehat{Cov}(a_i, b_i)$	1.1290	0.0375

We are also interested in determining whether the ROC curves for MRA to detect significant carotid stenosis is the same for different radiologists. Data from the MRA study for radiologists 3 and 4 are displayed in Table 5.6, in such a way that the dependence of the two ratings are noted. Using ROCKIT, the estimates of binormal parameters for radiologist 3 are $\widehat{a}_3 = 1.3548$, $\widehat{b}_3 = 0.5170$, and for radiologist 4 they are $\widehat{a}_4 = 1.9372$, $\widehat{b}_4 = 0.8500$. The estimated variance covariance matrix for these parameters is in Table 5.7. We note that the parameter estimates for radiologist 4 are slightly different from those shown in Chapter 4, because ROCKIT simultaneously estimates parameters for both radiologists. We can compute $\widehat{a}_{34} = -0.5824$, $\widehat{b}_{34} = -0.3333$. Using the estimated variance-covariance matrix in Table 5.7, the necessary variances estimates are $\widehat{Var}(\widehat{a}_{34}) = 0.0801 + 0.0898 - 2 \times 0.0348 = 0.1003$; $\widehat{Var}(\widehat{b}_{34}) = 0.0529 + 0.0409 - 2 \times 0.0082 = 0.0774$; and $\widehat{Cov}(\widehat{a}_{34}, \widehat{b}_{34}) = 0.0495 + 0.0443 - 0.0092 - 0.0111 = 0.0735$. The test statistic is

$$X^2 =$$

$$\frac{(-0.5824)^2 \times 0.1003 + (-0.3330)^2 \times 0.0774 - 2 \times 0.5824 \times 0.3330 \times 0.0735}{0.1003 \times 0.0774 - 0.0735^2}$$

$$= 5.97.$$

The test statistic has a p-value of 0.0505, which is not quite less than 0.05. With a strict interpretation of the Type I error, the two ROC curves would not be considered significantly different, but this conclusion may be open to interpretation.

5.2.2   Comparing ROC Curves at a Particular Point

The opposite extreme to comparing two ROC curves at every point is to compare the curves at a specific point along the curve. It is easy to compare two ROC curves at a specific point along the curve. Since the sensitivities for a particular FPR can be written as $Se_i = \Phi(a_i + b_i \Phi^{-1}(FPR))$, a comparison

Table 5.6   Paired Test Results for MRA Detection of Significant Carotid Stenosis

| | No Significant Carotid Stenosis | | | | | | | Significant Carotid Stenosis | | | | | |
| | Radiologist 4 | | | | | | | Radiologist 4 | | | | | |
Rad 3	1	2	3	4	5	Total	Rad 3	1	2	3	4	5	Total
1	36	20	8	6	0	70	1	1	2	2	2	1	8
2	0	3	3	1	0	7	2	0	0	0	0	2	2
3	0	1	0	4	0	5	3	0	0	0	2	0	2
4	0	0	2	3	2	7	4	0	0	0	2	0	2
5	2	1	2	5	2	12	5	0	0	1	8	39	48
Total	38	25	15	19	4	101	Total	1	2	3	14	42	62

Table 5.7   Variance Covariance Matrix of Parameter Estimates for MRA Example

	a_3	b_3	a_4	b_4
a_3	0.0801			
b_3	0.0495	0.0529		
a_4	0.0348	0.0111	0.0898	
b_4	0.0092	0.0082	0.0443	0.0409

at the point $FPR = e$ involves the difference

$$D(e) = (a_1 + b_1\Phi^{-1}(e)) - (a_2 + b_2\Phi^{-1}(e)) = a_{12} + b_{12}\Phi^{-1}(e). \quad (5.23)$$

The variance of the estimated difference is

$$Var[\widehat{D}(e)] = Var(\widehat{a}_{12}) + [\Phi^{-1}(e)]^2 Var(\widehat{b}_{12}) + 2\Phi^{-1}(e)Cov(\widehat{a}_{12}, \widehat{b}_{12}), \quad (5.24)$$

where $Var(\widehat{a}_{12})$, $Var(\widehat{b}_{12})$, and $Cov(\widehat{a}_{12}, \widehat{b}_{12})$ can be estimated as in equations (5.17)-(5.19) for unpaired data or (5.20)-(5.22) for paired data.

If $\widehat{a}_i$ and $\widehat{b}_i$ are MLEs, then the difference, $D(e)$, should asymptotically have a normal distribution. Thus we can test for differences between the TPRs at $FPR = e$ by testing the hypothesis $H_0 : D(e) = 0$ vs $H_1 : D(e) \neq 0$ by using the test statistic

$$Z = \frac{\widehat{D}(e)}{\sqrt{Var[\widehat{D}(e)]}}. \quad (5.25)$$

If this ratio is large, it is unlikely that the TPRs will be the same at this particular FPR. In fact, this test statistic should follow a standard normal distribution, so the value of the ratio can be compared to an appropriate critical value of the normal distribution.

A comparison of two sensitivities when a decision threshold has been estimated from ordinal- or continuous-scale data proceeds a bit differently. The estimation of the sensitivity and the corresponding variance for a single test in such a situation was discussed in Chapter 4, Subsection 4.3.6. The test statistic will be, according to the equation (5.1)

$$Z = \frac{\widehat{Se}(\widehat{T}_{1Sp}) - \widehat{Se}(\widehat{T}_{2Sp})}{\sqrt{\widehat{Se}(\widehat{T}_{1Sp}) - \widehat{Se}(\widehat{T}_{2Sp})}}, \quad (5.26)$$

which follows a normal distribution asymptotically. If the two sensitivities we wish to compare are from independent samples, the denominator will be simply the square root of the sum of the variances for each of the two diagnostic tests. The equation (4.109) can be used to estimate the sensitivity; equations (4.110)-(4.113) or the bootstrap method can be used to estimate the variance for each sample. The validity of the above methods relies on the normal assumption of the test statistics. Qin and Zhou (2006) proposed nonparametric bootstrap-based intervals for the difference between sensitivities of two diagnostic tests at a fixed value of specificity.

If the samples are dependent (paired), however, the variance in the denominator must incorporate the dependence between the samples. Linnet (1987) provided the following nonparametric estimate of the variance of the difference:

$$
Var[\widehat{Se}(\widehat{T}_{1Sp}) - \widehat{Se}(\widehat{T}_{2Sp})] = \frac{m_{110} + m_{101}}{n_1^2} + \frac{Sp(1-Sp)}{n_0}\left\{\left(\frac{\widehat{f}_1(\widehat{T}_{1Sp})}{\widehat{f}_0(\widehat{T}_{1Sp})}\right)^2\right.
$$

$$
\left.+\left(\frac{\widehat{f}_1(\widehat{T}_{2Sp})}{\widehat{f}_0(\widehat{T}_{2Sp})}\right)^2\right\} - \frac{2\widehat{f}_1(\widehat{T}_{1Sp})\widehat{f}_1(\widehat{T}_{2Sp})}{n_0\widehat{f}_0(\widehat{T}_{1Sp})\widehat{f}_0(\widehat{T}_{2Sp})}\left\{\frac{m_{111}}{n_0} - (1-Sp)^2\right\}, \qquad (5.27)
$$

where $\widehat{f}_i$ is the estimated probability density of the distribution at the decision threshold, as in the equation (4.112); n_0 and n_1 are the number of patients without and with the condition respectively, and m_{1ij} are as in Table 5.2.

5.2.2.1 Comparing ROC Curves at a Particular Point: Head Trauma Data

Looking at the head trauma data, if we ignore the fact that the two ROC curves may be identical, we can compare the sensitivity at a FPR of 0.10. At that FPR, the sensitivity for the younger patients is estimated to be 0.5160; for the older patients, 0.7414. We can compare these two sensitivities statistically. We have $\Phi^{-1}(0.1) = -1.28$; thus $\widehat{D} = 1.8935 + 1.0032 \times (-1.28) = 0.6094$. The variance is

$$
\widehat{Var}[\widehat{D}(0.1)] = 1.8401 + (-1.28)^2 \times 1.6487 + 2 \times (-1.28) \times 1.1665 = 1.555.
$$

The test statistic is

$$
\frac{0.6094}{\sqrt{1.555}} = 0.4887,
$$

which is not greater than the critical value of the normal distribution (1.96); we do not reject the null hypothesis. We cannot reject the possibility that the sensitivity at a FPR of 0.10 is the same for both age groups.

5.2.3 Determining the Range of FPRs for which TPRs Differ

Suppose that we are interested in comparing the TPRs for two tests and that we have performed a global test of the equality of the two ROC curves according to the method of Metz and colleagues (Metz and Kronman, 1980; Metz et al., 1984), as described in Subsection 5.2.1. If we reject the null hypothesis that the two ROC curves are identical, we still would want to consider the relative merits of the two medical tests other than that they do not produce identical ROC curves. We recognize that the results of this test do not imply that the TPRs show a statistically significant difference for every FPR (i.e., at every point along the curve). In fact, we can actually determine if there exists a range of FPRs for which the two curves differ and another range for which they do not differ significantly (McClish, 1990) .

We derive both ranges as follows: Because the difference between TPRs can be assessed with $D(e) = a_{12} + b_{12}\Phi^{-1}(e)$ as in the equation (5.23), we can determine for which value of e the difference $D(e)$ is statistically different from zero. One way of doing this is to construct a simultaneous confidence interval around $D(e)$ and determine where the confidence interval includes zero and where it does not. For any particular point e, when the confidence interval does not contain zero, we can say with $100(1 - \alpha)\%$ confidence that $D(e) \neq 0$ (i.e., that the $TPRs$ are significantly different). The locus of all such points e gives us the set of $FPRs$ for which the two ROC curves (i.e., $TPRs$) differ.

The simultaneous $100(1 - \alpha)\%$ confidence interval has the following form:

$$\widehat{D}(e) \pm K\sqrt{Var[\widehat{D}(e)]}, \tag{5.28}$$

where we set $K = \sqrt{2F_{2,N-4,\alpha}}$; F is the critical value for the upper $\alpha\%$ of the F distribution with 2 and $N - 4$ degrees of freedom, and N is the total sample size.

At any point e, the confidence interval does not include zero if the lower bound is greater than zero; that is if

$$\widehat{D}(e) - K\sqrt{Var[\widehat{D}(e)]} > 0 \tag{5.29}$$

or if the upper bound is less than zero; that is

$$\widehat{D}(e) + K\sqrt{Var[\widehat{D}(e)]} < 0. \tag{5.30}$$

We can write the condition for the confidence bands to not include zero more succinctly because this condition occurs when

$$[\widehat{D}(e)]^2 - K^2 Var[\widehat{D}(e)] > 0. \tag{5.31}$$

Substituting for $\widehat{D}$ and doing some algebraic manipulations, we have that the confidence interval will exclude zero whenever

$$(\widehat{b}_{12}^2 - K^2\widehat{V}_{b12})[\Phi^{-1}(e)]^2 + 2(\widehat{a}_{12}\widehat{b}_{12} - K^2\widehat{C}_{12})\Phi^{-1}(e) + (\widehat{a}_{12}^2 - K^2\widehat{V}_{a12}) > 0$$

where for convenience we write $\widehat{V}_{a12} = \widehat{Var}(\widehat{a}_{12}), \widehat{V}_{b12} = \widehat{Var}(\widehat{b}_{12})$ and $\widehat{C}_{12} = \widehat{Cov}(\widehat{a}_{12}, \widehat{b}_{12})$.

Thus we can determine the appropriate set of $FPRs$ by finding the two values for which $\Phi^{-1}(e)$ is actually zero, which provide the boundaries of the regions of interest

$$\Phi^{-1}(e) = \frac{K^2\widehat{C}_{12} - \widehat{a}_{12}\widehat{b}_{12}}{\widehat{b}_{12}^2 - K^2\widehat{V}_{b12}}$$

$$\pm \frac{\sqrt{(\widehat{a}_{12}\widehat{b}_{12} - K^2\widehat{C}_{12})^2 - (\widehat{b}_{12}^2 - K^2\widehat{V}_{b12})(\widehat{a}_{12}^2 - K^2\widehat{V}_{a12})}}{\widehat{b}_{12}^2 - K^2\widehat{V}_{b12}}. \tag{5.32}$$

We denote these two roots as $\Phi^{-1}(e_L^*)$ and $\Phi^{-1}(e_U^*)$. We can make the following observations.

1. If $\widehat{b}_{12}^2 - K^2\widehat{V}_{b12} > 0$, the two ROC curves will be different for $\Phi^{-1}(e) < \Phi^{-1}(e_L^*)$ and for $\Phi^{-1}(e) > \Phi^{-1}(e_U^*)$. In the original metric, the two ROC curves are different for $FPR < e_L^*$ and for $FPR > e_U^*$.

2. If $\widehat{b}_{12}^2 - K^2\widehat{V}_{b12} < 0$, the two ROC curves will be different between $\Phi^{-1}(e_L^*)$ and $\Phi^{-1}(e_U^*)$. In the original metric, the curves are different for $e_L^* < FPR < e_U^*$.

If the quantity under the square root sign is negative, that is,

$$(\widehat{a}_{12}\widehat{b}_{12} - K\widehat{C}_{12})^2 - (\widehat{b}_{12}^2 - K^2\widehat{V}_{b12})(\widehat{a}_{12}^2 - K^2\widehat{V}_{a12}) < 0,$$

there will be no real roots. If $\widehat{b}_{12}^2 - K^2\widehat{V}_{b12} < 0$, the region of significance will be the null set, and the TPRs will be similar for all FPRs. But if $\widehat{b}_{12}^2 - K^2\widehat{V}_{b12} > 0$, the region of significance will be all FPRs (i.e., the entire curve).

5.2.3.1 *Estimating Portions of the ROC Curves that Differ: Head Trauma Data and Cancer Biomarkers* Considering the head trauma example again, we have already determined that the ROC curves for the older and younger patients do not differ significantly, so it does not make sense for us to look for a range of FPRs where the two curves differ. In fact, if we look at the value under the square root, we find that it is negative (-45.8); hence there will be no real roots. Checking the value $\widehat{b}_{12}^2 - K^2\widehat{V}_{b12}$, we see that it is negative (-9.4), which verifies that the region of significance is the null set.

As another example, we consider data from a study of the relative accuracy of two biomarkers for pancreatic cancer: CA 125 and CA19-9 (Wieand et al., 1989). These data are described in Chapter 8 and appear in Table 8.1.2. Assuming binormality, we find that the area under the ROC curve for CA19-9 is 0.8627 and for CA125 is 0.70441. These two areas are significantly different. Using the methods above, we find that $\Phi^{-1}(e_L^*) = 0.3089, (e_L^* = 0.62)$ and $\Phi^{-1}(e_U^*) = 1.706, (e_U^* = 0.956)$. Since $\widehat{b}_{12}^2 - K^2\widehat{V}_{b12} = 0.36 > 0, TPR$s will be higher for CA19-9 as compared to CA125 when FPRs are less than 0.62 or very close to 1 (technically, when FPRs are greater than 0.95).

5.2.4 Comparison of the Area or Partial Area

For independent samples, if we assume binormality, the areas or partial areas under the two ROC curves can be easily compared using the equation (5.1), substituting the estimates of areas and partial areas and their variances as presented in Chapter 4 (the equation (4.52) or (4.53) for the estimate of area and the equations (4.54)-(4.58) for the estimate of the variance). Because the design is unpaired, the variance of the difference between the two area estimates will simply be the sum of the variances of individual areas.

The comparison of medical tests for the paired-sample design requires the covariance of the two area estimates. Early work on this subject was done by Hanley and McNeil (1983), who provided a (lookup) table to estimate the covariance of the two areas based on the average of those two areas and the average correlation between the test results for patients without the condition. Although this correlation estimate assumes binormality and equal numbers of patients with and without the condition, it has been used with both parametric and nonparametric area estimates.

A more accurate (but more computationally intensive) estimate of covariance of the area or partial area for binormal data is available. If we assume binormality, the covariance can be estimated as

$$Cov[A_{(e_1 \leq FPR_1 \leq e_2)}, A_{(e_1 \leq FPR_2 \leq e_2)}] = \widehat{f}_1 \widehat{f}_2 Cov(\widehat{a}_1, \widehat{a}_2) + \widehat{g}_1 \widehat{g}_2 Cov(\widehat{b}_1, \widehat{b}_2)$$
$$+ \widehat{g}_1 \widehat{f}_2 Cov(\widehat{b}_1, \widehat{a}_2) + \widehat{f}_1 \widehat{g}_2 Cov(\widehat{a}_1, \widehat{b}_2), \tag{5.33}$$

where, as we saw in Chapter 4, for $j = 1, 2$ (bounds) and $i = 1, 2$ (tests)

$$f_i = \frac{e^{-a_i^2/2(1+b_i^2)}}{\sqrt{2\pi(1+b_i^2)}}[\Phi(h_{2i}) - \Phi(h_{1i})], \tag{5.34}$$

$$g_i = \frac{e^{-a_i^2/2(1+b_i^2)}}{2\pi(1+b_i^2)}[e^{-h_{i1}^2/2} - e^{-h_{i2}^2/2}]$$
$$- \frac{a_i b_i e^{-a_i^2/2(1+b_i^2)}}{\sqrt{2\pi(1+b_i^2)^3}}[\Phi(h_{i2}) - \Phi(h_{i1})], \tag{5.35}$$

and

$$h_{ij} = [\Phi^{-1}(e_j) + a_i b_i/(1+b_i^2)]\sqrt{1+b_i^2}. \tag{5.36}$$

When we are interested in the area under the entire curve, this expression simplifies somewhat, in that

$$f_i = \frac{e^{-a_i^2/2(1+b_i^2)}}{\sqrt{2\pi(1+b_i^2)}}, \quad g_i = -\frac{a_i b_i e^{-a_i/2(1+b_i^2)}}{\sqrt{2\pi(1+b_i^2)^3}}. \tag{5.37}$$

Wieand et al. (1989) suggested an alternative to comparing area under the ROC curve for binormal data. They noted that since the total area was $A_i = \Phi(\delta_i)$ where $\delta_i = (\mu_{i1} - \mu_{i0})/\sqrt{\sigma_{i0}^2 + \sigma_{i1}^2}$, testing whether $A_1 = A_2$ was equivalent to testing whether $\delta_1 = \delta_2$. The variance of δ_i was written

$$Var(\delta_i) = \frac{1}{n_{i0} + n_{i1}} \frac{1}{\sigma_i^2} \left[\frac{\sigma_{i0}^2}{n_{i0}} + \frac{\sigma_{i1}^2}{n_{i1}}\right] + \frac{\delta_i^2}{2\sigma_i^4}\left\{\frac{\sigma_{i0}^4}{n_{i0}} + \frac{\sigma_{i1}^4}{n_{i1}}\right\}, \tag{5.38}$$

where $\sigma_i^2 = \sigma_{i0}^2 + \sigma_{i1}^2, i = 1, 2$ was the sum of the variances for those with and without condition for the i-th medical test being compared. If the medical tests were assessed on the same subjects (i.e., dependent samples) then $n_{10} =$

$n_{20} = n_0$ and $n_{11} = n_{12} = n_1$. It was also necessary to know the covariance of δ_1 and δ_2

$$Cov(\delta_1, \delta_2) = \frac{1}{\sigma_1 \sigma_2}\left(\frac{C_0}{n_0} + \frac{C_1}{n_1}\right) + \frac{1}{2}\frac{\delta_1 \delta_2}{\sigma_1^2 \sigma_2^2}\left(\frac{C_0^2}{n_0 - 1} + \frac{C_1^2}{n_1 - 1}\right), \qquad (5.39)$$

where $C_i = Cov(T_{1ij}, T_{2ij}), i = 0, 1, j = 1, 2, \cdots, n_i$. Sample estimates of all parameters above can be used in equations to provide consistent estimators and equations (5.2)-(5.3) with $\theta = \delta$ can be used for hypothesis testing.

Regression methods, as discussed in detail in Chapters 8 and 9, can be used to compare ROC curve areas by including a covariate that is an indicator of whether the area is from test 1 or test 2.

Occasionally, the design of a study of medical tests is only partially paired. In other words, even though some or most of the cases are evaluated by both tests, the remainder of the cases are evaluated only by a single test. To estimate the binormal parameters, Metz et al. (1998) suggested a likelihood function that was the sum of the likelihood for independent samples and the likelihood of dependent samples. The method assumed that the data were binormal, that both paired and unpaired cases for each medical test were representative of the same population, and that the unpaired cases were not biased samples. ROCKIT implements the methods for partially paired data.

The comparisons of areas and partial areas described above require the assumption of normality. As noted in Chapter 4, the logit transformation has been recommended in a number of studies as a transformation that makes the area better conform to the normal distribution, produces good coverage of the ROC curve, etc. Since the hypotheses:

$$H_0 : logit(A_1) = logit(A_2) \text{ vs } H_1 : logit(A_1) \neq logit(A_2)$$

are equivalent to hypotheses comparing the two areas directly (i.e., untransposed), the logit transformation can be used in equations (5.1)-(5.2) to test for equality of the ROC curve areas . To calculate the variance of the difference in the equation (5.2) we use the variance in the equation (4.66). For dependent samples the covariance term is also needed. That covariance is estimated as

$$Cov(logit(\widehat{A}_1), logit(\widehat{A}_2)) = \frac{Cov(\widehat{A}_1, \widehat{A}_2)}{\widehat{A}_1 \widehat{A}_2 (1 - \widehat{A}_1)(1 - \widehat{A}_2)}, \qquad (5.40)$$

where A_i is taken here to represent either the area or partial area.

Other transformations could also be used. In particular, for partial areas in the upper portion of the ROC curve the estimator presented in the equation (4.70) performs well when two ROC curves are compared. Recall that this estimator is

$$\ln\left[\frac{A_{mx} + \widehat{A}_{e_1, e_2}}{A_{mx} - \widehat{A}_{e_1, e_2}}\right],$$

where A_{mx} is an estimate of the maximum of the area between $FPRs$ e_1 and e_2. The variance of this transformation is given in the equation (4.69). The covariance between estimated areas that have been so transformed is

$$\frac{4A_{mx}^2}{(A_{mx}^2 - \widehat{A}_1)(A_{mx}^2 - \widehat{A}_2^2)} Cov(\widehat{A}_1, \widehat{A}_2), \tag{5.41}$$

where

$$\widehat{A}_i = \widehat{A}_{(e_1 \leq FPR_i \leq e_2)}, i = 1, 2$$

is the area between $FPRs$ e_1 and e_2 for the ith ROC curve.

If continuous-scale test data do not follow a normal distribution, a transformation could be applied to produce such. As described in Chapter 4, one such transformation is a Box-Cox transformation ψ, to achieve normality:

$$\psi(T) = \frac{(T)^\lambda - 1}{\lambda} \text{ for } \lambda \neq 0 \tag{5.42}$$

or

$$\psi(T) = \ln(T) \text{ for } \lambda = 0. \tag{5.43}$$

Molodianovitch et al. (2006) and Zou (2001) both used Box-Cox type transformations applied to paired data to compare ROC curves, but their implementations were different. Zou used maximum likelihood methods to estimate a single Box-Cox transformation parameter λ to apply to data from both medical tests. She assumed that after the transformation, the paired data from patients without the condition followed a bivariate normal distribution with mean μ_{i0}, common variance σ_0^2, and correlation ρ_{T_0} where the subscript i indexed the test. Similarly, the paired data from patients with the condition followed a bivariate normal distribution with mean μ_{i1}, common variance σ_1^2, and correlation ρ_{T_1}. Zou presented a log-likelihood function to estimate the set of parameters $(\mu_{10}, \mu_{20}, \sigma_0^2, \rho_{T_0}, \mu_{11}, \mu_{21}, \sigma_1^2, \rho_{T_1}, \lambda)$. The usual binormal parameters were then estimated for each of the two medical tests from these MLEs: $b = \sigma_1/\sigma_0$ and $a_i = (\mu_{i1} - \mu_{i0})/\sigma_0$. The estimated variances of the ROC curve parameter estimates were

$$\widehat{Var}(\widehat{a}_i) = \frac{1}{n_0} + \frac{1 + \widehat{\rho}_{T_0}^2 \widehat{a}_i^2}{4n_1} + \frac{\widehat{b}^2}{n_1}, \tag{5.44}$$

$$\widehat{Var}(\widehat{b}) = \frac{[(n_1 + 1)\widehat{\rho}_{T_0}^2 + (n_0 + 1)\widehat{\rho}_{T_1}^2]\widehat{b}^2}{4n_0 n_1}, \tag{5.45}$$

$$\widehat{Var}(\widehat{a}_1, \widehat{a}_2) = \frac{\widehat{\rho}_{T_0}}{n_0} + \frac{(1 + \widehat{\rho}_{T_0}^2)\widehat{a}_1 \widehat{a}_2}{4n_0} + \frac{\widehat{\rho}_{T_1}\widehat{b}^2}{n_1}, \tag{5.46}$$

and

$$\widehat{Var}(\widehat{a}_i, \widehat{b}) = \frac{(1 + \widehat{\rho}_{T_0}^2)\widehat{a}_i \widehat{b}}{4n_0}. \tag{5.47}$$

A few important assumptions were made here. First, Zou assumed that a single common transformation could be used for both continuous-scale tests from cases with and without the condition. Both tests had to provide results in the same metric. If the measurements for the tests were in different metrics, she suggested standardizing the data and then exploring the possibility of a common transformation.

Second, she assumed that after transformation, the distribution of the test results for patients without the condition had different means but the same variance. Similarly, the distribution of results for the two tests for patients with the condition had different means but the same variance (although the variance could have been different for patients with and without the disease). Because of this assumption, the parameters for both tests had to be estimated simultaneously. The assumption of equal variance (implying that $b_1 = b_2$) also means that a test of equality of various ROC curve measures (the entire curve, area, partial area, or specific sensitivities) could be accomplished by simply testing whether parameters a_1 and a_2 were the same, using the test statistic:

$$Z = \frac{\widehat{a}_1 - \widehat{a}_2}{\sqrt{\widehat{Var}(\widehat{a}_1) + \widehat{Var}(\widehat{a}_2) - 2\widehat{Cov}(\widehat{a}_1, \widehat{a}_2)}}, \tag{5.48}$$

which has, asymptotically, a normal distribution.

Molodianovitch et al. (2006) considered a similar Box-Cox transformation procedure, but without assuming $b_1 = b_2$ or $\lambda_1 = \lambda_2$. They also used maximum likelihood methods to simultaneously estimate the two Box-Cox parameters (λ_1, λ_2), one for each medical test. Without the assumption on b, the comparison of medical tests did not simplify to a comparison of the parameters a_i. Instead, Molodianovitch et al. (2006) suggested transforming the data using the estimated transformation parameters $\widehat{\lambda}_1$ and $\widehat{\lambda}_2$, then using the method of Wieand et al. (1989) for binormal data to compare areas. They acknowledged that this method ignored the variability introduced by the estimation of the λ's, but noted that their simulation indicated that this did not hurt the size or power of the test. Their research found that this method generally worked as well as or better than the nonparametric methods of DeLong et al. (1988) or assuming normality without transformation.

Zou (2001) also presented a semiparametric method in which she assumed that the data were transformed to follow a binormal distribution using an unspecified monotonic transformation. She developed a likelihood function based on the ranks of a binormal distribution to estimate the binormal parameters. Estimation of the area and their variances and covariances followed directly as a function of the parameters. Computer software for estimating ROC curve parameters by using the transformation methods can be obtained from Zou (2001).

We may prefer to use a nonparametric approach to analyze data. The most commonly used nonparametric method for comparing ROC curve areas is that of DeLong et al. (1988). Their estimates of ROC curve area and variance were presented in Chapter 4 (section 4.2.5). If our design involves tests on independent groups of subjects, we can substitute the appropriate estimates into equations (5.1)-(5.2) as detailed in equations (4.77)-(4.82).

For paired data, it is necessary to know the covariance of the area estimates. DeLong et al. (1988) presented a method for estimating the covariance term, which extends the results that we first introduced in Chapter 4, Subsection 4.2.5. This covariance term is

$$Cov(\widehat{A}_{1DL}, \widehat{A}_{2DL}) = \frac{1}{n_1}S_{10} + \frac{1}{n_0}S_{01}, \tag{5.49}$$

where S_{10} and S_{01} are covariance terms:

$$S_{10} = \frac{1}{n_1 - 1}\sum_{j=1}^{n_1}[V_{10}(T_{11j}) - \widehat{A}_{1DL}][V_{10}(T_{21j}) - \widehat{A}_{2DL}], \tag{5.50}$$

$$S_{01} = \frac{1}{n_0 - 1}\sum_{j=1}^{n_0}[V_{01}(T_{10j}) - \widehat{A}_{1DL}][V_{01}(T_{20j}) - \widehat{A}_{2DL}] \tag{5.51}$$

and the V_{10} and V_{01} are as defined in equations (4.77) and (4.78) in Chapter 4. Software to compute the components, the covariance matrices, and the test statistics for the full area under the curve, is available in SAS and Stata, among other programs.

If we are interested in the partial area, rather than the entire area under the curve, then, following He and Escobar (2008), the covariance can be similarly derived as follows:

$$Cov[A_{N(e_1<FPR_1<e_2)}, A_{N(e_1<FPR_2<e_2)}] = (\frac{n_p}{n})^2\{\frac{1}{n_p}S_{10} + \frac{1}{n_1}S_{01}\}, \tag{5.52}$$

where

$$S_{01} = \sum_{j=1}^{n_1}\{V_{01}(T_{11j}) - \widehat{\tau}_1\}\{V_{01}(T_{21j}) - \widehat{\tau}_2\}, \tag{5.53}$$

and

$$S_{10} = \frac{1}{n_p - 1}\sum\{V_{10}(T_{11i}) - \widehat{\tau}_1\}\{V_{10}(T_{11i}) - \widehat{\tau}_2\}, \tag{5.54}$$

The latter summation is limited to $T_{10i} \in [c_{11}, c_{12}]$ and $T_{20i} \in [c_{21}, c_{22}]$, n_p is the number of subjects that have both the sets $T_{10j} \in (c_{11}, c_{12})$ and $T_{20j} \in (c_{21}, c_{22})$, $c_{ji} = \bar{F}_j^{-1}(e_i), i, j = 1, 2$ and the V_{01} and V_{01} and τ_i are defined in Chapter 4, Section 4.3.4.

Other nonparametric methods, not covered here, include a nonparametric method for comparing the ROC curve areas of two tests in a study with a partially paired design developed by Zhou and Gatsonis (1996); and permutation methods such as have been presented by Bandos et al. (2005b), Bandos et al. (2005a) and Braun and Alonzo (2008).

Finally, we consider the comparison of two medical tests when the data are clustered. The bootstrap approach (Rutter, 2000) can be used to compare areas or partial areas, for either the binormal model or nonparametric approaches. For a less computer intensive approach, explicit variance formulae are available for the nonparametric estimates of variances and covariances. Estimates of the area and variances are as given in Chapter 4, Subsection 4.2.6. The covariance estimate for two estimated ROC curve areas is:

$$Cov(\widehat{A}_{1C}, \widehat{A}_{2C}) = \frac{S_{10}^{1,2}}{n_1} + \frac{S_{01}^{1,2}}{n_0} + \frac{S_{11}^{1,2}}{n_1 n_0} + \frac{S_{11}^{2,1}}{n_1 n_0}, \qquad (5.55)$$

where

$$S_{10}^{1,2} = \frac{I_{10}}{(I_{10}-1)n_1} \sum_{i=1}^{I_{10}} [V_{10}(T_{11i.}) - n_{1i}\widehat{A}_{1C}][V_{10}(T_{21i.}) - n_{1i}\widehat{A}_{2C}], \quad (5.56)$$

$$S_{01}^{1,2} = \frac{I_{01}}{(I_{01}-1)n_0} \sum_{i=1}^{I_{01}} [V_{01}(T_{10i.}) - n_{0i}\widehat{A}_{1C}][V_{01}(T_{20i.}) - n_{0i}\widehat{A}_{2C}], \quad (5.57)$$

$$S_{11}^{1,2} = \frac{I}{I-1} \sum_{i=1}^{I} [V_{10}(T_{11i.}) - n_{1i}\widehat{A}_{1C}][V_{01}(T_{20i.}) - n_{0i}\widehat{A}_{2C}], \qquad (5.58)$$

and

$$S_{11}^{2,1} = \frac{I}{I-1} \sum_{i=1}^{I} [V_{10}(T_{21i.}) - n_{1i}\widehat{A}_{2c}][V_{01}(T_{10i.}) - n_{0i}\widehat{A}_{1c}]. \qquad (5.59)$$

Here $V_{10}(T_{r1i.})$ and $V_{01}(T_{r0i.})$ denote the sums of the T_1 and T_0 components of the ith cluster for the rth test. Note that we need the latter two terms to account for the correlation between affected and unaffected units within a cluster.

5.2.4.1 Comparing ROC Curve Areas: Head Trauma Data and Case Study 3

The area under the ROC curve for the head trauma data can be calculated separately for the younger and older patients. As calculated by ROCKIT, we have the area for the younger patients estimated as 0.7656 with a standard error (SE) of 0.0886; for older patients, the area estimate is 0.9238, with a SE of 0.0858. These two patient groups are independent; thus the covariance between the two areas is zero, and we can easily calculate the test statistic to compare the two area as

$$Z = \frac{0.9238 - 0.7656}{\sqrt{0.0886^2 + 0.0858^2}} = 1.28.$$

The test statistic is not greater than 1.96, so for $\alpha = 0.05$, we cannot reject the null hypothesis that the area under the ROC curve for older and younger patients is the same.

In Chapter 4, Section 4.2.6.1, we learned that the MRA data were actually captured as clustered data, because MRA was performed on both the right and left carotid artery. Earlier, we compared results for radiologists 3 and 4 for the left carotid only. A better way to compare the accuracy of the two radiologists would be to include results from both left and right carotids. We already saw that for radiologist 4, $\widehat{A}_{4C} = 0.9141$, $\widehat{V}(\widehat{A}_{4C}) = 0.000293539$. Similarly, $\widehat{A}_{3C} = 0.8558$, $\widehat{V}(\widehat{A}_{3C}) = 0.000517455$ for radiologist 3. To be able to compare the two areas, we also need the covariance between them. We use the methods described above (equations 5.55-5.59) to get $S_{10}^{12} = 0.017694$, $S_{01}^{12} = 0.013196$, $S_{11}^{12} = 0.23303$, $S_{11}^{21} = -0.19182$; the covariance is 0.000205051. The test statistic for the comparison is

$$Z = \frac{0.9141 - 0.8558}{\sqrt{0.000517455 + 0.000293539 - 2 \times 0.000205051}} = \frac{0.0583}{0.02002} = 2.91.$$

The area under the ROC curve is significantly different for the two radiologists.

Comparison of radiologist 2 with radiologist 4, though, gives us a different result

$$Z = \frac{0.9141 - 0.9014}{\sqrt{0.000332028 + 0.000293539 - 2 \times 0.000154182}} = \frac{0.0127}{0.0178} = 0.713.$$

There is no statistically significant difference between the ROC curve areas. We have insufficient evidence to conclude that the accuracy of MRA, as interpreted by radiologists 2 and 4, are different.

5.3   TESTS OF EQUIVALENCE

Most of this chapter has focused on the question of whether the accuracy of two diagnostic tests differs. It may not be an appropriate question of interest in all situations, however. New technology is often more conservative than existing technology in terms of invasiveness or amount of radiation. When the issue of comparison arises, the more appropriate question may be whether new technology is comparable to, though not necessarily better than, the standard existing technology. For example, when comparing the accuracy of mammography using a digitized workstation to that of plain film, the real question may be not whether the two methods are different (the hypothesis that we have considered so far in this chapter) but, rather, whether the digitized workstation produces results similar to those of standard plain film, or perhaps, whether the digitized film is as good as the standard plain film.

Another possible question may be whether 3-dimensional time-of-flight MR angiography (MRA) can replace catheter angiography (CA) as a presurgical tool for carotid endarectomy. Even if MRA does not have a sensitivity or specificity as high as CA, the possible poorer accuracy should be considered in light of the risks (morbidity and mortality) associated with CA.

Most studies of diagnostic tests address the question of whether new technology is diagnostically superior to existing technology. Statistical tests are performed (as was done earlier in this chapter) to detect differences. If we do not detect a statistically significant difference (because p value > 0.05) we tend to draw the incorrect conclusion that this lack of difference must imply two diagnostically equivalent tests. Unfortunately, this conclusion is incorrect, partly because the SE's are not likely to be negligible and the concept of equivalence has not been specifically defined.

Let us consider this: when we test for differences, the probability exists that we will not find the difference statistically significant (p value > 0.05), even when the accuracy of the tests is truly different. This mistake is called a Type II error. In general (all things being equal), the larger the study, the smaller the Type II error. Often, however, studies are relatively small, so the Type II error may be as large as 20%. Thus to conclude that not rejecting the null hypothesis of equal accuracy means the same as finding the accuracy of the two tests to be actually equal is to assume that an error perhaps as high as 20% is negligible. Statisticians emphasize that the appropriate conclusion to draw when we do not reject the null hypothesis is simply that there is insufficient evidence of a difference smaller than a specific amount.

A clinically relevant difference is the difference between two tests that has clinical implications. Let $(\triangle_L, \triangle_U)$ denote an interval that allows two tests to be considered equivalent (i.e., the difference is clinically ignorable) if the difference in accuracy is between the lower bound, $\triangle_L$ and the upper bound $\triangle_U$. Clinically important are differences less than or equal to $\triangle_L$ and differences greater than or equal to $\triangle_U$.

There are many ways to perform equivalence testing. Here, we follow the method of Schuirmann (1987) as presented in Obuchowski (1997b). To test the equivalence of two tests statistically, we must be able to state formal null and alternative hypotheses. The null hypothesis will be

$$H_0 : \theta_1 - \theta_2 \leq \triangle_L \text{ or } \theta_1 - \theta_2 \geq \triangle_U \tag{5.60}$$

and the alternative hypothesis will be

$$H_1 : \triangle_L < \theta_1 - \theta_2 < \triangle_U, \tag{5.61}$$

both of which contrast with the null and alternative hypotheses for differences stated in equations (5.1) and (5.2).

Once the values of $(\triangle_L, \triangle_U)$ are known, the hypotheses are well stated; then a statistical test can be performed, which actually consists of two tests:

$$Z_1 = \frac{(\widehat{\theta}_1 - \widehat{\theta}_2) - \triangle_L}{\sqrt{Var(\widehat{\theta}_1 - \widehat{\theta}_2)}} \text{ and } Z_2 = \frac{\triangle_U - (\widehat{\theta}_1 - \widehat{\theta}_2)}{\sqrt{Var(\widehat{\theta}_1 - \widehat{\theta}_2)}}. \tag{5.62}$$

We reject the null hypothesis if both tests statistics, Z_1 and Z_2 are larger than the appropriate standard normal critical value of a 1-sided test at level α. In the literature this is called the TOST (Two One Sided Test) method. Note that the Type I error for this test would conclude that the tests are equivalent (the alternative is true) when, in fact, they are not. By setting $\alpha = 0.05$, we can keep the probability of making such an error to a minimum.

A related issue in comparing two diagnostic tests is whether one test is at least as good as the other. That is, although we think that a new test may be better than the standard test, we would be satisfied to discover that the new test is not really worse than the standard test, a condition that is referred to as non-inferiority. We can write the hypothesis as follows: The null hypothesis will be

$$H_0 : \theta_1 - \theta_2 \geq \triangle_M \tag{5.63}$$

and the alternative hypothesis will be

$$H_1 : \theta_1 - \theta_2 < \triangle_M, \tag{5.64}$$

where θ_1 can be regarded as the standard test, θ_2 as the new test we are considering, and $\triangle_M$ is the smallest difference in accuracy that we will not consider equivalent. For this set of hypotheses, the Type I error rate is the probability of concluding that the new test is "equivalent" when the standard test is more accurate. The Type II error is the probability of concluding that the standard test is more accurate when, in actuality, the new test is no worse than, and possibly even better than, within $\triangle_M$ from the standard (i.e., $\theta_2 + \triangle_M > \theta_1$).

This approach is really a variant of a 1-sided test. The test statistic is

$$Z_{NI} = \frac{\widehat{\theta}_2 + \triangle_M - \widehat{\theta}_1}{\sqrt{\widehat{V}ar(\widehat{\theta}_2 - \widehat{\theta}_1)}}. \tag{5.65}$$

The null hypothesis is rejected if the test statistic for noninferiority, Z_{NI}, is large than the critical value of the standard normal distribution (1-sided test at level α).

5.3.1   Testing Whether ROC Curve Areas are Equivalent: Case Study 3

We saw in the previous section that there was no significant difference in the accuracy of MRA as interpreted by radiologists 2 and 4, when the entire area under the curve was considered. Our conclusion was correct that we had insufficient evidence to conclude that the ROC curve areas were different. However, with an equivalence test we can confirm now that the two Radiologists had equivalent accuracy. We saw in the previous section that $\widehat{A}_{2C} = 0.9014$ and $\widehat{A}_{4C} = 0.9141$, and the standard error of the difference was 0.0178. If we set $\triangle_L = -0.05$ and $\triangle_U = 0.05$, our two test statistics are

$$Z_1 = \frac{(0.9141 - 0.9014) + 0.05}{0.0178} = 3.52$$

and

$$Z_2 = \frac{0.05 - (0.9141 - 0.9014)}{0.0178} = 2.10.$$

Since our Type I error, $\alpha = 0.05$, our critical value is 1.645, to which we must compare each test statistic. Both Z_1 and Z_2 are greater than the critical value; thus we can conclude that the two radiologists have equivalent diagnostic accuracy.

CHAPTER 6

SAMPLE SIZE CALCULATIONS

A well-designed study with an adequate sample size is important. It ensures a scientifically interesting result - whether the result supports or disputes the expectations of the study's investigators. A positive result supports the study investigators' expectation about the accuracy of a new test or comparison of two tests. A negative result allows the investigators to conclude that the new test does not have adequate accuracy or there is no clinically important difference between two tests. In contrast, if a study does not include enough patients, then underpowered results cannot be distinguished from clinically insignificant results, and the investigators have wasted time and resources and potentially exposed patients to risks and discomforts, with no potential scientific gain (Eng, 2004). In this chapter, we describe and illustrate how to compute sample size for some common diagnostic accuracy studies. We discuss studies assessing the accuracy of one diagnostic test and studies comparing the accuracies of diagnostic tests. We present sample size formulae for a variety of measures of accuracy, including sensitivity and specificity, the full and partial area under the ROC curve, and sensitivity at a fixed FPR. We consider diagnostic tests with quantitative results and both single- and multiple-reader studies of tests requiring subjective interpretation.

Statistical Methods in Diagnostic Medicine,
Second Edition. By Xiao-Hua Zhou, Nancy A. Obuchowski, Donna K. McClish
Copyright © 2011 John Wiley & Sons, Inc.

6.1 STUDIES ESTIMATING THE ACCURACY OF A SINGLE TEST

We begin with studies whose goal is to estimate the accuracy of a diagnostic test. For these studies the sample size must be adequate to ensure that the test's accuracy is estimated with good precision. That is, we want to construct a confidence interval (CI) for the test's accuracy and we want the confidence interval to be reasonably narrow. We denote L as the desired length of one-half of the CI.

6.1.1 Sample Size Calculations for Estimating Sensitivity and/or Specificity - Case Study 1

Suppose we are planning a study to measure the sensitivity of single photon emission computed tomography (SPECT) for detecting diseased parathyroid glands (Case Study 1). We will recruit patients who, based on clinical signs and the results of biochemical tests, have been scheduled to undergo parathyroid surgery. Prior to surgery, patients will be imaged with SPECT. A positive SPECT result will be defined as an area of increased activity that persists over time. Otherwise, the SPECT result will be considered negative. Findings at surgery will be considered the gold standard. We plan to estimate the sensitivity of SPECT and construct a CI for the true sensitivity. We want to know how many patients with a diseased gland are needed for the study.

Let θ denote the true accuracy of a test. Two formulae are given for determining the sample size. The first formula gives the number of patients needed for a study so that, with probability of $1 - \beta$, the width of a two-sided CI for the accuracy of the test will be 2L or less (Flahault et al., 2005).

$$n = \frac{[(z_{\alpha/2} + z_\beta)\sqrt{V(\hat{\theta})}]^2}{(L)^2}, \tag{6.1}$$

where $1 - \alpha$ is the size of the desired confidence interval, $z_{\alpha/2}$ is the upper $\alpha/2$ percentile of a standard normal distribution, z_β is the upper β percentile of a standard normal distribution where 1-β is the desired power, and L is the desired width of one-half of the CI. $V(\hat{\theta})$ is the variance function (McCullagh and Nelder, 1989). We assume that the variance of $\hat{\theta}$ can be written as $V(\hat{\theta})/n$, where $V(\hat{\theta})$ does not depend on n, and n is the required sample size. In our SPECT example, n is the required number of patients with a diseased parathyroid gland.

The second formula gives the number of patients needed for a two-sided CI of width roughly equal to 2L or less.

$$n = \frac{[(z_{\alpha/2})\sqrt{V(\hat{\theta})}]^2}{(L)^2}. \tag{6.2}$$

We now discuss application of both formulae.

Continuing with our SPECT example, suppose that we want to construct a 95% CI; then α equals 0.05 and $z_{\alpha/2}$ is 1.96. When the measure of accuracy is a proportion, like a test's sensitivity or specificity, the variance function is $V(\hat{\theta}) = Se \times (1 - Se)$ where Se is the conjectured sensitivity of the test (Arkin and Wachtel, 1990). To compute sample size we need a rough estimate of the (unknown) sensitivity of SPECT. Suppose there is one paper in the literature describing the sensitivity of SPECT for detecting parathyroid disease. That paper reports a sensitivity of 0.80 with 95% CI for the true sensitivity of 0.65 to 0.95. Using the 0.80 estimate initially, $\hat{V}(\hat{Se}) = 0.16$. In our study we want to estimate sensitivity more precisely than previously reported in the literature. To estimate sensitivity to within ±0.05, we set L=0.05.

Suppose we want our study to have 80% power (i.e. β is 0.20) to estimate the sensitivity to a precision of ±0.05. For a 95% CI the required number of patients with a diseased parathyroid gland is $\frac{[(1.96+0.84)\sqrt{0.16}]^2}{(0.05)^2} = 501.76 = 502$. The true sensitivity, however, may be as low as 0.65 or as high as 0.95. Thus, the sample size required to estimate the sensitivity of PET to within ±0.05 is between 149 and 714.

Alternatively, in a phase I exploratory study a CI of width about ±0.05 may be adequate. We use the equation (6.2), yielding a sample size in the range of 73-350 (based on the upper and lower bounds, respectively, of the published CI).

The formulae in equations (6.1) and (6.2) work well for sensitivities (or specificities) that are not close to one. For studies with expected sensitivities (or specificities) close to one, Flahault et al. (2005) provide tables for determining sample size using exact equations based on the binormal distribution.

In our illustration of equations (6.1) and (6.2) we assumed a retrospective study design such that, based on the surgical results, we could select the required number of patients with diseased parathyroid glands for our study. In a prospective study, however, patients are recruited for the study before the gold standard is performed, so the precise number of patients with a diseased parathyroid gland is not known at the time the study sample is composed. We might make the assumption that the prevalence of the condition in the sample will be identical to the prevalence of the condition in the population; however, because of random sampling, about 50% of the time we will have too few patients with the condition in the sample. A better approach is to specify a high probability of obtaining at least the needed number of patients with the condition for the study. Suppose we have determined that we need 350 patients with a diseased parathyroid gland for the study. We might specify that we want to recruit enough patients so that there is a 90% chance that our sample will have at least 350 patients with a diseased parathyroid gland. The following equation can be solved for N_{total}, the total number of patients that should be recruited (including patients both with and without the condition), so that there is $1 - \beta$ probability that at least n patients with the condition are included:

$$\frac{(N_{total} \times Prev_p) - n}{\sqrt{N_{total} \times Prev_p \times (1 - Prev_p)}} = z_\beta, \tag{6.3}$$

where $Prev_p$ is the prevalence of the condition in the population, and z_β equals 1.645 for 95% probability, 1.28 for 90% probability, and 0.84 for 80% probability.

Suppose we expect that 80% of presurgical patients have a diseased parathyroid gland. We substitute into the equation (6.3): $Prev_p = 0.8$, n=350, and $z_\beta = 1.28$. With 452 or more total patients, we can be 90% confidence that we will have at least 350 patients with a diseased parathyroid gland in the sample.

Note that if N_{total} is small and $Prev_p$ is near zero, then the formula in the equation (6.3) may underestimate N_{total}. For these studies, Flahault et al. (2005) provide a formula for determining N_{total} using the binormal distribution. Also, note that the methods described here for determining sample size for studies measuring the sensitivity of a test are also applicable to studies measuring the specificity of a test.

6.1.2   Sample Size for Estimating the Area Under the ROC Curve - Case Study 2

Suppose we are planning a study to assess a reader's accuracy in detecting colon polyps on computed tomography colonography (CTC) (Case Study 2). We will retrospectively review the CTC scans of all patients who subsequently underwent optical colonoscopy. The optical colonoscopy results will serve as the gold standard. We plan to randomly select a certain number, n, of patients with colon polyps and an equal number of patients without colon polyps. We will present the reader will all 2n CTC images in random order. We will ask the reader to mark the location of any polyps detected and score the polyp on a scale from 2 (probably not a polyp) to 5 (definitely a polyp). Any true polyps missed by the reader will be assigned a score of 1 (definitely not a polyp). We plan to estimate the ROC curve, its area, and a 95% CI for the ROC area. We want to know how large n should be.

We use the sample size formula in the equation (6.2). Here θ is the area under the ROC curve and n is the number of patients with the condition (i.e. with one or more colon polyps as determined by the gold standard) needed for the study. Since ROC curves are functions of sensitivity and specificity, we need to make sure we have sufficient numbers of patients with and without the condition. Let R denote the ratio of the number of patients without the condition to patients with the condition in the study sample. The total number of patients needed for the study is n(1+R).

To use equations (6.1) or (6.2) we need an estimate of the variance function for the ROC area. Hanley and McNeil (1982) proposed an estimate of the variance of the area under the ROC curve, based on an exponential distribution. (That is, the unobserved, underlying test results follow an exponential distribution, but the observed test results, either continuous or ordinal, do not necessarily have an exponential distribution.) For sample size calculations, we write the variance function as

$$\hat{V}(\hat{A}) = Q_1/R + Q_2 - A^2[1/R + 1], \qquad (6.4)$$

where $Q_1 = A/(2 - A)$, $Q_2 = 2A^2/(1 + A)$, and A is the conjectured area under the ROC curve.

It has been shown that the variance function in (6.4) often underestimates the variance when the test results are recorded as ordinal values from an underlying binormal distribution (Obuchowski, 1994). An alternative estimator of the variance function based on an underlying binormal distribution for the test results was proposed by Obuchowski (1994). (The assumption is that the unobserved, underlying test results follow a binormal distribution, but the observed test results, either continuous or ordinal, do not necessarily have a binormal distribution.)

$$\hat{V}(\hat{A}) = (0.0099 \times e^{-a^2/2}) \times ([5a^2 + 8] + [a^2 + 8]/R), \qquad (6.5)$$

where $a = \Phi^{-1}(A) \times 1.414$ and Φ^{-1} is the inverse of the cumulative normal distribution function. The variable a in the equation (6.5) is parameter a from a binormal distribution (parameter b is set to one in the derivation for a conservative estimate of sample size). The estimator in (6.5) works reasonably well for tests with ordinal or continuous results when either parametric or nonparametric estimates of the ROC area are used (Obuchowski and McClish, 1997).

Suppose we conjecture that the reader's ROC curve area, A, is about 0.80. We want to estimate the ROC area to within ±0.10; thus, L=0.10. The sample prevalence is 50% by design, so R=1.0. For the equation (6.5) we need to know the value of the binormal parameter a. Parameter a can be calculated using the above formula, or using Table 6.1.

Table 6.1   Pairs of Binormal Parameters for Different Values of the ROC Area

ROC Area	a,b	a,b	a,b	a,b	a,b
0.6	0.27,0.33	0.28,0.50	0.36,1.0	0.57,2.0	0.80,3.0
0.7	0.55,0.33	0.59,0.50	0.74,1.0	1.17,2.0	1.66,3.0
0.8	0.89,0.33	0.94,0.50	1.19,1.0	1.88,2.0	2.66,3.0
0.9	1.35,0.33	1.43,0.50	1.82,1.0	2.87,2.0	4.05,3.0
0.95	1.73,0.33	1.84,0.50	2.33,1.0	3.68,2.0	5.20,3.0

From the third row of Table 6.1 (where parameter b is one), we find that for an ROC area of 0.80, $a = 1.19$. Then, in the equation (6.5): $\hat{V}(\hat{A}) =$

$(0.0099 \times e^{-1.19^2/2}) \times ([5 \times 1.19^2 + 8] + [1.19^2 + 8]/1.0) = 0.11946$. For a 95% CI for the ROC area, the required number of patients with a colon polyp is 46 (from the equation (6.2)). The total sample size required for the study (i.e. number of patients with and without polyps) is n(1+R), or 92.

The formulae for $\hat{V}(\hat{A})$ in equations (6.4) and (6.5) were derived from specific models for the unobserved, underlying distribution of the test results, i.e. the exponential and binormal distributions, respectively. Blume (2009) provides the variance function for calculating 1) the sample size that would be applicable for the distribution that would yield the smallest sample size and 2) the smallest sample size that would be applicable for *all* distributions. The latter formula is important because it provides an upper bound on the required sample size for a study where usually little is known about the underlying distribution of the test results. The variance function that is applicable for all underlying distributions is:

$$\hat{V}(\hat{A}) = A(1 - A). \tag{6.6}$$

Note that this variance function is not a function of R, the ratio of patients without the condition to those with the condition. The variance function in the equation (6.6), when used in the equation (6.1) or (6.2) to determine sample size, yields the sample size for the smaller of the number of patients with and without the condition. In our CTC example, $R = 1$, but when $R < 1$, the formula gives the number of patients without the condition, and when $R > 1$, the formula gives the number of patients with the condition.

In our CTC example, using the variance function in the equation (6.6), we obtain n=62 and the total sample size of 124. Thus, the largest sample size needed for the study for any underlying distribution of the test results is 124.

In the special situation where the observed test results are on a truly continuous scale and follow a binormal distribution (or can be transformed to a binormal distribution), there is a more efficient estimator for the variance function (Obuchowski and McClish, 1997): $\hat{V}(\hat{A}) = (0.0099 \times e^{-a^2/2}) \times ([5a^2 + 8] + [a^2 + 8]/R) - (0.0398 \times a^2 e^{(-a^2/2)})$. This variance function should only be used for this special case.

6.1.3   Studies with Clustered Data

Consider now the situation where there could be multiple diseased parathyroid glands or multiple colon polyps in the same patient ("clustered data"). As we discussed in Chapter 3, there are several possible strategies with clustered data. Consider the CTC example. One strategy might be to use the highest confidence score assigned by the reader to any correctly located polyps as the test result for that patient. As we have seen in the previous section, we would need 46 patients with one or more polyps and 46 patients without polyps.

Another strategy, which often requires a smaller sample size, is to divide the colon into clinically relevant segments and define a test result for each segment. Segments with polyps are used in the calculation of sensitivity, while segments without polyps are used in the calculation of specificity (See Chapter 3 for details). In this strategy, we must account for the correlation, however small, between segments from the same patient.

Obuchowski (1997a) described an upper bound on the sample size required for such a design. The formula can be used to adjust the sample size for any study with clustered data, regardless of the measure of test accuracy.

$$n_C = n \times [1 + (s - 1)r], \tag{6.7}$$

where n_C is the number of observations required for the study, n is the number of patients that would be required if each patient had only one observation (which we computed as 46 using the variance function in (6.5)), s is the average number of observations per patient, and r is the average correlation between test results of observations from the same patient.

Suppose we expect 1.5 segments to have polyps, on average, among patients with polyps. In the design phase of a study, we do not know the correlation between test results of segments from the same patient; thus, we will assume moderate correlation of 0.5. In equation (6.7): s=1.5, r=0.5, and n=46 (using the variance function based on the binormal distribution). The number of segments with polyps required for the study is then 57.5. Therefore, we need about 39 patients with one or more polyps for the study. Now consider the segments without polyps. Patients with polyps will contribute, on average, 4.5 segments without polyps, while patients without polyps will contribute 6 segments; the average is s=5.25. We again assume moderate correlation between test results of segments from the same patient: r=0.5. From the equation (6.7), the number of segments without polyps required for the study is 143.75. Note that the 39 patients with polyps will contribute about 175 segments without polyps, so one might argue that no additional patients are needed. However, we recommend that the ratio of patients with and without the condition be maintained at R=1; thus, we recommend 39 patients with polyps and a similar number of patients without polyps. We reduced the total sample size for the study by 14 patients (92-78=14, 15% savings).

6.1.4 Testing the Hypothesis that the ROC Area is Equal to a Particular Value

In some studies we are interested in testing the hypothesis that the diagnostic accuracy of a test is equal to some pre-determined value, denoted as θ_o. For example, we might want to test the null hypothesis that a reader using CTC to detect colon polyps has an accuracy of 0.5, versus the alternative hypothesis that the accuracy is better than 0.5. The null and alternative hypotheses can be written as

$$H_0: \theta = \theta_o$$

$$H_1: \theta > \theta_o \text{ (one-tailed version)}$$

$$H_1: \theta \neq \theta_o \text{ (two-tailed version)}.$$

For sample size calculations we must specify a value for θ under the alternative hypothesis. We denote the conjectured value of θ under the alternative hypothesis as θ_1. A general formula for computing sample size for a study testing these hypotheses is

$$n = \frac{[z_{\alpha/2}\sqrt{V_o(\hat{\theta})} + z_\beta\sqrt{V_A(\hat{\theta})}]^2}{(\theta_o - \theta_1)^2}, \tag{6.8}$$

where α is the type I error rate, and β is the type II error rate (or 1-power). $V_o(\hat{\theta})$ is the variance function of $\hat{\theta}$ under the null hypothesis, and $V_A(\hat{\theta})$ is the variance function of $\hat{\theta}$ under the alternative hypothesis.

For our CTC example, $\hat{V}_o(\hat{A}) = 0.1584$ (i.e. setting $A = A_o = 0.5$ in the equation (6.5)). For a study with a 5% type I error rate (two-tailed) and 80% power (20% type II error rate) and setting A_1 at 0.80, the sample size requirements are n=13 patients with polyps and 13 patients without polyps (assuming one polyp per patient).

6.1.5 Sample Size for Estimating Sensitivity at Fixed FPR - Case Study 2

Continuing with our CTC example, suppose we would like to estimate the sensitivity of CTC at a FPR of 0.10 (i.e. sensitivity at which 10% of subjects undergoing colon cancer screening are unnecessarily called back for further testing). We want to determine the sample size required to estimate sensitivity to within ± 0.10.

We use the sample size formula in the equation (6.2), where θ is now the sensitivity at a fixed FPR of e ($e=0.10$ for our example, $Se_{FPR=0.10}$). n is the number of patients with a polyp needed for the study (assume one polyp per patient), and n(1+R) is the total number of patients needed. Obuchowski and McClish (1997) presented an estimator of variance of the sensitivity at a fixed FPR e, based on an underlying binormal distribution. (To clarify, Obuchowski and McClish assumed that the unobserved, underlying test results follow a binormal distribution, but the observed test results, either continuous or ordinal, do not necessarily have a binormal distribution.) They first define the z-transformed sensitivity at a FPR of e as

$$z[Se_{FPR=e}] = a + b\Phi^{-1}(e), \tag{6.9}$$

where a and b are the parameters of the assumed underlying binormal distribution and Φ^{-1} is the inverse of the cumulative normal distribution function. Note that the transformation is needed because the distribution of $Se_{FPR=e}$

is not normal. The variance function of the z-transformed sensitivity at fixed FPR e which is used for sample size calculation is

$$\hat{V}(z[\hat{Se}_{FPR=e}]) = [1 + b^2/R + a^2/2] + g^2[b^2(1 + R)/(2R)], \qquad (6.10)$$

where $g = \Phi^{-1}(e)$ and R is defined as it was in the equation (6.5).

To use the equations (6.9) and (6.10), we need to know the shape of the ROC curve, as defined by the parameters a and b. We usually do not know the shape of the ROC curve at the planning phase of the study; thus, we might consider different values for parameters a and b. Table 6.1 summarizes pairs of parameters a and b for ROC curves with different areas and shapes. For example, if we expected the test to have moderate ROC area, say 0.80, then from Table 6.1, we might consider values for a and b of (0.89, 0.33), (0.94,0.50), (1.19, 1.0), (1.88, 2.0), or (2.66, 3.0). In the first pair, the variability in test scores is three times as great for patients with the condition than without (i.e. b=0.33); in the second pair, the variability in test scores is two times greater for patients with the condition than without (b=0.5); in the last pair the variability is three times greater among patients without the condition than patients with the condition (b=3.0).

To compute n from the equation (6.2) we need to determine L in terms of the transformed value of $Se_{FPR=e}$, i.e. $z[Se_{FPR=e}]$. For example, for the ROC curve specified by $a=1.19$ and $b=1$, we first calculate the sensitivity at a FPR of 0.10 by solving for sensitivity in the equation (6.11):

$$a = b\Phi^{-1}(1.0 - FPR) - \Phi^{-1}(1.0 - Se). \qquad (6.11)$$

We obtain a value of 0.54 for the sensitivity of CTC at a FPR of 0.10. We desire a CI for the sensitivity no longer than 0.44 to 0.64 (that is, 0.54 ± 0.10 in terms of the untransformed values). We use the equation (6.11) again to determine the values of parameter a that correspond with sensitivities of 0.44 and 0.64 (fixing $b=1.0$ and FPR=0.10). The corresponding parameter a's are 1.13 and 1.64, respectively. From the equation (6.9) the z-transformed values of sensitivity are -0.15 and 0.36, respectively. The width of the CI for $z[Se_{FPR=e}]$ is $(0.36 - -0.15) = 0.51$; thus, $L = 0.255$ (in terms of the transformed values). From the equation (6.10), the variance function of the z-transformed sensitivity is as follows, setting $R = 1$: $[1 + 1/1 + 1.19^2/2] +$ $(-1.28)^2[1(1 + 1)/(2)] = 4.346$. Finally, from equation 6.2, the number of patients with colon polyps required for the study is n=257 and the total number of patients needed for the study is n(1+R)=514.

Note that the sample size can vary dramatically depending on the shape of the ROC curve. So, one might calculate sample size for ROC curves of different shapes and choose a sample size that covers the likely range of shapes. Alternatively, it might be worthwhile to conduct a small pilot study to estimate parameter b, then choose a sample size appropriate for the shape of the curve.

In the special situation where the observed test results are on a truly continuous scale and they follow a binormal distribution (or can be transformed to a binormal distribution), there is a more efficient estimator for the variance function. Obuchowski and McClish (1997) proposed the following estimator of the variance function for the sensitivity at a fixed FPR:
$\hat{V}(z[\hat{Se}_{FPR=e}]) = [1 + b^2/R + a^2/2] + g^2[b^2(1 + R)/(2R)] + g[ab]$.

For computing sample size for a study using the specificity at a fixed FNR as a measure of accuracy, one can simply switch definitions of sensitivity and specificity and use these same formulae. For example, suppose we want to construct a CI for the specificity of CTC at a fixed FNR=0.10 (i.e. 10% of subjects with polyps are incorrectly called "polyp-free"). For sample size calculations, we would redefine sensitivity as the proportion of normal patients correctly called "polyp-free" and specificity as the proportion of patients with polyps where polyps are correctly detected. With these definitions, the measure of accuracy is once again the sensitivity at a FPR=0.10, and the calculations are the same as those illustrated above.

6.1.6 Sample Size for Estimating the Partial Area Under the ROC Curve - Case Study 2

Continuing with the CTC example, suppose we are interested in designing a study to estimate the average sensitivity of CTC in the FPR range of 0.0 to 0.10. Suppose we want to estimate the average sensitivity to within ±0.10. We want to determine how many patients are needed for the study. Note that for ease in interpretation we have described the example in terms of the *average sensitivity* in a FPR range (i.e. $A_{e_1 \leq FPR \leq e_2}/(e_2 - e_1)$), but we will derive the sample size for this example in terms of the partial area under the ROC curve (i.e. $A_{e_1 \leq FPR \leq e_2}$) (See Chapter 2 for a distinction between these two).

We use the equation (6.2) to compute the required sample size. Here, θ is the partial area under the ROC curve in the FPR range of e_1 to e_2 (i.e. $A_{e_1 \leq FPR \leq e_2}$), and n is the number of patients with colon polyps needed for the study (we assume one polyp per patient). Obuchowski and McClish (1997) proposed an estimator of the variance for the partial area which can be used for sample size calculation. It is appropriate for tests with either ordinal or continuous test results where the underlying distribution is binormal. (The assumption is that the unobserved, underlying test results follow a binormal distribution, but the observed test results, either continuous or ordinal, do not necessarily have a binormal distribution.) The variance function of the partial area in the FPR range of e_1 to e_2 is

$$\hat{V}(\hat{A}_{e_1 \leq FPR \leq e_2}) = f^2[1 + b^2/R + a^2/2] + g^2[b^2(1 + R)/(2R)], \qquad (6.12)$$

where f and g are functions of binormal parameters a and b and the FPR range of interest, as follows:

$$f = (expr_1) \times [2\pi(expr_2)]^{-1/2} \times (expr_3)$$

and

$$g = (expr_1) \times [2\pi(expr_2)]^{-1} \times (expr_4) - (ab) \times (expr_1) \times [2\pi(expr_2)^3]^{-1/2} \times (expr_3),$$

where $expr_1 = e^{(-a^2/(2[1+b^2]))}$, $expr_2 = (1+b^2)$, $expr_3 = \Phi(e_2') - \Phi(e_1')$, Φ is the cumulative normal distribution function, $expr_4 = e^{(-e_1'')} - e^{(-e_2'')}$, $e_i' = [\Phi^{-1}(e_i) + (ab) \times (1+b^2)^{-1}] \times (1+b^2)^{1/2}$, and $e_i'' = (e_i')^2/2$.

We first calculate the partial area under the ROC curve in the FPR range of 0.0-0.10 using the integral for a binormal distribution given in Chapter 4 (see the equation (4.52)). For illustration, we use the same binormal parameters as in the previous example: $a=1.19$ and $b=1.0$. The resulting partial area is 0.0303. The average sensitivity in a FPR range is computed by dividing the partial area by the range for the FPRs (See Chapter 2). The average sensitivity in the FPR range of 0.0 to 0.10 is $0.0303/0.10 = 0.303$. The values of f and g are: f=0.0328127 and g=-0.0543776. From equation 6.12 we calculate the variance function as: $\hat{V}(\hat{A}_{0.0 \le FPR \le 0.1}) = (0.0328127)^2[1 + (1)^2/(1) + (1.19)^2/2] + (-0.0543776)^2[(1)^2(2)/(2)] = 0.005873$

We want to estimate the average sensitivity to within ±0.10. In terms of the partial area under the ROC curve, $L = 0.10 \times (e_2 - e_1)$. Thus, in the equation (6.2), L=0.01. The number of patients with polyps needed for the study is 226, and n(1+R)=452 total patients are needed.

The sample size requirements for the partial area under the ROC curve will vary depending on the shape of the ROC curve. Investigators should consider the sample size requirements for a range of values for parameter b before deciding on the sample size for their study.

In the special situation where the observed test results follow a binormal distribution, and thus, a and b can be estimated directly from the sample mean and sample variance, Obuchowski and McClish (1997) offered the following alternative estimator of the variance function for the partial area under the ROC curve. We warn that this estimator should only be used in this special case. $\hat{V}(\hat{A}_{e_1 \le FPR \le e_2}) = f^2[1 + b^2/R + a^2/2] + g^2[b^2(1+R)/(2R)] + fg[ab]$.

6.2 SAMPLE SIZE FOR DETECTING A DIFFERENCE IN ACCURACIES OF TWO TESTS

The goal of many diagnostic accuracy studies is to test whether the accuracies of two or more diagnostic tests (or display modes, or reading formats, etc.) are different. For these studies the sample size must be adequate to ensure that, if the tests truly have different accuracies, then the study has a high probability (power) of detecting a difference. For sample size calculation we can specify the minimum difference in accuracy between the tests that is clinically important to detect. Often, however, this minimum difference is very small; thus, the study requires an enormous sample. Another strategy is to specify the suspected difference in accuracy between the tests. The suspected difference is usually larger than the clinical minimum difference; thus, the required sample size is more reasonable. We denote the suspected difference in accuracy between the two tests as Δ_1. We now discuss sample size methods for testing for differences between tests for a variety of measures of test accuracy.

6.2.1   Sample Size Software

There are several software programs for computing sample size for studies comparing the accuracies of two tests. Some general software packages compute sample size for a limited number of situations. For example, PASS (available at www.ncss.com/pass _ procedures.html) computes sample size for studies comparing two tests' ROC areas from a paired design. There are some specialized software programs designed just for diagnostic test studies that offer more options. Metz and his colleagues have a FORTRAN program ROCPWR (www-radiology.uchicago.edu/krl/KRL _ ROC/software _ index6.htm) that computes power for studies of the comparison of two diagnostic tests' ROC areas, their sensitivities at a fixed FPR (or specificities at a fixed FNR), and the two tests' ROC curves. Another FORTRAN program is DESIGNROC (www.lerner.ccf.org/qhs/software/roc _ analysis.php) which computes sample size or power for studies comparing two diagnostic tests' ROC areas, their sensitivities at a fixed FPR (or specificities at a fixed FNR), and their partial areas at fixed FPR ranges (or fixed FNR ranges). In a simulation study, Obuchowski and McClish (1997) showed that ROCPWR and DESIGNROC yield very similar estimates of study power.

Software is also available directly from many of the authors of papers on sample size.

6.2.2   Sample Size for Comparing Tests' Sensitivity and/or Specificity - Case Study 1

In the SPECT study (Case Study 1), suppose we want to compare the sensitivity of SPECT to SPECT and Computed Tomography interpreted together (SPECT/CT). We suspect that the sensitivity of SPECT/CT will exceed that of SPECT. We want to test this hypothesis.

The null and alternative hypotheses are

$$H_0\colon \theta_1 = \theta_2$$

$$H_1\colon \theta_1 \neq \theta_2,$$

where θ_1 is the diagnostic accuracy of SPECT and θ_2 is the diagnostic accuracy of SPECT/CT. For sample size calculations we must specify, Δ_1, a value for the difference between θ_1 and θ_2 under the alternative hypothesis. A general formula for computing sample size for such a study is

$$n = \frac{[z_{\alpha/2}\sqrt{V_o(\hat{\theta}_1 - \hat{\theta}_2)} + z_\beta\sqrt{V_A(\hat{\theta}_1 - \hat{\theta}_2)}]^2}{(\Delta_1)^2}, \tag{6.13}$$

where $z_{\alpha/2}$ is the upper $\alpha/2$ percentile of a standard normal distribution, α is the type I error rate (two-tailed test in our example), z_β is the upper β percentile of a standard normal distribution, and β is the type II error rate (or 1-power). $V_o(\hat{\theta}_1 - \hat{\theta}_2)$ is the variance function of the estimated difference in accuracy between the two tests under the null hypothesis, and $V_A(\hat{\theta}_1 - \hat{\theta}_2)$ is the variance function of the estimated difference in accuracy between the two tests under the alternative hypothesis. We assume that the variance of $\hat{\theta}_1 - \hat{\theta}_2$ can be written as $V(\hat{\theta}_1 - \hat{\theta}_2)/n$, where $V(\hat{\theta}_1 - \hat{\theta}_2)$ does not depend on n. As we will see, n in the equation (6.13) takes on different meanings depending on the application.

The variance functions $V_o(\hat{\theta}_1 - \hat{\theta}_2)$ and $V_A(\hat{\theta}_1 - \hat{\theta}_2)$ take the general form:

$$V(\hat{\theta}_1 - \hat{\theta}_2) = V(\hat{\theta}_1) + V(\hat{\theta}_2) - 2C(\hat{\theta}_1, \hat{\theta}_2), \tag{6.14}$$

where $C(\hat{\theta}_1, \hat{\theta}_2)$ is the covariance function of $\hat{\theta}_1$ and $\hat{\theta}_2$. $C(\hat{\theta}_1, \hat{\theta}_2)$ equals zero for studies where different patients are evaluated by the two tests (i.e. unpaired study design), and often takes a positive value when the same patients are evaluated by both tests.

Beam (1992) presented formulae for determining the sample size of studies comparing the sensitivity and/or specificity of two tests. When the same patients will undergo both tests (i.e. paired study design), Beam recommends the equation (6.13) be used, where the variance functions are given by

$$V_o(\hat{Se}_1 - \hat{Se}_2) = \psi$$
$$V_A(\hat{Se}_1 - \hat{Se}_2) = \psi - \Delta_1{}^2, \tag{6.15}$$

where

$$\psi = Se_1 + Se_2 - 2 \times Se_2 \times P(T_1 = 1|T_2 = 1), \tag{6.16}$$

Se_1 and Se_2 are the conjectured values of sensitivity from the alternative hypothesis, and $P(T_1 = 1|T_2 = 1)$ is the probability that the first test is positive given that the second test is positive (Connor, 1987). The value of ψ ranges from Δ_1 (when there is perfect correlation between the test results) to $Se_1 \times (1 - Se_2) + (1 - Se_1) \times Se_2$ (when the correlation between the test results equals zero) (Beam, 1992). The variance functions are similar for specificity.

In our example, we suspect that the difference in sensitivity between SPECT and SPECT/CT is 0.10; thus, we set $\Delta_1 = 0.10$. Under the null hypothesis we set $Se_1 = Se_2 = 0.75$. Under the alternative hypothesis we set $Se_1 = 0.80$ and $Se_2 = 0.70$. We will compare the sample size requirements for unpaired and paired study designs with type I error rate of 5% and power of 80%.

The value of ψ in the equation (6.16) ranges from 0.10 (paired design where there is perfect correlation in the results of SPECT and SPECT/CT) to 0.38 (zero correlation between the test results, or unpaired design). Substituting into the equation (6.13), n ranges from 77 to 296. For a study using an unpaired design, a total of 592 patients with a diseased parathyroid gland are needed (i.e. 296 to undergo SPECT and 296 to undergo SPECT/CT). With a paired design we may need as few as 77 patients and as many as 296 patients with a diseased parathyroid gland, depending on the correlation in the test results of SPECT and SPECT/CT. In the paired design all n patients undergo both SPECT and SPECT/CT; thus, the paired design offers a savings of 296 to 515 patients over the unpaired study design. Without any information about the value of the correlation between the results of SPECT and SPECT/CT, it is advisable to use a sample size closer to 296 to ensure adequate power. It may be cost-effective to perform a pilot study to estimate the correlation and thus hopefully justify a smaller sample size.

In unpaired study designs there are situations where the sample size for one test is fixed (e.g. the study has already been performed for one test) and one needs to compute the sample size for the other test. Let n_1 denote the fixed sample size for one of the tests and n_2 the unknown sample size for the other test. Arkin and Wachtel (1990) recommend the following formula for computing n_2 (Cohen, 1977)

$$n_2 = (n \times n_1)/(2n_1 - n), \tag{6.17}$$

where n is the sample size from the equation (6.13).

6.2.3 Sample Size for Comparing Tests' Positive and Negative Predictive Values - Case Study 1

Suppose we want to compare the positive predictive value (PPV) and negative predictive value (NPV) of SPECT and SPECT/CT for detecting diseased parathyroid glands. As we discussed in Chapter 3, PPV and NPV are affected by the prevalence of the condition in the sample. Since Case Study 1 was originally designed as a prospective trial, we assume that the prevalence of the condition in our sample will be generalizable to a clinical population.

Moskowitz and Pepe (2006) describe a method of computing sample size for prospective studies comparing two tests where the tests are performed on all patients (paired design); sample size calculations for unpaired designs are given by Pepe (2003).

Moskowitz and Pepe (2006) define the relative predictive values of two tests, A and B, as follows:

$$rPPV = \frac{PPV_1}{PPV_2} \quad and \quad rNPV = \frac{NPV_1}{NPV_2},$$

where PPV_1 and NPV_1 are the positive and negative predictive values of test 1. To test that the PPV of test 1 is superior to test 2, we write the null hypothesis as: $H_o : rPPV \leq \delta$, where $\delta = 1$. To test that the PPV of test 1 is not equal to test 2, we write the hypothesis as: $H_o : rPPV = \delta$ and $H_A : rPPV \neq \delta$, where δ would be one.

The required sample size for rPPV is:

$$n = [\frac{z_\beta + z_\alpha}{log(\gamma/\delta)}]^2 \times [(p_5 + p_6)(p_5 + p_7)]^{-1} \times \{2(p_7 + p_3)\gamma PPV_2^2 +$$

$$(-p_6 + p_5(1 - \gamma))PPV_2 + p_6 + p_7(1 - 3\gamma PPV_2)\}, \tag{6.18}$$

where $(1 - \alpha)$ is the level of the confidence interval for rPPV (for a two-tailed test, this would be $(1 - \alpha/2)$) and the study power is $(1 - \beta)$. γ is a specific value of interest for rPPV under the alternative hypothesis.

Similarly, for rNPV the required sample size is:

$$n = [\frac{(z_\beta + z_\alpha)^2}{log(\gamma/\delta)}]^2 \times [(p_2 + p_4)(p_3 + p_4)]^{-1} \times \{-2(p_4 + p_8)\gamma NPV_2^2 +$$

$$(-p_3 + p_4 - \gamma(p_2 - p_4))NPV_2 + p_2 + p_3\}, \tag{6.19}$$

where γ is a specific value of interest for rNPV under the alternative hypothesis.

For patients without the condition, p_1 is the proportion of patients testing positive on both tests, p_2 is the proportion testing positive on test 1 and negative on test 2, p_3 is the proportion testing positive on test 2 and negative on test 1, and p_4 is the proportion testing negative on both tests. For patients with the condition, p_5 is the proportion of patients testing positive on both tests, p_6 is the proportion testing positive on test 1 and negative on test 2, p_7 is the proportion testing positive on test 2 and negative on test 1, and p_8 is the proportion testing negative on both tests. The formulae require estimates of these proportions. Moskowitz and Pepe (2006) recommend a small pilot study to estimate these proportions.

We will use the data from Case Study 1 as pilot study data to plan a bigger trial. Let PPV_1 and PPV_2 denote the PPVs of SPECT/CT and SPECT, respectively. The hypotheses are $H_o : rPPV = 1$ and $H_A : rPPV \neq 1$. Under the alternative hypothesis, we conjecture that the PPV of SPECT will be 0.8 and the PPV of SPECT/CT will be 10% greater; thus, we set $\gamma = 1.1$. Suppose we want a study with 80% power and 5% type I error rate (two-tailed). From the pilot study, we estimate the following proportions: p_1=0.04, p_2=0.0, p_3=0.52, and p_4=0.44; p_5=0.70, p_6=0.0, p_7=0.10, and p_8=0.20.

The required sample size is: $n = [\frac{0.84+1.96}{0.04139}]^2 \times [(0.70+0.0)(0.70+0.10)]^{-1} \times [2(0.10+0.52)(1.1)(0.64)+(-0.0+0.70(-0.1))(0.8)+0.0+0.10(1-3(1.1)(0.8))] = 5337$. With patients from a similar population as in the pilot study, a total of 5337 patients are needed; thus, it takes a very large study to detect a rather small difference, i.e. a 10% difference, in the PPVs of SPECT and SPECT/CT.

6.2.4 Sample Size for Comparing Tests' Area Under the ROC Curve - Case Study 2

We return to the CTC cancer screening study. Suppose we are designing a study to compare the ROC areas of a reader using CTC vs. the same reader using CTC with a computer aided detection (CAD) algorithm to aid the reader in finding polyps. The reader will review each image and assign a percent confidence score to each detected polyp. Under the null hypothesis, we assume that the reader has a ROC area of 0.80 with just CTC and that the reader's accuracy is not affected by the CAD marks. Under the alternative hypothesis, we conjecture that the reader's ROC area improves to 0.90 with CAD; thus, $\Delta_1 = 0.10$. We want to determine the required sample size for the study.

Obuchowski and McClish (1997) use the general sample size formula in the equation (6.13) to compute sample size for studies comparing the areas under two ROC curves. For indices associated with the ROC curve, n in the equation (6.13) is the number of patients with the condition; the total sample size required (i.e. patients with and without the condition) is $n(1+R)$, where R is the ratio of sample sizes of patients without to with the condition in the sample. The variance function of the difference in accuracies of two tests is given in the equation (6.14). An estimate of $V(\hat{A}_i)$, which assumes an underlying binormal distribution for the test results, was given in the equation (6.5). $C(\hat{A}_1, \hat{A}_2)$ should be set to zero for an unpaired study design. For a paired study design, Obuchowski and McClish recommend the following estimator for $C(\hat{A}_1, \hat{A}_2)$ for sample size estimation; note that it assumes an underlying bivariate binormal distribution for the test results:

$$\hat{C}(\hat{A}_1, \hat{A}_2) = \frac{e^{(-[a_1^2+a_2^2]/4)}}{12.5664} \times [r_D + \frac{r_N}{R} + \frac{r_D^2 a_1 a_2}{2}]$$
$$+ \frac{e^{(-[a_1^2+a_2^2]/4)}}{50.2655} \times [\frac{a_1 a_2(r_N^2 + R r_D^2)}{2R}]$$
$$- \frac{e^{(-[a_1^2+a_2^2]/4)}}{25.1327} \times [r_D^2 a_1 a_2], \tag{6.20}$$

where a_i is binormal parameter a for the i-th diagnostic test, r_D is the correlation of the underlying bivariate binormal distribution for patients with the condition, and r_N is the correlation of the underlying bivariate binormal distribution for patients without the condition.

Metz (1989) offer a similar approach to computing sample size in their FORTRAN program ROCPWR. Like the method of Obuchowski and McClish (1997), ROCPWR assumes an underlying bivariate binormal distribution for the test results. In both approaches one must specify the parameters of this assumed bivariate binormal distribution. One major difference between these two approaches is that ROCPWR takes into consideration the values of the decision threshold used to obtain the ordinal test results, while the approach of Obuchowski and McClish does not. In a Monte Carlo simulation study, Obuchowski and McClish found that both ROCPWR and their approach work reasonably well for either ordinal or continuous test results.

In our CTC example, under the null hypothesis, we specify $b_1 = b_2 = 1.0$ and $a_1 = a_2 = 1.19$, corresponding to an ROC area of 0.80. For the alternative hypothesis, we specify $b_1 = b_2 = 1.0$, $a_1 = 1.19$, and $a_2 = 1.82$, corresponding to ROC areas of 0.80 and 0.90, respectively (from Table 6.1). We assume that, by design, there will be equal numbers of patients with and without colon polyps; thus, R=1.0. We consider correlations for the underlying bivariate binormal distribution (i.e. $r_D = r_N$) of zero for an unpaired design and 0.50, corresponding to a typical value for the correlation between tests in a paired design (Rockette et al., 1999). Then, using the FORTRAN program DESIGNROC, for the unpaired design for 80% power and 5% (two-tailed) type I error rate, 173 patients with colon polyps need to be interpreted with CTC alone and 173 patients with colon polyps need to be interpreted with CTC and the aid of CAD; similarly, 173 patients without polyps need to be interpreted with CTC alone and 173 patients without polyps need to be interpreted with CTC and the aid of CAD (total of 692 patients). In contrast, for a paired design, 114 patients with colon polyps and 114 patients without colon polyps are needed (total of 228 patients).

For comparison, for a design with twice as many patients without polyps as with polyps (i.e. R=2.0), a total of 840 patients are needed for the unpaired design and 288 for the paired design.

Blume (2009) provide the variance functions for comparing two tests such that the sample size will be the smallest needed for a study with *any* underlying distribution of the test results.

$$V_o(\hat{\theta}_1 - \hat{\theta}_2) = \theta_1(1 - \theta_1) + \theta_1(1 - \theta_1) - 2r\sqrt{\theta_1(1 - \theta_1)\theta_1(1 - \theta_1)}$$

$$V_A(\hat{\theta}_1 - \hat{\theta}_2) = \theta_1(1 - \theta_1) + \theta_2(1 - \theta_2) - 2r\sqrt{\theta_1(1 - \theta_1)\theta_2(1 - \theta_2)}, \quad (6.21)$$

where r is the correlation between the tests because of the paired design. Continuing with the CTC example, with R=1, the total sample size that would ensure that the study had power of $(1 - \beta)$ regardless of the underlying test distribution is 936 for the unpaired design (compared to 692 assuming a bivariate binormal distribution) and 238 for the paired design (compared to 228 assuming a bivariate binormal distribution).

6.2.5   Sample Size for Comparing Tests with Clustered Data

For studies with clustered data, e.g. multiple polyps in the same patient, we can use the equation (6.7) to determine the number of segments with polyps needed for the study, after adjusting for the correlation between segments from the same patient. Suppose we expect 1.5 segments with polyps per patient, on average, and we assume moderate correlation of 0.5 between segments from the same patient. In the equation (6.7): s=1.5, r=0.5, and n=114 (using the variance function based on the binormal distribution for a paired design). The number of segments with polyps required for the study is then 142.5; therefore, we need about 95 patients with one or more polyps for the study. We can perform a similar calculation to determine the number of segments without polyps needed for the study; however, we recommend maintaining the ratio of R=1 patients without to with polyps as we discussed in section 6.1.3. Thus, about 190 total patients are needed with a clustered study design, as compared to 228 for a study that treats each patient as the unit of observation (17% savings).

Liu et al. (2005) also describe estimation of the sample size for clustered data when comparing two tests' ROC areas. They consider the special case where the test results are continuous and follow a normal distribution. Their formula includes estimates of the correlation between diseased lesions from the same patient, correlation between non-diseased lesions from the same patient, correlation between non-diseased and diseased lesions from the same patient, and correlation between the two tests with a paired design. They illustrate their method for a colon cancer study where the lesion's size as measured on the CT will be compared to metabolic uptake as measured on PET, both tests measured on truly continuous scales. Note that this method is not applicable in our CTC example because confidence levels rarely follow normal distributions. Interested readers should consult Liu's manuscript for details and illustrations.

6.2.5.1 Determining an Appropriate Value for the Difference in ROC Areas It is often difficult to determine a reasonable value for the difference in ROC areas between two tests, i.e. Δ_1, yet this value is critical to the sample size calculation. The difference in ROC areas tells us the *average* difference in sensitivity between the two tests over all false positive rates. The difference in sensitivity can vary considerably, however, over the range of false positive rates. For example, consider two ROC curves that are parallel; one with an ROC area of 0.7 and the other with an ROC area of 0.72. The average difference in sensitivity between the two tests over all FPRs is 0.02, but this difference varies from a difference near zero at very low and very high FPRs, to larger values in the middle of the curve. In the clinically relevant range of FPRs of 0.05 to 0.15, the difference in sensitivity is 0.03 to 0.04. Consider a second example where the difference is large between the two ROC curves' areas. For two parallel ROC curves, one with ROC area of 0.85 and one with area of 0.95, the *average* difference in sensitivity is 0.10, but in the FPR range of 0.05 to 0.20, the difference in sensitivity ranges from 0.20 to 0.33 (Obuchowski, 2003). The differences can be much larger, even changing the direction of the difference, for ROC curves that are not parallel.

For sample size calculations, we may have some pilot data on the difference in sensitivity between two tests at a common FPR, or we may just be able to conjecture the difference in sensitivity between two tests. We recommend that the effect size, in terms of the difference in ROC areas, Δ_1, be a value less than this difference in sensitivity. For small differences in sensitivity, e.g. ≤ 0.05, one might choose an effect size for the ROC area of ≤ 0.025. For larger differences in sensitivity, e.g. 0.10-0.20, one might choose an effect size of < 0.10 for the ROC area.

6.2.6 Sample Size for Comparing Tests' Sensitivity at Fixed FPR - Case Study 2

In the CTC study, suppose we want to compare the sensitivity of the reader with CTC alone vs. with CAD at a fixed FPR of 0.10. Obuchowski and McClish (1997) proposed a method for sample size estimation for studies comparing the sensitivities of two tests at a fixed FPR of e. The method is based on an underlying bivariate binormal distribution for the test results. To calculate sample size, we transform the sensitivities using the equation (6.9). Then the formula in the equation (6.13) is used, where $V(\hat{\theta}_1 - \hat{\theta}_2)$ is given in (6.14), n is the number of patients with the condition needed for the study, and the total sample size required is n(1+R). An estimate of $V((\hat{Se}_{FPR=e})_i)$ was given in the equation (6.10), and an estimate of $C((\hat{Se}_{FPR=e})_1, (\hat{Se}_{FPR=e})_2)$ appropriate for sample size estimation is

$$\hat{C}((\hat{Se}_{FPR=e})_1, (\hat{Se}_{FPR=e})_2) = [r_D + \frac{r_N b_1 b_2}{R} + \frac{r_D^2 a_1 a_2}{2}]$$

$$+ g^2 \times [\frac{b_1 b_2 (r_N^2 + R r_D^2)}{2R}]$$

$$+ \frac{g r_D^2}{2} \times [a_1 b_2 + a_2 b_1], \tag{6.22}$$

where $g = \Phi^{-1}(e)$.

Returning to our example, under the null hypothesis we assume that $a=1.19$ and $b=1.0$ for both ROC curves. Under the alternative hypothesis, we assume that $a=1.19$ and $b=1.0$ for the reader with just CTC and $a=1.82$ and $b=1.0$ when the reader has CAD as an aid. This corresponds to a difference in ROC areas of 0.10, and a difference in sensitivities of $\Delta_1=0.17$ (at a FPR of 0.10) (from the equation (6.11)). For an unpaired study with equal numbers of patients with and without polyps (R=1), using the software DESIGNROC, 178 patients with polyps are needed for interpretation with CTC alone and 178 patients with polyps are needed for interpretation with CAD. Similar numbers of patients without polyps are needed. For a paired design with $r_D=r_N=0.5$, 130 patients with polyps and 130 patients without polyps are needed.

We again point out that both the shape of the ROC curve (as defined by binormal parameter b) and the FPR value affect the sample size. In general, as the FPR value increases (i.e. moving closer to the middle of the same ROC curve), the sample size requirements decrease. For example, for a paired design at a FPR of 0.05, 167 patients with and without polyps are needed; at a FPR of 0.20, 97 patients with and without polyps are needed. The reduction in sample size requirement as the FPR increases is due, at least in part, to an increase in the difference in the sensitivities. Although we are comparing the same two ROC curves (a=1.19, b=1.0 versus a=1.82, b=1.0), the difference in their sensitivities changes for different FPRs. At a FPR=0.10, the difference in sensitivity is 0.17 and 260 total patients were needed (for a paired design); at a FPR=0.20, the difference in sensitivity is 0.20 and 194 total patients were needed.

The effect of the ROC curve shape on the sample size is less predictable, depending on whether the curves cross or not and their specific shapes.

Finally, we note that ROCPWR (Metz, 1989) also computes power for studies comparing the sensitivities of two tests at a fixed FPR. In a simulation study, Obuchowski and McClish (1997) found that both ROCPWR and DESIGNROC work reasonably well for continuous test results; however, both may underestimate the sample size required for studies with ordinal test results.

6.2.7   Sample Size for Comparing Tests' Partial Area Under the ROC Curve - Case Study 2

Continuing with the CTC study, suppose we want to compare the average sensitivity of the reader with CTC versus the same reader with the aid of CAD. Suppose we are interested in comparing sensitivities in the prespecified FPR range of 0.0 to 0.20. How large of a sample is needed for such a study?

Obuchowski and McClish (1997) proposed a method for sample size estimation for studies comparing the partial areas of two tests. Their method is based on an underlying bivariate binormal distribution for the test results. The formula in the equation (6.13) is used, where n is the number of patients with the condition needed for the study, n(1+R) is the total sample size needed, $V(\hat{\theta}_1 - \hat{\theta}_2)$ is given in (6.14), an estimate of $V((\hat{A}_{e_1 \leq FPR \leq e_2})_i)$ was given in equation (6.12), and an estimate of $C((\hat{A}_{e_1 \leq FPR \leq e_2})_1, (\hat{A}_{e_1 \leq FPR \leq e_2})_2)$ is

$$\hat{C}((\hat{A}_{e_1 \leq FPR \leq e_2})_1, (\hat{A}_{e_1 \leq FPR \leq e_2})_2) = f_1 f_2 \times [r_D + \frac{r_N b_1 b_2}{R} + \frac{r_D^2 a_1 a_2}{2}]$$

$$+ g_1 g_2 \times [\frac{b_1 b_2 (r_N^2 + R r_D^2)}{2R}]$$

$$+ f_1 g_2 \times \frac{[r_D^2 a_1 b_2]}{2} + f_1 g_2 \times [r_D^2 a_2 b_1], \tag{6.23}$$

where f_1 and g_1 are functions of a_1, b_1, e_1, and e_2, and f_2 and g_2 are functions of a_2, b_2, as well as e_1 and e_2 (See the equation (6.12) for definitions of these functions).

Under the null hypothesis we assume that $a=1.19$ and $b=1.0$ for both ROC curves. Under the alternative hypothesis, we assume that $a=1.19$ and $b=1.0$ for the reader with just CTC and $a=1.82$ and $b=1.0$ when the reader has CAD as an aid. This corresponds to a difference in ROC areas of 0.10, and a difference in the partial area under the ROC curve of $\Delta_1=0.0448$. For an unpaired study with equal numbers of patients with and without polyps ($R=1$), using the program DESIGNROC, 184 patients with polyps are needed for interpretation with CTC alone and 184 patients with polyps are needed for interpretation with CAD. Similar numbers of patients without polyps are needed. For a paired design with $r_D=r_N=0.5$, 135 patients with polyps and 135 patients without polyps are needed.

As with the sensitivity at a fixed FPR, the sample size required for a study comparing tests' partial areas under the ROC curves depends on the shapes of the ROC curves and the false positive rate ranges. For example, for a paired design in the FPR range of 0.0 to 0.10, 148 patients with and without polyps are needed; in the FPR range of 0.0 to 0.30, 128 patients with and without polyps are needed.

6.2.7.1 Comparison of Sample Size Requirements for ROC Area, Sensitivity at Fixed FPR, and Partial Area

We complete this section with a comparison of the sample size required with seven different measures of accuracy: 1) ROC area, 2) sensitivity at a fixed FPR of 0.01, 3) sensitivity at a fixed FPR of 0.10, 4) sensitivity at a fixed FPR of 0.20, 5) average sensitivity in the FPR range of 0.0 to 0.10, 6) average sensitivity in the FPR range of 0.0 to 0.20, and 7) average sensitivity in the FPR range of 0.10 to 0.20. For consistency across measures, we use the sample size approach of Obuchowski and McClish (1997). For each measure of accuracy we will use the same values for the parameters of the bivariate binormal distribution. Under the null hypothesis, we assume $b_1 = b_2 = 1.0$ and $a_1 = a_2 = 1.46$. Under the alternative hypothesis we assume $b_1 = b_2 = 1.0$, $a_1 = 1.46$, and $a_2 = 0.95$. We set $r_N = r_D = 0.25$. We specify a two-tailed test with $\alpha = 0.05$ and $\beta = 0.20$.

Table 6.2 summarizes the number of patients with the condition required for each measure of accuracy for two values of R: 0.176 and 1.0. The table also gives the detectable difference in accuracy (i.e. Δ_1) for each measure. The sample size requirements for the different measures of accuracy vary considerably. The sample size requirement is smallest for a study using the ROC area and largest for a study using the sensitivity at a FPR of 0.01. In general, studies using the ROC area will require smaller sample sizes than studies using these other measures. To compare the sample size requirements for studies using the partial area and studies using the sensitivity at a fixed FPR, consider $Se_{FPR=0.10}$ versus $Se_{0.10 \leq FPR \leq 0.20}$. The detectable differences, Δ_1, are similar yet the required sample size is considerably smaller for the partial area measure. Although it may be tempting to choose a measure of accuracy after considering the required sample size, this strategy is ill-advised. The measure of accuracy should be chosen based on the clinical questions that the study will attempt to answer; however, consideration of the sample size, cost, and duration of the study may influence the clinical questions that can be addressed.

Table 6.2   Number of Patients with the Condition Required for Comparing the Same Two ROC Curves But Using Different Measures of Accuracy.

		SAMPLE SIZE	
Measure	Δ_1	*R=0.176*	*R=1.0*
ROC Area	0.100	358	139
$Se_{FPR=0.01}$	0.108	1394	465
$Se_{FPR=0.10}$	0.201	675	246
$Se_{FPR=0.20}$	0.276	496	191
$A_{0.0 \leq FPR \leq 0.10}/(e_2 - e_1)$	0.167	1031	361
$A_{0.0 \leq FPR \leq 0.20}/(e_2 - e_1)$	0.182	722	261
$A_{0.10 \leq FPR \leq 0.20}/(e_2 - e_1)$	0.198	515	192

6.3   SAMPLE SIZE FOR ASSESSING NON-INFERIORITY OR EQUIVALENCY OF TWO TESTS

A common goal of diagnostic accuracy studies is to assess whether the accuracies of two diagnostic tests (or display modes, or reading formats, etc.) are equivalent or whether the accuracy of a new test (which might have fewer complications) is non-inferior to an existing test. For these studies, the sample size must be adequate to ensure that, if the two tests' accuracies truly are equivalent (or non-inferior), then the study has a high probability (power) of showing their equivalence. For sample size calculation we need to specify the smallest difference in accuracy which would not be considered equivalent (or not considered non-inferior). We denote this unacceptable difference by Δ_M. We now discuss sample size methods for testing for equivalency or non-inferiority. We present general formulae appropriate for any measure of test accuracy; the formulae can be used by substituting in the appropriate variance functions described in previous sections of this chapter.

Suppose we are designing a study to determine whether or not the diagnostic accuracy of 3-dimensional (3D) mammography is as good as (i.e. non-inferior to) the diagnostic accuracy of conventional, 2-dimensional (2D) mammography. We are particularly interested in the ability of the two image formats to distinguish malignant from benign lesions. A single mammographer will interpret the 3D and 2D images from the same patients during separate, masked, reading sessions. The area under the ROC curve will be used as the measure of accuracy. We have determined that the ROC area of the 3D image cannot be 0.05 lower than the ROC area for 2D. That is, if the ROC area with 2D is 0.90, then the ROC area of the 3D image must be better than 0.85 to be considered non-inferior. We want to determine the number of patients required for this study.

The null and alternative hypotheses are

$$H_0: (\theta_S - \theta_E) \geq \Delta_M$$

$$H_1: (\theta_S - \theta_E) < \Delta_M \ ,$$

where θ_S is the true accuracy of the standard test (i.e. 2D), θ_E is the true accuracy of the experimental test (i.e. 3D images), and Δ_M is the smallest difference in accuracy which is not acceptable. For our example, $\Delta_M = 0.05$. For this set of hypotheses the Type I error rate is the probability of concluding that the experimental test is not inferior, when in truth the standard test is more accurate. The Type II error rate is the probability of concluding that the standard test is more accurate, when in truth the experimental test is not inferior to the standard test.

For sample size calculations we must specify values for θ_S and θ_E under the alternative hypothesis. Note that θ_S and θ_E do not have to take the same value, but $\theta_S - \theta_E$ must be less than Δ_M. We apply the sample size formula for testing non-inferiority given by Blackwelder (1982).

$$n = \frac{(z_\alpha + z_\beta)^2 V_A(\hat{\theta}_S - \hat{\theta}_E)}{(\theta_S - \theta_E - \Delta_M)^2}, \tag{6.24}$$

where θ_S and θ_E are the conjectured accuracies of the two tests under the alternative hypothesis, z_α is the upper α percentile of a standard normal distribution, α is the type I error rate (one-tailed test), z_β is the upper β percentile of a standard normal distribution, β is the type II error rate (or 1-power), $V_A(\hat{\theta}_E - \hat{\theta}_S)$ is the variance function for the difference in accuracy of the two tests under the alternative hypothesis, and n is the number of patients with the condition required (for paired designs) or the number of patients with the condition required for each test (unpaired design). $V_A(\hat{\theta}_E - \hat{\theta}_S)$ is a function of R, the ratio of the sample sizes of patients without to with the condition. Thus, the total sample size required is $n(1+R)$. As in the equation (6.1), (6.2) and (6.13) we assume that the variance of $(\hat{\theta}_E - \hat{\theta}_S)$ can be written as $V(\hat{\theta}_E - \hat{\theta}_S)/n$, where $V(\hat{\theta}_E - \hat{\theta}_S)$ does not depend on n.

Estimates of $V(\hat{\theta}_S - \hat{\theta}_E)$ for various measures of diagnostic accuracy have been presented and illustrated in section 6.2. For our mammography example, we use the equation (6.14) where the estimator of the variance function for the ROC area is given in the equation (6.5) and the estimator of the covariance function in given in the equation (6.20).

We suspect that the accuracy of the 3D images is slightly less than that of 2D. The conjectured accuracy of 2D is $\theta_S = 0.90$; the conjectured accuracy of the 3D images is $\theta_E = 0.88$. We will assume moderate correlation in the underlying distributions for 2D and the 3D images, i.e. $r_D = r_N = 0.5$ in the equation (6.20). We will randomly sample patients from a list of all patients undergoing biopsy. We will sample an equal number of patients with malignant and benign conditions, i.e. R=1.0.

From the equation (6.5) $\hat{V}(\hat{\theta}_S) = 0.0686$, $\hat{V}(\hat{\theta}_E) = 0.0812$, and from the equation (6.20) $\hat{C}(\hat{\theta}_S, \hat{\theta}_E) = 0.0209$. For a study with 5% type I error rate and 80% power, n in the equation (6.24) is 742. Thus, the mammographer needs to interpret both the 2D and 3D images of 742 patients with cancer and 742 patients with a benign lesion in order to test whether the 3D images are non-inferior to 2D.

Suppose instead we want to test whether or not the diagnostic accuracy of 3D mammography is equivalent to 2D mammography. The null and alternative hypotheses are

$$H_0:\ (\theta_S - \theta_E) \le \Delta_L \text{ or } (\theta_S - \theta_E) \ge \Delta_U$$

$$H_1:\ \Delta_L < (\theta_S - \theta_E) < \Delta_U\ ,$$

where Δ_L and Δ_U are the prespecified lower and upper clinical limits for equivalence. Tu (1997) gave sample size formulae for testing equivalence for the case where $-\Delta_L = \Delta_U$. If $\theta_S - \theta_E > 0$ then

$$n = \frac{(z_\alpha + z_\beta)^2 V_A(\hat{\theta}_S - \hat{\theta}_E)}{(\Delta_U - (\theta_S - \theta_E))^2}. \tag{6.25}$$

If $\theta_S - \theta_E < 0$ then

$$n = \frac{(z_\alpha + z_\beta)^2 V_A(\hat{\theta}_S - \hat{\theta}_E)}{(\Delta_U + (\theta_S - \theta_E))^2}. \tag{6.26}$$

If $\theta_S - \theta_E = 0$ then

$$n = \frac{(z_\alpha + z_{\beta/2})^2 V_A(\hat{\theta}_S - \hat{\theta}_E)}{(\Delta_U)^2}. \tag{6.27}$$

Using the same conjectured values as in the previous example and setting Δ_L and Δ_U equal to -0.05 and 0.05, respectively, we determine that for a study with 5% type I error rate and 80% power, n in the equation (6.25) is 742. This estimated sample size is the same as the test for non-inferiority, a result that is a little surprising but is based on the assumption that the power from the other tail is near zero (Tu, 1997). For conjectured values of θ_E of 0.90 and 0.92, the required sample sizes from equations (6.27) and (6.26) are 343 and 598, respectively.

Alonzo and Pepe (2002) describe an alternative approach for testing non-inferiority and/or superiority; their method is applicable for studies where the measures of test accuracy are sensitivity and specificity. They define the relative accuracies of two tests, 1 and 2, by their relative true and false positive rates, as follows:

$$rTPR = \frac{TPR_1}{TPR_2} \;\; and \;\; rFPR = \frac{FPR_1}{FPR_2}, \tag{6.28}$$

where TPR_1 and FPR_1 are the sensitivity and false positive rate of test 1. Joint confidence intervals for rTPR and rFPR are constructed; the null hypotheses are rejected if the joint confidence intervals do not contain specified values of interest, denoted as Δ. For example, suppose you want to test whether the TPR of test 1 is superior to 2 and the FPR of test 1 is non-inferior to test 2. The null hypotheses are $H_o : rTPR \leq \Delta_1$ and $H_o : rFPR > \Delta_2$, where $\Delta_1 = 1$ and Δ_2 is a value greater than one, perhaps 1.2 so that test 1's FPR must not be more than 20% greater than test 2's.

For a paired study, the sample size needed for testing the rTPR parameter is (Alonzo and Pepe, 2002):

$$n = [\frac{z_\beta + z_{\alpha^*}}{log(\gamma/\Delta_1)}]^2 [\frac{(\gamma + 1)TPR_2 - 2TPPR}{\gamma TPR_2^2}], \tag{6.29}$$

where $(1 - \alpha)$ is the level of the joint confidence interval for rTPR and rFPR and $\alpha^* = 1 - \sqrt{(1 - \alpha)}$ which is needed to adjust for the two simultaneous hypotheses. The study has power of $(1-\beta)$. γ is a specific value of interest for rTPR under the alternative hypothesis and TPPR is the probability that both tests 1 and 2 are positive for patients with the condition. A range of values for TPPR should be considered under the constraint that $(1+\gamma)TPR_2 - 1 \leq TPPR \leq TPR_2$. A similar calculation can be performed for rFPR.

In a retrospective study, to ensure adequate numbers of patients with and without the condition, the power should be set to $1 - \beta^* = \sqrt{(1 - \beta)}$. In prospective studies, however, where the prevalence of the condition is usually low, the sample size of the study can be driven by including enough patients to test rTPR, assuming that the prevalence of the condition is much less than 50%.

Alonzo and Pepe (2002) also consider studies with unpaired designs, studies where the gold standard is performed only for patients positive on at least one of the tests, and studies where the gold standard is imperfect. Interested readers should consult the manuscript directly for these types of studies.

Finally, we note that the method described in section 6.2 for comparing two tests' PPV and NPV can also be used to test for non-inferiority. Moskowitz and Pepe (2006) define the relative predictive values of two tests, 1 and 2, as:

$$rPPV = \frac{PPV_1}{PPV_2} \;\; and \;\; rNPV = \frac{NPV_1}{NPV_2},$$

where PPV_1 and NPV_1 are the positive and negative predictive values of test 1. To test that the PPV of test 1 is non-inferior to test 2, we write the null hypothesis as: $H_o : rPPV \leq \Delta$, where Δ would be a value less than but close to one. For example, Δ might be set to 0.9 so that test 1's PPV must not be 10% less than test 2's. Equations (6.18) and (6.19) can be used to determine sample size.

6.4   SAMPLE SIZE FOR DETERMINING A SUITABLE CUTOFF VALUE

A less common goal in diagnostic accuracy studies is to identify a suitable cutoff value of the test result, given specifications on the required accuracy at the cutoff (note that this assumes that a suitable cutoff exists). For these studies the sample size must be adequate to ensure that the chosen cutoff meets the minimum requirements for sensitivity and specificity. For sample size calculation we need to specify both the minimum sensitivity (denoted as SE') and minimum specificity (SP') in order for the cutoff to be useful.

A digital imaging algorithm has been developed to identify patients whose implanted artificial heart valve has fractured. One measure potentially useful in distinguishing fractured from intact valves is the width of the gap between the strut legs of the valve. The larger the gap, the more likely it is that the valve has fractured. Suppose you want to perform a study to determine a cutoff value for the gap measure such that patients with a gap value greater than this cutoff will undergo surgery to replace the valve; patients with a gap value less than this cutoff will not undergo surgery. Surgery is risky. We have determined that we can tolerate a FPR of no more than 0.10. Thus, we specify that a cutoff value for gap will be suitable only if the FPR is no more than 0.10. Once we identify a suitable cutoff value such that we are certain that the FPR is no more than 0.10, we will estimate the sensitivity at this cutoff. How many patients are needed for this study?

Schafer (1989) derived a sample size formula for this problem. To compute sample size one must specify the minimum specificity required at the cutoff (which we denote by SP'), the conjectured sensitivity at the cutoff (denoted by $SE_{SP'}$), and the sensitivity at which the cutoff value for the test would no longer be useful (denoted by SE'). The method requires numerical minimization, but Schafer offers the following upper bound, which he indicates is a good approximation for many applications

$$N \leq \frac{(\sqrt{2}\Phi^{-1}(\sqrt{1-\alpha}) + \Phi^{-1}(1-\beta))^2(v_x + v_y)^2}{\lambda^2}. \qquad (6.30)$$

N is the total sample size (i.e. patients with and without the condition). The optimal ratio of patients with the condition to without the condition is v_y/v_x. Under the assumption of binormality for the test results,

$$\lambda = \Phi^{-1}(SE_{SP'}) - \Phi^{-1}(SE')$$

$$v_x = b\sqrt{1 + \frac{1}{2}(\Phi^{-1}(SP'))^2}$$

$$v_y = \sqrt{1 + \frac{1}{2}(\Phi^{-1}(SE'))^2}. \qquad (6.31)$$

In planning a study we assume that a cutoff exists such that the sensitivity at the specified FPR exceeds the minimum threshold for sensitivity, i.e. $\Phi^{-1}(SE_{SP'}) > \Phi^{-1}(SE')$. The choice of α determines an overall confidence probability of $1 - \alpha$ for the statement "the specificity at the chosen cutoff is at least SP'." The choice of $1 - \beta$ determines the probability of finding such a cutoff, when such a cutoff truly exists.

For our heart valve example, SP' equals 0.90. We speculate that at a FPR of 0.10, the sensitivity will be about 0.60, but we have determined that the sensitivity must be at least 0.50 in order for the test to be useful. Thus, $SE_{SP'} = 0.60$, $SE' = 0.50$, and $\lambda = 0.25$. We want to be 95% confident in the statement, "at the chosen cutoff, the specificity is at least 0.90", and we want power of 0.80 to find a suitable cutoff, if it exists. Thus, $\alpha = 0.05$ and $\beta = 0.20$. The shape of the ROC curve for the gap measure is unknown, so we consider different values for the binormal parameter b: 0.5, 1.0, and 2.0. From the equation (6.31), v_x equals 0.674, 1.349, and 2.698, respectively, and $v_y = 1.0$. Then, from the equation (6.30) a total sample size of 568, 1118, and 2772, respectively, is needed for the study.

Now suppose in the heart valve imaging study we specify that a cutoff value for gap will be suitable only if both the FPR is no more than 0.10 and the sensitivity is no less than 0.50. In this situation, where the cutoff point is determined based on a prespecified specificity *and* sensitivity, Schafer (1989) proposes using the equation (6.30) but $-2\Phi^{-1}(\sqrt{\alpha/2})$ is substituted for $\sqrt{2}\Phi^{-1}(\sqrt{1-\alpha})$. Then, for binormal parameter b equal to 0.5, 1.0, and 2.0, the required total sample size is 362, 713, and 1765, respectively. Here, the choice of α determines an overall confidence probability of $1 - \alpha$ for the statement "the specificity at the chosen cutoff is at least SP' and the sensitivity at the chosen cutpoint is at least SE'." Schafer points out that if the cutoff value is based on both a desired sensitivity and specificity, then the required sample size is reduced by up to one-third.

6.5 SAMPLE SIZE DETERMINATION FOR MULTI-READER STUDIES

In this section we describe and illustrate how to compute sample size for multiple-reader diagnostic accuracy studies. As we discussed in Chapter 3, multiple-reader studies are needed for tests that must be interpreted by a trained reader because the accuracy of the test depends on the reader interpreting it. Readers naturally have different abilities and different training and experiences. In the diagnostic imaging literature, multiple-reader multiple-case (MRMC) studies are quite common. Typically, several readers interpret the test results of a sample of patients and the readers' average accuracy is used to describe the test's accuracy. Here, we describe how to calculate sample size (both the number of patients and the number of readers) for studies comparing two tests' accuracies. Our examples involve the ROC area as the measure of test accuracy, but other measures of test accuracy can also be used.

We discuss two common situations: computation of the required sample sizes when there is no pilot data available to estimate the various parameters needed for the calculations, and computation of the required sample sizes when there is a pilot study with similar patients and readers as proposed for the pivotal study. A pilot study is highly recommended because there are many parameters needed for the sample size calculation of a MRMC study, and these parameters are difficult to estimate without pilot study. Furthermore, the methods that are available for scaling up a pilot study for a pivotal trial will often yield estimates of sample size that better reflect the trial's needs.

6.5.1   MRMC Sample Size Software

We are aware of several SAS programs for calculating sample size for MRMC studies. They are available at www.lerner.ccf.org/qhs/software/roc_analysis.php and perception.radiology.uiowa.edu/SampleSize/tabid/182/Default.aspx.

6.5.2   MRMC Sample Size Calculations with No Pilot Data

Suppose we are planning a study to compare the accuracy of two mammography lesion enhancement algorithms for distinguishing benign and malignant breast tumors. We plan to randomly sample patients from a registry of patients with lesions who have undergone biopsy. The biopsy results will serve as the gold standard. We will sample equal numbers of patients with benign lesions and patients with malignant lesions (i.e. stratified sampling). The films of the patients will be digitized and the algorithms applied to the digitized images. From our institution and affiliated hospitals, we will sample up to eight board-certified mammographers who are willing to participate in the study. The mammographers will record their percent confidence in the presence of a malignancy (i.e. a 0-100% scale where 0%=no confidence in the presence of a malignancy and 100%=complete confidence in the presence of a malignancy). Each reader will interpret the images from a particular enhancement algorithm on one occasion only (i.e. no rereading of the images).

We will use the area under the ROC curve as the measure of accuracy. We expect that the average ROC area of readers will be 0.85. We would like to be able to detect a difference in average ROC areas of 0.10 in the two enhancement algorithms (two-tailed test, with $\alpha = 0.05$). We want to determine the combinations of reader and patient sample sizes which could be used for such a study. We would also like to consider several study designs.

The null and alternative hypotheses are

$$H_0\colon v_1 = v_2$$

$$H_1: v_1 \neq v_2$$

where v_i is the mean accuracy of enhancement algorithm i for the population of readers. Obuchowski (1995) described a sample size approach for such studies based on a mixed-effects model for the diagnostic accuracy of a reader j using a particular diagnostic test i on reading occasion q:

$$\hat{\theta}_{ijq} = \mu + \mu_i + r_j + (\mu r)_{ij} + \epsilon_{ijq}.$$

Here, $v_i = \mu + \mu_i$ is the mean accuracy of diagnostic test i (fixed effect) (where $\sum \mu_i = 0$), r_j is a random reader effect reflecting differences in diagnostic accuracy due to different reader abilities (j=1, ..., J), $(\mu r)_{ij}$ is an interaction term for readers and tests (random effect), and ϵ_{ijq} is an error term. $\hat{\theta}_{ijq}$ can be any measure of diagnostic accuracy (e.g. ROC area, partial area, sensitivity at a fixed FPR). This model is discussed in more detail in Chapter 9.

For hypothesis testing and sample size determination, Obuchowski and Rockette (1995) assume that the diagnostic accuracies of the J readers of the two tests follow a multivariate normal distribution. An F-statistic with 1 and (J-1) df is used for testing the null hypothesis that the mean diagnostic accuracies of the tests are equal. The non-centrality parameter of the noncentral F-distribution must be determined in order to compute power and/or sample size. There are several variance components and correlation coefficients which must be known or estimated in order to compute the noncentrality parameter. These parameters are defined in Table 6.3. The estimated noncentrality parameter is

$$\hat{\lambda} = \frac{J(v_1 - v_2)^2}{2(\hat{\sigma}_b^2(1 - \hat{\rho}_b) + (\hat{\sigma}_w^2/Q) + \hat{\sigma}_c^2[(1 - \hat{\rho}_1) + (J - 1)(\hat{\rho}_2 - \hat{\rho}_3)])}. \quad (6.32)$$

The estimated power of a study with J readers is $power = Prob(F_{1,(J-1);\lambda} > F_{1-\alpha;1,(J-1)})$, where $F_{1,(J-1);\lambda}$ denotes a random variable having a noncentral F distribution with dfs 1 and (J-1) and noncentrality parameter λ, and $F_{1-\alpha;1,(J-1)}$ is the $(1 - \alpha)$ 100th percentile of a central F distribution with dfs 1 and $(J - 1)$.

The values of the different parameters in the equation (6.32) depend on the study design used (Obuchowski and Rockette, 1995). The most common multi-reader study design is the paired-patient, paired-reader design, where the same J readers interpret the test results of all patients in both tests. Other designs, however, exist and have various advantages and disadvantages (See Chapter 3). Table 6.4 describes the parameterizations for the various study designs.

Obuchowski (1995) suggests that one first consider several potential sample sizes for the patients, then estimate the corresponding value of σ_c^2. For the ROC area measure, one possible estimate of σ_c^2 can be obtained from equation (6.5) by dividing the variance function given in the equation (6.5) by n; for the sensitivity at a fixed FPR, an estimate of σ_c^2 can be obtained from the

Table 6.3   Parameters Needed for Planning Multi-Reader ROC Study

Parameters	Description
$\hat{\sigma}_b{}^2$	The estimated variability in $\hat{\theta}$s from different readers interpreting the results of the same patients using the same test
$\hat{\sigma}_w{}^2$	The estimated variability in $\hat{\theta}$s from the same reader interpreting the results of the same patients using the same test on different occasions
$\hat{\sigma}_c{}^2$	The estimated variability in $\hat{\theta}$s from different samples of patients
$\hat{\rho}_1$	The estimated correlation between $\hat{\theta}$s when the same patients are evaluated by the same reader using different tests
$\hat{\rho}_2$	The estimated correlation between $\hat{\theta}$s when the same patients are evaluated by different readers using the same test
$\hat{\rho}_3$	The estimated correlation between $\hat{\theta}$s when the same patients are evaluated by different readers using different tests
$\hat{\rho}_b$	The estimated correlation between $\hat{\theta}$s when the same readers evaluate patients using different tests
J	number of readers for each diagnostic test
Q	number of times each reader interprets the test results of each patient using the same test (often Q=1)

Table 6.4   Parameter Values in Various MRMC Study Designs

Design	Parameter Values
Paired-patient, Paired-reader	$\rho_1 \geq \rho_2 \geq \rho_3 \geq 0$, $\rho_b \geq 0$
Unpaired-patient, Paired-reader	$\rho_2 \geq \rho_1 = \rho_3 = 0$, $\rho_b \geq 0$
Paired-patient, Unpaired-reader	$\rho_2 \geq \rho_1 = \rho_3 \geq 0$, $\rho_b = 0$
Unpaired-patient, Unpaired-reader	$\rho_2 \geq \rho_1 = \rho_3 = 0$, $\rho_b = 0$
Paired-patient per reader, Paired-reader	$\rho_2 = \rho_3 = 0.0$, $\rho_1 \geq 0$, $\rho_b \geq 0$

equation (6.10) by dividing the variance function by n; and similarly for the partial area under the ROC curve, an estimate of $\sigma_c{}^2$ can be obtained from the equation (6.12). The estimate of $\sigma_c{}^2$ is substituted into the equation (6.32). For our mammography example we estimate $\sigma_c{}^2$ from the estimator in the equation (6.5). We consider n equal to 50 and 100. From the equation (6.5), $\hat{\sigma}_c{}^2$ corresponds to 0.00196 and 0.00098, respectively. The sample size n here is interpreted differently for the various study designs. For the paired-patient study designs n is the total number of patients with a malignant lesion needed for the study. For unpaired-patient designs n is the number of patients with a malignant lesion needed per diagnostic test. For the paired-patient per reader design (i.e. hybrid design), n patients with a malignant lesion are needed for each of the J readers.

Next, we determine suitable values for the other variance components in Table 6.3. The inter-reader variability, σ_b^2, describes the variability in accuracy when different readers interpret the results of the same sample of patients using the same test. Rockette et al. (1999) reviewed the published studies of 32 multi-reader ROC studies and has summarized the estimates of σ_b^2 in terms of the ROC area for three diseases (interstitial disease, lung nodules, and pneumothorax) and a fourth "other" category. The estimates of σ_b^2 for the ROC area ranged from 0.000004 (for lung nodules) to 0.0014 (for simulated interstitial disease). In mammography, large inter-observer variability has been reported in a study by Beam et al. (1996). They reported a range in ROC areas of 0.21 for 108 mammographers. Perhaps the simplest way to estimate the reader variability is to speculate on the range of accuracies for the readers in the sample. For example, we might conjecture that with eight mammographers, the range in ROC areas might be as much as 0.10. Using the relationship between the sample range and the standard deviation of a normal distribution (Harter, 1960) (Nelson, 1975), we multiple the range, 0.10, by the factor 0.3512 (Steen, 1982) to get our estimate of σ_b; thus, $\hat{\sigma}_b^2 = 0.00123$. Another approach is to estimate the range of accuracies for a population of readers; then an estimate of the variability can be obtained by assuming that the range includes 4 standard deviations (about 95% of readers' accuracies). Using the range estimated in the Beam et al. (1996) study, we obtain that $\hat{\sigma}_b^2 = [(range)/4]^2 = [(0.21)/4]^2 = 0.002756$.

Similarly, we expect a reader will vary somewhat in accuracy even when interpreting the same sample of mammograms on different occasions (i.e. intra-observer variability). Powell et al. (1999) reported the intra-observer variability of 5 mammographers who interpreted the same set of 60 films on two reading occasions. The ROC areas differed by as little as 0.01 to as much as 0.09. We conjecture that over three reading occasions, the average range in ROC areas might be 0.05. We multiple the range, 0.05, by the factor 0.5908 (Steen, 1982) to get our estimate of σ_w^2: $\hat{\sigma}_w^2 = 0.00087$.

Now we consider the four correlations in Table 6.3. The correlation ρ_1 describes the correlation between the accuracy estimates from the same reader using different diagnostic tests, that is, $\hat{\theta}_{1jq}$ and $\hat{\theta}_{2jq'}$. The larger the value of ρ_1, the smaller the required sample size. When the two tests evaluate different patient samples (i.e. unpaired-patient study design), $\rho_1 = 0.0$. The best way to determine the value of ρ_1 for sample size calculations is to estimate it from a pilot study or from a similar study. (See Chapter 5 for various methods of estimating the covariance and/or correlation between two ROC indices.) However, when this is not practical, one might consider the range of values of ρ_1 reported by Rockette et al. (1999) for the ROC area. The value of ρ_1 ranged from 0.35 (for pneumothorax) to 0.59 (for alveolar infiltrates); the average value of ρ_1 was 0.47. For illustration, we set $\rho_1 = 0.5$.

The correlation ρ_2 describes the correlation between the accuracy estimates from different readers using the same diagnostic test; that is, $\hat{\theta}_{ijq}$ and $\hat{\theta}_{ij'q'}$. The correlation ρ_3 describes the correlation between the accuracy estimates from different readers using different diagnostic tests; that is, $\hat{\theta}_{ijq}$ and $\hat{\theta}_{i'j'q'}$. For the unpaired-patient study design, $\rho_3 = 0.0$. For the so-called "hybrid" study design (Obuchowski, 1995), where each reader interprets a different sample of patients but the same patients are studied under both tests, both ρ_2 and ρ_3 equal zero. The noncentrality parameter in the equation (6.32) is a function of the difference between ρ_2 and ρ_3. The larger the difference, the larger the required sample size. ρ_2 and ρ_3 can be estimated from a pilot study or similar study. If a pilot study is not practical, then we might consider the range of values for $(\rho_2 - \rho_3)$ reported by Rockette et al. (1999) for the ROC area: -0.0196 (for pneumothorax) to +0.0139 (for alveolar infiltrates). Rockette et al suggest that a value of zero for $(\rho_2 - \rho_3)$ is reasonable for sample size calculations when no pilot data are available. For illustration, we set $\rho_2 = 0.3$ and $\rho_3 = 0.25$.

Lastly, ρ_b describes the correlation between the estimated accuracies obtained when the same readers evaluate the patients' test results using different enhancement algorithms. In particular, it describes the tendency for the reader with the highest accuracy on test 1 to also have one of the highest accuracies on test 2, and likewise for the reader with the lowest accuracy on test 1 to also have one of the lowest accuracies on test 2. ρ_b differs from ρ_1 in that ρ_b is attributable to having the same readers interpret both tests, while ρ_1 is attributable to having the same patients studied by both tests. ρ_b can be nonzero even when the patients in the two tests are unpaired (i.e. $\rho_1 = 0.0$). When the readers are unpaired, $\rho_b = 0.0$, while ρ_1 is not necessarily zero; with unpaired readers, ρ_1 is equivalent to ρ_3. The larger the value of ρ_b, the smaller the required sample size. We expect that the mammographers who perform the best on one enhancement algorithm will also perform the best on the other enhancement algorithm, thus we expect ρ_b to be large. However, in other studies where readers might have considerably different experiences with the two tests, such as a comparison of film to filmless reading, ρ_b may be near zero. ρ_b can be estimated from a pilot study or a similar study by estimating the Pearson correlation coefficient between the estimated accuracies obtained by the readers in the first test and the estimated accuracies obtained by the readers in the second test. From the review article by Rockette et al. (1999), the value of ρ_b for the ROC area ranged from 0.44 (for rib fractures) to 0.86 (for lung nodules); they suggested that a value of 0.80 is reasonable for sample size estimation when no pilot study data are available. For illustration, we set $\rho_b = 0.75$.

Finally, we specify a range of possible reader sample sizes to be considered. For our mammography study we have up to eight readers. We now compute the noncentrality parameter in the equation (6.32) and determine the associated power of the study for each possible value of J. If the power is inadequate for the largest reader sample size, then we must choose a larger patient sample size and recompute the noncentrality parameter. This approach emphasizes the inherent trade-off between the number of readers and number of patients required for such a study.

Table 6.5 summarizes the value of the noncentrality parameter and the corresponding power for various MRMC study designs with n=50 and 100, and the number of readers per test (J) equal to 4, 6, and 8. We computed the power for each value of J and λ using the PROBF function in SAS (SAS Institute Inc. Cary, N.C.).

The paired-patient per reader, paired-reader (hybrid) design, where each reader interprets a different sample of patients, is the most powerful. With six readers and 50 benign and 50 malignant patients per reader (600 total patients for the study), the study has an estimated 84% power to detect differences in ROC area of 0.10. The traditional paired-patient, paired-reader design offers slightly less power. With six readers and 200 total patients or eight readers and 100 total patients, the study has an estimated 88-89% power. The least powerful study is the unpaired-patient, unpaired-reader design.

For our mammography example, since there are a limited number of patients with biopsy-verified lesions and only eight possible readers, the paired-patient, paired-reader design is the most reasonable. With 50 patients with benign lesions and 50 patients with malignant lesions and eight readers, we have good power with this design (i.e. 89% power). Such a study would require a total of 1600 image interpretations, 200 from each reader.

Obuchowski et al. (2000) provide tables for the number of patients and readers required for various endpoints (e.g. ROC area, sensitivity at a false positive rate ≤ 0.10, and specificity at a false negative rate ≤ 0.10), for various accuracy values, differences in accuracy, different levels of reader variability, and ratios of patients without to patients with the condition. Although the tables do not cover all scenarios for MRMC studies, they do provide a quick, rough estimate of the numbers of patients and readers required of MRMC studies. For example, with a four-reader MRMC study, there are many combinations of accuracy values, differences, and reader variability that are not feasible with just four readers. Even with ten readers, if the reader variability is large, the study may not be feasible.

6.5.2.1 Fixed-Reader MRMC Designs

In the mammography example described above, the study readers were assumed to be a random sample from the population of board-certified mammographers; thus, the study results would be generalizable to this population. This design is the most common for MRMC studies. In contrast, investigators may be interested in the average performance of a specific group of readers (e.g. the particular residents at an institution); thus, the study results are generalizable to these readers only. Sample size calculations are different for the latter design. Blume (2009) suggests using the variance function given in the equation (6.21) for the difference between two tests' ROC areas, then multiplying the quantity from (6.21) by the following quantity which deflates the variance function according to the number of readers included in the study:

$$\hat{V}(v_1 - v_2) = \hat{V}(\hat{\theta}_1 - \hat{\theta}_2)(1/J + (J-1)\rho_{dr}/J), \qquad (6.33)$$

where ρ_{dr} is the correlation between different readers on the difference in ROC areas. $\hat{V}(v_1 - v_2)$ is then substituted into the following equation to determine the sample size for the fixed-reader MRMC design

$$n = \frac{[z_{\alpha/2}\sqrt{\hat{V}_o(\hat{v}_1 - \hat{v}_2)} + z_\beta\sqrt{\hat{V}_A(\hat{v}_1 - \hat{v}_2)}]^2}{(v_1 - v_2)^2}. \qquad (6.34)$$

Obuchowski (1995) suggests a similar approach for the fixed-reader design. The variance function for the difference between the readers' average accuracy is given by

$$\hat{V}(v_1 - v_2) = \hat{V}(\hat{\theta}_1 - \hat{\theta}_2)(1/J + (J-1)(\hat{\rho}_2 - \hat{\rho}_3)/J),$$

where ρ_2 and ρ_3 are defined in Table 6.3 and $\hat{V}(\hat{\theta}_1 - \hat{\theta}_2)$ is computed from substituting values from equations (6.5) and (6.20) into the equation (6.14).

Continuing with the mammography example, suppose we are interested in the average performance of six particular residents at our institution. Under the null hypothesis, we expect that the average ROC area of these readers will be 0.85 with both algorithms; under the alternative hypothesis we expect average ROC areas of 0.80 and 0.90 (two-tailed test, with $\alpha = 0.05$). We assume equal numbers of patients with benign and malignant lesions. All six readers will interpret the images of the same sample of patients (paired-reader, paired-patient design). We use the variance function of Blume (2009) to determine an upper bound on the number of patients needed for such a study. Assuming modest correlation between the two algorithms (i.e. r=0.5 in the equation 6.21), $\hat{V}_o(\hat{\theta}_1 - \hat{\theta}_2) = 0.1275$ and $\hat{V}_A(\hat{\theta}_1 - \hat{\theta}_2) = 0.13$. From the equation (6.33) and arbitrarily setting $\rho_{dr} = 0.05$, $\hat{V}_o(v_1 - v_2) = 0.02656$ and $\hat{V}_A(v_1 - v_2) = 0.02708$. From the equation (6.34), for a study with 80% power, n=21 patients with malignant lesions and 21 patients with benign lesions are needed (total number of patients required is 42).

We compare this result with the sample size requirement for a random sample reader design (Section 6.5.2). From the first row of Table 6.5 we observe that with six readers and 160 total patients, the estimated power is 77% and with 200 total patients the estimated power is 88%. In general, the fixed reader design will demand considerably fewer patients/readers than the random sample reader design.

6.5.3 MRMC Sample Size Calculations with Pilot Data

Hillis and Berbaum (2004) present a method for power and sample size estimation for MRMC studies when data from a pilot study or previous study, similar to the planned study, are available. The method is based on the Dorfman-Berbaum-Metz MRMC method (see Chapter 9) but can be used for study planning for any MRMC study. The authors note that it is important that the pilot or previous study is comparable to the planned study with respect to the diagnostic tests, reader expertise, patient selection, and the ratio of patients without to with the condition.

Hillis and Berbaum (2004) describe a four-step process for estimating power for a planned study with J readers and N total patients, while the pilot or prior study used J* and N* readers and patients, respectively. The four steps are as follows:

Step 1: Specify the effect size, i.e. the difference in ROC areas between the two diagnostic tests, which we have been denoting as $v_1 - v_2$.

Step 2: Analyze the pilot or previous study using the DBM method (see chapter 9). From this analysis, obtain estimates of the modality-by-reader interaction mean squares (MS_{TR}), the modality-by-patient interaction mean squares (MS_{TP}), and the modality-by- reader-by-patient interaction mean squares (MS_{TRP}) based on the J* readers and N* patients in the pilot study.

Step 3: Estimate the following quantities:

$$\widehat{\sigma}^2 = MS_{TRP}$$

$$\widehat{\sigma}^2_{TR} = \frac{MS_{TR} - MS_{TRP}}{N^*}$$

and

$$\widehat{\sigma}^2_{TP} = \frac{MS_{TP} - MS_{TRP}}{J^*}.$$

If an estimate of variance is negative, set it to zero for the remaining step.

STEP 4: Compute the denominator degrees of freedom for the noncentral F distribution:

$$df2 = \begin{cases} (J-1) & \text{if } \widehat{\sigma}^2_{TP} = 0 \\ \frac{[N\widehat{\sigma}^2_{TR}+J\widehat{\sigma}^2_{TP}+\widehat{\sigma}^2]^2}{(N\widehat{\sigma}^2_{TR}+\widehat{\sigma}^4/(J-1)+(J\widehat{\sigma}^2_{TP}+\widehat{\sigma}^2/(N-1)+(\widehat{\sigma}^2))/(J-1)(N-1)} & \text{if } \widehat{\sigma}^2_{TP} > 0. \end{cases}$$

The noncentrality parameter, λ, is given by

$$\lambda = \frac{(v_1 - v_2)^2}{(2/JN)[N\widehat{\sigma}^2_{TR} + J \times \widehat{\sigma}^2_{TP} + \widehat{\sigma}^2]}]. \tag{6.35}$$

The estimated power of a study with J readers and N total patients is *power* = $Prob(F_{1,df2;\lambda} > F_{1-\alpha;1,df2})$, where $F_{1,df2;\lambda}$ denotes a random variable having a noncentral F distribution with dfs 1 and df2 and noncentrality parameter λ, and $F_{1-\alpha;1,df2}$ denotes the $(1 - \alpha)$ 100th percentile of a central F distribution with dfs 1 and df2. Hillis and Berbaum (2004) recommend that a variety of combinations of J and N be considered.

Hillis and Berbaum (2004) compute sample size using the Thoracic Aortic Dissection (TAD) example described in Chapter 9 as pilot data. In step 1, they set the effect size, $v_1 - v_2 = 0.05$. In step 2, from the pilot data, J^*=5, N^*=114 (45 with an aortic dissection and 69 without), $(MS_{TR}) = 0.110275$, $(MS_{TP}) = 0.150114$, and $(MS_{TRP}) = 0.068255$. In step 3, $\hat{\sigma}^2 = 0.068255$, $\hat{\sigma}^2_{TR} = 0.0003686$, and $\hat{\sigma}^2_{TP} = 0.016372$. In step 4, they determined that with 8 readers and 251 total patients (99 patients with an aortic dissection), the study has a power of 80%. Similarly, the study has 80% power with six readers and 401 total patients (158 patients with an aortic dissection), as well as 12 readers and 180 patients (71 patients with a dissection).

6.6 ALTERNATIVE TO SAMPLE SIZE FORMULAE

We have discussed a variety of sample size techniques for a variety of endpoints. Most of our examples were clear-cut; however, in clinical research, study designs are not always so clear-cut. Studies can be complicated by partially-paired designs, complicated correlation structures, missing data, uninterpretable results, etc. For studies where a sample size formula does not exist, simulation can be a powerful approach (Eng, 2004). Simulation can be applied to any study, regardless of its complexity. The general idea is that a mathematical model is used to generate hypothetical data that might be generated in the study being planned. The hypothetical data would include the same number of patients as the planned study. Many hypothetical data sets are then generated and a p-value is calculated for each. The estimated study power is then equal to the percentage of these data sets in which the null hypothesis is rejected. Eng (2004) describes the approach in more detail with illustrative examples.

Table 6.5 Estimated Power for Various MRMC Study Designs and Sample Sizes.

Study Design	J=4		J=6		J=8	
	n=50	n=100	n=50	n=100	n=50	n=100
Paired-Patient, Paired-Reader	$\lambda=8.16$ pwr=0.50	$\lambda=11.02$ pwr=0.61	$\lambda=11.33$ pwr=0.77	$\lambda=15.69$ pwr=0.88	$\lambda=14.07$ pwr=0.89	$\lambda=19.90$ pwr=0.97
Unpaired-Patient, Paired-Reader	$\lambda=4.08$ pwr=0.29	$\lambda=6.58$ pwr=0.42	$\lambda=4.94$ pwr=0.44	$\lambda=8.27$ pwr=0.64	$\lambda=5.51$ pwr=0.53	$\lambda=9.49$ pwr=0.75
Paired-Patient, Unpaired-Reader	$\lambda=5.31$ pwr=0.36	$\lambda=6.82$ pwr=0.44	$\lambda=7.57$ pwr=0.60	$\lambda=9.90$ pwr=0.71	$\lambda=9.62$ pwr=0.76	$\lambda=12.78$ pwr=0.86
Unpaired-Patient, Unpaired-Reader	$\lambda=3.43$ pwr=0.26	$\lambda=5.05$ pwr=0.35	$\lambda=4.29$ pwr=0.39	$\lambda=6.59$ pwr=0.54	$\lambda=4.89$ pwr=0.48	$\lambda=7.79$ pwr=0.67
Paired-Pt/Reader, Paired-Reader	$\lambda=9.27$ pwr=0.54	$\lambda=11.99$ pwr=0.64	$\lambda=13.90$ pwr=0.84	$\lambda=17.99$ pwr=0.92	$\lambda=18.54$ pwr=0.96	$\lambda=23.99$ pwr=0.99

CHAPTER 7

INTRODUCTION TO META-ANALYSIS FOR DIAGNOSTIC ACCURACY STUDIES

In this chapter, we focus on meta-analysis of studies assessing the accuracy of diagnostic tests. We describe important design issues that need to be considered when evaluating such a published meta-analysis, or conducting one yourself. Basic analytic methods for meta-analyses of diagnostic tests will be presented here, with more advanced methods described in Chapter 12. We highlight the issues by following a specific example from a meta-analysis by DeVries et al. (1996) concerning a comparison of the accuracy of two types of ultrasound for the detection of stenosis in peripheral arterial disease (PAD).

The term "meta-analysis" was first used by Glass (1976) to mean "the statistical analysis of a large collection of analysis results from individual studies for the purpose of integrating the findings." Such integration is particularly useful when results from different studies disagree, or when sample sizes are too small to provide accurate estimates from single studies alone.

There are a number of good references in the medical literature that explain the theory behind meta-analysis and how to perform a meta-analysis, most of which are concerned with the specifics for Randomized Controlled Trials (RCTs) (Sacks et al., 1987, 1996; L'Abbe et al., 1987; Chalmers et al., 1989; Wortman and Yeaton, 1987). More recently, as meta-analysis of diagnostic

Statistical Methods in Diagnostic Medicine,
Second Edition. By Xiao-Hua Zhou, Nancy A. Obuchowski, Donna K. McClish
Copyright © 2011 John Wiley & Sons, Inc.

tests has gained in importance, articles on how to perform such meta-analyses have become available (DeVille et al., 2002; Irwig et al., 1994, 1995; Vamvakas, 1998; Shapiro, 1995; Gatsonis and Paliwal, 2006; Leeflang et al., 2008). The Cochrane Collaborative has established the Cochrane Diagnostic Review of Test Accuracy Working Group which has a website with links to primary studies as well as a handbook for systematic reviews: http://www.srdta.cochrane.org.

A meta-analysis of diagnostic accuracy can do many things. Specifically, it can:

1) Identify the number, quality and scope of primary studies

2) Summarize diagnostic accuracy over the reported studies

3) Determine whether there is heterogeneity amongst the accuracy values across studies

4) Examine the relationship of diagnostic accuracy to study quality, patient characteristics and test characteristics

5) Compare diagnostic accuracy of related tests, increasing power as compared to individual comparative studies.

6) Examine the relationship between test comparisons and study quality, patient characteristics and test characteristics.

7) Provide directions for future research.

7.1 OBJECTIVES

A good meta-analysis should be conducted as a research study. As with any research study, the first step is to identify the objectives and scope of the meta-analysis. This is particularly important, as a meta-analysis is retrospective in nature, and thus subject to more potential biases. In particular, we have to determine the exact diagnostic test whose accuracy is to be assessed, patient subgroups of interest, the clinical setting(s) to which the results should apply, the condition for which the test is to be evaluated (being sure to consider the spectrum of disease), the reference standard(s) that could be used to measure the condition, perhaps even the evaluators of the test results. For example, do we only want to look at screening tests, or will follow-up tests also be of interest? Do we want to assess the utility of a test to identify metastatic cancer among all patients, or only those already known to have cancer? If we are assessing a new radiologic technique, do we want to assess the possible effects of the level of training of the radiologist on the results? These elements of the study objectives will be used as a guide to operationalize inclusion/exclusion criteria.

The meta-analysis reported by DeVries et al. (1996) was intended to evaluate and compare the diagnostic accuracy of duplex ultrasonography with and without color guidance for use in evaluating peripheral arterial disease. Specifically, the authors wanted to evaluate the accuracy of the diagnosis of stenosis of 50-99% or occlusion. An additional reason for the publication was to show how the SROC method could be used for meta-analysis of a diagnostic test, as a possible alternative to controlled experiments.

7.2 RETRIEVAL OF THE LITERATURE

The second step in a meta-analysis is to search the literature. Search strategies include: using computerized bibliographies, asking content experts, looking through textbooks, hand searching appropriate journals, looking at reference lists of articles obtained, adding to the search terms any index terms found in relevant articles, using the "related articles" feature in electronic databases.

Research indicates that more than one database should be searched to increase the likelihood of finding most published work (Song et al., 2002; Whiting et al., 2008). Databases available include those that are of general interest, such as MEDLINE, EMBASE or Current Contents, containing individual published studies as well as reviews and meta analyses. Other databases focus more specifically on diagnostic testing, or on reviews. BIO-SIS databases focus on the fields of biological and biomedical sciences. The MEDION Database (`http://www.mediondatabase.nl`), which is produced by researchers in the Department of General Practice of the University of Maasticht in the Netherlands and Leuven in Belgium includes systematic reviews of diagnostic studies, genetic tests, and methodologic studies of systematic reviews. The Committee on Evidence Based Laboratory Medicine (C-EBLM) also has a relevant website and database. The Centre for Reviews and Dissemination, a part of the National Institute for Health Research in Great Britain is a good source. It compiles databases such as the Health Technology Assessment (HTA) database, which contains abstracts of systematic reviews as well as many individual research studies, and DARE, which focuses on evaluations of the quality of systematic reviews. The latter could be particularly useful when attempting to assess tests that have previously been evaluated. DARE and HTA are also available through the Cochrane library of the Cochrane Collaboration. The Aggressive Research Intelligence Facility of the University of Birmingham compiles the ARIF review database (`http://www.arif.bham.ac.uk/databases.shtml`). As of Fall 2009, approximately 10% of reviews in the ARIF database(over 800) were systematic reviews of diagnostic test accuracy studies.

While the Cochrane Collaboration is currently focused on controlled trials, the Cochrane Collaboration Steering Group on the Register of Reports of Diagnostic Test Accuracy Studies is currently in the process of developing a register of reports of studies of diagnostic test accuracy. The initiative, referred to as the Cochrane Register for Diagnostic Test Accuracy Studies (CRDTAS) is work in conjunction with the Screening and Test Evaluation Program of the School of Public Health at the University of Sydney in Australia, and is being managed at the Cochrane Renal Group editorial base in Sydney. It is intended to be the equivalent to the Cochrane Central Register of Controlled Trials of the Cochrane Library. Intention is also to be able to add to Medline an appropriate "Publication Type" to be able to more easily identify appropriate studies.

Citation databases such as the ISI Web of Knowledge, which includes the Web of Science Cited Reference Search, provide access to citation indices for journals (such as Science Citation Index), books, reports and conference proceedings (such as Conference Proceeding Citation Index-CPCI) and can be used independently as well as to follow up on relevant studies/authors.

Other sources of unpublished work (grey literature) may include government reports, dissertations, or abstract books and proceedings of relevant scientific meetings. The National Technical Information Service(NTIS), is a source of information (published and unpublished) on science and technology based publications produced by US government agencies since 1990. BIOSIS data base (`http://www.biosis.org`) also can be used to access conference proceedings. Grey literature can also be accessed using OpenSIGLE from the Institute for Scientific and Technical Information – National Centre for Scientific Research (INIST-CNRS) in France which provides access to databases of grey literature in Europe and a website of the New York Academy of Medicine which has the Grey Literature Report (`http://www.nyam.org/library/grey.shtml`), a bimonthly listing of grey literature publications in public health. Dissertations and theses can be accessed using the ProQuest Dissertations and Thesis database (`http://www.proquest.co.uk/products_pq/descriptions/pqdt.shtml`) and Index to Theses in Great Britain and Ireland (`http//www.theses.com`)

Contrary to meta-analysis of interventions, where the keyword or index "randomized controlled trials" can be used to identify relevant studies, no key word or phrase currently used in electronic databases will consistently identify diagnostic accuracy studies. According to Leeflang et al. (2008), even terms such as "sensitivity and specificity" do not appear to be used in a consistent fashion. In addition, information on the accuracy of a diagnostic test may be contained within studies that were designed for other purposes, making the study reports harder to identify as relevant. To improve results, search strategies should use both subject headings as well as text word searches to maximize the chances of finding all relevant papers. Search terms should include the name of the disease in question (including as many synonyms as possible) and the name of the diagnostic test, along with words such as diagnosis, screening, diagnostic test, as well as various accuracy related terms such as accuracy, sensitivity, specificity, false positive or negative, predictive value, likelihood ratio, ROC, etc. Having more than one person screen the initial lists of citations for retrieval is also important to avoid missing papers (two seems to be sufficient, according to Doust et al. (2005)).

Unfortunately, many papers not relevant to the meta-analysis may need to be reviewed in order to find the appropriate set of papers. Some researchers have developed electronic search filters to use to search for appropriate studies in hopes of reducing the "number-needed-to-read" (Deville et al., 2000; Bachmann et al., 2002; Haynes and Wilcynski, 2004; Astin et al., 2008; Kastner et al., 2009). Other researchers, though, do not believe these filters to be successful, as they found that filters often miss articles, and do not significantly decrease the number of studies that need to be screened (Doust et al., 2005; Leeflang et al., 2008). Kastner et al. (2009) pointed out that many filters assessed only used a single database (generally Medline), while theirs uses multiple databases which may reduce the number of missed articles.

A particular concern with meta analyses is the influence of publication bias. Publication bias is a form of selection bias where not all relevant reports on a topic are published. It has been shown for clinical trials that there is a tendency for published studies to represent positive results (Easterbrook et al., 1991; Dickersin et al., 1992). Recent research suggests that, once submitted, studies with positive results are not more likely to be published than negative studies (Olson et al., 2002). Publication bias appears to be primarily a function of the decision by researchers to not submit manuscripts with negative results to journals for consideration (Easterbrook et al., 1991; Dickersin et al., 1992; Olson et al., 2002).

The strongest correlate with publication bias in RCTs has been shown to be sample size (Berlin et al., 1989; Dickersin et al., 1987). Effect sizes for published studies with small sample size tend to be considerably larger than effect sizes for published studies with large sample size. Berlin et al. (1989) suggest that this implies that small studies which are published should be viewed with skepticism, and perhaps excluded from literature reviews and formal meta analyses. While this advice may seem sound in an ideal world, many studies of diagnostic tests are based on small sample sizes (Bachmann et al., 2006). Eliminating such studies from consideration would leave few studies, perhaps making a meta-analysis impossible. Since decisions whether to use diagnostic tests have to be make regardless, we believe that exclusion of small studies is probably not realistic in most cases.

Meta-analyses of comparisons of diagnostic tests would likely be subject to similar kinds of publication bias as RCTs. That is, articles about new diagnostic tests that are significantly better, statistically, than the standard tests may be more likely to be published, while articles about new tests that are equivalent or worse may be less likely to be published. On the other hand, studies of the performance of individual diagnostic tests often do not involve comparisons and statistical testing, hence the decision by journals to publish will not be a function of statistical significance. The possibility that publication decisions might be a function of the level of accuracy (i.e. studies of test that have high accuracy may be more likely to be published than those with low accuracy) is still an open question. Song et al. (2004) showed that small studies are more likely to have higher diagnostic accuracy, which may reflect publication bias.

Funnel plots have been used to detect publication bias in meta-analysis of efficacy studies. Briefly, a funnel plot is a plot of a measure of precision such as sample size or variance versus effect size. In the context of diagnostic accuracy tests, the effect size most often used is the diagnostic odds ratio (DOR). Asymmetric funnel plots are considered to be indicative of publication bias. Deeks et al. (2005) have shown that some of the standard tests used to detect asymmetry of funnel plots of RCT meta analyses- Begg's rank correlation (Begg, 1994), Eggers regression (Egger et al., 1997) and Macaskills regression methods (Macaskill et al., 2001) do not work well for detecting asymmetry in meta-analyses of diagnostic tests. They suggest substituting $1/\sqrt{ESS}$ where $ESS = 4n_1 n_0 / (n_1 + n_0)$ for sample size or variance in funnel plots as well as in the aforementioned tests of asymmetry. In simulations, they found that their alternate tests were not heavily influenced by study design characteristics such as high values of DOR, prevalence of disease or heterogeneity of test accuracy.

For meta-analysis involving RCTs it is sometimes possible to check trial registries on topics, such as perinatal trials (Chalmers et al., 1986; Dickersin et al., 1985) and the Cochrane Controlled Trials Register (CCTR) which lists funded trials on particular topics. In fact, the CCTR was developed in part due to research (Dickersin et al., 1994) that indicated that existing bibliographic databases were not sufficient to identify all relevant studies. This helps to seek out studies regardless of publication status, allowing the meta-analyst to be as complete and up-to-date as possible. A similar registry is being developed in conjunction with the Cochrane Diagnostic Review of Test Accuracy Working Group. Information can be accessed through their previously mentioned website. While not available specifically for diagnostic tests, resources such as CRISP (Computer Retrieval of Information on Scientific Projects), a database of research ventures supported by the US Public Health Service, can be used. It is likely, though, that issues with searching the database to identify studies will mirror that of bibliographic databases. Another issue with registry development itself is that studies of diagnostic accuracy can be done on a smaller scale than RCTs, or with clinical databases, perhaps not even requiring formal IRB approval, so there may be no way to be aware of these studies to enter into a registry. In fact, the ability to do such retrospective analysis, and the fact that many published studies are retrospective in nature implies that authors may tend to publish only if they find encouraging results - resulting in more publication bias (Dinnes et al., 2005). Presently, the lack of comprehensive registries for diagnostic tests makes it difficult to adequately investigate methodologically the effect of publication bias on results of meta-analysis.

Exclusion of articles during the initial literature retrieval process should be made only for articles that clearly do not meet the objectives of the study. For example, material without original data would be automatically excluded. This includes editorials, letters to the editor and literature reviews.

A few *a priori* decisions have an effect on the search strategy itself. One such decision is whether to include only English language articles, or include articles in foreign languages also. Limiting articles to English has a practical aspect, as it may be difficult for the analyst to have the article translated. For RCTs it has been suggested (Gregoire et al., 1995; Egger et al., 1997; Moher et al., 1996) that there may be a bias in restricting research to articles published in English language journals, since researcher are more likely to publish RCTs in an English language journal if the results are statistically significant. While it has not been extensively investigated for studies of diagnostic test accuracy, Song et al. (2002) did not find important English-language bias in their study.

Another issue is whether to search and/or include material other than that appearing in peer reviewed journals. This would include articles published in journals that are not peer reviewed, as well as abstracts, government reports, book chapters, dissertations and conference proceedings. Some of the problems with this material, in addition to not having been subject to appropriate scrutiny, is that it may not include sufficient data to analyze. It may also be lacking in sufficient detail to assess the quality of the study. Of course, exclusion of this material may lead to publication bias. In fact, their inclusion does not guarantee that results are free of publication bias. There is research, for example, to suggest that acceptance of abstracts at scientific meetings also displays publication bias, being associated with positive results and large sample size, rather than on study design or quality aspects such as blinding and randomization (Callaham et al., 1998; Dundar et al., 2006). Even if non-peer reviewed articles are to be excluded, a search strategy might include grey literature in order to identify authors to contact, or for further searches. It is also possible to include non-peer reviewed data in a meta-analysis and then consider the effect of the peer review process on the accuracy results. This has been done by some authors, and no significant effect on accuracy was found (Loy et al., 1996). This would be similar to assessing the effect of other factors such as study design, patient and test characteristics. This is discussed further below.

7.2.1   Literature Search: Meta-analysis of Ultrasound for PAD

The primary method of literature retrieval used by DeVries et al. (1996) was a MEDLINE search of English language articles published between January 1984 and June 1994. Search terms included "peripheral vascular disease," "peripheral arterial disease," "arterial occlusive disease," "intermittent claudication," "arterial insufficiency," "lower limb ischemia," "ultrasonics," "ultrasonography," "diagnostic imaging," "hemodynamics," "noninvasive," "angiology," "angiologic," "blood flow velocity," and "human." No other bibliographic sources were used. Additional articles were found in the reference section of review articles and the original papers.

7.3   INCLUSION/EXCLUSION CRITERIA

Decisions need to be made *a priori* as to criteria for inclusion and exclusion of studies. These decisions usually revolve around definitions of the exact condition, reference standard and diagnostic test to include, as well as to the clinical setting. For example, we must decide either to include studies that only use a specific reference test, or allow studies with different reference tests, perhaps planning to analyze by subgroup (defined by reference test) later. Similarly, we must decide on the exact diagnostic test to be evaluated. Technology often changes over time, so consideration must be given whether to exclude early versions of the test. In radiologic evaluations, factors such as dosage and the contrast medium may be important to define the test. Exclusions may also apply to the clinical setting. For example, the scope of the analysis may include diagnostic tests assessed in adults only, used for screening purposes, or in tertiary care centers. These decisions should be enumerated initially in the objectives step of the analysis. Here, it is operationalized by way of specific inclusion/exclusion criteria.

In the case of a meta-analysis that will compare two or more diagnostic tests, a decision must be made whether to include only studies that assess all diagnostic tests on each patient, allow studies which assess all tests but randomly assign patients to tests (one test only), or be more inclusive and accept studies which do not include all tests. Irwig et al. (1994) feel strongly that comparisons between two studies should be made only when both tests are evaluated on the same set of subjects. They argue that statistical comparisons cannot control for differences in quality, study design and patient populations. Unfortunately, that may not be practical. For example, it may be impossible or even unethical to do more than one invasive tests on a subject. In addition, if the desired comparison is between more than two tests, it may be impractical to perform multiple tests on a single individual. Ignoring such information when comparing tests would likely make it impossible to compare tests and could introduce bias.

An important issue is whether to include or exclude articles that have less than excellent quality. Chapter 3 presents material on various biases that can effect study design and results. A few recent studies have shown empirically how certain quality issues may effect results of diagnostic accuracy studies (Lijmer et al., 1999; Whiting et al., 2008; Rutjes et al., 2006; Westwood et al., 2005). For example, Lijmer et al. (1999) found that case-control studies greatly over-estimated the diagnostic odds ratio (DOR) compared to studies using clinical cohorts. Using different reference tests for positive and negative test results also inflated DORs (Lijmer et al., 1999; Rutjes et al., 2006). Interpreting reference tests while knowing results of the index test, insufficient description of index or reference test or the population have been associated with modest increases in the DOR, while partial verification, retrospective data collection and selective inclusion of patients into the study showed no effect on DOR (Lijmer et al., 1999). In contrast, Whiting et al. (2008), looking separately at sensitivity and specificity, found that verification bias resulted in increased sensitivity with little effect on specificity. Lijmer et al. (1999) found no effect of retrospective data collection on accuracy measures, while Rutjes et al. (2006) found that retrospective studies had higher estimated relative accuracy. Decreased accuracy was found when patients were selected based on referral rather than clinical symptoms (Rutjes et al., 2006).

While a number of quality assessment tools for diagnostic studies exist, the vast majority have not been well-described and to date, only QUADAS (Quality Assessment of Diagnostic Accuracy Studies) has been validated. QUADAS provides a check list of 14 items, which include assessment of spectrum of disease of patients, adequacy of reference test, verification process, independence of the index and references tests, among other items. Reports of inter-rater reliability for individual items range from very poor (average kappa=0.22, Hollingworth et al. (2006)) to very good (average agreement between rater and consensus=90%, Whiting et al. (2005)). Nevertheless, it appears that QUADAS is becoming an accepted tool to evaluate quality. QUADAS is also being adapted to suit specific types of diagnostic data such as "-omics" data (genomics, proteomics, etc) (Lumbreras et al., 2008).

There are a few schools of thought on whether to exclude articles based on study quality. One is that only articles of the highest quality should be included in a summary. This, in part, is the motivation behind restricting meta-analysis of therapeutic interventions to RCTs. While this has its virtue, it may not be practical. A number of investigators (Reid et al., 1995; Irwig et al., 1994; Cooper et al., 1988; Rutjes et al., 2006; Lijmer et al., 1999; Smidt et al., 2005; Zafar et al., 2008) have found research, or at least published reports of research, to be sorely wanting in terms of quality. While it is tempting to ignore these articles, there would not be many articles left to base needed decisions regarding the accuracy and hence use of tests. In addition, publication bias could result.

It may not be clear whether a study was done poorly, or the article is simply missing important detail. The STARD guidelines (Bossuyt et al., 2003) and other reporting guidelines such as MIAME (Brazma et al., 2001) for microarray studies and MIAPE (Taylor, 2006) for proteomics should improve the situation, but the transition to using these guidelines appears to be slow (see, for example, Coppus et al. (2006) on studies in reproductive medicine, Zafar et al. (2008) on diabetic retinopathy studies, and Cook (2007) on orthopedics). These guidelines suggest that articles include information on the type of study (prospective or retrospective), the study population, method of patient recruitment, sampling method, description of the gold standard and index test including how and by whom they were interpreted, the number of eligible patients that did and did not undergo the diagnostic test(s) and gold standard, the time interval between diagnostic test and gold standard, the distribution of disease severity and comorbidities in the study sample, any adverse events of the test or gold standard, estimates of test accuracy with 95% CIs, the number and handling of indeterminate test results, variability in test results for subgroups of patients, and estimates of test reproducibility. Once journals begin to insist that STARD be used for reporting, there may also be a concomitant improvement in the quality of the studies themselves, knowing that the details of study design and implementation will be made known.

An alternative to excluding studies of questionable quality is to include the articles, taking care that they be noted and handled in some special manner. For example, it is possible to incorporate such articles into the meta-analysis using quality scores as weights during analysis. But weighting by quality score may be inappropriate since some quality items cause under-estimates while others over-estimate of accuracy, making a total score meaningless, or worse, misleading (Whiting et al., 2004; Westwood et al., 2005). Thus we do not recommend doing adjustments on a total quality score. A better approach is to do subgroup analysis or sensitivity analysis, where the meta-analysis is repeated excluding certain quality defined subgroups, or meta-regression with individual quality items entered. These methods allow for the examination of the relationship between individual quality items and results.

Most analysts take a middle road, leaning towards being more inclusive in their choice of primary studies. Nevertheless, certain items might cause a study to be excluded. For example, studies must include a reference standard. Also, if insufficient data are presented to determine sensitivity and specificity, then the article cannot be included in any quantitative analysis. Even still, the study should be described initially, prior to exclusion.

Another criteria for exclusion could be small sample size. Research on meta-analysis of RCTs have found that studies are more likely to be published if they are larger, regardless of the results (Begg, 1994; Dickersin et al., 1987, 1992). As mentioned above in the discussion on publication bias, in the case of studies of diagnostic accuracy, small studies are more likely to have higher sensitivity and/or specificity (Song et al., 2004). Thus to limit studies to a larger size would be an attempt to limit this bias. Exclusion based on sample size, though, would dramatically reduce the number of meta-analysis that could be completed, as many studies of diagnostic tests are based on small sample sizes (Bachmann et al., 2006). In addition, some researchers speculate that smaller studies might be better than very large studies, because the very large studies may be from databases that are not products of well designed studies of diagnostic accuracy.

7.3.1   Inclusion/Exclusion Criteria: Meta-analysis of Ultrasound for PAD

DeVries et al. (1996) limited the studies included in the meta-analysis to those which used a single gold standard - contrast angiography, where the lesion of interest had to represent an arterial diameter reduction of 50-100%. Otherwise, inclusion criteria were not very strict, the authors choosing instead to collect data on study design and quality with the possibility of looking at the effect of these characteristics on the accuracy of duplex ultrasonography. Both diagnostic tests (duplex and color guided duplex ultrasonography) did not have to be done on the same individuals, nor be part of the same study. In fact, each test was performed on separate individuals. DeVries et al. (1996)

comment in their introduction that an experimental comparison where both forms of duplex sonography were performed on the patient would take over two hours of imaging time, which would be impractical to do in the same laboratory.

7.4   EXTRACTING INFORMATION FROM THE LITERATURE

Once articles have been retrieved, information must be extracted and coded. The choice of data to extract depends on the inclusion/exclusion criteria, the measures of quality to be assessed, etc. Of course, sufficient data need to be collected to determine whether the study meets the criteria for the meta-analysis.

Literature on meta-analyses for RCTs suggests that a detailed protocol and data collection form should be used (Wortman and Yeaton, 1987; Chalmers et al., 1989). In addition, it has been suggested that at least two people perform the extraction independently, with disagreements settled either by a third person or by consensus (L'Abbe et al., 1987; Sacks et al., 1996; Chalmers et al., 1989). Some even suggest that the data abstractors be blinded to authorship of the manuscripts, and, until it is decided whether or not to accept an article for analysis, that the abstractors also be blinded to the results. The blinding is intended to protect against any bias in assessment (Sacks et al., 1987; Wortman and Yeaton, 1987; Chalmers et al., 1989). Irwig et al. (1994) comment that there is no evidence with studies of diagnostic tests that blinding results in decreased bias. On the other hand, the need for more than one abstractor in diagnostic assessment studies was substantiated by Reid et al. (1995). In their study, two reviewers performed a blinded review of methodological standards for 12 articles on diagnostic test. Agreement was not perfect, with kappa scores about 0.75. Examination of the source of disagreement showed that the criteria related to work-up (verification) bias seemed to give the most difficulty.

There are a number of data items that should be collected to assess quality. The exact items may be a function of any specific quality assessment tool being used. At the very least, sufficient information must be extracted to assess reviewer bias, verification bias, and spectrum bias. To assess reviewer bias, data need to be abstracted regarding the exact method and ordering of the diagnostic test and reference standard. In addition, we must determine whether the tests were assessed independently, or whether knowledge of the results of one test influenced the results of the other in any way.

To assess the possibility of work up or verification bias, information must be abstracted relative to how patients were chosen for verification of the diagnostic test. This includes whether the reference standard was assessed on all patients receiving the diagnostic test, a random sample of those subjects, or neither. If only a random sample of subjects were assessed by the reference standard, the percent sampled of test positive and negative should be determined.

Data need to be collected concerning the population that was evaluated by the diagnostic study in order to determine the possible existence and extent of spectrum bias. This should include demographic variables such as age, sex, and race/ethnicity, clinical factors such as presenting symptoms, stage or severity of the condition, length of illness prior to testing, and important comorbid factors. If possible, this information should be collected for those with and without the condition, in order to determine the spectrum for each sample. This information will also be useful to assess the generalizability of the test.

Other important descriptors (and indicators of possible bias) include the practice setting, such as whether the patients are being seen in a primary or tertiary care setting, as inpatients or outpatients, and what previous tests or other evaluations occurred prior to the patients being referred for the test in question. Prevalence of the condition in the sample of patients evaluated by each test may be useful to help amplify the spectrum, setting and generalizability.

Technical details of the diagnostic test need to be collected. This may include the type of biochemical method used or whether computerized techniques or human assessment was used for test evaluation. For "-omics" based technologies (genomics, proteomics, etc.) details of the test will include sources, collection and handling of samples/specimens. For radiologic tests, we might need to note such details as the imaging method, contrast media, dose or imaging time. Particularly for subjective tests, details describing readers such as education or level of experience should also be obtained, if possible. Year of study may be relevant information to collect, as it may affect the details of the specific diagnostic test. For example, the study year can indicate the version of the machine used or how experienced people might be with the technology. Since it is often not possible to determine the exact year of the study, the year of publication may be a reasonable proxy.

Similar information needs to be abstracted regarding the reference standard. In addition, it should be determined whether the final diagnosis was based on a specific test or routine, or involved monitoring the patient clinically over time to determine whether the condition developed. Certainly, if more than one reference standard is allowed, the type of reference standard should be recorded.

Finally, we need to collect data that allows calculation of the accuracy measures. If data are presented in ordered categories, the frequency of these categories for those positive and negative on the reference standard should be collected. If data are binary, as is most often the case, raw data needs to be collected that includes true and false positives and negatives. It is best to record the raw numbers rather than the published sensitivity and specificity or other accuracy values to be compared later, as these might be incorrectly calculated. Loy et al. (1996) found in a meta-analysis that eight of 20 articles contained arithmetic errors in calculations of sensitivity and specificity. If raw data are not presented, then sensitivity and specificity can be used along with numbers positive and negative on the reference standard to estimate true and false positives and negatives on the diagnostic test. If data are also available on any patient subsets, these should also be abstracted. If possible, the explicit thresholds used to define a positive (or, if ordered categories are provided, the thresholds for each) should be abstracted. In addition, the percent of subjects excluded because the test either could not be done or provided indeterminate results should be recorded.

In comparative analyses, some additional information must be ascertained pertaining to assignment of tests to patients. In particular, we must determine whether all tests were performed on each patient, the patients were randomly assigned to have different diagnostic tests, all tests were performed in each study, but without random allocation, or studies did not evaluate all tests.

7.4.1 Data Abstraction: Meta-analysis of Ultrasound for PAD

In the meta-analysis by DeVries et al. (1996), data were extracted onto standardized forms. Neither the number of reviewers, nor blinding of review were discussed, so it is likely there was only one reviewer and that s/he was not blinded. Data collected on the study population included the number of patients, the age, sex, clinical indications (defined as the percent of patients with claudications, critical ischemia and other diagnoses), and the anatomic sites studies (percent of aortoiliac segments used).

Data collected relative to study design included the technique used for the angiogram, (biplane or single projection), whether the interpretation of the angiogram and/or the duplex sonography were blinded, whether there was verification bias, and whether or not the number of segments used was the most available (i.e., all segments from all limbs used). Finally, the imaging time, in minutes, was collected. These detailed data on patient and study characteristics were not universally available. For example, age was only available in eight of 14 studies, and the technique used for the angiogram was also available in only eight studies. Criteria used to define a positive ultrasound was available in all the manuscripts.

7.5 STATISTICAL ANALYSIS

7.5.1 Binary-Scale Data

If diagnostic test data are truly binary, then the goal of a meta-analysis will be to summarize the sensitivity or specificity of the test. Since sensitivity and specificity are proportions, standard methods developed for meta-analysis of proportions can be used. If one assumes homogeneity of studies, and if only sensitivity, or only specificity are of interest (so one does not need to be concerned about the correlation between the two accuracy measures) these proportions can be combined as simple weighted averages (which are fixed effect, maximum likelihood estimates). If we let θ_i represent the sensitivity or specificity of the ith of G studies, then a summary estimate for the meta-analysis would be

$$\widehat{\theta} = \frac{\sum_{i=1}^{G} \widehat{\theta}_i / \widehat{\sigma}_i^2}{\sum_{i=1}^{G} 1/\widehat{\sigma}_i^2}, Var(\widehat{\theta}) = \frac{1}{\sum_{i=1}^{G} 1/\widehat{\sigma}_i^2},$$

where σ_i^2 is the variance of the estimate of θ_i.

If it is not reasonable to assume homogeneity, as is most often the case, then methods that take into account random variation between studies should be used. The methods presented by DerSimonian and Laird (1986), which assumes errors are normally distributed are most often cited. These methods, though, have been shown to provide biased estimates. More on these issues and alternative methods of estimation will be discussed in Chapter 12. We will not discuss this further here.

7.5.2 Ordinal- or Continuous- Scale Data

Very often, studies of diagnostic tests only report a single sensitivity and specificity pair, even if the diagnostic test can produce results in several ordinal classes or is continuous. Thus most meta-analyses of diagnostic tests involve summarizing information on sensitivity and specificity. Studies often show widely different estimates for these values. The appropriate model for summarizing the accuracy of the diagnostic test depends on the assumptions that you make. The most restrictive is to assume that all studies use the same decision threshold and have the same level of accuracy (i.e., ability to discriminate those with and without the condition of interest). For the latter to be true, it would likely require that the studies applied the diagnostic test to the same population. Then the variation seen in sensitivity and specificity over studies would simply be due to random variation and a mean sensitivity and specificity might be appropriate summarization. This is the method used by most early meta-analyses, although no effort was generally made to assure that the appropriate assumptions were met, and they were most likely not!

A somewhat more realistic assumption is that the accuracy of the diagnostic test is the same across studies, but that the decision threshold varies between studies. That is, the sensitivity, specificity pairs from different studies actually lie on the same ROC curve, but at different locations along the curve. In Chapter 2 we talked about how the sensitivity and specificity are linked through the decision threshold. For a single study, these tradeoffs can be represented by an ROC curve. Likewise, for a meta-analysis, we can plot the values of true positive rate (=sensitivity) and false positive rate (=1-specificity) from each study on an axis to produce what has been called a summary ROC curve (denoted SROC). For example, Figure 7.1 represents such an SROC curve of 17 studies of LAG to detect lymph node metastases

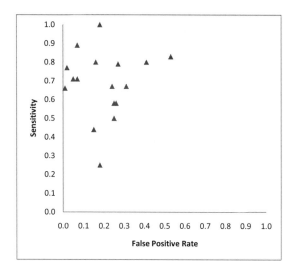

Figure 7.1   Empirical SROC Curve of LAG to Detect Lymph Node Metastases in Cervical Cancer Patients.

in cervical cancer patients (Scheidler et al., 1997). Analysis that assumes that the sensitivity, specificity pairs all lie on the same ROC curve involve what is often referred to as "fixed effect" modeling.

When studies use different decision thresholds, summarizing sensitivity and specificity with a mean will result in values that are too small. As an illustration, we revisit an example from Chapter 2, concerning the accuracy of gap measurements from digital imaging to identify fractured heart valves. Suppose that three different researchers had assessed the accuracy of the gap measurements and that the results of each study were identical to the data in Table 2.4, except that different decision thresholds were used to report sensitivity and specificity. If the three decision thresholds used were > 0.13, > 0.07 and > 0.03, the (FPR, TPR) pairs would be $(0.0, 0.5)$, $(0.2, 0.6)$ and $(0.4, 0.9)$ respectively (see Table 2.5). Assuming these 3 studies were the basis of a meta-analysis and the mean sensitivity and specificity were computed, we would have as summary values $FPR = 0.2$, $TPR = 0.67$. But we know that the study results are really just 3 points from a single ROC curve and that they represent the same underlying accuracy, varying due to the different thresholds. If we were to graph these points as in Figure 2.3.1 and fit a smooth ROC curve, the estimated TPR corresponding to a FPR of 0.20 (the mean FPR) is actually 0.78. This is a considerably higher value than the mean TPR of 0.67! Thus it is important to use analytic methods that capture the differences in thresholds.

Under the assumption that the ROC curve of the test is the same across studies, we can plot the TPR and FPR from each study on an axis to obtain an empirical summary ROC curve. To produce a smooth SROC curve for the test, we need to use the concept of a latent variable. Let us assume that FPR and TPR are for the continuous-scale latent response corresponding to a particular cutoff point chosen in a particular study. Kardaun and Kardaun (1990) were the first authors to suggest that the smooth SROC curve be generated through the transformation of (FPR, TPR) to (U, V) space, where

$$U = \text{logit}(FPR) \text{ and } V = \text{logit}(TPR). \tag{7.1}$$

Here $\text{logit}(p) = \ln[p/(1 - p)]$. They assumed that U and V follow a logistic distribution, which implies that the SROC curve is linear in (U, V) space.

More popular is the approach suggested by Moses et al. (1993). Their approach transforms the values from (FPR, TPR) space to (S, B) space where S and B are defined as

$$B = V - U \text{ and } S = U + V, \tag{7.2}$$

and U and V are the logits of FPR and TPR, as defined above. If the distributions of the latent test values for those with and without the condition of interest follow a 2-parameter logistic distribution then the SROC curve will be exactly linear in (S, B) space. Because the logistic distribution is similar to the normal distribution, and because many authors (Swets, 1986a; Hanley, 1988) have shown that the binormal model is reasonable for the construction of the ROC curve (see Chapter 4), the bilogistic distribution should be reasonable. Moses et al. (1993) postulate a linear relationship between B and S for all possible thresholds:

$$B = \phi_0 + \phi_1 S, \tag{7.3}$$

where ϕ_0 and ϕ_1 are unknown parameters.

Note that $B = V - U$ is just the log of the odds ratio (often referred to as the diagnostic odds ratio, in meta-analysis literature), i.e., the odds of a positive test result given the condition compared to the odds of a positive test result given a person is without the condition. The variable S can be interpreted as a measure of the effect of the decision threshold. The value S is 0 when sensitivity and specificity are equal. When the sensitivity is greater than specificity, the value of S is positive and increases as the discrepancy between sensitivity and specificity increases (i.e. as the decision threshold gets increasingly more lax). Likewise, when the sensitivity is less than specificity, the value of S is negative and becomes more negative as the value of sensitivity decreases (i.e., the decision threshold gets increasingly strict).

The parameter ϕ_0 represents the value of the log odds ratio (B) when $S = 0$, which we know is a measure of discrimination. The parameter ϕ_1 measures how strongly the decision threshold influences the log-odds ratio. If ϕ_1 is close to 0, it may be reasonable to assume that the discrimination ability of the diagnostic test (as measured by the odds ratio) is the same at all values of the decision threshold. The closeness also implies that there is an odds ratio common to all the studies, which is equal to ϕ_0. This common value for the odds ratio can also be estimated according to standard methods for combining odds ratios found in the epidemiology literature and in meta-analyses of randomized clinical trials, such as that of Mantel-Haenzel (assuming fixed effects) or DerSimonian and Laird (1986) (assuming random effects).

The relationship between S and B implies a relationship between Se and FPR which provides us with a formula for the latent smooth SROC curve. For $\phi_1 \neq 0$ we have

$$SROC(FPR) = \left[1 + e^{-\phi_0/(1-\phi_1)}\left(\frac{1-FPR}{FPR}\right)^{(1+\phi_1)/(1-\phi_1)}\right]^{-1}. \qquad (7.4)$$

If $\phi_1 = 0$, so that the diagnostic odds ratio is not dependent at all on the threshold value and $B = \phi_0$, the SROC can be written more simply as

$$SROC(FPR) = \left[1 + e^{-\phi_0}\frac{1-FPR}{FPR}\right]^{-1}. \qquad (7.5)$$

Note that the SROC curve in the latter circumstance is symmetric around the anti-diagonal ($y = 1 - x$). When $\phi_1 \neq 0$, the SROC curve is asymmetrical. Walter (2002) has shown that for extreme values of ϕ_1 (greater than $+/-1$) the SROC curve shows a negative relationship between TPR and FPR, which is implausible.

Moses et al. (1993) and Shapiro (1995) made many suggestions regarding the estimation of ϕ_0 and ϕ_1. First, they suggested adding 0.5 to the numerator and denominator in the estimates of U and V. Doing so avoids an attempt to take the logarithm of 0, but produces a slightly pessimistic bias in the SROC curve. Second, they suggested limiting the values of sensitivity and specificity used to estimate the equation to a "relevant region." The reasons given were concerns that (1) extreme values had an unreasonable effect on the estimates of the regression parameters and (2) these extreme values were not likely values of sensitivity and/or specificity for a reasonable test. Shapiro (1995) showed that defining the relevant region to be $TPR \geq 0.5$ and $FPR \leq 0.5$ improved the robustness against the non-linearity in the true ROC curve. However, Irwig et al. (1995) presented an opposing view, arguing that it was difficult to know what constituted a clinically relevant region, as this region might differ with the clinical context. In addition, even if one can specified a range a priori, a sensitivity and specificity pair from a study might appear outside the range, and hence be excluded, simply because of random variation.

Three methods to estimate ϕ_0 and ϕ_1 have been suggested: (1) the method of equally weighted least squares (EWLS), (2) the method of weighted least squares (WLS) and (3) the robust method. The EWLS method is appropriate where intra-study variation is very small compared to inter-study variation. When intra-study variation is dominant, the WLS method may be more appropriate (Stuart et al., 1999). The weights, W_i, are generally estimated as the reciprocal of the estimated variance of $\widehat{B}_i$; that is

$$\widehat{W}_i = \frac{1}{\widehat{Var}(\widehat{B}_i)} = \left[\frac{1}{r_{1i}+0.5} + \frac{1}{r_{0i}+0.5} + \frac{1}{s_{1i}+0.5} + \frac{1}{s_{0i}+0.5}\right]^{-1}, \quad (7.6)$$

where s_{1i}, r_{0i}, r_{1i} and s_{0i} are the number of true-positive, true-negative, false-positive and false-negative patients in the ith study, respectively. Most standard statistical packages should include regression modules that can be used to obtain either the weighted or unweighted estimates using least squares.

Shapiro (1995) showed that in the absence of inter-study variation, the difference in MSE for the two least squares methods was relatively small compared to other effects. Thus, unless it is known that a fixed effects, intra-study variation model is exactly correct, it is reasonable to recommend the equally weighted least squares as the method of choice.

Moses et al. (1993) also proposed estimating the line in (B, S) space using robust modeling. The authors suggested using the 3-group robust-resistant method, or median-fit line. Since the robust method does not lend itself easily to tests of hypotheses and incorporating covariates, it is not often used; see Moses et al. (1993) for details.

While the SROC curve is a graphic representation of the accuracy of a diagnostic test, a summary measure would also be useful. It is possible to obtain a summary measure of the accuracy of a diagnostic test, the area under the curve, by numerically integrating the equation for the SROC curve in Eq. (7.4). In the homogenous case, when $\phi_1 = 0$ and the simpler Eq. (7.5) applies, Walter (2002) showed that an exact formula for the area in terms of the common odds ratio (OR) was

$$A_{hom} = \frac{OR}{(OR-1)^2}[(OR-1) - \ln(OR)], \qquad (7.7)$$

with standard error

$$SE(\widehat{A}_{hom}) = \frac{OR}{(OR-1)^3}[(OR+1)lnOR - 2(OR-1)]SE(\widehat{\phi}_0), \qquad (7.8)$$

where $OR = exp(\phi_0)$. In fact, Walter (2002) showed that the area estimate was an upper bound for the area when studies are heterogeneous, and was actually a fairly good approximation in that case.

Some issues have been raised about using the area under the entire SROC. As with the pjROC curve for a single study, the area under the full ROC curve includes ranges of FPRs that are not clinically relevant. Another issue, unique to the SROC curve, is that the full SROC curve involves extrapolating beyond the range of sensitivities and specificities provided by the studies in the meta-analysis. As an alternative, the partial area under the SROC curve could be used, corresponding to any particular range of false positives of interest. This could be a clinically relevant FPR range, or limiting the SROC and hence the area to the range of FPRs covered by the studies in the meta-analysis. Since the SROC curve is not derived from the binormal model of the classical ROC curve, the methods of Chapter 4 cannot be used directly. Nevertheless, numerical integration could be used with (7.4), and, if $\phi_1 = 0$, integration of (7.5) between limits e_1 and e_2 yields the explicit formula for partial area between FPR rates e_1 and e_2

$$\frac{OR}{(OR-1)^2}\Big[(OR-1)(e_2-e_1)-\ln\Big(\frac{1+e_2(OR-1)}{1+e_1(OR-1)}\Big)\Big]. \tag{7.9}$$

Standard error estimates, which are somewhat complicated, can be found in Walter (2005).

Walter (2005) explored the properties of the partial SROC curve, and found that contrary to the full SROC area, the partial area was sensitive to the range of interest, as well as to the degree of heterogeneity or dependence of the results on the threshold value (ϕ_1). The latter would also imply that the "shortcut" method of using the closed form solution (7.9) as an approximation for the partial area when $\phi_1 \neq 0$, would not provide good estimates, particularly when $e_1 = 0$ and e_2 is small.

As an alternative to the SROC curve area, Moses et al. (1993) suggested as a summary measure the statistic Q, which is the TPR at the point of intersection of the SROC curve with the line $Se - Sp = 0$ (i.e., the negative diagonal). At this point, the sensitivity and specificity are equal. The measure Q operates in a manner similar to that of the full SROC-curve area in that for any reasonable test (i.e. one such that $TPR \neq FPR$), Q takes on values between 0.5 and 1.0. The measure Q is close to 1 when the SROC curve is near the upper northwest corner, and it is close to 0.5 when the SROC curve is near the chance diagonal. Moses et al. (1993) showed that Q can be estimated as

$$\widehat{Q} = [1 + e^{-\widehat{\phi}_0/2}]^{-1}, \tag{7.10}$$

with standard error derived using the method of differentials as

$$SE(\widehat{Q}) = \frac{SE(\widehat{\phi}_0)}{8 \times [\cosh(\widehat{\phi}_0/4)]^2}, \tag{7.11}$$

where $\cosh(z)$ is a hyperbolic cosine function, defined as $\cosh(z) = [\exp(z) + \exp(-z)]/2$. Moses et al. (1993) suggested that if there were at least 10 studies used to estimate the regression equation, Q would be approximately normally distributed. Thus Q could also be used to compare two SROC curves.

To compare Q for dependent samples, it is necessary to have an estimate of the covariance of the Q. Although Moses et al. (1993) did not provide an estimate of the covariance between $\widehat{Q}_1$ and $\widehat{Q}_2$, the delta method can be used to derive it:

$$Cov(\widehat{Q}_1, \widehat{Q}_2) = \frac{Cov(\widehat{\phi}_{01}, \widehat{\phi}_{02})}{64 \times [\cosh(\widehat{\phi}_{01}/4)\cosh(\widehat{\phi}_{02}/4)]^2}. \tag{7.12}$$

Values of Q can be used to compare different diagnostic tests or to evaluate the effect of quality issues on accuracy (and/or to determine the effect of study design, test or patient characteristics). For example, if we want to determine the effect of verification bias on accuracy, we could estimate SROC curves separately for those studies with and without verification bias, and then compare the resulting values of Q. Similarly this comparison can be done for tests used as screening vs follow-up, as well as for other tests.

Some issues concerning the basic SROC method of Moses et al. (1993) have been raised. First, the three estimation methods discussed in the preceding text are fixed effects methods and thus tacitly assume that ϕ_0 and ϕ_1 do not vary across studies. That is, variation is a function only of the threshold and within-study sampling variability. It is likely that this assumption regarding sensitivity and specificity pairs from various studies is unrealistic. In particular, while the decision threshold might vary from one study to another, so might the level of accuracy. In fact, a number of recent studies have focused on heterogeneity of accuracy in diagnostic studies (Dinnes et al., 2005; Lijmer et al., 2002; Leeflang et al., 2008; Rutjes et al., 2006; Whiting et al., 2004). An implication of this is that more than one ROC curve exists for the diagnostic test. The different levels of accuracy might be functions of specific patient or study characteristics, levels of quality or even other unmeasured features. If the accuracy varies by measurable characteristics, then in theory, separate SROC curves can be plotted (assuming there are sufficient studies within subgroup). Thus we might plot separate SROC curves corresponding to different age groups, or representing studies with and without verification bias. One can both visually and formally (through methods such as meta-regression) determine whether there are differences among these subgroups.

Let $X_1, \cdots, X_M$ be M study-level covariates. A fixed-effects regression model assumes the following relationship between B and S in the presence of study covariates, extending Eq. (7.3)

$$B = \phi_0 + \phi_1 S + \sum_{j=1}^{M} \eta_j X_j. \tag{7.13}$$

We rewrite this as

$$B = \phi_0 + \sum_{j=1}^{M} \eta_j X_j + \phi_1 S = \phi_0^* + \phi_1 S, \tag{7.14}$$

where $\phi_0^* = \phi_0 + \sum_{j=1}^{M} \eta_j X_j$ can be thought of as a study-specific intercept, giving each study its own SROC curve which is a function of the characteristics of the studies. Either of the least square methods discussed earlier easily accommodate this model. Significance tests on the individual parameters address hypotheses concerning the effect that corresponding study-level covariates have on the accuracy of the test. Because most meta-analyses do not include large numbers of studies, we should generally not include many variables in a single equation. In fact, Irwig et al. (1995) suggest that only one characteristic be considered at a time, both because of sample size considerations and because different factorss might have an effect in different directions.

Table 7.1   Data for 14 Studies of Duplex and Color Guided Duplex Ultrasonography to Detect Serious Stenosis.

	Test	TP	FN	TN	FP
Study 1	Duplex	78	28	516	20
Study 2	Duplex	59	8	89	12
Study 3	Duplex	75	23	235	5
Study 4	Duplex	89	20	262	22
Study 5	Duplex	118	14	488	9
Study 6	Duplex	48	7	48	3
Study 7	Duplex	39	2	156	14
Study 8	Duplex	121	31	376	12
Study 9	Color	134	15	347	3
Study 10	Color	45	0	20	0
Study 11	Color	187	26	236	4
Study 12	Color	25	3	89	6
Study 13	Color	49	7	173	9
Study 14	Color	108	5	375	13

Residual variation in accuracy between studies due to unmeasured sources can also be accounted for in analysis using random effects methods (see Chapter 12). Ignoring this variability using a fixed effects model can give biased estimates of parameters, and usually underestimates standard errors.

Another important issue with the basic SROC methodology is that the three fixed effects estimation methods discussed in the preceding text do not account for sampling errors in $\widehat{S}$. Therefore, the good statistical properties associated with least-squares estimators in a linear model (e.g., unbiasedness) may be lost for the estimators $\widehat{\phi}_0$ and $\widehat{\phi}_1$. The sampling error may also effect the estimate of the standard error. Increased sampling error could result in the misleading conclusion that $\phi_1 = 0$ (and thus saying studies are homogeneous). In addition, since most meta-analyses include a small number of studies, small sample properties of the methods need to be explored (Walter, 2002).

Another issue is that the estimation procedures ignore the correlation between B and S. It is not clear what the effect of this is on results. Methods to handle this correlation are described in Chapter 12.

7.5.2.1 Analysis: Meta-analysis of Ultrasound for Detection of PAD   DeVries et al. (1996) used simple SROC curve methods to compare the diagnostic accuracy of duplex ultrasonography (US) with and without color guidance, for use in the diagnosis of stenosis of 50-99% or occlusion. Table 7.1 has data necessary to create the SROC curve, while Figure 7.2 has a scatter plot of the data and Figure 7.3 has the smooth SROC for each test. While both curves

show excellent accuracy, with the curves in the upper northwest corner, the SROC curve for color duplex is even closer to the corner.

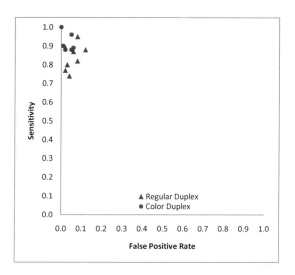

Figure 7.2   Empirical SROC Curves of Regular Duplex and Color-Guided Duplex Ultrasound.

Table 7.2 is a worksheet which has the data from DeVries et al. (1996) needed to construct SROC curves for regular and color guided duplex ultrasonography. The values of U and V were estimated by first adding 0.5 to each data point. Thus for example, for the first reference, we have

$$\widehat{V} = \ln\left[\frac{78 + 0.5}{28 + 0.5}\right] = \ln(2.75) = 1.01,$$

and

$$\widehat{U} = \ln\left[\frac{20 + 0.5}{516 + 0.5}\right] = \ln(0.040) = -3.23.$$

To determine whether there was a difference in the two ultrasound methods, DeVries et al. (1996) fit the following model:

$$B = \phi_0 + \phi_1 S + CX,$$

where $X = 1$ if color duplex ultrasonography was used and $X = 0$ if simple duplex ultrasonography was used. No decision needed to be made about restricting the points used to estimate the equation, as the sensitivity and specificity values were all high. DeVries et al. (1996) performed a weighted least squares regression analysis. Table 7.3 summarizes the regression results

Table 7.2   Worksheet to Construct SROC Curves for Comparing Duplex and Color Guided Duplex Ultrasonography to Detect Serious Stenosis.

	Test	FPR	TPR	U	V	B	S	Variance	Weight
Study 1	Duplex	0.04	0.74	-3.23	1.03	-4.24	-2.12	0.10	10.1
Study 2	Duplex	0.12	0.88	-1.97	1.95	-3.91	-0.02	0.23	4.4
Study 3	Duplex	0.02	0.77	-3.76	1.17	-4.92	-2.59	0.24	4.1
Study 4	Duplex	0.08	0.82	-2.46	1.47	-3.93	-0.98	0.11	9.2
Study 5	Duplex	0.02	0.89	-3.94	2.10	-6.04	-1.84	0.18	5.4
Study 6	Duplex	0.06	0.87	-2.63	1.87	-4.49	-0.76	0.46	2.2
Study 7	Duplex	0.08	0.95	-2.38	2.76	-5.14	0.38	0.50	2.0
Study 8	Duplex	0.03	0.80	-3.40	1.35	-4.75	-2.05	0.12	8.2
Study 9	Color	0.01	0.90	-4.63	2.16	-6.79	-2.47	0.36	2.8
Study 10	Color	0.00	1.00	-3.71	4.51	-8.22	0.80	4.07	0.2
Study 11	Color	0.02	0.88	-4.00	1.96	-5.96	-2.05	0.27	3.7
Study 12	Color	0.06	0.89	-2.62	1.99	-4.61	-0.64	0.49	2.0
Study 13	Color	0.05	0.88	-2.90	1.89	-4.79	-0.02	0.26	3.8
Study 14	Color	0.05	0.96	-3.02	2.98	-6.0	-0.03	0.27	3.7

for both a weighted and unweighted analysis. The parameter estimates are similar for both analyses, whereas the standard errors are larger for the unweighted least squares. This difference in standard errors is consistent with the idea that the unweighted method takes into account inter-study differences. In both weighted and unweighted cases, though, the conclusions are the same. The coefficient of the US indicator is statistically significant ($p = 0.02$, for weighted, $p = 0.04$ for unweighted analysis) implying that the two SROC curves are different. Although both curves show excellent accuracy, with curves in the upper northwest corner, the color duplex US is even closer to the corner. It might be noted that ϕ_1, the coefficient of S, is not statistically significant. Even though this lack of significance may indicate that the log odds ratio is not a function of threshold, it seems unlikely, for we know that the criteria for positivity varies among the studies. Because the number of studies is so small, with corresponding low power, it makes sense to keep S in the model, even though its coefficient is not significant statistically.

The mean sensitivity for the 8 studies using duplex ultrasonography was 0.84 with a mean specificity of 0.94 ($FPR = 0.06$). Looking at the 6 studies of color guided duplex ultrasonography, the mean sensitivity was 0.92 and the mean specificity was 0.97 ($FPR = 0.03$). For the duplex ultrasound, at the mean FPR of 0.06, the estimated sensitivity from the SROC curve was 0.85, which was slightly higher than the mean sensitivity. For the color duplex,

Table 7.3 Results of Estimating Regression Equation for Comparing Regular and Color-Guided Duplex US to Detect Serious Stenosis

	$\widehat{\phi}_0$	$Se(\widehat{\phi}_0)$	p	$\widehat{\phi}_1$	$Se(\widehat{\phi}_1)$	p	$\widehat{C}$	$Se(\widehat{C})$	p
Weighted	4.19	0.44	< 0.01	-0.25	0.24	0.29	1.26	0.47	0.02
Unweighted	4.80	0.51	< 0.01	0.09	0.27	0.74	1.39	0.58	0.03

the sensitivity on the SROC curve corresponding to $FPR = 0.03$ was 0.996, which was also higher than the mean.

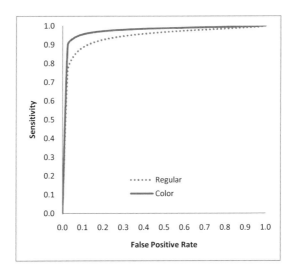

Figure 7.3 Smooth ROC Curve of Regular Duplex and Color-Guided Duplex Ultrasound.

DeVries et al. (1996) also performed additional regression analyses to assess the effect of patient and study design characteristics on the ultrasonography results. For each of the characteristics taken individually, an additional co-variate was added to the previous model. For example, we could look at the possible effect of verification bias on the comparison of the two methods of ultrasound. According to DeVries et al. (1996) studies 1, 8, 10, 11, 13 and 14 were free of verification bias. We let X_1 be the ultrasound variable as defined above and define a new variable X_2 which equals 1 if there is no verification bias, and 0 if there is possible or definite verification bias, and fit the equation

$$B = \phi_0 + \phi_1 S + \eta_1 X_1 + \eta_2 X_2.$$

DeVries et al. (1996) fit this model equation using both EWLS and WLS methods. The estimated value for η_2 and the associated p values were 0.18 and 0.78, respectively, using the unweighted analysis; -0.35 and 0.47, respectively, using the weighted analysis. Although the estimated values from the unweighted and weighted analyses were different, their p values all led to the same conclusion: that verification bias did not significantly affect the accuracy of the test. DeVries et al. (1996) found no other covariates to be statistically significant. They concluded that none of the covariates affected the diagnostic accuracy, although they admitted that the small number of studies limited the power to assess such effects.

Another way to compare the two ultrasound methods is to calculate and compare the summary measure, Q. Although DeVries et al. (1996) did not do this in their paper, it can be easily accomplished. Two separate regressions need to be estimated - one for the regular US, the other for color-guided duplex US. The estimates of the parameter ϕ_{0i} are $\widehat{\phi}_{01} = 4.49$ for regular duplex US and $\widehat{\phi}_{02} = 6.47$ for color-guided duplex US. The corresponding standard error of estimates are $SE(\widehat{\phi}_{01}) = 0.42$ and $SE(\widehat{\phi}_{02}) = 0.77$, respectively. Using Eqns (7.10) and (7.11), we obtain an estimate of Q for regular duplex as

$$\widehat{Q}_1 = [1 + e^{-4.49/2}]^{-1} = 0.90$$

with standard error

$$\widehat{SE}(\widehat{Q}_1) = \frac{0.42}{8 \times [\cosh(-4.49/4)]^2} = \frac{0.42}{23.1} = 0.018.$$

Similarly, for the color-guided duplex US, we obtain an estimate for Q as $\widehat{Q}_2 = 0.96$ with an estimated standard error 0.014. Both types of duplex US have high values of Q, indicating that the overall accuracy of each is excellent. Nevertheless, color-guided duplex US appears to be slightly better. These two values can be compared statistically (albeit, the sample size is small) assuming a normal distribution.

$$Z = \frac{0.96 - 0.90}{\sqrt{(0.018)^2 + (0.014)^2}} = \frac{0.06}{0.023} = 2.62,$$

which has a p value of less than 0.01. The test agrees with the earlier results, showing that the overall accuracy of color-guided duplex US is significantly better than that of the regular duplex US.

One can also estimate and compare the area under the SROC curves for each type of US. Using the homogeneous approximation and Eqns (7.7), and (7.8) we have that

$$\widehat{A}_1 = \frac{e^{4.49}}{(e^{4.49} - 1)^2}[(e^{4.49} - 1) - \ln(e^{4.49})] = 0.95982,$$

$$\widehat{SE}(\widehat{A}_1) = \frac{e^{4.49}}{(e^{4.49}-1)^3}[(e^{4.49}+1)\ln(e^{4.49}) - 2(e^{4.49}-1)](0.42) = 0.012494.$$

Similarly, we find $\widehat{A}_2 = 0.99150$ and $\widehat{SE}(\widehat{A}_2) = 0.005373$. Comparing these areas, we have

$$Z = \frac{0.99510 - 0.95982}{\sqrt{0.012494^2 + 0.005373^2}} = 2.33,$$

which has a p value less than 0.01. The results are similar to that with Q.

7.5.3 Area Under the ROC Curve

If the results of a diagnostic test are ordinal or continuous and the investigator reports the results with such measures as the ROC curve area or partial area, then different methods can be used to summarize these findings over studies.

Suppose that G studies investigate the accuracy of the same diagnostic test. Each study has different patient samples. Let A_i denote the true area ROC curve for the ith study. An estimate for A_i may be derived either by nonparametric method or parametric methods, as described in Chapter 4.

If we assume that there is a common value of ROC curve area and that each study provides an estimate of this common area (i.e., $A_1 = \cdots = A_G = A$), then a reasonable estimate of the common area, A, is the weighted mean of the areas of the individual studies, where we choose weights which are the reciprocal of the variance, i.e., $W_i = 1/Var(\widehat{A}_i)$. Then

$$\widehat{A} = \frac{\sum_{i=1}^{G} W_i \, \widehat{A}_i}{\sum_{i=1}^{G} W_i} \tag{7.15}$$

with its variance being

$$Var(\widehat{A}) = \frac{\sum_{i=1}^{G} W_i^2 Var(\widehat{A}_i)}{(\sum_{i=1}^{G} W_i)^2} = \frac{1}{\sum_{i=1}^{G} W_i}, \tag{7.16}$$

where $Var(\widehat{A}_i)$ is assumed to be known from the ith study.

The area under the ROC curve is approximately normally distributed; thus $\widehat{A}$ will also be normally distributed. A 2-sided $100(1-\alpha)\%$ confidence interval for $\widehat{A}$ can be constructed with limits

$$\widehat{A} \pm z_{1-\alpha/2}\sqrt{Var(\widehat{A})}. \tag{7.17}$$

Before assuming the existence of a common ROC curve area across studies, it is necessary to test this assumption. Formally, we test the null hypothesis

$$H_0 : A_1 = \cdots = A_G \text{ vs } H_1 : A_i \neq A_j \text{ for at least some } i \neq j.$$

The test for equality of ROC curve areas is the sum of squared deviations of the individual areas from the mean area, weighted by the variances:

$$\chi_{homogeneous}^2 = \sum_{i=1}^{G} W_i(\widehat{A}_i - \widehat{A})^2. \tag{7.18}$$

This test statistic has a χ^2 distribution with $G - 1$ degrees of freedom. This test may suffer from lack of power if the number of studies is small (McClish, 1992).

If we reject the null hypothesis, it will not be appropriate to consider $\widehat{A}$ as an estimate of the common area under the ROC curve, although one could consider $\widehat{A}$ as an estimate of an average value of the areas. That may or not be meaningful. A better alternative is to use a method that specifically incorporates inter-study variation. Such methods will be described in Chapter 12, section 12.3.

Note that the method discussed in this section can be used whether the ROC curve is estimated parametrically or nonparametrically. The method can be extended easily to accommodate the partial area should that information be published. For this extension, however, we would need to consider whether the partial areas across studies are from the same part of the ROC curve. These methods are fixed effect methods, which assume that differences in ROC curve areas can be attributed completely to within-study variation. As for the SROC curve, it is likely that this assumption is violated. Other methods which take into account other sources of variability are discussed in Chapter 12.

7.5.3.1 Analysis: Meta-analysis of DST

We present an example based on an evaluation of the dexamethasone suppression test (DST), a simple laboratory assessment of pituitary-adrenal dysregulation. Use of this simple test has been suggested for the diagnosis of and differentiation between various psychiatric disorders, including psychotic depression, schizophrenia and mania. A paper by Mossman and Somoza (1989) summarized the ROC curve analysis, including the area under the ROC curve, of seven studies of DST. These results are in Table 7.4 along with the needed weights.

We can calculate the mean value of the area estimates using Eq. (7.15)

$$\widehat{A} = \frac{307.8 \times 0.789 + 1600.0 \times 0.724 + \cdots + 692.54 \times 0.652}{307.8 + 1600.0 + \cdots + 692.5} = \frac{4278.9}{5479.9} = 0.781$$

with estimated variance

$$\widehat{Var}(\widehat{A}) = \frac{1}{307.8 + 1600.0 + \cdots + 692.5} = \frac{1}{5479.9} = 0.0001825.$$

Note that this differs from the composite value of 0.792 determined by Mossman and Somoza (1989). For the composite they used the (unweighted) arithmetic mean of the maximum likelihood estimates of slope (b_i) and intercept (a_i). No estimate of variance was given by Mossman and Somoza (1989).

Before interpreting the estimate $\widehat{A}$ as the common underlying area, we should test whether the seven studies all estimate a single common value. Using the equation (7.18) we find

$$\chi^2_{homogeneous} = 307.8 \times (0.789 - 0.781)^2 + \ldots + 692 \times (0.652 - 0.781)^2 = 35.71,$$

Table 7.4 Summary of Seven Studies of the Dexamethasone Suppression Test.

Reference	$\hat{A}$	$Se(\hat{A})$	Number of Subjects With Condition	Without Condition	W
Study 1	0.789	0.057	34	33	307.8
Study 2	0.724	0.025	215	152	1600.0
Study 3	0.851	0.028	119	79	1275.6
Study 4	0.876	0.029	54	41	1189.1
Study 5	0.782	0.102	52	49	96.1
Study 6	0.702	0.056	65	31	318.9
Study 7	0.652	0.038	111	77	692.5

which is highly significant ($p < 0.0001$) when compared with a chi-square distribution with 6 degrees of freedom. Hence we should reject the null hypothesis of homogeneity; that is, the individual ROC curve areas across studies are not the same. Thus the estimated ROC curve area from the seven studies are subject to both within- and between-study variation, and more complex methods such as will be presented in Chapter 12 will be more appropriate.

7.5.4 Other Methods

More advanced methods of data analysis for meta-analyses of diagnostic tests, which expand upon the simple methods presented in this chapter, are found in Chapter 12. These methods will accommodate heterogeneity in accuracy, and include procedures to specifically incorporate random effects when combining information on sensitivity and specificity. When data are reported in an ordinal or continuous manner, other advanced techniques will involve random effects methods for summarizing ROC curves and the area under them.

7.6 PUBLIC PRESENTATION

Reporting requirements for meta-analysis of observational studies and RCTs have been published (Moher et al., 1999; Stroup et al., 2000). At this writing, such reporting requirements have not yet been published for meta-analysis of diagnostic tests. Meta-analyses being submitted to appear in the Cochrane Database of Systematic Reviews must follow a specific format that is outlined in Chapter 4 of their handbook. General suggestions that would apply to publication in most journals follows.

Since a meta-analysis is a scientific endeavor, the standard format for scientific presentation should be used, i.e., introduction, methods, results, discussion. Authors should strive to include as much detail of the process and results of the meta-analysis as possible. Presentation of this detail allows others to determine if they agree with the authors on the interpretation of the items such as the design characteristics. It also allows other researchers to redo the analysis using different methods or with different subsets. Finally, it makes it easier to add studies for future meta-analyses on the same topic.

The introduction should provide a clear statement of the objectives and scope of the study. The methods section should provide a detailed description of the literature retrieval process. This should include the date of the literature search, a list of key words used to search the electronic literature, the languages used and the years of publication considered. Inclusion/exclusion criteria should be clearly stated, as the results of any meta-analysis may be highly dependent on these decisions. The method of data abstraction should be described including the number of abstractors, method of resolution of disagreements (if more than one abstractor) and whether (and how) the abstraction was blinded. Methods for assessing quality of included studies, if used, should be described. Statistical analysis should be described including methods used to summarize results, as well as methods used to assess existence and sources of heterogeneity amongst studies. If publication bias is explored the methods should also be described.

The results section should include findings for each aspect of the meta-analysis. The number of potentially relevant articles accessed, screened and excluded should be given, along with reasons for exclusions. In other types of meta-analyses this is generally presented in a figure. Design, test and patient characteristics of each study should be displayed. The preferred method, if space allows, would be to include a table which lists the study design, test and patient characteristics of each individual article. An alternative, which uses less space, would be to report frequencies of these characteristics; e.g., the number of studies that exhibit verification bias, the number published before a certain date, etc. Presentation of the quality of articles can be presented in a similar fashion. A table which lists each article along with an indication of the quality of selected items (perhaps a subset from QUADAS) would be best. An alternative would be a figure that shows the percent of included articles that achieve particular levels of quality, again for a selected set of quality items.

As much raw accuracy data should be presented as the journal allows. This should include sufficient information to determine sensitivity, specificity and likelihood ratios overall and possibly in subgroups such as categories of study design, patient or test characteristics, or quality. Sensitivities and specificities can be presented in tabular form or plotted on axes as a SROC curve. The former is easier to use in future studies, but the latter may more clearly convey the results, thus presentation of both would be optimal. Using both methods of presentation is preferable.

Analysis results presented should include findings related to heterogeneity of accuracy values, as well as any summary values which are calculated.

Findings illuminating the relationship of diagnostic accuracy to study quality should be presented, as well as relationship of accuracy results to patient and test characteristics.

An important goal of a meta-analysis is to assess the quality of information available on the diagnostic test in question. Thus the Discussion section should address the current state of knowledge and availability of information. This should be illuminated by a critical assessment of the research that was found, as well as what was lacking. Recommendations should be made relative to improvements of future research both in terms of design quality and in terms of any specific questions that remain to be answered. This may include recommendations to collect data on certain important subpopulations of specific variants of the diagnostic test.

7.6.1   Presentation of Results: Meta-analysis of Ultrasound for PAD

DeVries et al. (1996) clearly stated their study objectives. The Methods section listed the years of inclusion and the specific terms used in the MEDLINE search. While the authors did not list the excluded studies and their individual reasons for exclusion, they indicated that they would make such a list available on request. Summary reasons for exclusion were presented (e.g., nine of 34 excluded articles were reviews, 4 articles reported data already included in other articles). Study and patient characteristics were presented individually for each included article. The number of TP, FN, TN and FP observations were presented in tabular form and SROC curves were presented for both types of ultrasound. Details of the statistical analysis comparing the two ultrasounds were included in an appendix. Analysis investigating the effects of study design and patient characteristics were summarized in the results section without details such as levels of statistical significance. Additional analysis regarding the effect of individual studies on the meta-analysis (jackknife sensitivity analysis) was also mentioned briefly, with more detail presented in the Appendix.

In their discussion, DeVries et al. (1996) comment on the heterogeneity they found in the literature on duplex ultrasonography. They also point out the problems performing the meta-analysis due to the lack of detail found in many of the articles. They indicated that this lack of detail could be at least partially responsible for failing to show a relationship between some of the design characteristics and the accuracy of the tests.

PART II

ADVANCED METHODS

CHAPTER 8

REGRESSION ANALYSIS FOR INDEPENDENT ROC DATA

In previous chapters, we discussed how to estimate a receiver operating characteristic (ROC) curve for a single diagnostic test and how to compare the ROC curves for different diagnostic tests. Recall from Chapters 2 and 3 that patient covariates, such as the severity of disease and age of a patient, may affect the accuracy of a diagnostic test. The methods we have discussed thus far cannot accommodate patient covariates. In this chapter, we introduce two regression models that can be used to study covariate effects on the accuracy of a diagnostic test. These regression models allow us not only to study the simultaneous or independent effects of covariates on the accuracy of a test, but also to compare the accuracy of different tests while controlling for potential confounders. Our focus is on regression models for the ROC curves of continuous- and ordinal-scale tests. When the response is binary, standard logistic regression (Agresti, 1990) can be used to model a test's sensitivity and/or specificity; this will not be covered here.

In the literature, three regression models for ROC analysis have been proposed. The first approach fits a regression model for the distribution of test responses for patients with the condition and a separate regression model for the distribution of test responses for patients without the condition; then,

Statistical Methods in Diagnostic Medicine,
Second Edition. By Xiao-Hua Zhou, Nancy A. Obuchowski, Donna K. McClish
Copyright © 2011 John Wiley & Sons, Inc.

it assesses covariate effects on the induced ROC curves (Tosteson and Begg, 1988). The second approach directly models covariate effects on ROC curves (Pepe and Thompson, 2000; Alonzo and Pepe, 2002). The third approach first computes a summary measure, such as the area under the ROC curve, for test accuracy for each combination of covariates; then, it uses a regression model to assess covariate effects on the summary measure (Thompson and Zucchini, 1989). It is important to note that the first two approaches can be applied to both discrete and continuous covariates. However, the third method can only be applied when covariates are discrete and there are enough patients in each covariate combination to permit calculation of the summary accuracy measure. Because of these limitations with the third approach, we focus on the first two approaches in this chapter only.

Although it is important to assess the effects of covariates on diagnostic accuracy of a test, sometimes it may be also important to assess the overall diagnostic accuracy of a test and to compare overall accuracies of competing tests. When covariates affect the accuracy of diagnostic tests, unadjusted ROC curves may be misleading measures of the overall diagnostic accuracy of the tests. An appropriate measure for representing the overall diagnostic accuracy of a test should take into account covariates. Such an overall measure is called a covariate-adjusted ROC curve (Janes and Pepe, 2008a). In this chapter we will discuss the definition of covariate-adjusted ROC curves and how to estimate them.

In Section 8.1, we give four examples, which will be used to illustrate the proposed regression models in later sections. In Section 8.2, we introduce the regression models for ROC curves when the test response is continuous. In Section 8.3, we describe the regression models for ROC curves when the test response is ordinal. In Section 8.4, we define a covariate-adjusted overall measure of diagnostic accuracy and how to estimate it.

8.1 FOUR CLINICAL STUDIES

In this section, we describe four diagnostic accuracy studies that require the use of regression models. In the first three studies, the response of the test is continuous, and in the fourth study, the test response is ordinal. We present the analyses of the first three data sets in Sections 8.2.3, 8.2.4, and 8.2.5, respectively, and that of the fourth data set in Section 8.3.3. Of the four studies described in the text that follows, the second and third have an additional problem of correlated data. For the purpose of illustration, we assume independence among test-result observations. (We will discuss how to adjust for possible correlations in estimation in Chapter 9.)

8.1.1   Surgical Lesion in a Carotid Vessel Example

The first study is Case Study 3, described in Chapter 1, which considers the accuracy of magnetic resonance angiography (MRA) for detection of a significant surgically resectable lesion in the left carotid vessel. A significant surgically resectable lesion was established by conventional catheter angiography, which was considered as the gold standard. The reader of the MRA image reported his interpretation on a 0% to 100% scale for the percentage of the vessel blocked by stenosis. The study included both symptomatic and asymptomatic patients. A patient was called *asymptomatic* if he or she underwent MRA for screening purposes and *symptomatic* if he or she underwent MRA for diagnostic purposes (i.e., he or she recently had a stroke). Because the accuracy of MRA may depend on the age of a patient and whether the patient is symptomatic or asymptomatic, we must account for the continuous covariate (age) and the binary covariate (the symptomatic indicator) when assessing the accuracy of MRA.

8.1.2   Pancreatic Cancer Example

The second study was taken from Wieand et al. (1989) at the Mayo Clinic concerning the relative accuracy of two biomarkers for pancreatic cancer. One biomarker, called CA125, was a cancer antigen; the other, called CA19-9, was a monoclonal antibody with a carbohydrate antigenic determinant. The study collected serum concentrations of the two biomarkers from 51 control patients with pancreatitis and 90 case patients with pancreatic cancer. The responses of the biomarkers are continuous; thus, by creating a binary indicator for the biomarker type, we can then compare the relative accuracy of the two biomarkers in a regression framework. Of course, these two biomarkers could also be compared using methods from Chapter 5.

8.1.3   Hearing Test Example

The third data set was taken from a study conducted by Stover et el. (Stover et al., 1996) on the accuracy of the distortion product otoacoustic emission (DPOAE) test to separate normal-hearing from hearing-impaired ears and the effect of primary stimulus level on the test's accuracy. For each ear, the DPOAE test was applied under nine different settings for the input stimulus. Each setting was defined by a particular frequency (f) and intensity (L) of the auditory stimulus. The response of the ear to the stimulus could be affected by the stimulus parameters, as well as by the hearing status of the ear. Among hearing-impaired ears the severity of hearing impairment, as measured by the true hearing threshold, would be expected to affect the results of the DPOAE test. A total of 103 normal-hearing and 107 hearing-impaired subjects were included in the study. Following the same notation as in Pepe (Pepe, 1998), we define the test result, T, as the negative signal-to-noise ratio response, to coincide with a convention that higher values are associated with hearing impairment. The disease variable, D, is hearing impairment of 20 decibels(dB) or more on their pure tone thresholds at any of the nine stimulus frequencies. In this study we have two covariates, frequency and intensity levels of the stimulus, which are common to both diseased and non-diseased subjects: (1) $X_f = $ frequency/100, which is measured in Hertz, and (2) $X_L = $ intensity/10, which is measured in dB. We also use a disease-specific covariate, $Z_d = $ (hearing threshold $- 20$)/10, which is measured in decibels, taking values that are greater than 0 dB for hearing-impaired ears and undefined for normal-hearing ears. We are interested in assessing how these three covariates affect the accuracy of the DPOAE test.

8.1.4   Staging of Prostate Cancer Example

The fourth dataset was a subset taken from a multicenter study on the accuracy of magnetic resonance imaging (MRI) and transrectal ultrasound (US) in detecting periprostatic invasion in patients with known prostate cancer. For a detailed description of the entire study, see Rifkin et al. (1990). Before their induction into the study, all patients had carcinoma confirmed on biopsy and were clinically deemed to have localized cancers, and therefore, felt to be candidates for surgical resection of the prostate gland. Treatment options for a patient with prostate cancer depend on whether the patient has an advanced stage of the disease. If invasion of the gland's capsule has occurred, the patient is best managed with a radiation therapy-hormonal therapy combination, but if the lesion is contained within the gland, the patient has a high likelihood of surgical cure. Therefore, the critical issue is the presence or absence of periprostatic invasion.

All patients enrolled in the study were examined preoperatively with MRI and transrectal US. The MRI and US examination were interpreted separately by two different groups of radiologists - one for the MRI studies and the other for the US studies. After the radiologists read the films, they were asked to provide information about periprostatic fat infiltration and the presence, size and location of tumors. The radiologists used a 5-point ordinal scale to rate their degree of confidence that periprostatic invasion had occurred. The gold standard on periprostatic invasion was established by pathology analysis of the patient's specimens obtained from surgery.

The subset contains the results from the institution with the largest number of patients - 117 patients with periprostatic invasion and eight patients without periprostatic invasion. The ordinal-scale data are given in Table 8.1 We are interested in assessing the accuracy of US in detecting periprostatic invasion. Because the accuracy of US is different with different radiologists, we account for reader effects on the accuracy of US in a regression model with three indicators for the four readers.

Table 8.1 Ultrasound Rating Data By the Four Radiologists

Reader	Disease*	Ordinal-scale response				
		1	2	3	4	5
1	0	11	0	4	9	4
1	1	15	0	4	18	6
2	0	7	0	5	3	2
2	1	8	3	5	20	7
3	0	14	0	4	7	1
3	1	10	0	6	21	3
4	0	2	1	3	3	0
4	1	4	2	4	1	0

*Disease $=1$ if a patient has periprostatic invasion;
*Disease $=0$ if a patient does not have periprostatic invasion.

8.2 REGRESSION MODELS FOR CONTINUOUS-SCALE TESTS

Assume that T is the continuous-scale response of a diagnostic test for a patient. Let X denote the vector of covariates that can potentially affect the test accuracy. For example, in the first clinical study described in Section 8.1, T represents the reader's interpretation of the MRA, and X includes the patient's age and an indicator for presence or absence of symptoms. We further assume that each sampled patient has a confirmed condition status determined independently of the test result and denoted by D, where $D = 1$ for a patient with the condition and 0 for a patient without the condition. Let $\bar{F}_{d,x}(t)$ be the survival function of T given $D = d$ and $X = x$; that is,

$$\bar{F}_{d,x}(t) = P(T > t | D = d, X = x).$$

Then, the ROC curve for T among patients with the vector of covariates' value x is a plot of $\bar{F}_{1,x}(t)$ versus $\bar{F}_{0,x}(t)$ for $-\infty < t < \infty$. If we define the inverse function of $\bar{F}_{d,x}(t)$ by

$$\bar{F}_{d,x}^{-1}(p) = \sup\{t : \bar{F}_{d,x}(t) \geq p\},$$

we can write the ROC curve as

$$ROC_x(p) = \bar{F}_{1,x}(\bar{F}_{0,x}^{-1}(p)), \tag{8.1}$$

where $p = \bar{F}_{0,x}(t)$, the false-positive rate (FPR) corresponding to a cutoff point t in the domain of the survival distribution function $\bar{F}_{0,x}$. That is, the ROC curve is a plot of $ROC_x(p)$ versus p for $0 \leq p \leq 1$.

From (8.1) we see that the ROC curve for T depends on the survival functions, $\bar{F}_{1,x}$ and $\bar{F}_{0,x}$, of the populations of patients with and without the condition, respectively. Therefore, one way to assess the covariate effects on the ROC curve is to model the covariate effects on $\bar{F}_{1,x}$ and $\bar{F}_{0,x}$, and then use (8.1) to derive the covariate effects on the ROC curve. We describe this indirect regression approach in Section 8.2.1. An alternative approach is to directly model the covariate effects on the ROC curve, which is the topic of Section 8.2.2.

8.2.1   Indirect Regression Models for ROC Curves

We propose the following heteroscedastic linear regression model for the test result T:

$$T = \mu(D, X; \beta) + \sigma(D, X; \alpha)\epsilon, \tag{8.2}$$

where ϵ is the residual term with mean 0 and variance 1 but with an unknown distribution function $G_0(.)$. Here, β is the vector of location parameters, representing the effects of D and X on the mean of T, and α is the vector of scale parameters, representing the effects of D and X on the variance of T. The proposed model (8.2) is an extension of the homoscedastic linear model proposed by Pepe (1998).

Let $\bar{G}_0 = 1 - G_0$ be the survival function of ϵ. Under model equation (8.2), we can show that

$$\bar{F}_{d,x}(t) = \bar{G}_0(\frac{t - \mu(d, x; \beta)}{\sigma(d, x; \alpha)}). \tag{8.3}$$

Therefore, the ROC curve among patients with covariates $X = x$ is given by

$$ROC_x(p) = \bar{G}_0[b(x; \alpha)\bar{G}_0^{-1}(p) - a(x; \beta, \alpha)], \tag{8.4}$$

where $\bar{G}_0^{-1}$ is the inverse function of $\bar{G}_0$,

$$a(x; \beta, \alpha) = \frac{\mu(1, x; \beta) - \mu(0, x; \beta)}{\sigma(1, x; \alpha)}, \text{ and } b(x; \alpha) = \frac{\sigma(0, x; \alpha)}{\sigma(1, x; \alpha)}. \tag{8.5}$$

To see how the covariates x affect the ROC curve, $ROC_x(p)$, we consider a simple example with 1-dimensional X (e.g., age). In this example, we take mean $\mu(\text{d,x}; \beta)$ and variance $\sigma^2(\text{d,x}; \alpha)$ to be

$$\mu(d, x; \beta) = \beta_0 + \beta_1 d + \beta_2 x + \beta_3(d * x) \text{ and } \sigma^2(d, x; \alpha) = \sigma^2(d), \tag{8.6}$$

respectively, wherein the variance does not depend on the value x. Under this simple model, the ROC curve associated with $X = x$ is given by

$$ROC_x(p) = \bar{G}_0[b(x; \alpha)\bar{G}_0^{-1}(p) - a(x; \beta, \alpha)], \tag{8.7}$$

where $a(x; \beta, \alpha) = \beta_1/\sigma(1) + (\beta_3/\sigma(1))x$ and $b(x; \alpha) = \sigma(0)/\sigma(1)$. Let $a_1 = -(\beta_3/\sigma(1))$. From (8.7), we see that the effect of x on the corresponding ROC curve is quantified by a_1, which is a function of β_3 and $\sigma(1)$. Because $\bar{G}_0$ is a survival function, a positive value of a_1 results in a decrease in the ROC curve, whereas a negative a_1 results in an increase in the ROC curve.

We now introduce a two-stage procedure for estimating the ROC curves that are defined by (8.4), an extension of Pepe's method (Pepe, 1998) for the homoscedastic linear regression model. In the first stage, we use the method of generalized estimating equations (GEE) for estimating β and α in (8.2), denoted by $\hat{\beta}$ and $\hat{\alpha}$, respectively. In the second stage, we use the residuals to estimate the baseline function $\bar{G}_0$ and, hence, the ROC curve, $ROC_x(p)$. The estimating equation in the first stage is based on the observation that the mean and variance of T are $\mu(d, x; \beta)$ and $\sigma^2(d, x; \alpha)$, respectively. Let us rearrange our sample so that subjects with the condition appear first, and let T_i and x_i be the values of T and X for the ith patient with the condition (where $i = 1, \ldots, n_1$) and T_j and x_j be the values of X and T for the jth patient without the condition (where $j = n_1 + 1, \ldots, N = n_1 + n_0$). The estimating equations have the following forms:

$$\sum_{i=1}^{n_1} \frac{\partial \mu(1, x_i; \beta)}{\partial \beta} \frac{T_i - \mu(1, x_i; \beta)}{\sigma^2(1, x_i; \alpha)} + \sum_{j=n_1+1}^{N} \frac{\partial \mu(0, x_j; \beta)}{\partial \beta} \frac{T_j - \mu(0, x_j; \beta)}{\sigma^2(0, x_j; \alpha)} = 0,$$

$$\sum_{i=1}^{n_1} (T_i - \mu(1, x_i; \beta))^2 - \sigma^2(1, x_i; \alpha) + \sum_{j=n_1+1}^{N} (T_j - \mu(0, x_j; \beta))^2 - \sigma^2(0, x_j; \alpha) = 0.$$

To estimate the ROC curve, we need to estimate the unknown baseline function, $\bar{G}$; to estimate this baseline function, we define the following standardized residuals:

$$\hat{\epsilon}_i = \frac{T_i - \mu(1, x_{1i}; \hat{\beta})}{\sigma(1, x_i; \hat{\alpha})} \text{ and } \hat{\epsilon}_j = \frac{T_j - \mu(0, x_j; \hat{\beta})}{\sigma(0, x_j; \hat{\alpha})}, \tag{8.8}$$

where $i = 1, \ldots, n_1$, and $j = n_1 + 1, \ldots, N$. Our estimator is then defined as follows:

$$\widehat{\bar{G}}_0(t) = N^{-1} \{ \sum_{i=1}^{n_1} I_{[\hat{\epsilon}_i \geq t]} + \sum_{j=n_1+1}^{N} I_{[\hat{\epsilon}_j \geq t]} \}, \tag{8.9}$$

where $I_{(\hat{\epsilon} \geq t)}$ is an indicator variable, equaling 1 if $\hat{\epsilon} \geq t$ and 0 otherwise. We estimate the ROC curve corresponding to the covariate value x by

$$\widehat{ROC}_x(p) = \widehat{\bar{G}}_0 [b(x; \hat{\alpha}) \widehat{\bar{G}}_0^{-1}(p) - a(x; \hat{\beta}, \hat{\alpha})], \tag{8.10}$$

where $a(x; \beta, \alpha)$ and $b(x; \alpha)$ are defined by (8.5).

See Liu and Zhou (2011b) for a detailed discussion on the variance of the estimated ROC curve and asymptotic properties of the resulting estimators. Since the asymptotic variance of the estimated ROC curve involves unknown density functions, to avoid non-parametric density estimation, we can use a bootstrap method to derive the variances for the estimated ROC curve

(Davison and Hinkley, 1997). To describe the bootstrap method, we need additional notation. Let T_k, d_k, and x_k be the values of T, D, and X for the ith patient, where $k = 1, \ldots, N$. The bootstrap method is based on the assumption that it is appropriate to treat D and X as being random. Under such an assumption, we can consider the observed data, (T_k, d_k, x_k), $k = 1, \ldots, N$, as an independent and identically distributed (i.i.d.) sample from the joint distribution of T, D, and X. Each bootstrap sample is generated by sampling with replacement from (T_k, d_k, x_k), $k = 1, \ldots, N$. We summarize the first bootstrap method for estimating the variance of $\widehat{ROC}_x(p)$ in the following steps:

1. Sample $(k_1^*, \ldots, k_N^*)$ with replacement from $(1, \ldots, N)$.

2. Set $T_k^* = T_{k_k^*}$, $d_k^* = d_{k_k^*}$, and $x_k^* = x_{k_k^*}$, for $k = 1, \ldots, N$.

3. Apply the proposed 2-stage procedure to the bootstrap sample-(T_k^*, d_k^*, x_k^*), $k = 1, \ldots, N$-to get $\widehat{\beta}^*$, $\hat{\alpha}^*$, and $\widehat{G}_0^*$.

4. Obtain a bootstrap estimate for the ROC curve $ROC_x(p)$ by substituting the bootstrap estimates into (8.10),

$$\widehat{ROC}_x^*(p) = \hat{G}_0^*[-a(x; \hat{\beta}^*, \hat{\alpha}^*) + b(x; \hat{\alpha}^*)(\hat{G}_0^*)^{-1}(p)].$$

5. Repeat steps 1-4 B times to obtain B bootstrap estimates, $\widehat{ROC}_{bx}^*(p)$, $b = 1, \ldots, B$.

6. Estimate the variance of $\widehat{ROC}_x(p)$ by

$$(S^*)^2 = \frac{1}{R-1} \sum_{b=1}^{B} [\widehat{ROC}_{bx}^*(p) - \overline{\widehat{ROC}}_x^*(p)]^2, \qquad (8.11)$$

where

$$\overline{\widehat{ROC}}_x^*(p) = (1/B) \sum_{b=1}^{B} \widehat{ROC}_{bx}^*(p). \qquad (8.12)$$

After obtaining a variance estimate for $\widehat{ROC}_x(p)$ with the aforementioned bootstrap method, we can now construct a confidence interval (CI) for $ROC_x(p)$ at a fixed p. If we can assume normality for $(\widehat{ROC}_x(p) - ROC_x(p))/S^*$, we can obtain a two-sided $(1 - \delta)100\%$ CI for $ROC_x(p)$ as follows:

$$(\widehat{ROC}_x(p) - z_{1-\delta/2}S^*, \widehat{ROC}_x(p) + z_{1-\delta/2}S^*), \qquad (8.13)$$

where z_δ is the δth percentile of the standard normal distribution.

Without assuming normality for $(\widehat{ROC}_x(p) - \widehat{ROC}_x(p))/S^*$, we can use another bootstrap sampling method, which is called a *double* bootstrap, to obtain a bootstrap CI for $ROC_x(p)$ (Hall, 1998). Although the double boot-strap method is more robust than the standard bootstrap method, it can increase computational time considerably.

We can also use the bootstrap method to make inferences about the area under the ROC curve. The area under the ROC curve for patients with $X = x$ can be calculated by

$$A_x = \int_0^1 ROC_x(p)dp.$$

Thus an estimate for the ROC curve area is given by

$$\hat{A}_x = \int_0^1 \widehat{ROC}_x(p)dp,$$

where $\widehat{ROC}_x(p)$ is given by (8.10). For example, if G_0 in the model (8.2) is the standard normal distribution, then $\hat{A}_x$ has the following explicit form:

$$\hat{A}_x = \Phi\left(\frac{a(x; \hat{\beta}, \hat{\alpha})}{\sqrt{1 + (b(x; \hat{\alpha}))^2}}\right),$$

where $a(x; \beta, \alpha)$ and $b(x; \alpha)$ are defined by (8.5).

To estimate the variance of $\hat{A}_x$, we first use the same bootstrap sampling methods as described in the preceding text to obtain R bootstrap estimates for the area under the ROC curve, $\hat{A}_{rx}^*$, for $r = 1, \ldots, B$. Then, we obtain the bootstrap variance estimate for the estimated area under the ROC curve, $\hat{A}_x$, as follows:

$$(\hat{\sigma}_A^*)^2 = \frac{1}{B-1} \sum_{r=1}^B (\hat{A}_{rx}^* - \bar{\hat{A}}_x^*)^2,$$

where $\bar{\hat{A}}_x^* = (1/B) \sum_{r=1}^B \hat{A}_{rx}^*$. With this variance estimate, we can obtain a CI for the ROC curve area A_x. Assuming normality for $(\hat{A}_x - A_x)/\hat{\sigma}_A^*$, we obtain a 2-sided $(1 - \delta)100\%$ CI for the ROC curve area A_x as follows:

$$(\hat{A}_x - z_{1-\delta/2}\hat{\sigma}_A^*, \hat{A}_x + z_{1-\delta/2}\hat{\sigma}_A^*).$$

Without assuming normality for $(\hat{A}_x - A_x)/\hat{\sigma}_A^*$, we can use the double boot-strap method to obtain a bootstrap CI for A_x (Hall, 1998).

One main disadvantage of regression model (8.2) is the interpretability of its parameters. Although its regression parameters have simple inter-pretations on the distribution of the test responses, it is difficult to inter-pret its regression parameters on the ROC curves. In the next section, we introduce the second regression method that directly models covariate ef-fects on the smooth ROC curves, simplifying interpretation of the regres-sion parameters on ROC curves. We have implemented this direct regres-sion method in R, and the R code can be downloaded from the website, http://faculty.washington.edu/azhou/books/diagnostic.html.

8.2.2   Direct Regression Models for ROC Curves

The direct regression model allows one to estimate the ROC curve without specifying parametric distributions for the test results of patients with and without the condition.

Let X be a vector of covariates common to both a patient with the condition and one without the condition, and let X_D denote a vector of covariates specific to the patient with the condition. The common covariates X and condition-specific covariates X_D may affect the corresponding ROC curve. In practice, most studies focus on the common covariates. For example, in the first, second, and fourth studies described in Section 8.1, we were interested in the common covariates. In the third study, however, we have both the common and condition-specific covariates. We define $Z = (X', X_D')'$.

Let T_1 and T_0 be the test results of a patient with and without the condition, respectively; let $\bar{F}_{1,z}$ be the survival function of T_1 given $Z = z$ and $\bar{F}_{0,x}$ be the survival function of T_0, given $X = x$. We also let $F_{1,z} = 1 - \bar{F}_{1,z}$ and $F_{0,x} = 1 - \bar{F}_{0,x}$. Then, the smooth ROC curve corresponding to $z = (x', x_D')'$ can be defined as

$$ROC_z(p) = \bar{F}_{1,z}[\bar{F}_{0,x}^{-1}(p)], \tag{8.14}$$

where $p \in (0,1)$, and the resulting ROC curve can be interpreted as one that compares the test response of a patient with the condition to a patient without the condition at the same common covariate value. Of course, we can also write the ROC curve as

$$ROC_z(p) = 1 - F_{1,z}[F_{0,x}^{-1}(1-p)],$$

where $F_{0,x}^{-1}$ is the inverse function of $F_{0,x}$.

We model the effects of x and x_D on $ROC_z(p)$ using the following regression model:

$$ROC_z(p) = F\{\beta'z + H(p)\}, \tag{8.15}$$

where p is the false positive rate, which varies from 0 to 1; X is a covariate vector; F is a link function; and H is a baseline monotone increasing function that satisfies the conditions, $H(0) = -\infty$ and $H(1) = +\infty$. Model (8.15) includes the classic binormal model when $F(\cdot) = \Phi(\cdot)$ and $H(\cdot) = \alpha_0 + \alpha_1\Phi^{-1}(\cdot)$, as discussed in Chapter 4.

Note that the regression ROC model (8.15) above assumes that the covariate effect on the ROC curve is the same at all false-positive rates p, and hence, the ROC curves corresponding to different values of the covariates do not intersect. We can relax this restriction by including interactions between functions of p and the covariates, x and x_D. For example, we can assume the following ROC regression model:

$$ROC_z(p) = F\{\beta'z + \alpha'\eta(p)z + H(p)\}, \tag{8.16}$$

where $\eta(.)$ is some known function.

In the next three sections, we focus on the model (8.15) without any inter-actions between false positive rates and the covariates. However, the methods discussed in these sections can also be easily applied to a model with some interactions between false positive rates and the covariates.

Compared to the indirect ROC regression methods, the direct regression approach is more attractive, since it directly models the effect of covariates on the test's accuracy; hence, the direct regression ROC model is more easily interpreted. Another difference between the two models is that the direct ROC regression model only makes an assumption about a functional form of the ROC curve but avoids making any additional assumptions about the distributions of test results. Thus, the direct ROC regression model enjoys a certain degree of robustness (Hanley, 1988; Metz et al., 1998). In addition, the direct regression model has the property of invariance, a fundamental property of a ROC curve. Finally, directly modeling ROC curves enables one to (a) easily make inferences about ROC curves in a restricted range of false-positive rates, (b) easily incorporate interactions between covariate and false-positive rates, and (c) compare ROC curves of tests with different numerical scales.

Next, we show that the regression ROC model (8.15) is equivalent to a transformation regression model. We first note that

$$P(\bar{F}_{0,x}(T_1) \leq p \mid Z = z) = P(1 - F_{0,x}(T_1) \leq p \mid Z = z) =$$

$$P(T_1 > F_{0,x}^{-1}(1 - p) \mid Z = z) = ROC_z(p).$$

Let us then define

$$Y = \bar{F}_{0,x}(T_1), \tag{8.17}$$

which is called the placement value in the literature (Pepe and Cai, 2004). We can show that the regression model (8.15) is equivalent to the following transformation model:

$$H(Y) = -\beta'z + \varepsilon, \tag{8.18}$$

where ε is a random error with distribution function F. This equivalence can be easily seen by noting the following equalities under the models (8.15) and (8.18):

$$P(Y \leq p) = P(H(Y) \leq H(p)) = P(\varepsilon \leq \beta'z + H(p)) = F(\beta'z + H(p)).$$

If we assume that both F and H are known, then the model (8.15) becomes a parametric ROC regression model. Alonzo and Pepe (2002) and Pepe and Cai (2004) proposed a generalized linear model-based estimation and a quasi-likelihood estimation method for such parametric regression models; however, the mis-specification of the baseline function can lead to biased estimates of the ROC curves. To reduce bias, Cai (2004) extended the parametric regression ROC model to a semi-parametric regression model by assuming a parametric form for the link function G but allowing the baseline function

H to be nonparametric. Lin et al. (2011) showed by simulation that a mis-specified link function of G could also lead to substantially biased ROC curve estimates and the new nonparametric model (8.15), in which both the baseline and link functions are unknown. Next, we discuss these models in detail.

8.2.2.1 Parametric ROC regression models   By assuming that the link function $F(.)$ is known and that the baseline function $H(.)$ depends on only a vector of parameters α, $H(u) = H_\alpha(u)$, the model (8.15) becomes the following parametric ROC regression model proposed by Pepe and Cai (2004):

$$ROC_z(p) = F\{\beta'z + H_\alpha(p)\}. \tag{8.19}$$

In this model, we assume that the effect of covariates and the FPR on the F-transformed ROC curve is additive.

Let T_i, x_i, and x_{Di} be the values of the test result, common covariates, and condition-specific covariates for the ith patient with the condition, respectively, where $i = 1, \ldots, n_1$, and T_j and x_j be the values of the test result and common covariates for the jth patient without the condition, where $j = n_1 + 1, \ldots, N$. We then calculate the placement value of the ith patient with the condition, $Y_i = \bar{F}_{0,x}(T_{1i})$, $i = 1, \ldots, n_1$. We note that $P(Y_i \leq p \mid Z = z) = ROC_z(p)$. Hence, the density function of Y_i at p, conditional on $Z = z$, is given by $f(\beta'z_i + H_\alpha(p))h_\alpha(p)$, where $f(p)$ and $h_\alpha(p)$ are the derivatives of $F(p)$ and $H_\alpha(p)$ with respect to p, respectively. Therefore, we can write the log-likelihood function, based on $Y_i's$, as follows:

$$l(\beta, \alpha) = \sum_{i=1}^{n_1} \log f(\beta'z_i + H_\alpha(Y_i))h_\alpha(Y_i). \tag{8.20}$$

However, because the likelihood function above involves the unknown survival function $\bar{F}_{0,x_i}$, it cannot be used to estimate β and α. We first need to estimate $\bar{F}_{0,x_i}$, based on the sample of subjects without the condition, (T_{0j}, x_j), $j = n_1 + 1, \ldots, N$. For example, we can use the location and scale model (8.2) in Section 8.2.1 to estimate $\bar{F}_{0,x_i}$, based on data from subjects without the condition. This estimator can be written as follows:

$$\widehat{\bar{F}}_{0,x}(p) = \widehat{G}_0\left(\frac{t - \widehat{\mu}(x)}{\widehat{\sigma}(x)}\right), \tag{8.21}$$

where $\widehat{\sigma}(x) = \sigma(0, x; \widehat{\alpha})$. Substituting $\widehat{\bar{F}}_{0,x_i}$ for $\bar{F}_{0,x_i}$ in the placement value, defined by (8.17), we can then obtain the following estimated placement values:

$$\widehat{Y}_i = \widehat{\bar{F}}_{0,x_i}(T_{1i}). \tag{8.22}$$

Replacing Y_i by the new variable $\widehat{Y}_i$, the resulting $\tilde{l}(\beta, \alpha)$ is no longer a likelihood function but a quasi-likelihood function, which is given as follows:

$$\widehat{l}(\beta, \alpha) = \sum_{i=1}^{n_1} \log f(\beta'z_i + H_\alpha(\widehat{Y}_i))h_\alpha(\widehat{Y}_i). \tag{8.23}$$

By maximizing the quasi-likelihood function (8.23) above with respect to β and α, we obtain the maximum quasi-likelihood estimators $\widehat{\beta}$ and $\widehat{\alpha}$. It can be shown that the vector $\widehat{\beta}$ is consistent and asymptotically normally distributed (Pepe and Cai, 2004). We can then estimate the ROC curve corresponding to the covariates $z = (x', x'_D)'$ at a fixed FPR, p, by

$$\widehat{ROC}_x(p) = F\{\widehat{\beta}'z + H_{\widehat{\alpha}}(p)\}. \tag{8.24}$$

In some applications, we may be interested in partial ROC curves over a range of FPRs, say, the interval $[p_0, p_1]$. We can easily accommodate such cases in estimation of the ROC curves by using the following modified quasi-likelihood function:

$$
\begin{aligned}
\widehat{l}(\beta, \alpha) &= \sum_{i=1}^{n_1} \{ I_{[\widehat{Y}_i < p_1]} \log F(\beta' z_i + H_\alpha(p_1)) \\
&+ I_{[p_0 \leq \widehat{Y}_i \leq p_1]} \log f(\beta' z_i + H_\alpha(\widehat{Y}_i)) h_\alpha(\widehat{Y}_i) \\
&+ I_{[\widehat{Y}_i > p_0]} \log(1 - F(\theta' z_i + H_\alpha(p_0))).
\end{aligned} \tag{8.25}
$$

By maximizing the above quasi-likelihood function with respect to β and α, we would obtain the maximum quasi-likelihood estimators $\widehat{\beta}$ and $\widehat{\alpha}$. We can then estimate the partial ROC curve on the interval $[p_0, p_1]$ corresponding to the covariates $z = (x, x_D)$ by

$$\widehat{ROC}_z(p) = F\{\widehat{\beta}'z + H_{\widehat{\alpha}}(p)\}, \tag{8.26}$$

where $p \in [p_0, p_1]$. Since the formulas for the variances of the estimated ROC curves are not available, we can use the same bootstrap methods as discussed in Section 8.2.1 to derive the variances for the estimated ROC curve.

Alternatively, we may model $H_\alpha(p)$ by a linear model of known basis functions,

$$H_\alpha(p) = \alpha_1 H_1(p) + \ldots + \alpha_q H_q(p), \tag{8.27}$$

where $H_1(p), \ldots, H_q(p)$ are known functions. To estimate regression parameters in the model (8.27), Alonzo and Pepe (2002) used the method of estimating equations, which is based on the following indicator variables of the placement values:

$$\tilde{U}_{ip} = I_{[Y_i \geq p]} \text{ for } i = 1, \cdots, n_1. \tag{8.28}$$

Alonzo and Pepe (2002) showed that the conditional mean and variance of $\tilde{U}_{ip}$, given $z_i = (x_{1i}, x_{Di})$, are

$$E(\tilde{U}_{ip} \mid Z_i = z_i) = ROC_{z_i}(p),$$

and

$$\text{Var}(\tilde{U}_{ip} \mid Z_i = z_i) = ROC_{z_i}(p)(1 - ROC_{z_i}(p)),$$

respectively. Let Γ be a finite set of FPRs. Alonzo and Pepe (2002) proposed the following estimating equation for estimating θ:

$$\sum_{i=1}^{n_1}\sum_{p\in\Gamma} W(\theta,p)(\tilde{U}_{ip} - \eta_i(\theta,p)) = 0, \tag{8.29}$$

where $\theta = (\beta', \alpha')'$, $\eta_i(\theta,p) = ROC_{z_i}(p) = F(\beta'z_i + \alpha_1 H_1(p) + \ldots + \alpha_q H_q(p))$,

$$W_i(\theta,p) = \frac{(\partial/\partial\theta)\eta_i(\theta,p)}{\eta_i(\theta,p)(1 - \eta_i(\theta,p))},$$

and $\partial/\partial\theta$ is the derivative operator with respect to θ.

However, because $\tilde{U}_{ip}$ involves the unknown placement value Y_i, it cannot be used to estimate θ. Using the same estimated placement value as given by (8.22), we can obtain the following new binary variable:

$$\widehat{U}_{ip} = I_{[\hat{Y}_i \geq p]}. \tag{8.30}$$

Replacing $\tilde{U}_{ip}$ by the new binary variable $\widehat{U}_{ip}$, we obtain the following estimating equation:

$$\sum_{i=1}^{n_1}\sum_{p\in\Gamma} W_i(\theta,p)[\widehat{U}_{ip} - \eta_i(\theta,p)] = 0. \tag{8.31}$$

Because the proposed ROC curve model belongs to a class of GLMs, we can utilize standard statistical software packages for GLMs to solve the system of equations (8.31).

Alonzo and Pepe (2002) summarized the algorithm in the following steps:

1. Choose a set of FPRs, $\Gamma = (p)$.

2. Find a $\sqrt{n_0}$-consistent estimator $\widehat{\bar{F}}_{0,x}$ for the survival function of the test result for a patient without the condition, $\bar{F}_{0,x}$, based on data from patients without the condition-$(T_{0j}, x_{0j}), j = 1, \ldots, n_0$. This can be done by using empirical survival function estimates (when applicable) or quantile regression (Koenker and Basset, 1978; Heagerty and Pepe, 1999).

3. Compute binary variables $\widehat{U}_{ip} = I_{[\hat{Y}_i \geq p]}$ for each i and $p \in \Gamma$, where $i = 1, \ldots, n_1$.

4. Fit a binary GLM to $\widehat{U}_{ip}$ and $E(\widehat{U}_{ip}) = F\{\widehat{\beta}'z_i + \alpha_1 H_1(p) + \ldots + \alpha_q H_q(p)\}$; then estimate θ by solving the estimating equation (8.31).

If we are only interested in a partial ROC curve over a range of FPRs, say, less than or equal to p_0, we can accommodate such cases in estimation of the

ROC curves by including only those observations U_{ip} for which $p \leq p_0$, and the resulting estimation equations are given by

$$\sum_{i=1}^{n_1} \sum_{p \in \Gamma} I_{[p \leq p_0]} W_i(\theta, p)[\widehat{U}_{ip} - \eta_i(\theta, p)] = 0. \tag{8.32}$$

A key step in the above estimation algorithm is to specify Γ, the set of FPRs. One possibility is to set $\Gamma = (j/n_0, j = 1, \ldots, n_0)$, corresponding to the cutoff points at every observed patient without the condition. With such a choice, the estimating equation (8.31) becomes

$$\sum_{i=1}^{n_1} \sum_{j=1}^{n_0} S_i(\theta, j/n_0) = 0, \tag{8.33}$$

where $S_i(\theta, p) = W_i(\theta, p)[\widehat{U}_{ip} - \eta_i(\theta, p)]$. If we take $\widehat{F}_{0,x}$ to be the empirical survival function, under some regularity conditions, the estimating equation (8.33) would be the same equation given in Alonzo and Pepe (2002). It is also worth noting that when $\widehat{F}_{0,x}$ is the empirical survival function, the foregoing choice of Γ gives the maximal set of FPRs. From the estimating equation (8.31), we see that the larger the set Γ, the more efficient the parameter estimation. However, greater efficiency is achieved at the expense of computational time, particularly when n and m are large. For example, in the third study described in Section 8.1.3, the sample sizes from the populations with and without the condition are $n_1 = 535$ and $n_0 = 3287$, respectively. Therefore, the application of the foregoing estimation algorithm to this dataset requires fitting a binary GLM model to more than 1.7 million observations (i.e., n_1 times n_0), which is impractical. To find a computationally less intensive algorithm, Alonzo and Pepe (2002) conducted a simulation study and found that a relatively small number of FPRs in Γ can achieve similar efficiency as the one based on the maximal set of FPRs.

After obtaining the estimator, $\hat{\theta}$, for θ, we can estimate the ROC curve corresponding to the covariates x and x_D at a fixed FPR, p, by

$$\widehat{ROC}_z(p) = F\{\hat{\beta}'z + +\hat{\alpha}_1 H_1(p) + \ldots + \hat{\alpha}_q H_q(p)\}. \tag{8.34}$$

With the choice of the observed FPRs, Pepe and Thompson (2000) showed consistency and asymptotic normality for the estimated ROC curve $\widehat{ROC}(p)$ in the special case of no covariates.

We next introduce a bootstrap method for estimating the variance of $\widehat{ROC}_z(p)$ and constructing a CI for the ROC curve at a fixed FPR. The bootstrap method treats (T_i, x_i, x_{Di}), for $i = 1, \ldots, n_1$, as an i.i.d. sample from a joint distribution of T, X, and X_D of a subject with the condition; it treats (T_j, x_j), for $j = 1 + n_1, \ldots, N$, as another i.i.d. sample from the joint distribution of T and X of a subject without the condition, respectively.

We can then use the following steps to estimate the variance of $\widehat{ROC}_z(p)$ and construct a CI for $ROC_z(p)$:

1. Sample (T_i^*, x_i^*, x_{Di}^*), $i = 1, \ldots, n_1$, with replacement from the original sample of patients with the condition, $\{(T_i, x_i, x_{Di})\}$, and sample (T_j^*, x_j^*), $j = n_1 + 1, \ldots, N$, with replacement from the original sample of patients without the condition, $\{(T_j, x_j)\}$.

2. Obtain bootstrap estimates, $\hat{\gamma}^*$ and $\hat{\beta}^*$, for γ and β by solving the estimating equation (8.31) based on the bootstrap sample, (T_i^*, x_i^*, x_{Di}^*) and (T_j^*, x_j^*), where $i = 1, \ldots, n_1; j = n_1 + 1, \ldots, N$.

3. Obtain a bootstrap estimate $\widehat{ROC}_z^*(p)$ for the ROC curve using (8.34) with the bootstrap estimates $\hat{\gamma}^*$, $\hat{\beta}^*$, and $\hat{\beta}_D^*$.

4. Repeat steps 1-3 B times to obtain B bootstrap estimates, $\widehat{ROC}_{r,z}^*(p)$, $r = 1, \ldots, B$, for the ROC curve.

5. Estimate the variance of $\widehat{ROC}_z(p)$ by

$$(S^*)^2 = \frac{1}{B-1} \sum_{r=1}^{B} (\widehat{ROC}_{r,z}^*(p) - \widehat{ROC}^*(p))^2,$$

where

$$\widehat{ROC}(p)^* = (1/B) \sum_{r=1}^{B} \widehat{ROC}_{r,z}^*(p).$$

6. Assuming normality for $[\widehat{ROC}_z(p) - ROC_z(p)]/S^*$, we obtain a two-sided $(1 - \delta)100\%$ CI for $ROC_z(p)$ as

$$[\widehat{ROC}_z(p) - z_{1-\delta/2}S^*, \widehat{ROC}_z(p) + z_{1-\delta/2}S^*]. \tag{8.35}$$

Without assuming normality for $[\widehat{ROC}_z(p) - ROC_z(p)]/S^*$, we can use a double bootstrap method to obtain a bootstrap CI for $ROC_z(p)$ (Hall, 1998).

We now discuss how to construct a CI for the area under the ROC curve for patients with the condition at the covariate values x and x_D, and patients without the condition at the covariate value x. This ROC curve area is defined by

$$A_z = \int_0^1 ROC_z(p)dp,$$

where $z = (x, x_D)$, and $ROC_z(p)$ is defined by (8.16). We estimate the area under the ROC curve by

$$\hat{A}_z = \int_0^1 \widehat{ROC}_z(p)dp,$$

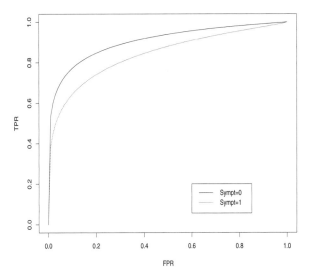

Figure 8.1 Fitted ROC Curves for 60 Year-Old Patients

where $\widehat{ROC}_z(p)$ is given by (8.34). Using a similar procedure as described in Section 8.2.1, we can obtain a bootstrap estimate for the standard error (SE) of $\hat{A}_z$, denoted by $\hat{\sigma}_A^*$. By assuming normality for $(\hat{A}_z - A_z)/\hat{\sigma}_A^*$, we obtain a two-sided $(1 - \delta)100\%$ CI for A_z as follows:

$$(\hat{A}_z - z_{1-\delta/2}\hat{\sigma}_A^*, \hat{A}_z + z_{1-\delta/2}\hat{\sigma}_A^*).$$

Without assuming normality for $(\hat{A}_z - A_z)/\hat{\sigma}_A^*$, we can use a more computationally intensive double bootstrap method to derive a bootstrap CI for A_z (Hall, 1998).

8.2.2.2 *Analysis of the MRA Data in Case Study 3* In this section, we apply the direct parametric regression approach to analyze the MRA data as described in Section 8.1.1. We are interested in assessing the accuracy of MRA in detecting a surgical lesion in the left carotid vessel, and in how the accuracy changes with two covariates: patient age and patient symptom. The dataset consists of 29 patients with surgical lesions ($n_1 = 29$) and 43 patients without surgical lesions ($n_0 = 43$). Because MRA accuracy may depend on the patient's age and whether the patient is symptomatic or asymptomatic, we need to account for the continuous covariate age, denoted by X_1, and the binary-indicator covariate for symptom status, denoted by X_2, when we assess the MRA accuracy. Let $X = (X_1, X_2)$ and $ROC_x(p)$ denote the ROC curve for patients with $X = x$. We model the covariate effects on the corresponding

ROC curve by the following regression:

$$ROC_x(p) = \Phi[\gamma_1 + \gamma_2\Phi^{-1}(p) + \beta_1 x_1 + \beta_2 x_2]. \tag{8.36}$$

To apply the estimation algorithm outlined in Section 8.2.2, we must estimate the covariate-specific pth quantile, $\bar{F}_{0,x}^{-1}(p)$, and choose Γ, a set of FPRs. Using quantile regression (Koenker and Basset, 1978) based on the data for patients without the condition, we obtain an estimator $\widehat{\bar{F}}_{0,x}^{-1}(p)$ for $\bar{F}_{0,x}^{-1}(p)$. Based on the simulation study in Alonzo and Pepe (2002), we chose 50 equally spaced FPRs, $\Gamma = \{1/51, \ldots, 50/51\}$. The resulting estimates, $\hat{\gamma}_1$, $\hat{\gamma}_2$, $\hat{\beta}_1$, and $\hat{\beta}_2$, for γ_1, γ_2, β_1, and β_2 are -2.349, 0.631, 0.065, and -0.377, respectively. Therefore, the estimated ROC curve is given by

$$ROC_x(p) = \Phi[-2.349 + 0.631\Phi^{-1}(p) + 0.065x_1 - 0.377x_2]. \tag{8.37}$$

The positive coefficient for age, $\hat{\beta}_1$, indicates that the older the patient, the more accurate MRA is in detecting surgical lesions. The negative coefficient for the symptomatic indicator implies that MRA is less accurate in detecting surgical lesions among patients with symptoms than among patients without symptoms. To visualize the effect of the binary covariate (the symptom indicator) on the corresponding ROC curve, we plot in Figure 8.1 the two ROC curves for 60-year-old patients: one curve for patients with symptoms, and another for patients without symptoms.

In Figure 8.1, we see that the ROC curve of MRA among patients without symptoms is above that of MRA among patients with symptoms, implying that MRA is more accurate in detecting surgical lesions among the former group.

8.2.2.3 Biomarkers for Detection of Pancreatic Cancer As discussed in Section 8.1.2, Wieand et al. (1989) reported a study on the relative accuracy of the two biomarkers, CA125 and CA19-9, for pancreatic cancer. The study collected serum concentrations of CA125 and CA19-9 from 51 control patients with pancreatitis and 90 case patients with pancreatic cancer (See Table A.6 in Appendix A).

In this example, the condition is referred to as a case; hence the numbers of patients with and without the condition are $m = 90$ and $n = 51$, respectively. To visually compare the accuracy of the two biomarkers, we plot the empirical ROC curves of the biomarkers as well as the portion of the empirical ROC curves when the FPRs are restricted to be ≤ 0.20 (see Figure 8.2).

From the plots in Figure 8.2, we see that the ROC curve for CA19-9 is above that for CA125 when the FPRs are less than 0.85 and below that for CA125 when the FPRs are greater than 0.85. Furthermore, when the FPRs are less than 0.20, the partial ROC curve for CA19-9 is substantially above that for CA125.

To assess whether or not the ROC curves for the two biomarkers are different, we define a binary indicator X for the biomarker type, where $X = 1$ for the CA19-9 biomarker and $X = 0$ for the CA125 biomarker. Let $ROC_x(p)$ denote the ROC curve for patients with $X = x$. From Figure 8.2, we note that the relative accuracy of the two biomarkers may depend on the range of FPRs. Hence, we chose the following parametric regression model to allow different covariate effects over different ranges of FPRs:

$$ROC_x(p) = \Phi[\gamma_1 + \gamma_2\Phi^{-1}(p) + \beta_1 x + \beta_2 x * \Phi^{-1}(p)]. \qquad (8.38)$$

where $ROC_1(p)$ represents the ROC curve of the CA19-9 biomarker, and $ROC_0(p)$ represents the ROC curve of CA125. In fact, this regression model is equivalent to having two separate parametric binormal ROC curves for the two biomarkers. Define $\theta = (\gamma_1, \gamma_2, \beta_1, \beta_2)'$. To emphasize the dependence of $ROC_x(p)$ on the vector of parameters θ, we write $ROC_x(p) = ROC_x(\theta, p)$.

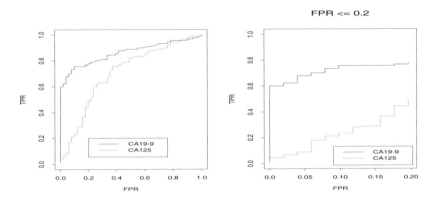

Figure 8.2 Empirical ROC Curves for the Two Biomarkers

Before we can apply the estimation algorithm outlined in Section 8.2.2 to the data set, we first need to choose Γ, the set of FPRs, and then need to estimate $\bar{F}_{0,0}^{-1}(p)$ and $\bar{F}_{0,1}^{-1}(p)$, the pth quantiles of the survival functions of the CA 125 and CA 19-9 for a patient without the condition, respectively. We chose Γ to be $\Gamma = \{1/n, \ldots, 50/n\}$, which gave us 50 equally spaced FPRs, and used empirical quantile functions $\widehat{\bar{F}}_{0,x}^{-1}(p)$ for $\bar{F}_{0,x}^{-1}(p)$, where $x = 0, 1$.

Let T_{1i} and x_{1i} be the test result and the value of X for the ith patient with the condition, where $i = 1, \ldots, 90$. We then define $U_{ip} = I_{[T_{1i} \geq \widehat{\bar{F}}_{0,x_{1i}}^{-1}(p)]}$. The estimating equation for the regression parameters in (8.38) is given by

$$\sum_{i=1}^{90}\sum_{p\in\Gamma}(1, \Phi^{-1}(p), x_{1i}, x_{1i}\Phi^{-1}(p))'W_i(\theta, p)(U_{ip} - ROC_{x_{1i}}(\theta, p)) = 0, \qquad (8.39)$$

where

$$W_i(\theta, p) = \frac{\phi[\gamma_1 + \gamma_2\Phi^{-1}(p) + \beta_1 x_{1i} + \beta_2 x_{1i}\Phi^{-1}(p)]}{ROC_{x_{1i}}(\theta, p)[1 - ROC_{x_{1i}}(\theta, p)]},$$

and $\phi(.)$ is the density function for the standard normal distribution. Solving the estimating equation (8.39), we obtain the resulting estimates for γ_1, γ_2, β_1, and β_2 as 0.82, 1.04, 0.40, and -0.58, respectively.

To investigate the partial ROC curve in the range of FPRs of ≤ 0.20, we can restrict our estimation of the ROC curve to this domain by including only the observations with $p \leq 0.2$ in the estimating equation (8.39). The resulting estimates for γ_1, γ_2, β_1, and β_2 are 0.95, 1.23, 0.15, and -0.89, respectively.

Replacing the parameters in (8.38) by their estimates, we obtain the fitted ROC curves for CA19-9 and CA125, as displayed in Figure 8.3.

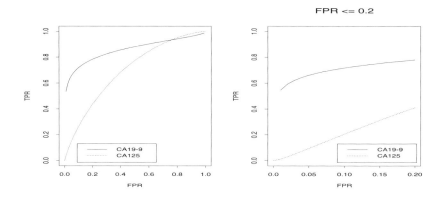

Figure 8.3 Fitted ROC Curves for the Two Biomarkers

From the plots, we see that the CA19-9 biomarker appears much more accurate than CA125 when the FPRs of each are restricted to ≤ 0.2. Because the test results for the two biomarkers on the same patients are correlated, we may use a bootstrap method to compute the SEs and CIs for parameter estimates.

8.2.2.4 Semi-parametric ROC regression models With the unknown baseline function $H(.)$, model (8.15) becomes the following semi-parametric ROC regression model, proposed by Cai (2004):

$$ROC_z(p; \alpha) = F\{\beta'z + H(p)\}, \tag{8.40}$$

where $F(.)$ is a known function, and $H(.)$ is an unknown monotone increasing function with a continuous first derivative. Let $\widehat{Y}_i$ be the estimated placement value of Y_i as given by (8.22), and define $Z_i = (X'_{i1}, X'_{Di})'$. Cai (2004) proposed the following estimating equations to estimate β, β_D, and $H(.)$ simultaneously:

$$\sum_{i=1}^{n_1} w(Z_i, p)[\widehat{U}_{ip} - F\{\beta'Z_i + H(p)\}] = 0, \text{ for } p \in [p_0, p_1], \tag{8.41}$$

and

$$\sum_{i=1}^{n_1} \int_{p_0}^{p_1} w(Z_i, p) Z_i [\widehat{U}_{ip} - F\{\beta' + H(p)\}] d\widehat{\nu}(p) = 0. \tag{8.42}$$

Let $\widehat{H}(p)$ and $\widehat{\beta}$ be the solutions to the system of equations (8.41) and (8.42). Then, we can estimate the ROC curve corresponding to the covariates z at a fixed FPRs p by

$$\widehat{ROC}_z(p) = F\{\widehat{\beta}'z + +\widehat{H}(p)\}. \tag{8.43}$$

Under the assumption that the covariates X and X_D are bounded and $H(.)$ has the continuous first derivative, Cai (2004) showed that $\widehat{ROC}_z(p)$ had an asymptotically normal distribution with the mean, $ROC_z(p)$, when $p \in [p_0, p_1]$.

8.2.2.5 Non-parametric ROC regression models   If we allow both the link function $F(.)$ and baseline function to be unknown, the model (8.14) becomes the following non-parametric ROC regression model proposed by Lin et al. (2011):

$$ROC_z(p) = F\{\beta'z + H(p)\}. \tag{8.44}$$

Model (8.44) continues to hold if H, θ and ε are replaced by $cH, c\theta$, and $c\varepsilon$ for any positive constant c. Model (8.44) also holds if H and ε are replaced by $H+c$ and $\varepsilon+c$ for any constant c. Therefore, scale and location normalization are needed to make the model identifiable. Here we set $H(t_0) = a_0$, and $E[\varepsilon] = 0$ for some finite constant a_0. To begin derivation of the estimator of H, we observe that in transformation model (8.44), Y depends on X only through the index $W = \theta'X$.

Let $G(\cdot|w)$ be the cumulative distribution function (CDF) of T conditional on $W = w$. Assume that H, F, and G are differentiable with respect to all their arguments. Define $h(t) = dH(t)/dt$, $f(t) = dF(t)/dt$, $p(t|w) = dG(t|w)/dt$, and $g(t|w) = dG(t|w)/dw$. Model (8.44) implies that $G(t|w) = F(H(t) + w)$. Therefore, $p(t|w) = f(H(t) + w)h(t)$ and $g(t|w) = f(H(t) + w)$. So, $g(t|w)h(t) = p(t|w)$. Denote $g(t, w) = g(t|w)p(w)$ and $p(t, w) = p(t|w)p(w)$, where $p(\cdot)$ is the density function of W. We then obtain the following equation:

$$g(t, w)h(t) = p(t, w). \tag{8.45}$$

Define $W_i = X_i'\theta$. Replacing w in (8.45) by W_i and summing over all subjects with the condition, we get $\sum_{i=1}^{n_1} g(t, W_i)h(t) = \sum_{i=1}^{n_1} p(t, W_i)$. Therefore we obtain the following expression for $h(t)$:

$$h(t) = \frac{\sum_{i=1}^{n_1} p(t, W_i)}{\sum_{i=1}^{n_1} g(t, W_i)}. \tag{8.46}$$

Hence, integrating the both sides of (8.46) with respect to t gives us the following expression for $H(t)$:

$$H(t) = a_0 + \int_{t_0}^{t} \frac{\sum_{i=1}^{n_1} p(u, W_i)}{\sum_{i=1}^{n_1} g(u, W_i)} du. \tag{8.47}$$

To construct an estimator H_n of H, we need to estimate $G(t|w)$ and its derivatives. Let K_0 and K_1 be one-dimensional density functions, and let b_0 and b_1 be bandwidths. We estimate $p(\cdot)$ by the following kernel estimator:

$$p_n(w) = \frac{1}{n_1 b_0} \sum_{i=1}^{n_1} K_0 \left(\frac{W_i - w}{b_0} \right). \tag{8.48}$$

We can then estimate $G(t|w)$ by the following kernel estimator:

$$G_n(t|w) = \frac{1}{n_1 b_0 p_n(w)} \sum_{i=1}^{n_1} I(T_i \leq t) K_0 \left(\frac{W_{ik} - w}{b_0} \right), \tag{8.49}$$

where $Y_i = S_{\bar{d}, Z_i}(T_i)$, $= 1, \ldots, n_1$. We obtain an estimate of $g(t|w)$ by differentiating $G_n(t|w)$ with respect to w,

$$g_n(t|w) = \partial G_n(t|w)/\partial w. \tag{8.50}$$

Although $p(t|w) = \partial G(t|w)/\partial t$, we cannot use $\partial G_n(t|w)/\partial t$ to estimate $p(t|w)$, because $G_n(t|w)$ is a step function of t. Instead, we estimate $p(t|w)$ by the following kernel density estimator:

$$p_n(t|w) = \frac{1}{n_1 b_0 b_1 p_n(w)} \sum_{i=1}^{n_1} K_1 \left(\frac{Y_i - t}{b_1} \right) K_0 \left(\frac{W_{ik} - w}{b_0} \right). \tag{8.51}$$

The estimator H_n of H is obtained by substituting (8.48), (8.50), and (8.51) into (8.47).

Without imposing a parametric structure on F, it is natural to estimate θ by a solution to the following estimating equation:

$$\sum_{i=1}^{n_1} (H(Y_i) + X_i'\theta) X_i = 0. \tag{8.52}$$

When given H, the estimator of θ has the following closed-form:

$$\theta_n = -\left(\sum_{i=1}^{n_1} X_i X_i' \right)^{-1} \sum_{i=1}^{n_1} X_i H(T_i). \tag{8.53}$$

Implementation

We outline the algorithm for estimating θ, $H(\cdot)$, and $F(\cdot)$ as follows:

1. Derive the estimated placement value, $\hat{Y}_i$, of the ith subject with the condition, using (8.22).

2. Specify an initial value of θ. We obtain such an initial value by an estimate of θ using the maximum rank correlation (MRC) method proposed by Han (1987). This method allows us to estimate θ without

knowing $H(.)$. That is, estimating θ with $\tilde{\theta} = \operatorname{argmax}_\theta W_n(\theta)$, where $W_n(\theta) = \sum_{i \neq j}\{\hat{Y}_i < \hat{Y}_{j\ell}\}\{X_i'\theta > X_j'\theta\}$.

3. Repeat (a) and (b) below until two successive values of θ do not differ significantly.

(a) Given θ, estimate H using (8.47), (8.48), (8.50), and (8.51), with Y_i replaced by $\hat{Y}_i$.

(b) Given H, estimate θ using (8.53) with T_i replaced by $\hat{T}_i$.

Denote $\hat{H}$ and $\hat{\theta}$ to be the final results from the algorithm above.

4. Estimate F using the empirical distribution function of $\hat{U} = \hat{H}(\hat{T}) + \hat{\theta}'X$, denoted by $\hat{F}$.

5. The ROC curve for a test with covariates x can be estimated by $\hat{ROC}(t, x) = \hat{F}\{\hat{\theta}'x + \hat{H}(t)\}$.

Lin et al. (2011) established the asymptotic properties for $\hat{\theta}$, $\hat{H}(\cdot)$, $\hat{F}(\cdot)$, and $\hat{ROC}(t, x)$; they have also shown that $\hat{ROC}(t, x)$ has an asymptotically Gaussian process and converges to the true value at a rate of $n_1^{-1/2}$.

8.2.2.6 Accuracy of Hearing Test   In this section, we apply all three direct regression methods, described in Section 8.2.2, to the data in the third clinical study on the accuracy of the hearing test, as described in Section 8.1.3. We fit the following model to the data, using the parametric, semi-parametric, and non-parametric methods, respectively:

$$ROC_{X_L,X_f,Z_d}(u) = F(H(u) + \theta_1 X_L + \theta_2 X_f + \theta_3 Z_d).$$

For the parametric method, described in Section 8.2.2.1, we chose $F = \Phi$ and $H = \alpha_0 + \alpha_1 \Phi^{-1}$. For the semi-parametric method, described in Section 8.2.2.2, we only chose $F = \Phi$ and left H unspecified. For the non-parametric method, described in Section 8.2.2.3, we left both F and H unspecified, and we estimated the non-parametric function H using the bandwidth selection method in Lin et al. (2011).

Table 8.2 presents the coefficient estimates and their bootstrap standard errors using the parametric quasi-likelihood, semi-parametric, and non-parametric methods. The test appears to perform better when the stimulus used has a low intensity and a higher frequency. The estimate of θ_3 clearly indicates that it is easier to detect hearing-impairment among severe hearing impaired patients than mildly impaired patients.

Table 8.2 shows that the parameter estimates in absolute value using the non-parametric method are smaller than those using the existing single semi-parametric and parametric methods. The estimated ROC curves at $X_L = 6.0$, $X_f = 14.16$, and $Z_d = 0.5$ using the three methods are plotted in Figure 8.2.2.6.

Table 8.2   Estimated Parameters and Standard Errors in the Hearing Test Example

	Non-parametric Estimate (SD)	Semi-parametric Estimate (SD)	Parametric quasi-likelihood Estimate (SD)
θ_1	-0.4951(0.1137)	-0.5525(0.1136)	-0.5435(0.0955)
θ_2	0.0401(0.0157)	0.0394(0.0173)	0.0370(0.0171)
θ_3	0.3740(0.0462)	0.4241(0.0483)	0.3819(0.0484)

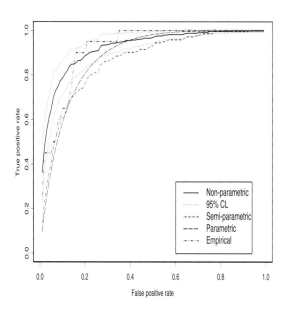

Figure 8.4   The Estimated ROC Curves of the Hearing Test at $X_L = 6.0, X_f = 14.16, Z_d = 0.5$

From Figure 8.4, we see that the estimated ROC curve, using the non-parametric method, is higher than those from the other two methods. Table 8.3 and Figure 8.4 also show that the non-parametric estimates are closer to those using the parametric method than those from the semi-parametric method. The conclusion is consistent with the simulation studies; that is, the semi-parametric estimates may be less robust than the parametric methods in some cases. The estimated ROC curve from the non-parametric method in Figure 8.4 is different from the ROC curves estimated by the other two methods. To see if the estimated ROC curve from the non-parametric method is acceptable, we display the empirical ROC curve in Figure 8.4, based on 147 non-diseased patients with $X_L = 6.0$, $X_f = 14.16$ and 20 diseased patients with $X_L = 6.0, X_f = 14.16$, and $Z_d = 0.5$. From this figure, we see that the non-parametric estimate coincides with the empirical ROC curve, while the other two estimates are below the empirical curve, suggesting that the semi-parametric and parametric estimators may be biased.

8.3   REGRESSION MODELS FOR ORDINAL-SCALE TESTS

In the previous section, we discussed how to model covariate effects on ROC curves of continuous-scale tests. In this section, we introduce regression models for assessing covariate effects on ROC curves of ordinal-scale tests. For an ordinal scale test, the ROC curve can be defined in two ways: (1) the discrete ROC curve and (2) the smooth ROC curve of a latent continuous-scale variable. For estimating the covariate effects on discrete ROC curves, we can apply the indirect and direct regression methods for the continuous-scale test, as discussed in Section 8.2, to the ordinal-scale test; this will not be covered here. Unlike a continuous-scale test, which can directly produce a smooth ROC curve, we cannot directly derive a smooth version of the ROC curve for an ordinal-scale test. We propose to use a latent variable model, as discussed in Chapter 4, to produce the latent smooth ROC curve.

Let T be the ordinal-scale response of the test for a patient, ranging from 1 to W, where $T = 1$ indicates complete confidence in the absence of the condition, and $T = W$ indicates complete confidence in the presence of the condition. Due to the discrete nature of the test response, T, in order to produce a smooth ROC curve for T, we need to consider T as a categorization of the latent continuous variable T^* such that if $c_{w-1} < T^* \le c_w$, then the outcome $T = w$ is observed, $w = 1, \ldots, W$, and if $T^* \ge c_W$, $T = W$ is observed, where $c_0 = -\infty$, and $c_W = +\infty$. Here we assume that the cutoff points, $c_1, \ldots, c_{W-1}$, do not depend on any covariates. It is possible to extend the proposed models to the case in which the c_w depend on covariates.

Next, we define the latent smooth ROC curve for the ordinal-scale test, T. Let X be a vector of covariates that are common to patients with and without the condition. Let $\bar{F}_{d,x}(.)$ be the survival function of the latent variable T^*

given $D = d$ and $X = x$. Then, the latent smooth ROC curve for patients with $X = x$ is defined by the same formula as in (8.1).

Like regression models for continuous-scale tests, we also propose both the indirect and direct regression models for the latent smooth ROC curves of ordinal-scale tests. We present the indirect regression models in Section 8.3.1 and the direct regression models in Section 8.3.2.

8.3.1   Indirect Regression Models for Latent Smooth ROC Curves

Similar to the indirect regression model for a continuous-scale test, as discussed in Section 8.2.1, we first model the effects of x on the two latent survival functions, $\bar{F}_{0,x}$ and $\bar{F}_{1,x}$ and then use (8.1) to derive the covariate effects on the induced latent smooth ROC curve.

Tosteson and Begg (1988) took such an approach, and they proposed to model $\bar{F}_{D,x}(y)$ by the following ordinal regression model:

$$g(\bar{F}_{d,x}(y)) = \frac{y - h_1(d, x; \beta)}{\exp(h_2(d, x; \alpha))}, \tag{8.54}$$

where the link function g is a monotone function. In the model (8.54), terms $h_1(d, x; \beta)$ and $h_2(d, x; \alpha)$ represent the effects of the covariates X and D on the location and scale of the survival function, $\bar{F}_{d,x}(y)$, respectively, and the corresponding parameter vectors β and α are called the location and scale parameters, respectively.

To make the scale parameters in (8.54) identifiable, McCullagh (McCullagh, 1980) imposed the constraint that

$$\sum_{i=1}^{N} h_2(d_i, x_i; \alpha) = 0,$$

where x_i and d_i are the values of X and D for the ith patient. (See McCullagh (1980) for a detailed discussion on the issue of parameter identifiability.) One of the most commonly chosen forms for h_2 is

$$h_2(d, x; \alpha) = \alpha_1(d - \bar{d}) + \alpha_2'(x - \bar{x}),$$

where $\bar{d} = \sum_{i=1}^{N} d_i/N$ and $\bar{x} = \sum_{i=1}^{N} x_i/N$.

After specifying the regression model (8.54) for $\bar{F}_{d,x}(.)$, we can then derive the induced latent smooth ROC curve for patients with the covariates $X = x$. This induced ROC curve is given by

$$ROC_x(p) = g^{-1}[b(x; \alpha)g(p) - a(x; \beta, \alpha)], \tag{8.55}$$

where

$$
\begin{aligned}
a(x; \beta, \alpha) &= \frac{h_1(1, x; \beta) - h_1(0, x; \beta)}{\exp(h_2(1, x; \alpha))}, \\
b(x; \alpha) &= \exp(h_2(0, x; \alpha) - h_2(1, x; \alpha)).
\end{aligned} \tag{8.56}
$$

If we include the condition status, d, as the only covariate in regression model (8.54), then we obtain $h_1(d, x; \beta) = \beta d$ and $h_2(d, x; \alpha) = \alpha(d - \bar{d})$. Hence, $a(x; \beta, \alpha) = \beta \exp(-\alpha(1 - \bar{d}))$ and $b(x; \alpha) = \exp(-\alpha)$. The resulting ROC curve is the well-known "binormal ROC model" proposed by Dorfman and Alf (1969).

From (8.55), we see that the ROC curve, $ROC_x(p)$, is determined by the two parameters $a(x; \beta, \alpha)$ and $b(x; \alpha)$. Hence, the effects of parameters α and β in the latent regression model (8.54) on the ROC curve, $ROC_x(p)$, are through the parameters $a(x; \beta, \alpha)$ and $b(x; \alpha)$.

To illustrate the effects of α and β on $ROC_x(p)$, we now consider a simple model for (8.54) with two indicator covariates, x_1 and x_2. Denote $x = (x_1, x_2)$. We model $h_1(d, x; \beta)$ and $h_2(d, x; \alpha)$ by a linear function of β and α, respectively,

$$h_1(d, x; \beta) = \beta_0 d + \beta_1 x_1 + \beta_2 x_2 + \beta_3(d * x_1)$$

and

$$h_2(d, x; \alpha) = \alpha_0(d - \bar{d}) + \alpha_1(x_1 - \bar{x}_1) + \alpha_2(x_2 - \bar{x}_2) + \alpha_3((d - \bar{d}) * (x_1 - \bar{x}_1)).$$

Under this model, the two parameters that determine $ROC_x(p)$ are

$$a(x; \alpha, \beta) = \frac{\beta_0 + \beta_3 x_1}{\exp(\alpha_0(1 - \bar{d}) + (\alpha_1 + \alpha_3)(x_1 - \bar{x}_1) - \alpha_3 \bar{d}(x_1 - \bar{x}_1) + \alpha_2(x_2 - \bar{x}_2))}$$

and

$$b(x; \alpha) = \exp(-\alpha_0 - \alpha_3(x_1 - \bar{x}_1)).$$

From these expressions, we conclude that the location parameter, β_2, does not affect the ROC curve; it only shifts the cutoff points uniformly on the same ROC curve. The other two location parameters, β_0 and β_3, would shift the ROC curve up or down. As for the effect of the scale parameters on the ROC curve, α_2 can only affect the location of the ROC curve, whereas α_0 and α_3 can affect both the location and shape of the ROC curve. From the above discussion, we see that even with just two covariates, it is difficult to interpret parameters in regression model (8.54).

One desired property of an ROC curve is concavity, which ensures that the ROC curve is always above the 45° diagonal line. The resulting ROC curve is called a "regular" curve (Altham, 1973; Swets, 1986b). In general, we cannot guarantee that the induced ROC curve, defined by (8.55), has a concave shape unless $h_2(d, x; \alpha) = 0$ (Tosteson and Begg, 1988). If a non-concave ROC curve is obtained, then it is important to make a judgment about the appropriateness of the proposed model and the validity of the gathered ordinal-scale data. We further discuss the latter point when we analyze the ultrasound ordinal-scale data in Section 8.3.3.

After specifying ordinal regression model (8.54), we can use the method of maximum likelihood (ML) to estimate the unknown regression parameters, α and β. To derive the ML estimates, we first need to obtain the log-likelihood function for the observed data. Let T_i, d_i, and x_i be the test result, the true condition status, and the covariate value for the ith patient, where $i = 1, \ldots, N$, and N is the total number of patients in the sample. Let Y_{iw} be an indicator variable, equaling to one if the ith patient's test response is w; that is, $Y_{iw} = 1$ if $T_i = w$ and 0 otherwise. Denote the conditional probability that $Y_{iw} = 1$ given $D = d_i, X = x_i$ by $\pi_w(d_i, x_i) = P(Y_{iw} = 1 \mid D = d_i, X = x_i)$. Note that we can consider the observation from the ith patient, $(Y_{i1}, \ldots, Y_{iW})$, as a single multinomial observation with the corresponding probabilities $(\pi_1(d_i, x_i), \ldots, \pi_W(d_i, x_i))$, where $\sum_{w=1}^{W} \pi_w(d_i, x_i) = 1$. From the relationship between the observed ordinal-scale test, T, and the latent variable, T^*, we see that

$$P(T \leq w \mid D = d_i, X = x_i) = P(T^* \leq c_w \mid D = d_i, X = x_i).$$

Hence, under the model (8.54), we can show that

$$\pi_w(d_i, x_i) = g^{-1}\left(\frac{c_w - h_1(d_i, x_i; \beta)}{\exp(h_2(d_i, x_i; \alpha))}\right) - g^{-1}\left(\frac{c_{w-1} - h_1(d_i, x_i; \beta)}{\exp(h_2(d_i, x_i; \alpha))}\right) \text{ for } w < W,$$

and

$$\pi_W(d_i, x_i) = 1 - g^{-1}\left(\frac{c_W - h_1(d_i, x_i; \beta)}{\exp(h_2(d_i, x_i; \alpha))}\right).$$

Therefore, we can write the log-likelihood function as

$$l = \sum_{i=1}^{N} \sum_{w=1}^{W} Y_{kw} \log \pi_w(d_i, x_i), \tag{8.57}$$

which is a function of c_w's, α, and β.

By maximizing log-likelihood function (8.57) over these parameters, we can obtain the ML estimates for c_w's, α, and β, and their corresponding covariance matrix can be obtained as the inverse of Fisher's information matrix. Unfortunately, there are no explicit expressions for these ML estimates, so an iterative algorithm has to be used. An interactive computer program, called PLUM, was developed by Peter McCullagh at the University of Chicago using the Newton-Raphson method with Fisher scoring. Replacing the unknown parameters, α and β, in (8.55) with their ML estimates, we obtain the following ML estimator for the induced smooth ROC curve in the subpopulation of patients with $X = x$:

$$\widehat{ROC}_x(p) = g^{-1}(b(x; \hat{\alpha})g(p) - a(x; \hat{\beta}, \hat{\alpha})), \tag{8.58}$$

for $0 \leq p \leq 1$. Using the first bootstrap method as described in Section 8.2.1, we can obtain a bootstrap estimate for the variance of $\widehat{ROC}_x(p)$ and construct a confidence interval for the latent smooth ROC curve at a fixed p, $ROC_x(p)$.

Because the regression parameters α and β can only affect $ROC_x(p)$ through $a(x; \alpha, \beta)$ and $b(x; \beta)$, indirect modeling makes the interpretation of the covariate effects on the ROC curves difficult. Next, we introduce a regression method that directly models the covariate effects on the smooth ROC curves.

8.3.2   Direct Regression Model for Latent Smooth ROC Curves

Let $\bar{F}_{1,z}$ denote the survival function of the latent variable, T^*, given $D = 1$, $X = x$ and $X_D = x_D$ and $\bar{F}_{0,x}$ denote the survival function of T^* given $D = 0$ and $X = x$. Then, the latent smooth ROC curve corresponding to (z), $ROC_z(p)$, is defined by the same formula as the one given in (8.14).

Using the same notation and idea as in Section 8.2.2, we model the effects of x and x_D on the latent ROC curve, $ROC_z(p)$, by the following parametric regression model:

$$ROC_z(p) = G(\beta' z + H_\alpha(p)), \qquad (8.59)$$

where $G(.)$ is a known function, and $H_\alpha(.)$ is a parametric function.

Let T_i, x_i, and x_{D_i} be the ordinal test result, common and condition-specific covariates for the ith patient with the condition, respectively, where $i = 1, \ldots, n_D$. Let T_j and x_j be the ordinal test result and value of common covariates for the jth patient without the condition, where $j = n_1 + 1, \ldots, N$. Although we can write the ROC curve, $ROC_z(p)$, as the conditional probability, $P(T^* \geq \bar{F}_{0,x}^{-1}(p) \mid D = 1, X = x, X_D = x_D)$, we cannot directly use the indicator variables, as defined in Section 8.2.2, since T^* is unobserved. We define the following indicator variables that are based on observed ordinal-scale test results and involve double arrays to estimate θ in the model (8.59):

$$U_{ij} = I_{[T_i \geq T_j]}, \text{ for } i = 1, \cdots, n_1; j = n_1 + 1, \ldots, N. \qquad (8.60)$$

The reason for using the above binary indicator variables is that if we let $p_{ij} = \bar{F}_{0,x_{1i}}^{-1}(c_{T_j-1})$, we can show that

$$E(U_{ij} \mid x_{1i}, x_{Di}) = ROC_{x_{1i}, x_{Di}}(p_{ij}),$$

and

$$\text{Var}(U_{ij} \mid x_{1i}, x_{Di}) = ROC_{x_{1i}, x_{Di}}(p_{ij})(1 - ROC_{x_{1i}, x_{Di}}(p_{ij})).$$

We can see this equation by first noting that

$$P(T_i \geq w \mid X_i = x_i, X_{Di} = x_{Di}) = P(T_i^* \geq c_{w-1} \mid X_{1i} = x_i, X_{Di} = x_{Di}),$$

for $k = 1, \ldots, W$. Hence, we obtain that

$$P(T_i \geq T_j \mid X_{1i} = x_i, X_{Di} = x_{Di})$$

$$= \sum_{w=1}^{W} P(T_i \geq w \mid X_{1i} = x_i, X_{Di} = x_{Di}) P(T_j = w)$$

$$= \sum_{w=1}^{W} P(T_i^* \geq c_{w-1} \mid X_{1i} = x_i, X_{Di} = x_{Di}) P(T_j = w)$$

$$= P(T_i^* \geq c_{T_j-1} \mid X_{1i} = x_i, X_{Di} = x_{Di}).$$

Thus, we see that the expectation of U_{ij} is the ROC curve at the FPRs, p_{ij}.

Applying a similar idea as discussed in Section 8.2.2 to the binary variables U_{ij}, we propose the following algorithm to estimate θ:

1. Fit an ordinal regression model, as discussed above, to ordinal test response data from patients without the condition to obtain the estimates, $\hat{\bar{F}}_{0,x}$ and $\hat{c}_j$, for $\bar{F}_{0,x}$ and c_j, respectively.

2. Estimate p_{ij} by $\hat{p}_{ij} = \hat{\bar{F}}_{0,x_i}(\hat{c}_{T_{0j}-1})$.

3. Compute binary variables $U_{ij} = I_{[T_i \geq T_j]}$ for i and j, where $i = 1, \ldots, n_1$, and $j = n_1 + 1, \ldots, N$.

4. Estimate θ by solving the estimating equation,

$$\sum_{i=1}^{n_1} \sum_{j=n_1+1}^{N} I_{[\hat{p}_{ij}>0]} W_i(\theta, \hat{p}_{ij})(U_{ij} - \eta_i(\theta, \hat{p}_{ij})) = 0, \qquad (8.61)$$

where $\eta_i(\theta, p) = G(\beta' z + H_\alpha(p))$, and

$$W_i(\theta, p) = \frac{(\partial/\partial\theta)\eta_i(\theta, p)}{\eta_i(\theta, p)(1 - \eta_i(\theta, p))}.$$

The solution to the equation (8.61), $\hat{\theta}$, is an estimate for θ.

Then, an estimator for the latent smooth ROC curve corresponding to (z) is given by

$$\widehat{ROC}_z(p) = G(\hat{\beta}' z + H_{\hat{\alpha}}(p)). \qquad (8.62)$$

Following the same bootstrap steps as discussed in Section 8.2.2, we can obtain confidence intervals for the latent smooth ROC curve at a fixed value of p, $ROC_z(p)$, and the area under the latent smooth ROC curve.

8.3.3 Detection of Periprostatic Invasion with Ultrasound

In this section, we apply the indirect and direct regression methods to analyze the data from a study about the diagnostic accuracy of ultrasound readers in detecting periprostatic invasion in patients with prostate cancer, as described in Section 8.1.4. Table 8.1 summarizes ordinal-scale responses of the four ultrasound readers. To assess the effects of the four ultrasound readers on the ROC curves, we define three binary indicators, X_1, X_2, and X_3, for each patient, where (X_1, X_2, X_3) is $(1, 0, 0)$ if the patient's image was interpreted by the first reader, $(0, 1, 0)$ if the patient's image was interpreted by the second reader, $(0, 0, 1)$ if the patient's image was interpreted by the third reader, and $(0, 0, 0)$ if the patient's image was interpreted by the fourth reader. Let T and D denote the test result and the true disease status of a patient. We consider the ordinal regression model that includes main effects of D and X, as well as their first-order interactions, $X_4 = X_1 * D$, $X_5 = X_2 * D$, and $X_6 = X_3 * D$.

Table 8.3   Parameter Estimates and the Associated Standard Deviations in the Ordinal Regression Model for Ultrasound Rating Data

Parameter	Estimate	Standard deviation
c_1	-0.7081	0.182
c_2	-0.5683	0.179
c_3	0.2257	0.175
c_4	3.118	0.399
β_1	-0.4231	0.349
β_2	0.1827	0.668
β_3	-0.2603	0.707
β_4	-0.7225	0.595
β_5	0.8026	0.819
β_6	1.788	0.817
β_7	1.880	0.704
α_1	-0.4627	0.572
α_2	1.249	0.501
α_3	1.051	0.541
α_4	0.9773	0.518
α_5	0.3910	0.650
α_6	0.3577	0.680
α_7	0.2686	0.667

Denote $X = (X_1, X_2, X_3)'$. Let $\bar{F}_{d,x}$ be the survival function of T given $D = d$ and $X = x$.

Using the notation in PLUM (Tosteson and Begg, 1988), we write the indirect regression model as the following ordinal regression model:

$$P(T \leq w \mid D = d, X = x) = 1 - \bar{F}_{d,x}(c_w) = \Phi(\frac{B_1}{B_2}), \qquad (8.63)$$

where

$$\begin{aligned} B_1 \;=\; & c_w - \beta_1(d - \bar{d}) - \beta_2(x_1 - \bar{x}_1) - \beta_3(x_2 - x_2) - \beta_4(x_3 - \bar{x}_3) \\ & - \beta_5(x_4 - \bar{x}_4) - \beta_6(x_5 - \bar{x}_5) - \beta_7(x_6 - \bar{x}_6), \end{aligned}$$

and

$$\begin{aligned} B_2 \;=\; & \exp(\alpha_1(d - \bar{d}) + \alpha_2(x_1 - \bar{x}_1)) \\ & \times\; \exp(\alpha_3(x_2 - \bar{x}_2) + \alpha_4(x_3 - \bar{x}_3)) \\ & \times\; \exp(\alpha_5(x_4 - \bar{x}_4) + \alpha_6(x_5 - \bar{x}_5) + \alpha_7(x_6 - \bar{x}_6)). \end{aligned}$$

Here $\bar{d}$ and $\bar{x}_1, \ldots, \bar{x}_6$ are the sample means of covariates $d, x_1, \ldots, x_6$, respectively. We use the computer program PLUM to fit this ordinal regression model. We report the resulting estimates of the regression parameters, β and α, and the cutoff points, c_w's, in Table 8.4, which also includes the estimates for the associated SDs.

After obtaining the estimates for β and α, we obtain an estimate for the ROC curve corresponding to the covariates $X = x$, using (8.55) and (8.56), and this estimated ROC curve is given by

$$ROC_x(p) = \Phi(b(x)\Phi^{-1}(p) - a(x)), \qquad (8.64)$$

where

$$a(x) \quad = \quad \frac{B_1}{B_2},$$

$$B_1 \quad = \quad 0.42 - 0.80(x_1 - 0.25) - 1.79(x_2 - 0.25) - 1.88(x_3 - 0.25),$$

$$
\begin{aligned}
B_2 \quad = \quad & \exp(-0.23 + 1.25(x_1 - 0.25) + 1.05(x_2 - 0.25)) \\
\times \quad & \exp(0.98(x_3 - 0.25) + 0.39(x_4 - 0.16) + 0.36(x_5 - 0.13)) \\
\times \quad & \exp(0.27(x_6 - 0.13)),
\end{aligned}
$$

and

$$b(x) \quad = \quad \exp(0.46 - 0.39x_1 - 0.36x_2 - 0.27x_3).$$

Based on this fitted model, we plot the ROC curves for the four ultrasound readers; the resulting ROC curves are displayed in Figure 8.5.

From the fitted ROC curves, we conclude that the ROC curves for the four ultrasound readers are different. It is worth noting that the ROC curve for Reader 4 is below the 45° diagonal line, meaning that this reader has an accuracy even lower than that of tossing a fair coin. When examining the ordinal-scale data in Table 8.1, we see that Reader 4 tends to give a higher response for a patient without the disease than for one with the disease. This observation leads us to suspect that Reader 4 may have intentionally or unintentionally switched the meanings of $D = 1$ with that of $D = 0$.

Next, we fit the following direct regression method to this data set:

$$
\begin{aligned}
ROC_x(p) = \quad & \Phi\left(\alpha_0 + \alpha_1\Phi^{-1}(p) + \beta_1 X_1 + \beta_2 X_2 + \beta_3 X_3 \right. \qquad (8.65) \\
& \left. + \beta_4 X_1 \times \Phi^{-1}(p) + \beta_2 X_2 \times \Phi^{-1}(p) + \beta_3 X_3 \times \Phi^{-1}(p)\right).
\end{aligned}
$$

The results of the regression model are shown in Figure 8.6. The results also suggest that Reader 3 had better discrimination than the rest of the readers, with Reader 4 performing most poorly. Based on this fitted direct regression model, we plot the ROC curves for the four US readers; the resulting ROC curves are displayed in Figure 8.6.

8.4   COVARIATE ADJUSTED ROC CURVES OF CONTINUOUS-SCALE TESTS

As discussed in the previous sections, when some covariates affect the accuracy of diagnostic tests, we need to adjust for covariates in estimating the overall

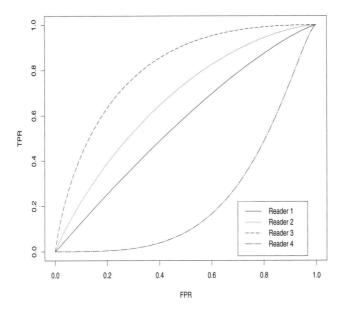

Figure 8.5   Fitted ROC Curves for the Four Ultrasound Readers Using the Indirect ROC Regression Method

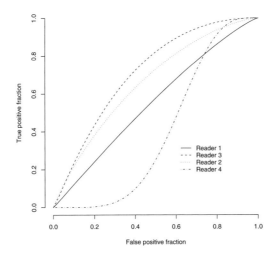

Figure 8.6   Fitted ROC Curves for the Four Ultrasound Readers Using the Direct ROC Regression Method

diagnostic accuracy of the tests. Unadjusted or pooled ROC curves can be misleading in representing the overall diagnostic accuracy and comparing the relative accuracy of two diagnostic tests. Janes and Pepe (2008a) illustrated this point in an example shown in their Figure 3, where T^1 and T^2 are two tests measured on the same set of subjects. Although T^1 and T^2 have the same covariate-specific ROC curve for a binary-scale covariate Z, the distribution of T^1 is affected by Z, whereas that of T^2 is not. Using unadjusted or pooled ROC curves of T^1 and T^2, we would wrongly conclude that T^2 outperforms T^1 when the covariate-adjusted overall ROC curves of T^1 and T^2 are the same (Janes and Pepe, 2008a).

Using the same notations as in Section 8.2, we let T and X be the continuous-scale response of a diagnostic test and vector of covariates for a patient. To allow possibly different distributions of covariates for a diseased and non-diseased subject, we let X_1 and X_0 be the vector of covariates for a diseased subject and non-diseased subject, respectively. Mathematically, the covariate-adjusted ROC curve (AROC) is given as follows:

$$AROC(v) = E_{X_1}\{ROC(v \mid X_1)\} = \int ROC(v \mid x)dF_1(x), \qquad (8.66)$$

where $ROC(v|x)$ is the ROC curve of the test in the subpopulation with covariate value x, the expectation is taken with respect to X_1, and F_1 is the c.d.f of X_1. From the expression for the AROC curve, we conclude that when X_1 does not affect the ROC curve of the test, the adjusted ROC curve is the same as the common covariate-specific ROC curve. When X_1 affects the ROC curve of the test, the AROC curve is a weighted average of covariate-specific ROC curves over the distribution of X_1.

To estimate the AROC curve, we can re-write it as follows:

$$AROC(v) = P\{T_1 > \bar{F}_{0,X_1}^{-1}(v)\}, \qquad (8.67)$$

where $\bar{F}_{0,x}(t)$ is the survival function of T_0 among the non-diseased subjects with $X_1 = x$, and T_1 is the test result of a diseased subject. When X is a single covariate, Janes and Pepe (2009) proposed both nonparametric and semi-parametric estimators for the AROC curves. From the equation (8.67), we see that if we obtain an estimator for $\bar{F}_{0,1}^{-1}(v)$, $\widehat{\bar{F}}_{0,x}^{-1}(v)$, we can then estimate the AROC curve as follows:

$$\widehat{AROC}(v) = \frac{1}{n_1} \sum_{i=1}^{n_1} I_{T_{1i} > \widehat{\bar{F}}_{0,X_{1i}}^{-1}(v)},$$

where X_{1i} is the value of the covariate for the ith diseased subject. Janes and Pepe (2009) have provided the asymptotic distribution theory for this estimator for the AROC curve.

CHAPTER 9

ANALYSIS OF MULTIPLE READER AND/OR MULTIPLE TEST STUDIES

In this chapter, we describe and illustrate statistical methods for analyzing studies comparing multiple tests, often with multiple readers, and sometimes with important covariates. The common characteristic of these studies is a complicated correlation structure which must be handled appropriately for unbiased estimation and inference.

In Section 9.1 we discuss the analysis of studies comparing multiple tests on the same sample of patients (paired design) when there are important covariates to account for. In these studies, the test results from the same patient are correlated, but the test results from different patients can be assumed to be independent. We illustrate the methods using data from two clinical studies on prostate cancer.

In Section 9.2 we focus on multiple-reader, multiple-case, so-called MRMC, studies designed to assess and compare two or more tests that rely on human observers for interpretation. In these studies there are two samples - a sample of patients and a sample of observers - which may be treated as random observations from respective populations. In Section 9.2.1. we describe three real-world MRMC studies to motivate the development of statistical methods. In Section 9.2.2 we introduce four methods for analyzing MRMC data, and in

Statistical Methods in Diagnostic Medicine,
Second Edition. By Xiao-Hua Zhou, Nancy A. Obuchowski, Donna K. McClish
Copyright © 2011 John Wiley & Sons, Inc.

Section 9.2.3 we apply these four statistical methods to one of the real-world examples described in Section 9.2.1. Finally, in Section 9.2.4 we summarize the similarities and differences between these four statistical methods.

In Section 9.3 we describe the challenges associated with analyzing studies of diagnostic tests designed to locate and detect lesions. These tests are common in diagnostic imaging, for example, for diagnosing suspicious lesions in the lung, colon, and breast, and require special statistical methods.

9.1   STUDIES COMPARING MULTIPLE TESTS WITH COVARIATES

We present two regression models that allow us not only to estimate the ROC curves at different occasions and their summary measures of diagnostic accuracy, but also to study covariate effects on the ROC curves and their summary measures. These two regression models are extensions of the indirect and direct regression models for independent ROC data, as discussed in Chapter 8, to correlated ROC data.

9.1.1   Two Clinical Studies

In this section we describe two diagnostic accuracy studies that require the use of regression models for comparing the relative accuracy of correlated diagnostic tests. In the first study, the response of the test is continuous, while in the second study, the test response is ordinal.

9.1.1.1   MR Imaging on Prostate Cancer Staging Example   Prostate cancer is a common malignancy in men. Early detection is very important in patient management because complete cure is more likely for patients in the early stage of prostate cancer. Tempany et al. (1994) conducted a multi-center clinical study to investigate the relative accuracies of MR imaging with a conventional body coil, fat suppression, and an endorectal coil. MR imaging was performed on 213 patients with prostate cancer with these three techniques. All patients were supposed to undergo a prostate biopsy prior to entry into the study. Pathologic examination of biopsy specimens was used as the gold standard to establish the true disease status (localized versus advanced stage cancer) of patients. On each image, a radiologist gave an ordinal-scale score to describe his/her confidence level in the presence of advanced state prostate cancer: 0 for definitely or almost definitely localized stage prostate cancer, 1 for probably localized stage prostate cancer, 2 for possibly advanced stage prostate cancer, 3 for probably advanced stage prostate cancer, and 4 for definitely or almost definitely advanced stage prostate cancer. There were four hospitals involved in this study. Due to the differences in patient case-mix across the four hospitals, the accuracy of the MR imaging techniques may depend on the hospital types. Hence, we need to adjust for this covariate in comparing the relative accuracy of the MR imaging techniques.

9.1.1.2 PSA on Prostate Cancer Screening Example   Ellis et al. (2001) at Fred
Hutchinson Cancer Research Center conducted a case-control study to assess
the relative accuracy of the free-to-total prostate specific antigen (PSA) ratio
and complexed total PSA in detecting prostate cancer. The gold standard
for the diagnosis of prostate cancer was biopsy. This case-control study was
based on a large double-blind clinical study, called the β-Carotene and Retinol
Efficacy Trial (CARET) (Omenn et al., 1996), which was designed to assess
the chemopreventive efficacy and safety of β-carotene and retinol in a population at risk for lung cancer. Both the free-to-total PSA ratio and complexed
total PSA are continuous-scale. Since the accuracy of the PSA can depend on
the age of a patient, we need to adjust for age in comparison of the relative
accuracy of the PSA ratio and complexed total PSA in detecting prostate
cancer.

9.1.2   Indirect Regression Models for Ordinal-Scale Tests

We first define the covariate-specific smooth ROC curves of an ordinal-scale
test at a particular occasion. For example, in the accuracy study on MR
imaging for the prostate cancer staging, described in Section 9.1.1.1, we have
three ordinal-scale tests: conventional body coil MRI, fat suppression MRI,
and endorectal coil MRI, with one covariate indicating hospital type. Let T_q
be the ordinal-scale test response, ranging from 1 to W, at the qth occasion
for a patient, where $q = 1, \ldots, Q$. In our prostate cancer staging study, $Q = 3$,
and the three occasions correspond to the three MR imaging techniques. Here
$T_q = 1$ indicates the least suspicion of the condition and $T_q = W$ indicates
the strongest suspicion of the presence of the condition. To produce a smooth
ROC curve for the ordinal-scale variable T_q at the qth occasion, we consider
T_q as a discretization of a latent continuous variable T_q^* such that $T_q = w$ if
$c_{q(w-1)} < T_q^* \le c_{qw}$, for $w = 1, \ldots, W$, where $c_{q0} = -\infty$ and $c_{qW} = +\infty$.
Here we allow the cut-off points c_{qw} to depend on the qth occasion. Let D_q be
the true condition status of the patient at the qth occasion and X_q be a vector
of the patient's other covariates at the qth occasion that can potentially affect
the accuracy of the test. Usually, $D_q = D$. In our prostate cancer staging
example, $X_q = x$ if this patient is from the xth hospital, where $x = 1, 2, 3$.
Let $\bar{F}_{q,d,x}(.)$ be the survival function of T_q^* given $D_q = d$ and $X_q = x$. Then,
the smooth ROC curve for the test at the qth occasion among patients with
$X_q = x$ is defined by

$$ROC_{q,x}(p) = \bar{F}_{q,1,x}(\bar{F}_{q,0,x}^{-1}(p)), \qquad (9.1)$$

where $p = \bar{F}_{q,0,x}(t)$, the false positive rate corresponding to a cutoff point t
in the domain of the distribution function, $\bar{F}_{q,0,x}$.
    As discussed in Chapter 8, the indirect regression approach first fits marginal
regression models for $\bar{F}_{q,1,x}$ and $\bar{F}_{q,0,x}$, separately, and then uses (9.1) to derive the covariate effects on the ROC curve. Toledano and Gatsonis (1996)

took such an approach and proposed the following marginal regression model:

$$F_{q,d,x}(y) = \Phi \left[\frac{y - h_{1q}(d, x; \beta_q)}{\exp(h_{2q}(d, x; \alpha_q))} \right], \tag{9.2}$$

where $\Phi(.)$ is a probit link function, and $h_{1q}(.,.;.)$ and $h_{2q}(.,.;.)$ are two known functions. Under the model (9.2), we obtain the following marginal ordinal regression model for the observed ordinal-scale test response, T_q:

$$P(T_q \leq w \mid D_q = d, X_q = x) = \Phi \left[\frac{c_{qw} - h_{1q}(d, x; \beta_q)}{\exp(h_{2q}(d, x; \alpha_q))} \right]. \tag{9.3}$$

Under the model (9.3), we can show that the effects of covariates, x, on the smooth ROC curve, $ROC_{q,x}(p)$, are represented by the following model:

$$ROC_{q,x}(p) = 1 - \Phi \left[b_q(x; \alpha) \Phi^{-1}(1 - p) - a_q(x; \beta, \alpha) \right], \tag{9.4}$$

where

$$a_q(x; \beta, \alpha) = \frac{h_{1q}(1, x; \beta_q) - h_{1q}(0, x; \beta_q)}{\exp(h_{2q}(1, x; \alpha_q))}$$

and

$$b_q(x; \alpha) = \exp(h_{2q}(0, x; \alpha_q) - h_{2q}(1, x; \alpha_q)). \tag{9.5}$$

Under ROC curve model (9.4), we can derive an explicit form for the area under the ROC curve. If we denote the ROC curve area at the qth occasion by $A_{q,x}$, we can show that

$$A_{q,x} = \Phi \left(\frac{a_q(x; \beta, \alpha)}{\sqrt{1 + b_q^2(x; \alpha)}} \right). \tag{9.6}$$

Denote the parameters in the marginal ordinal regression model (9.3) by

$$B_q = (c_{q1}, \ldots, c_{q(K-1)}, \beta_q', \alpha_q')',$$

where the notation $'$ denotes the transpose operation. Let $B = (B_1', \ldots, B_Q')'$. Toledano and Gatsonis (1996) proposed the method of generalized estimating equations (GEE) for estimation of the vector of parameters, B, as follows.

Let $Y_{iqw} = I_{[T_{iq} \leq w]}$ be an indicator variable, equaling 1 if $T_{iq} \leq w$ and 0 otherwise, and μ_{iqw} be the expected value of Y_{iqw} given that $D_{iq} = d$ and $X_{iq} = x$; that is, $\mu_{iqw} = E(Y_{iqw} \mid D_{iq} = d, X_{iq} = x)$. Let Y_i be the vector whose elements consist of Y_{iqw}, $q = 1, \ldots, Q$, and $w = 1, \ldots, W-1$. Let μ_i be the vector whose elements consist of μ_{iqw}, $q = 1, \ldots, Q$, and $w = 1, \ldots, W-1$.

From (9.3) we see that μ_i is a function of B. To emphasize this dependence, we write $\mu_i = \mu_i(B)$. Although test responses from different patients are independent, test responses on the same patient are correlated. To complete a specification in the marginal model, we assume that the covariance matrix of Y_i is given by $V_i(\eta) = \Lambda_i^{1/2} R_i(\eta) \Lambda_i^{1/2}$, where Λ_i is a diagonal matrix whose non-zero entries are variances for Y_{iqw}'s, and $R_i(\eta)$ is an assumed correlation matrix for Y_i, called a "working" correlation matrix, which is allowed to depend on a vector of unknown parameters, η. Then, the estimating equations for B are given by

$$\sum_{i=1}^{N} (E_i(B))' V_i(\hat{\eta})^{-1} (Y_i - \boldsymbol{\mu}_i(B)) = 0, \tag{9.7}$$

where $E_i(B) = \frac{\partial \boldsymbol{\mu}_i(B)}{\partial B}$, $(E_i(B))'$ denotes the transpose of $E_i(B)$, and $\hat{\eta}$ is a $\sqrt{N}$-consistent estimator for η. An estimator $\hat{B}$ for B is the solution to (9.7). This estimator is called a robust estimator because it is a consistent estimator for B, regardless of whether the assumed working correlation $R_i(\eta)$ is the true correlation of Y_i.

Under some regularity conditions, Toledano and Gatsonis (1996) have shown that $\sqrt{N}(\hat{B} - B)$ has an asymptotically multivariate normal distribution with zero mean and covariance matrix given by

$$N [\sum_{i=1}^{N} (E_i(B))' V_i^{-1}(\eta) E_i(B)]^{-1} \{ \sum_{i=1}^{N} E_i(B)' V_i^{-1}(\eta) cov(Y_i) V_i^{-1}(\eta) E_i(B) \}$$

$$[\sum_{i=1}^{N} (E_i(B))' V_i^{-1}(\eta) E_i(B)]^{-1}, \tag{9.8}$$

where $cov(Y_i)$ denotes the true covariance matrix of Y_i.

Estimating $cov(Y_i)$ by $(Y_i - \boldsymbol{\mu}_i(\hat{B}))' (Y_i - \boldsymbol{\mu}_i(\hat{B}))$ and B by $\hat{B}$, Toledano and Gatsonis (1996) obtained the following estimator for the covariance matrix of $\hat{B}$:

$$[\sum_{i=1}^{N} (E_i(\hat{B}))' V_i^{-1}(\hat{\eta}) E_i(\hat{B})]^{-1}$$

$$\{ \sum_{i=1}^{N} (E_i(\hat{B}))' V_i^{-1}(\hat{\eta}) (Y_i - \boldsymbol{\mu}_i(\hat{B}))' (Y_i - \boldsymbol{\mu}_i(\hat{B})) V_i^{-1}(\hat{\eta}) E_i(\hat{B}) \}$$

$$[\sum_{i=1}^{N} E_i(\hat{B})' V_i^{-1}(\hat{\eta}) E_i(\hat{B})]^{-1}. \tag{9.9}$$

This covariance matrix estimator is consistent, regardless of whether the assumed working correlation $R_i(\eta)$ is the true correlation of Y_i. However, this covariance matrix estimator may not be efficient if the assumed working correlation $R_i(\eta)$ is different from the true correlation of Y_i.

Selection of a working correlation, $R_i(\eta)$, depends on the focus of our analysis. If we are only interested in estimation of B, we can take the working correlation matrix $R_i(\eta)$ to be the identity matrix. The resulting GEE estimator, $\hat{B}$, for B is still consistent. Such an estimator is less efficient than that with the correlation matrix correctly specified.

If we are also interested in estimation of the correlation matrix of Y_i in order to increase the efficiency of the estimators for β and allow the correlation to depend on patient covariates, then we need to correctly model the correlation matrix.

Note that for two different categories w and $\tilde{w}$ ($w \neq \tilde{w}$) and two different occasions q and $\tilde{q}$ ($q \neq \tilde{q}$),

$$cov(Y_{iqw}, Y_{iq\tilde{w}}) = P(T_{iq} \leq min(w, \tilde{w})) - \mu_{iqw}\mu_{iq\tilde{w}} = \mu_{iq(min(w,\tilde{w}))} - \mu_{iqw}\mu_{iq\tilde{w}}$$

and

$$cov(Y_{iqw}, Y_{i\tilde{q}\tilde{w}}) = P(T_{iq} \leq w, T_{i\tilde{q}} \leq \tilde{w}) - \mu_{iqw}\mu_{i\tilde{q}\tilde{w}}.$$

Hence, to model the correlation matrix of Y_i, we need to model the correlation between T_{iq} and $T_{i\tilde{q}}$.

One way to model the correlation between T_{iq} and $T_{i\tilde{q}}$ is to assume that pairs arise from a categorization of latent variables T_{iq}^* and $T_{i\tilde{q}}^*$ such that

$$P(T_{iq} < w, T_{i\tilde{q}} < \tilde{w}) = P(T_{iq}^* < c_w, T_{i\tilde{q}}^* < c_{\tilde{w}})$$

and that the joint distribution of the latent variables T_{iq}^* and $T_{i\tilde{q}}^*$ has a bivariate normal distribution with a correlation $\rho_{i,q\tilde{q}}$, which may depend on the value of covariates, x_i. Toledano and Gatsonis (1996) assumed the following form for the correlation:

$$\rho_{i,q\tilde{q}} = \frac{1 - \exp(x_i'\eta)}{1 + \exp(x_i'\eta)}.$$

To emphasize the dependence of $\rho_{i,q\tilde{q}}$ on the unknown parameter η, we write $\rho_{i,q\tilde{q}} = \rho_{i,q\tilde{q}}(\eta)$. Under this latent bivariate model and the marginal model (9.3), we can write the joint probability for test responses T_{iq} and $T_{i\tilde{q}}$ as follows:

$$\nu_{iqw\tilde{q}\tilde{w}} = P(T_{iq} < w, T_{i\tilde{q}} < \tilde{w}) = \Phi_2[\rho_{i,q\tilde{q}}(\eta), \Phi^{-1}(\mu_{iqw}), \Phi^{-1}(\mu_{i\tilde{q}\tilde{w}})], \quad (9.10)$$

where $\Phi_2(.,.,.)$ is the standard bivariate normal distribution function.

Denote $U_{iqw\tilde{q}\tilde{w}} = I_{[T_{iq} < w, T_{i\tilde{q}} < \tilde{w}]}$. Its expectation is $\nu_{iqw\tilde{q}\tilde{w}}$, defined by (9.10). Let U_i be a vector with elements $U_{iqw\tilde{q}\tilde{w}}$, $q, \tilde{q} = 1, \ldots, Q$, and $w, \tilde{w} = 1, \ldots, W - 1$. Let ν_i be a vector whose elements are $\nu_{iqw\tilde{q}\tilde{w}}$, $q, \tilde{q} = 1, \ldots, Q$, and $w, \tilde{w} = 1, \ldots, W - 1$. Then, the expectation of U_i is ν_i. If we denote Ω_i to be a working covariance matrix for U_i, we then obtain the following additional estimating equations for η:

$$\sum_{i=1}^{N} (\frac{\partial \nu_i(B)}{\partial \eta})' \Omega_i^{-1}(U_i - \nu_i) = 0. \quad (9.11)$$

By alternately solving (9.7) and (9.11), we obtain estimators $\hat{B}$ and $\hat{\eta}$ for B and η. We can still use the formula (9.9) to estimate the covariance matrix of $\hat{B}$. Toledano and Gatsonis (1996) have also provided a robust covariance estimator for the covariance matrix of $\hat{\eta}$.

Substituting the ML estimator $\hat{B}$ for B in (9.4) and (9.6), we obtain the ML estimators for the ROC curve at the false positive rate, p, and the area under the ROC curve, given by

$$\widehat{ROC}_{q,x}(p) = 1 - \Phi[b_q(x; \hat{\alpha}_q)\Phi^{-1}(1 - p) - a_q(x; \hat{\beta}_q, \hat{\alpha}_q)]$$

and

$$\hat{A}_{q,x} = \Phi\left(\frac{a_q(x; \hat{\beta}_q, \hat{\alpha}_q)}{\sqrt{1 + b_q^2(x; \hat{\alpha}_q)}}\right), \tag{9.12}$$

respectively, where $a_q(x; \hat{\beta}_q, \hat{\alpha}_q)$ and $b_q(x; \hat{\alpha}_q)$ are defined by (9.5). Using the multivariate delta method (Sen and Singer, 1993), we can obtain a consistent estimator for the covariance matrix of $(\hat{A}_{1,x}, \ldots, \hat{A}_{Q,x})'$.

9.1.2.1 Application to the Accuracy Study of MRI in Prostate Cancer Staging

In this section, we apply the indirect regression model for ordinal-scale tests, described in Section 9.1.2, to the accuracy example of three MRIs in detecting prostate cancer staging, described in Section 9.1.1.1. Although four institutions participated in the original study, two of the four institutions were only able to contribute a few patients to the study. Hence, to illustrate the method, we only use the data from the two hospitals with the largest numbers of patients who have all three MRI measurements and the pathology data available.

Our example data consist of 99 patients with 42 having advanced state prostate cancer and 57 having localized stage prostate cancer. Each patient has the three MR imaging measurements: conventional body coil MRI, fat suppression MRI, and endorectal coil MRI, denoted by csusp, fsusp, and esusp, respectively. Let D_i and X_i denote the true disease status (advanced versus localized stage) and the binary hospital indicator (of the ith subject ($X_i = 0$ for Hospital A; $X_i = 1$ for Hospital B).

We modeled the indirect ROC curve by the following regression:

$$P(T_{ik} \leq c \mid D_i = d, X_i = x) = \Phi\left(\frac{\theta_{ck} - (\beta_{1k}x + \beta_{2k}d + \beta_{3k}x * d)}{e^{\alpha_{1k}d}}\right), \tag{9.13}$$

where $d = 1$ for the advanced stage prostate cancer. The analysis was carried out using R. The estimated parameters are displayed in Table 9.1.

To assess the relative accuracies of the three MR imaging techniques, we also compute the confidence intervals for the differences of pairwise AUCs of the three MR imaging techniques and report the results in Table 9.2. From Table 9.2, we see that the conventional body coil MRI performs slightly better than the endorectal coil MRI in both hospitals. While the convention body coil MRI performs slightly better than the endorectal coil MRI in Hospital A, the

Table 9.1 Estimates for Cutoff Points, Location and Scale Parameters in Marginal Ordinal Regression Model (9.13)

Parameter	Conventional Body (k=1)	Suppression (k=2)	Endorectal (k=3)
Cutoff points			
θ_{1k}	1.109**	0.704*	0.751*
θ_{2k}	1.392***	1.054**	1.194***
θ_{3k}	1.963***	1.957***	2.319***
Location			
β_{1k}	0.844*	1.072**	0.349
β_{2k}	0.977	0.285	0.174
β_{3k}	−0.165	0.029	0.844
Scale			
α_{1k}	−0.319	0.056	0.490

$(^{***},^{**},^{*})$ =p-value$(< .001, < .01, < .05)$

Table 9.2 95% CI's for AUC's for the Three MR Imaging Techniques by Institution for the Prostate Cancer Example

	Hospital B		Hospital A	
	AUC Difference	95%CI	AUC Difference	95%CI
Csusp - esusp	0.159	(0.092,0.227)	0.208	(0.062,0.354)
Csusp - fsusp	0.042	(-0.082,0.166)	0.249	(0.144,0.354)
Esusp - fsusp	-0.117	(-0.223,-0.011)	0.041	(-0.001,0.084)

convention body coil MRI and endorectal coil MRI have similar performance in Hospital B.

To visualize the diagnostic performance of the three MR imaging techniques by the two hospitals, we plot the ROC curves with the associated AUCs, stratified by hospital, in Figure 9.1.

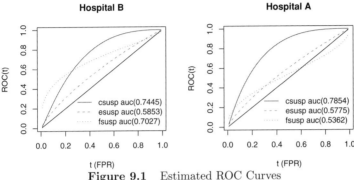

Figure 9.1   Estimated ROC Curves

From this plot we conclude that there is a hospital effect on the accuracy of the conventional body coil MRI, suppression MRI, and endorectal coil MRI; thus the relative accuracies of the conventional body coil MRI, fat suppression MRI, and endorectal coil MRI depend on the hospital type. Since our sample may not be a representative sample of the original sample and is used only for the illustrative purpose, we caution about the interpretation of the results in practice.

9.1.3   Direct Regression Models for Continuous-scale Tests

We can extend the direct regression models for independent ROC data, as discussed in Section 8.2 for continuous-scale tests, to correlated ROC data. In our example, we have two correlated continuous-scale test results on the same patient, the free-to-total PSA ratio and complexed total PSA, and the age of the patient, which may affect the relative accuracy of these two tests.

Let X be a vector of covariates common to both patients with and without the condition and X_D denote a vector of covariates that are specific to patients with the condition. For example, in the PSA on prostate cancer screening example, described in Section 9.1.1.2, we have one covariate, age, which is common to both patients with and without the prostate cancer, and have no disease-specific covariates. We denote $Z = (X', X_D')'$. Let T_{1q} be the continuous-scale test result for a patient with the condition at the qth occasion, and T_{0q} be the continuous-scale test result for a patient without the condition at the qth occasion, where $q = 1, \ldots, Q$. Again, in our prostate cancer screening example, occasion refers to a test, and $Q = 2$.

Let $\bar{F}_{1q,x,x_D}$ denote the survival function of T_{1q} given $X = x$ and $X_D = x_D$ and $\bar{F}_{0q,x}$ be the survival function of T_{0q} given $X = x$. Then the smooth ROC curve corresponding to $z = (x, x_D)$ at the qth occasion can be defined as

$$ROC_{q,z}(p) = \bar{F}_{1q,z}(\bar{F}_{0q,x}^{-1}(p)), \tag{9.14}$$

where $p \in (0, 1)$. As in Chapter 8, we model the effects of z

$$ROC_{q,z}(p) = G_q\{\beta' z + H(p)\}, \tag{9.15}$$

where G_q is a link function, and H is a baseline monotone increasing function that satisfies $H(0) = -\infty$ and $H(1) = +\infty$. If we denote A_{q,x,x_D} as the area under the ROC curve, $ROC_{q,x,x_D}(p)$, for $0 < p < 1$, we can use the following formula to compute the ROC curve area:

$$A_{q,x,x_D} = \int_0^1 G_q(\theta'(h(p)', x', x_D')')dp. \tag{9.16}$$

Similar to the indirect method, we assume that test responses from different patients are independent in order to use the method of GEE to estimate parameters θ. Let T_{0lq} and x_{0lq} be the values of T_{0q} and X for the lth patient without the condition at the qth occasion. Assume that $\widehat{\bar{F}}_{0q,x}$ is a consistent estimator for $\bar{F}_{0q,x}^{-1}$, based on the data, (T_{0lq}, x_{0lq}), for $l = 1, \ldots, n$, and $q = 1, \ldots, Q$. Let T_{1iq}, x_{1iq}, and x_{Diq} be the values of T_{1q}, X, and X_D for the ith patient with the condition at the qth occasion, $i = 1, \ldots, n_1$. For the ith patient with the condition at the qth occasion, Alonzo and Pepe (2002) define the following indicator variable:

$$U_{iqp} = I_{[T_{1iq} > \widehat{\bar{F}}_{0q,x_{1iq}}^{-1}(p)]}, \tag{9.17}$$

where $p \in \Gamma$, a finite set of false positive rates. Alonzo and Pepe (2002) proposed the following estimating equations for estimating θ:

$$\sum_{i=1}^{n_1} \sum_{q=1}^{Q} \sum_{p \in \Gamma} W_{iq}(\theta, p)(U_{iqp} - \eta_{iq}(\theta, p)) = 0, \tag{9.18}$$

where $\eta_{iq}(\theta, p) = ROC_{q,x_{1iq},x_{Diq}}(p) = G_q(\theta'(h(p)', x_{1iq}', x_{Diq}')')$, $\partial/\partial\theta$ is the derivative operator with respect to θ, and

$$W_{iq}(\theta, p) = \frac{(\partial/\partial\theta)\eta_{iq}(\theta, p)}{\eta_{iq}(\theta, p)(1 - \eta_{iq}(\theta, p))}.$$

Let $\hat{\theta}$ be the solution to the equation (9.18). By replacing θ in (9.15) by $\hat{\theta}$, we obtain an estimator for the ROC curve at the qth occasion, corresponding to the covariates (x, x_D),

$$\widehat{ROC}_{q,x,x_D}(p) = G_q(\hat{\gamma}'h(p) + \hat{\beta}'x + \hat{\beta}_D'x_D). \tag{9.19}$$

By substituting $\hat{\theta}$ for θ in (9.16), we can obtain an estimator for the area under the ROC curve at the qth occasion,

$$\hat{A}_{q,x,x_D} = \int_0^1 g_q(\hat{\theta}'(h(p)', x', x_D')')dp. \tag{9.20}$$

Denote $\hat{A}_{x,x_D} = (\hat{A}_{1,x,x_D}, \ldots, \hat{A}_{Q,x,x_D})'$, which is an estimator for $A_{x,x_D} = (A_{1,x,x_D}, \ldots, A_{Q,x,x_D})'$,

After obtaining the estimators for θ and A_{x,x_D}, $\hat{\theta}$ and $\hat{A}_{x,x_D}$, we introduce a bootstrap method for estimating their covariance matrices. Let $T_{0l} = (T_{0l1}, \ldots, T_{0lQ})'$, $x_{0l} = (x_{0l1}, \ldots, x_{0lQ})'$, $T_{1i} = (T_{1i1}, \ldots, T_{1iQ})'$, $x_{1i} = (x_{1i1}, \ldots, x_{1iQ})'$, and $x_{Di} = (x_{Di1}, \ldots, x_{DiQ})'$. The proposed bootstrap method treats (T_{1i}, x_{1i}, x_{Di})'s as an i.i.d. sample, and (T_{0l}, x_{0l})'s as another i.i.d. sample. We summarize the bootstrap method for estimating the covariance matrices for $\hat{\theta}$ and $\hat{A}_{x,x_D}$ in the following steps:

1. Sample $\{(T_{1i}^*, x_{1i}^*, x_{Di}^*), i = 1, \ldots, n_1\}$ with replacement from the original sample of patients with the condition, $\{(T_{1i}, x_{1i}, x_{Di}), i = 1, \ldots, n_1\}$ and sample $\{(T_{0l}^*, x_{0l}^*), l = 1, \ldots, n_0\}$ with replacement from the original sample of patients without the condition, $\{(T_{0l}, x_{0l}), l = 1, \ldots, n_0\}$.

2. Obtain the bootstrap estimator, $\hat{\theta}^*$, for θ by solving the estimating equations (9.18), using the bootstrap sample, $(T_{1i}^*, x_{1i}^*, x_{Di}^*)$ and (T_{0l}^*, x_{0l}^*), where $i = 1, \ldots, n_1$, and $l = 1, \ldots, n_0$.

3. Obtain the bootstrap estimate for the area under the ROC curve, $\hat{A}_{q,x,x_D}^*$, by replacing θ in (9.16) by the bootstrap estimate, $\hat{\theta}^*$, and the bootstrap estimate for A_{x,x_D} by $\hat{A}_{x,x_D}^* = (\hat{A}_{1,x,x_D}^*, \ldots, \hat{A}_{Q,x,x_D}^*)'$.

4. Repeat Steps 1-3 B times to obtain B bootstrap estimates for θ and A_{x,x_D}, $\hat{\theta}_r^*$ and $\hat{A}_{r,x,x_D}^*$, where $r = 1, \ldots, B$.

5. Estimate the covariance matrix for $\hat{\theta}$ by

$$\frac{1}{B-1} \sum_{r=1}^B (\hat{\theta}_r^* - \bar{\hat{\theta}}^*)(\hat{\theta}_r^* - \bar{\hat{\theta}}^*)',$$

where

$$\bar{\hat{\theta}}^* = (1/B) \sum_{r=1}^B \hat{\theta}_r^*,$$

and the covariance matrix for $\hat{A}_{x,x_D}$ by

$$(S^*)^2 = \frac{1}{B-1} \sum_{r=1}^B (\hat{A}_{r,x,x_D}^* - \bar{\hat{A}}^*)(\hat{A}_{r,x,x_D}^* - \bar{\hat{A}}^*)',$$

where

$$\bar{\hat{A}}^* = (1/B) \sum_{r=1}^{B} \widehat{A}^*_{r,x,x_D}.$$

After obtaining the bootstrap estimate, $(S^*)^2$, for the covariance matrix of $\widehat{A}_{x,x_D}$, we can use normal theory to compare the areas under the ROC curves across the Q occasions. For example, a two-sided $100(1 - \delta)\%$ confidence interval for the difference between the ROC curve areas at the qth and $\tilde{q}$th occasions $(q \neq \tilde{q})$, $A_{q,x,x_D} - A_{\tilde{q},x,x_D}$, is given as follows:

$$\widehat{A}_{q,x,x_D} - \widehat{A}_{\tilde{q},x,x_D} \pm z_{1-\delta/2} \sqrt{C'_{q\tilde{q}}(S^*)^2 C_{q\tilde{q}}},$$

where z_δ is the δth percentile of the standard normal distribution, $C_{q\tilde{q}}$ is a Q dimensional vector with elements equal to zero except at the qth and $\tilde{q}$th positions whose elements are +1 and -1, respectively.

9.1.3.1 Application to the accuracy study of PSA in prostate cancer screening

In this section we illustrate the application of the method described in Section 9.1.2, to the PSA on prostate cancer screening example. In this example we have two tests per patient, free PSA and total PSA. Thus $Q = 2$ per subject at each of the nine time points. We restrict our analysis to the first time point with one binary indicator covariate, X, which indicates whether the patient's age is 65 years old or younger. Let $ROC_{q,x}(p)$ be the ROC curve of the qth test among the subpopulation of subjects with $X = x$, where $q = 1, 2$, and $x = 0, 1$. Here, $X = 1$ for a patient who is 65 years old or younger. We model the covariate-specific ROC curve by the following equation:

$$ROC_{q,\mathbf{x}}(p) = \Phi[\gamma_{0q} + \gamma_{1q}\Phi^{-1}(p) + \beta_{1q}x + \beta_{2q}x\Phi^{-1}(p)].$$

Here γ_{0q} and γ_{1q} represent the intercept and shape of the inverse Probit function of the ROC curve of the qth test among the sub-population of subjects with $x = 0$, and $\gamma_{0q} + \beta_{1q}$ and $\gamma_{1q} + \beta_{2q}$ represent the intercept and shape of the inverse Probit function of the ROC curve of the qth test among the sub-population of subjects with $x = 1$. Hence, β_{1k} and β_{2k} represent the covariate effects on the intercept and the shape of the inverse Probit function of the ROC curve of the kth test, respectively.

The corresponding covariate-specific area under the ROC curve can be calculated as follows:

$$A_{q,x} = \int_0^1 \Phi[\gamma_{0q} + \gamma_{1q}\Phi^{-1}(p) + \beta_{1q}x + \beta_{2q}x\Phi^{-1}(p)]dp.$$

Using the estimation approach outlined in Section 9.1.2, as implemented in R, we obtain the parameter estimates with 95% confidence intervals. From the results in Table 9.3, we conclude that the age covariate (65 years old

Table 9.3 Parameter Estimates with Bootstrapped 95%CI

	Free PSA(k=1)	Total PSA(k=2)
γ_{0q}	0.90 (0.41,1.4)	1.18 (0.69,1.67)
γ_{1q}	0.73 (0.35,1.1)	0.71 (0.35,1.08)
β_{1q}	0.20 (-0.56,0.97)	0.04 (-1.26,1.33)
β_{2q}	-0.08 (-0.56,0.4)	-0.20 (-0.92,0.53)

or younger versus more than 65 years) has some effect but does not have a significant effect on the ROC curves.

To visualize the covariate effect, we also report the covariate-specific ROC curves for the two tests in Figure 9.2.

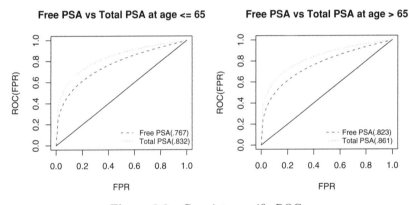

Figure 9.2 Covariate specific ROC curves

Table 9.4 reports the AUCs of the two tests and their differences among the various subpopulations defined by age. From these results we conclude

Table 9.4 Estimated AUC's and the Differences in AUC's with Bootstrapped 95%CI

	Free PSA(95%CI)	Total PSA(95%CI)	Diff (95%CI)
$age \leq 65$	0.767 (0.664,0.869)	0.832 (0.745,0.919)	0.065 (0.001,0.13)
$age > 65$	0.823 (0.71,0.936)	0.861 (0.751,0.971)	0.038 (-0.026,0.103)

that the total PSA is more accurate than the free PSA among patients 65 years old or younger and has a similar but smaller trend for older patients.

9.2 STUDIES WITH MULTIPLE READERS AND MULTIPLE TESTS

Radiographic images, such as mammograms and magnetic resonance imaging, rely on trained radiologists to interpret the features on the image to diagnose the patient. For these tests, diagnostic accuracy is not only a function of the characteristics of the machine (e.g. resolution, noise-to-signal ratio) but also the experience, training, and cognitive and perceptual abilities of the human readers. Thus, to describe and compare these tests' accuracies, we need to assess the performance of multiple readers using them.

MRMC studies can vary in size from four or five readers to 100 readers, and 50 to hundreds of patients. The patient and reader sample sizes are both important to the power of MRMC studies. We discussed the sample size for MRMC studies in Chapter 6. The primary goal of most MRMC studies is to compare the diagnostic accuracies of two or more tests. Stated more precisely, we want to assess readers' average diagnostic accuracy on each test and compare competing tests to assess i) superiority (i.e. a new test is better than an existing test), ii) equivalence (i.e. a new test has the same accuracy as an existing test), or iii) non-inferiority (i.e. a new test's accuracy is at least as good as the existing test). There are many important secondary objectives of MRMC studies, including identifying subgroups of readers where the differences between the tests vary (i.e. interaction between test and readers), identifying reader and patient characteristics that affect accuracy, and comparing between-reader variability of tests. The specialized statistical methods described in this section account for the multiple correlations between readers and patients that are common in MRMC studies.

9.2.1 Three MRMC Studies

First we describe three MRMC studies. In all of these examples, a traditional paired-reader, paired-patient design was used.

9.2.1.1 Interstitial Disease Example The first example is a subset from the study reported in Obuchowski et al. (2004). In this example, we are interested in comparing the relative accuracy of high and medium resolution chest images for the detection of interstitial disease. This data set consists of 40 patients with and 110 without interstitial disease. Five radiologists independently interpreted all of the images using a quasi-continuous 0% to 100% confidence scale.

9.2.1.2 Thoracic Aortic Dissection example The second study, originally analyzed by Obuchowski (1995), assessed the relative performance of conventional single Spin-Echo Magnetic Resonance (MR) imaging and MR imaging with a new CINE sequence for the detection of thoracic aortic dissection (TAD). Forty-five patients with an aortic dissection and 69 patients without a dissection participated in the study. Each patient was imaged by both MR sequences and evaluated independently by five radiologists who used a five-point ordinal-scale to rate their degree of confidence in the presence of TAD. We are interested in comparing the diagnostic accuracy of the conventional MR sequence (SP) and MR cine sequence (CN) in detecting the presence of TAD.

9.2.1.3 Breast Cancer Example   The third study examined whether computer-aided diagnosis (CAD) could improve radiologists' performance in breast cancer diagnosis. In this study, ten radiologists read mammograms of 104 patients with lesions, first without the aid of CAD and then with CAD. For the computer-aided diagnosis, the radiologists were given a computer-estimated likelihood of malignancy based on eight computer-extracted image features from the mammagrams. For each lesion the radiologists were asked to give their degree of suspicion that the lesion was malignant by reading the mammagrams and then placing a mark on a 5-cm line labeled benign at the left end and malignant on the right end. These marks were then converted to numerical scores with a ruler based on the distance of the mark from the "benign" end. These scores represent the observed test results. The true disease status of each patient was verified using a near-consecutive biopsy series. Among the 104 patients, 46 had malignant lesions and 58 had benign lesions. The objective was to compare the accuracy of readers unaided versus with the computer-aid.

9.2.2   Statistical Methods for Analyzing MRMC Studies

In this section, we describe three different approaches to analyzing MRMC studies. All three approaches address the complex correlation structure in the data. Ignoring the correlations, by using a simple paired t-test for example, leads to erroneous conclusions; thus all three methods are improvements over this naive approach. The first method is based on an analysis of variance (ANOVA) set-up on estimates of diagnostic summary measures modified for the multi-reader design; we present several approaches to estimating the parameters in this model. In the second method, a bootstrap method is used to estimate the variances in a MRMC design and to make inferences about the accuracies of the tests. In the third method, a marginal regression model is proposed for diagnostic summary measures, which can adjust for covariates as well. There are other, more specialized, MRMC methods that we do not discuss in the chapter. These other methods include Ishwaran and Gatsonis (2000) and Song (1997).

We first present some common notations for the three methods. In the paired-reader paired-patient design, J readers each independently examine a sample of N patients with each of I diagnostic tests on Q occasions. These test results are either continuous or ordinal-scale random variables, and they reflect the confidence level of a reader about the presence of the disease condition.

Without loss of generality, we assume that larger values of the test results indicate greater confidence level in the presence of the condition.

9.2.2.1   A Mixed-effects ANOVA Model for Summary Measures of Diagnostic Accuracy

Two main approaches were proposed for modeling a summary measure of the ROC curve (e.g. the area under the ROC curve) in multi-reader ROC studies. The first approach, proposed by Obuchowski and Rockette (1995) and known as the OR method, first calculates AUCs for different combinations of readers and tests and then applies a two-way mixed-effects ANOVA model to the estimated AUCs. Although these two methods appear to be different, Hillis et al. (2005) showed that the F statistics proposed in these two methods have the same form and produce similar results. Hillis (2007) has further shown that the DBM procedure can be considered as a particular application of the OR method. The second approach, proposed by Dorfman et al. (1992) and known as the DBM method, uses a jackknife method to compute pseudovalues for the summary ROC curve measure for each combination of patients, readers, and tests and then applies a three-way mixed-effects ANOVA model to these pseudovalues. We first introduce the OR method, followed by the DBM method.

Based on the same patient sample, we derive an estimator of a summary ROC measure, $\hat{\theta}_{kjq}$, for the kth test by the jth reader at the qth occasion, where $k = 1, \ldots, I, j = 1, \ldots, J$, and $q = 1, \ldots, Q$. For example, $\hat{\theta}_{kjq}$ could be the nonparametric or parametric estimator of the area under the ROC curve (Bamber, 1975; Dorfman and Alf, 1969). It is worth noting that the $\hat{\theta}_{kjq}$'s are correlated because they are estimated from the same patient sample. Usually there is no replication of the study; that is $Q = 1$, but to be more general, here we allow $Q > 1$.

Obuchowski and Rockette (1995) proposed a mixed-effects ANOVA model to account for the correlations among the $\hat{\theta}_{kjq}$'s in a MRMC study, in which tests were considered as fixed, and readers were considered as random. Their mixed-effects linear model is defined by

$$\hat{\theta}_{kjq} = \mu + \mu_k + r_j + (\mu r)_{kj} + \epsilon_{kjq}, \tag{9.21}$$

where $1 \leq k \leq K$, $1 \leq j \leq J$, and $1 \leq q \leq Q$. In this model, Obuchowski and Rockette (1995) made the following six assumptions: (1) The overall mean is μ. (2) The fixed effect corresponding to the kth test is μ_k. (3) The random effect due to the jth reader is r_j, which is normally distributed with mean 0 and variance σ_b^2. (4) The random effect due to the two-way interaction between the kth test and the jth reader is $(\mu r)_{kj}$, which is normally distributed with mean 0 and variance σ_{ab}^2. (5) The error term is ϵ_{kjq} with mean zero, and the $\epsilon = (\epsilon_{111}, \ldots, \epsilon_{KJQ})'$ vector of length (KxJxQ) has a multivariate normal distribution with the covariance matrix Σ,

$$E(\epsilon_{kjq}\epsilon_{\tilde{k}\tilde{j}\tilde{q}}) = \begin{cases} \sigma_c^2 & \text{if } k = \tilde{k}, j = \tilde{j}, q \neq \tilde{q} \\ \sigma_c^2 \rho_1 & \text{if } k \neq \tilde{k} \text{ and } j = \tilde{j} \\ \sigma_c^2 \rho_2 & \text{if } k = \tilde{k} \text{ and } j \neq \tilde{j} \\ \sigma_c^2 \rho_3 & \text{if } k \neq \tilde{k} \text{ and } j \neq \tilde{j} \end{cases},$$

where the indices k and $\tilde{k}$ refer to two different tests, the indices j and $\tilde{j}$ refer to two different readers, and the indices q and $\tilde{q}$ refer to two different occasions. (6) The random variables, r_j, $(\mu r)_{kj}$, and ϵ_{kjq}, are all independent.

Here, ρ_1, ρ_2, and ρ_3 represent, respectively, the correlation of error terms in diagnostic accuracies of the same reader in different tests, the correlation of error terms in diagnostic accuracies of different readers in the same test, and the correlation of error terms in diagnostic accuracies of different readers in different tests on the same patient. These correlations exist because the same patient sample is interpreted by all J readers in all K tests. It can be shown that $\sigma_c^2\rho_2$ and $\sigma_c^2\rho_3$ are the covariance in diagnostic accuracies of different readers in the same test and the covariance in diagnostic accuracies of different readers in different tests on the same patient, respectively.

We first focus our inferences on the accuracy of an individual diagnostic test. Denote

$$\hat{\theta}_{kj.} = \sum_{q=1}^{Q} \hat{\theta}_{kjq}/Q, \ \hat{\theta}_{k..} = \sum_{j=1}^{J}\sum_{q=1}^{Q} \hat{\theta}_{kjq}/(JQ), \text{ and } \xi = r_2\sigma_c^2/\sigma^2(\hat{\theta}_{kj.}),$$

where $\sigma^2(\hat{\theta}_{kj.})$ denotes the variance of $\hat{\theta}_{kj.}$. Let $\hat{\theta}_{k.} = (\hat{\theta}_{k1.}, \ldots, \hat{\theta}_{kJ.})'$ denote the vector of estimated accuracies for the kth test averaged over Q occasions. Under mixed-effects linear model (9.21), we can show that $\hat{\theta}_{k.}$ has a J-dimensional multivariate normal distribution with mean vector $(\mu+\mu_1, \ldots, \mu+\mu_J)'$ and covariance matrix Σ, which is equal to $\sigma^2(\hat{\theta}_{kj.})\{(1-\xi)I_J + \xi E_{JJ}\}$, where I_J is the identity matrix of rank J, and E_{JJ} denotes a $J x J$ matrix with all entries equal to one.

To construct a confidence interval for $\mu + \mu_k$, Obuchowski and Rockette (1995) used the following pivotal statistic:

$$t^* = \frac{1-\xi}{1+(J-1)\xi}t, \tag{9.22}$$

where t is the usual one-sample t-statistic and is defined by

$$t = \frac{\hat{\theta}_{k..} - (\mu + \mu_k)}{\sqrt{\sum_{j=1}^{J}(\hat{\theta}_{kj.} - \hat{\theta}_{k..})^2/(J(J-1))}}.$$

Bhat (1962) showed that t^* has a central Student's t-distribution with $(J-1)$ degrees of freedom when ξ is known.

Since ξ is unknown, it must be estimated in order to use the pivotal statistic t^*. With the assumption of equal correlation between readers, an estimator is computed as $\hat{\rho}_2\hat{\sigma}_c^2$ for $\rho_2\sigma_c^2$ by taking an average of all covariances between two reader pairs in the same test. Let $\hat{\sigma}^2(\hat{\theta}_{kj.})$ be an ANOVA-type estimator for $\sigma^2(\hat{\theta}_{kj.})$, which is defined by

$$\hat{\sigma}^2(\hat{\theta}_{kj.}) = \frac{1}{J-1}(\sum_{j=1}^{J}(\hat{\theta}_{kj.} - \hat{\theta}_{k..})^2) + \hat{\rho}_2\hat{\sigma}_c^2.$$

Then an estimator for ξ is given by $\hat{\xi} = \hat{\rho}_2\hat{\sigma}_c^2/\hat{\sigma}^2(\hat{\theta}_{kj.})$. Replacing ξ in (9.22) by $\hat{\xi}$, the following asymptotic statistic is obtained,

$$t^* = \frac{\hat{\theta}_{k..} - (\mu + \mu_k)}{\sqrt{\frac{1}{J(J-1)}\sum_{j=1}^{J}(\hat{\theta}_{kj.} - \hat{\theta}_{k..})^2 + \hat{\rho}_2\hat{\sigma}_c^2}}. \tag{9.23}$$

Assuming that t^* follows an approximately central Student's t-distribution with $J - 1$ degrees of freedom, Obuchowski and Rockette (1995) obtain the $(1 - \delta)100\%$ confidence interval for $\mu + \mu_k$ as

$$\hat{\theta}_{k..} \pm t_{\delta/2,J-1}\sqrt{\frac{1}{J(J-1)}\sum_{j=1}^{J}(\hat{\theta}_{kj.} - \hat{\theta}_{k..})^2 + \hat{\rho}_2\hat{\sigma}_c^2},$$

where $t_{\delta/2,J-1}$ is the $\delta/2$th quantile of the central Student's t-distribution with $(J\text{-}1)$ degrees of freedom.

Next we consider inferences on the relative accuracy of I tests. We first consider the null hypothesis that the accuracies of I tests are the same; that is, $H_0 : \mu_1 = \ldots = \mu_K$. Since the error terms in the mixed-effects linear ANOVA model (9.21) are not independent, the standard F tests may lead to grossly inaccurate results. Under the assumption of equal correlation in a mixed-effects ANOVA model, Pavur (1984) proposed a modified F statistic that can compensate for correlation. Obuchowski and Rockette (1995) have adopted this modified F test to the multi-reader ROC model defined by (9.21), and the resulting F^* statistic is a function of the usual F statistic and a quantity that corrects for the dependency in the observations. More specifically, let

$$\hat{\theta}_{...} = \sum_{k=1}^{K}\sum_{j=1}^{J}\sum_{q=1}^{Q}\hat{\theta}_{kjq}/(KJQ), \ \hat{\theta}_{.j.} = \sum_{k=1}^{K}\sum_{q=1}^{Q}\hat{\theta}_{kjq}/(IQ),$$

and $\hat{\sigma}_c^2\hat{\rho}_3$ be an estimator of the covariance in the estimated accuracies of different readers in different diagnostic tests. The following test and test $\times$ reader mean squares can be defined:

$$MS(T) = \frac{J}{K-1}\sum_{k=1}^{K}(\hat{\theta}_{k..} - \hat{\theta}_{...})^2,$$

$$MS(T * R) = \frac{1}{(J-1)(K-1)} \sum_{k=1}^{K} \sum_{j=1}^{J} (\hat{\theta}_{kj.} - \hat{\theta}_{k..} - \hat{\theta}_{.j.} + \hat{\theta}_{...})^2.$$

Then, the modified F^* statistic is defined as follows:

$$F^* = \frac{MS(T)}{MS(T * R) + max[J(\hat{\sigma}_c^2 \hat{\rho}_2 - \hat{\sigma}_c^2 \hat{\rho}_3), 0]}. \tag{9.24}$$

Obuchowski and Rockette (1995) treated F^* as having an approximate F distribution with the numerator degrees of freedom equal to $(K-1)$ and the denominator degrees of freedom equal to $(K-1)(J-1)$ under the null hypothesis that $\mu_1 = \ldots = \mu_K$. Using the F distribution, H_0 is rejected with the Type I error rate of δ if $F^* > F_{1-\delta, K-1, (K-1)(J-1)}$, where $F_{\delta, K-1, (K-1)(J-1)}$ is the δth quantile of the F distribution with $(K-1)$ degrees of freedom in the numerator and $(K-1)(J-1)$ degrees of freedom in the denominator.

Hillis (2007) showed that the above F^* test statistic has an approximate F distribution under H_0 with $(K-1)$ degrees of freedom in the numerator, but he proposed different degrees of freedom in the denominator from the one in Obuchowski and Rockette (1995). The degrees of freedom in the denominator proposed by Hillis (2007) has the following form:

$$\frac{(MS(T * R) + max[J(\hat{\sigma}_c^2 \hat{\rho}_2 - \hat{\sigma}_c^2 \hat{\rho}_3), 0])^2}{\frac{(MS(T))^2}{(K-1)(J-1)}}.$$

Hillis (2007) further showed that the new degrees of freedom improves the performance of F^* test, compared with the original denominator degrees of freedom, $(K-1)(J-1)$.

To compare the accuracies between diagnostic tests, we compute a confidence interval for the difference in mean diagnostic accuracies between the kth test and $\tilde{k}$th test, where $1 \leq k \neq \tilde{k} \leq I$. Obuchowski and Rockette (1995) obtained the following $100(1-\delta)\%$ confidence interval for $(\mu + \mu_k) - (\mu + \mu_{\tilde{k}})$:

$$(\hat{\theta}_{k..} - \hat{\theta}_{\tilde{k}..}) \pm$$

$$t_{\delta/2, J-1} \sqrt{\frac{1}{J(J-1)} \sum_{j=1}^{J} [(\hat{\theta}_{kj.} - \hat{\theta}_{\tilde{k}j.}) - (\hat{\theta}_{k..} - \hat{\theta}_{\tilde{k}..})]^2 + 2(\hat{\rho}_2 \hat{\sigma}_c^2 - \hat{\rho}_3 \hat{\sigma}_c^2)}. \tag{9.25}$$

Obuchowski and Rockette (1995) conducted a large simulation study to investigate finite-sample properties of the OR method. In their paper the authors reported the Type I error rate of the OR method when the patient sample size was small (25 patients with and 25 without the condition), the reader sample size was small (4-12 readers), and the correlations (that is, r_1, r_2, and r_3) differed for patients with and without the condition. The authors found that the Type I error rate is close to the nominal level when the number of readers is moderate or large (> 8 readers); with fewer readers the Type I error rate is conservative (i.e. below the nominal level). For small patient sample sizes (total N=50), the type I error rate rarely exceeded the nominal level. They found no effect on the Type I error rate when the correlations were not equivalent for patients with and without the condition. Finally, the OR method has also been extended to accommodate clustered data, e.g. two breasts from the same patient where the radiologists assign their confidence to each breast (Obuchowski, 1997a). In his simulation study, Hillis (2007) found that the OR method can be ultraconservative with significance levels considerably below the nominal level. A FORTRAN program to run the OR method is called OBUMRM2 and can be found at www.lerner.ccf.org/qhs/software/obumrm.php.

An alternative way to analyze data from a multi-reader study is to perform a standard analysis of the mixed-effects ANOVA on Tukey's jackknife pseudovalues. This approach was originally developed by Dorfman et al. (1992) and is commonly known as the Dorfman-Berbaum-Metz (DBM) method. The DBM method was originally proposed for a multi-reader study with no replications of the study; that is $Q = 1$.

We assume that the sample contains n_1 patients with the condition and $n_0 = N - m$ patients without the condition. Applying either the parametric or nonparametric method to data from the kth test by the jth reader, we obtain an estimator for the area under the ROC curve of the kth test by the jth reader, and denote the resulting estimator by $\hat{\theta}_{kj}$, where $k = 1, \ldots, K$, and $j = 1, \ldots, J$. Dorfman et al. (1992) proposed to apply the one-sample Jackknife method to compute pseudovalues for the test statistic $\hat{\theta}_{kj}$. Since there are N patients in the sample, this procedure re-computes $\hat{\theta}_{kj}$ N times. Let $\hat{\theta}_{kj(i)}$ denote the value of $\hat{\theta}_{kj}$ when the ith patient is deleted from the sample, $i = 1, \ldots, N$. Dorfman et al. (1992) calculated the jackknife pseudovalue for the kth test by the jth reader for the ith patient by

$$Y_{ijk} = \hat{\theta}_{kj} + (N-1)(\hat{\theta}_{kj} - \hat{\theta}_{kj(i)}). \tag{9.26}$$

By treating the Y_{ijk} as observed data, Dorfman et al. (1992) fitted a mixed-effects linear model for the jackknife pseudovalues Y_{ijk}'s in which readers and patients are random factors whereas tests are a fixed factor. Their model can be written as

$$Y_{ijk} = \mu + \mu_k + r_j + p_i + (\mu r)_{kj} + (\mu p)_{ik} + (rp)_{ji} + (\mu rp)_{ijk} + \epsilon_{ijk}, \tag{9.27}$$

where μ is the overall mean, μ_k is a fixed effect corresponding to the kth test, r_j is a random effect due to the jth reader, p_i is a random effect due to the ith patient, $(\mu r)_{kj}$ is a random effect due to the two-way interaction between the kth test and the jth reader, $(\mu p)_{ik}$ is a random effect due to the two-way interaction between the kth test and the ith patient, $(rp)_{ji}$ is a random effect due to the two-way interaction between the jth reader and the ith patient, $(\mu rp)_{ijk}$ is a random effect due to the three-way interaction among the ith patient, the jth reader and the kth test, and ϵ_{ijk} is a random error term. To complete the model, Dorfman et al. (1992) further assume that the random effects and error terms, r_j, p_i, $(\mu r)_{kj}$, $(\mu p)_{ik}$, $(rp)_{ji}$, $(\mu rp)_{ijk}$, and ϵ_{ijk} are independent and have normal distributions with zero means and variances σ_r^2, σ_p^2, σ_{tr}^2, σ_{tp}^2, σ_{rp}^2, σ_{rpt}^2, and σ_e^2, respectively.

One main null hypothesis we wish to test is that the fixed test effects are equal; that is, $H_0 : \mu_1 = \ldots = \mu_K$. If there are no interactions between test and reader and between test and patient, we can use a standard F test for treatment effects. This F test statistic is defined by $F = MS_T/MS_{TRP}$ (see Table 9.5), which has an F distribution with the numerator degrees of freedom equal to $K - 1$ and the denominator degrees of freedom equal to $(K-1)(J-1)(N-1)$ under the null hypothesis that $\mu_1 = \ldots = \mu_K$.

Table 9.5   Analysis of Variance Table for Mixed Effect Model (9.27)

Source	SS	df	MS	EMS
Test (T)	SST	K-1	MS_T	$\sigma_e^2 + \sigma_{rpt}^2 + J\sigma_{tp}^2 + N\sigma_{tr}^2 + JN\sigma_r^2$
Reader (R)	SSR	J-1	MS_R	$\sigma_e^2 + K\sigma_{tp}^2 + KN\sigma_r^2$
Patient (P)	SSP	N-1	MS_P	$\sigma_e^2 + K\sigma_{rp}^2 + KJ\sigma_p^2$
TxR	SSTR	(K-1)(J-1)	MS_{TR}	$\sigma_e^2 + \sigma_{rpt}^2 + N\sigma_{tr}^2$
TxP	SSTP	(K-1)(N-1)	MS_{TP}	$\sigma_e^2 + \sigma_{rpt}^2 + J\sigma_{tp}^2$
RxP	SSRP	(J-1)(N-1)	MS_{RP}	$\sigma_e^2 + \sigma_{rpt}^2 + K\sigma_{rp}^2$
TxRxP	SSTRP	(K-1)(J-1)(N-1)	MS_{TRP}	$\sigma_e^2 + \sigma_{rpt}^2$

If interactions between treatment and reader or between the treatment and patient exist, however, the above F test can no longer be used for testing $H_0 : \mu_1 = \ldots = \mu_K = 0$. Instead, we need to use the Satterthwaite approximate F test statistic for testing H_0 (Winer et al., 1991). The numerator and denominator of the Satterthwaite approximate F test statistic are constructed by two different linear combinations of independent mean squares such that the expected values of the two linear combinations are equal under the null hypothesis H_0, and the resulting test statistic is defined by

$$\tilde{F} = \frac{MS_T}{MS_{TR} + MS_{TP} - MS_{TRP}},$$

where MS_T, MS_{TR}, and MS_{TP}, and MS_{TRP} are mean squares defined in Table 9.5. It can be shown that $\tilde{F}$ has an F distribution with degrees of freedom for the numerator equal to $I - 1$ and degrees of freedom for the denominator equal to

$$\frac{(MS_{TR} + MS_{TP} - MS_{TRP})^2}{\frac{MS_{TR}}{(K-1)(J-1)} + \frac{MS_{TP}}{(K-1)(N-1)} + \frac{MS_{TRP}}{K-1}}.$$

Dorfman et al. (1992) also developed confidence intervals for the fixed test effect means and their differences by using the Satterthwaite procedure. We refer readers to Dorfman et al. (1992) for the detailed expressions for those confidence intervals.

From the above discussion, we see that in order to choose an appropriate test for the null hypothesis, $H_0 : \mu_1 = \ldots = \mu_K = 0$, we need to test whether the interactions between treatment and reader and between treatment and patient exist. Those two-way interactions can be represented by the following null hypotheses: $H_0 : \sigma_{tr}^2 = 0$ and $H_0 : \sigma_{tp}^2 = 0$, respectively. We use the statistic $F = MS_{TR}/MS_{TRP}$ to test the null hypothesis that $\sigma_{tr}^2 = 0$; the statistic has an F distribution with numerator degrees of freedom equal to $(K - 1)(J - 1)$ and denominator degrees of freedom equal to $(K - 1)(J - 1)(N - 1)$. Similarly we can use the statistic $F = MS_{TP}/MS_{TRP}$ to test the null hypothesis that $\sigma_{tp}^2 = 0$; the statistic has a F distribution with $(K - 1)(N - 1)$ degrees of freedom in the numerator and $(K - 1)(J - 1)(N - 1)$ degrees of freedom in the denominator. A computer program to run the DBM method is called MRMC and can be found at www-radiology.uchicago.edu/krl/KRL_ROC/software_index6.htm

Dorfman and Berbaum (1995), Roe and Metz (1997), and Dorfman et al. (1998) conducted some simulation studies to evaluate finite-sample performance of the DBM method and concluded that the DBM method performs well in general. However, in his simulation study, Hillis (2007) found that the DBM method can sometimes result in extremely wide confidence intervals. He then proposed a new estimator for the denominator degrees of freedom that can be used with both the DBM and OR procedures, which overcomes the problem of ultraconservative significance levels with the OR method and the problem of wide confidence intervals with the DBM method.

9.2.2.2 A Bootstrap Approach

Beiden et al. (2000) proposed an alternative bootstrap method for the analysis of multi-reader ROC studies. Let $\widehat{A}_{ijk}$ be the estimated area under the ROC curve for the kth test by the jth reader on the ith patient sample. Following Dorfman et al (1992), Beiden et al. (2000) considered the following mixed-effects linear model for $\widehat{A}_{ijk}$'s:

$$A_{ijk} = \mu_k + r_j + c_i + (\mu r)_{jk} + (\mu c)_{ik} + (rc)_{ij} + (\mu rc)_{ijk} + \epsilon_{ijk}. \qquad (9.28)$$

In the model (9.28), the term, μ_k, is a fixed effect due to the kth test; the terms, r_j and c_i, are random effects due to the jth reader and the ith patient sample, respectively; the terms with two subscripts, $(\mu r)_{jk}$, $(\mu c)_{ik}$, and $(rc)_{ij}$, are random effects due to the two-way interactions between test and reader, test and patient sample, and reader and patient sample, respectively; the term with three subscripts, $(\mu rc)_{ijk}$, is a random effect due to the three-way interaction among test, reader, and patient sample; and the last term, ϵ_{ijk}, is a random error in the experiment. Beiden et al. (2000) assumed that the random variables in the model (9.28), r_j, c_i, $(\mu r)_{jk}$, $(\mu c)_{ik}$, $(rc)_{ij}$, $(\mu rc)_{ijk}$, and ϵ_{ijk}, are independent and have zero mean and variances, σ_r^2, σ_c^2, σ_{mr}^2, σ_{mc}^2, σ_{rc}^2, σ_{mrc}^2, and σ_z^2, respectively.

Because in most studies there are no replications of a given experiment by readers, the terms σ^2_{mrc} and σ^2_z are not separable. Beiden et al. (2000) combined them into one single term, σ^2_ϵ; that is, $\sigma^2_\epsilon = \sigma^2_{mrc} + \sigma^2_z$. Under model (9.28), the variance of $\widehat{A}_{ijk}$ is given by

$$\sigma^2_r + \sigma^2_c + \sigma^2_{mr} + \sigma^2_{mc} + \sigma^2_{rc} + \sigma^2_\epsilon.$$

To emphasize that the model (9.28) treats tests as a fixed factor and both readers and patients as random factors, Beiden et al. (2000) wrote the variance of $\widehat{A}_{ijk}$ as $var(A_{RC|M})$, where subscripts that precede the vertical bar denote random factors, and subscripts that follow the vertical bar denote fixed factors. Hence,

$$var(A_{RC|M}) = \sigma^2_r + \sigma^2_c + \sigma^2_{mr} + \sigma^2_{mc} + \sigma^2_{rc} + \sigma^2_\epsilon. \tag{9.29}$$

Note that there are six variance components in (9.29). To uniquely identify the six variance components in (9.29), Beiden et al. (2000) considered an experiment for $\widehat{A}_{ijk}$'s in which both readers and tests are considered as fixed factors and in which patient samples remain a random factor. Under such an experiment, the corresponding mixed-effects linear model can be written as

$$A_{ijk} = \mu^{(2)}_k + r^{(2)}_j + c^{(2)}_i + (\mu r)^{(2)}_{jk} + (\mu c)^{(2)}_{ik} + (rc)^{(2)}_{ij} + (\mu rc)^{(2)}_{ijk} + \epsilon^{(2)}_{ijk}, \tag{9.30}$$

where $\mu^{(2)}_k$ and $r^{(2)}_j$ are fixed effects due to the kth test and the jth reader, respectively. The random effects variables $r^{(2)}_j$, $c^{(2)}_i$, $(\mu r)^{(2)}_{jk}$, $(\mu c)^{(2)}_{ik}$, $(rc)^{(2)}_{ij}$, and $(\mu rc)^{(2)}_{ijk}$ are assumed to have zero mean and variances, $(\sigma^{(2)}_r)^2$, $(\sigma^{(2)}_c)^2$, $(\sigma^{(2)}_{mr})^2$, $(\sigma^{(2)}_{mc})^2$, $(\sigma^{(2)}_{rc})^2$, $(\sigma^{(2)}_{mrc})^2$, and $(\sigma^{(2)}_z)^2$, respectively. Under mixed-effects linear model (9.30), one can show that the variance for $\widehat{A}_{ijk}$ is

$$var(A_{C|RM}) = (\sigma^{(2)}_c)^2 + (\sigma^{(2)}_{mc})^2 + (\sigma^{(2)}_{rc})^2 + (\sigma^{(2)}_\epsilon)^2. \tag{9.31}$$

To avoid confusion, it is important to use superscripts in mixed-effects linear model (9.30) because these factors have different interpretations than the ones in model (9.28). For example, even though both the symbols $(rc)_{ij}$ and $(rc)^{(2)}_{ij}$ represent a random effect due to the interaction between reader and patient sample, $(rc)_{jk}$ represents the random effect due to the interaction between two random factors, reader and patient sample while $(rc)^{(2)}_{jk}$ represents the random effect due to the interaction between a fixed factor, reader, and a random factor, patient sample. Therefore, the random-effect, $(rc)_{ij}$, should be different from the random effect, $(rc)^{(2)}_{ij}$. Hence, mixed effects linear model (9.30) has the six variance components that are, in general, different from those in (9.28).

To find a system of six equations that can be used to uniquely determine the six variance components in (9.28), as proposed by Beiden et al. (2000), one has to make the assumption that

$$\sigma_c = \sigma^{(2)}_c, \sigma_{mc} = \sigma^{(2)}_{mc}, \sigma_{rc} = \sigma^{(2)}_{rc}, \sigma_\epsilon = \sigma^{(2)}_\epsilon. \tag{9.32}$$

Under Assumption (9.32), Beiden et al. (2000) derived the six equations for

$$\sigma^2 = (\sigma_r^2, \sigma_c^2, \sigma_{mr}^2, \sigma_{mc}^2, \sigma_{rc}^2, \sigma_\epsilon^2)$$

from the models (9.28) and (9.30). Specifically, under the model (9.28) for two different tests M and $\tilde{M}$, Beiden et al. (2000) obtained the following equation:

$$var(A_{RC|M} - A_{RC|\tilde{M}}) = 2(\sigma_{mr}^2 + \sigma_{mc}^2 + \sigma_\epsilon^2). \tag{9.33}$$

Under the model (9.30) for two different tests M and $\tilde{M}$ and two different readers R and $\tilde{R}$, Beiden et al. (2000) obtained the following three equations:

$$var(A_{C|RM} - A_{C|\tilde{R}M}) = 2(\sigma_{rc}^2 + \sigma_\epsilon^2), \tag{9.34}$$

$$var(A_{C|RM} - A_{C|R\tilde{M}}) = 2(\sigma_{mc}^2 + \sigma_\epsilon^2), \tag{9.35}$$

and

$$var(A_{C|RM} - A_{C|\tilde{R}\tilde{M}}) = 2(\sigma_{rc}^2 + \sigma_{mc}^2 + \sigma_\epsilon^2). \tag{9.36}$$

Let

$$\mathbf{VAR} = (var(A_{RC|M}), var(A_{C|RM}), var(A_{RC|M} - A_{RC|\tilde{M}}),$$

$$var(A_{C|RM} - A_{C|\tilde{R}M}), var(A_{C|RM} - A_{C|R\tilde{M}}), var(A_{C|RM} - A_{C|\tilde{R}\tilde{M}}))'.$$

Beiden et al. (2000) re-wrote equations (9.29) to (9.36) as the following system of six linear equations:

$$\mathbf{VAR} = W\sigma^2, \tag{9.37}$$

where W is a matrix of known constants.

Since in practice **VAR** is unknown, Beiden et al. (2000) proposed to use a standard bootstrap method that is for an i.i.d. data structure to estimate **VAR**. The proposed bootstrap method consists of two sampling plans: in the first plan the original rating data are resampled with replacement over patients and readers, and in the second plan original rating data are resampled with replacement over patients. Specifically, for a given rating dataset, Beiden et al. (2000) used the first re-sampling plan to estimate $var(A_{RC|M})$ and $var(A_{RC|M} - A_{RC|\tilde{M}})$ and the second re-sampling plan to estimate $var(A_{C|RM} - A_{C|\tilde{R}M})$, $var(A_{C|RM} - A_{C|R\tilde{M}})$, and $var(A_{C|RM} - A_{C|\tilde{R}\tilde{M}})$. After obtaining the bootstrap estimator $\widehat{\mathbf{VAR}}^*$ for **VAR**, Beiden et al. (2000) obtain estimators for the six variance components by solving (9.37) with **VAR** replaced by $\widehat{\mathbf{VAR}}^*$.

9.2.2.3 A Marginal Model Approach

Song and Zhou (2005) proposed a marginal generalized linear model for the AUCs which allows inclusion of patient-specific and reader-specific covariates in the model (e.g. gender of a patient and the training level of a reader). This regression model is an extension of the marginal regression model for the AUCs for independent ROC data, proposed by Dodd and Pepe (2003), to multi-reader multi-test ROC data. Let X_i^1 denote a vector of covariates for diseased patient i $(i = n_0 + 1, \ldots, N)$, X_s^0 denote a row vector of covariates for non-diseased patient s $(s = 1, \ldots, n_0)$, and Q_j denote a vector of covariates for reader j $(j = 1, \ldots, J)$. Let $Z_k = (Z_{k1}, Z_{k2}, \ldots, Z_{kN})'$ $(k = 1, \ldots, K)$, where $Z_{kr} = I(k = r)$ is the indicator for test r. We define the covariate-specific AUC, A_{ijks}, as

$$A_{ijks} = E(\varphi_{ijks}|Z_k, Q_j, X_i^1, X_s^0) = P(Y_{kji} > Y_{kjs}|Z_k, Q_j, X_i^1, X_s^0).$$

Then Song and Zhou (2005) proposed the following regression model for A_{ijks}:

$$A_{ijks} = g(\beta_1' Z_k + \beta_2' Q_j + \beta_3' X_i^1 + \beta_4' X_s^0), \tag{9.38}$$

where $g(\cdot)$ is a monotone link function, and $\beta = (\beta_1', \beta_2', \beta_3', \beta_4')'$ is a vector of regression parameters. Under model (9.38), we have the regression model for φ_{ijks}:

$$\Pr\left(\varphi_{ijks} = 1|Z_k, Q_j, X_i^1, X_s^0\right) = g(\beta_1' Z_k + \beta_2' Q_j + \beta_3' X_i^1 + \beta_4' X_s^0). \tag{9.39}$$

For this marginal model, the set of "observations" is $\{(\varphi_{ijks}, Z_k, Q_j, X_i^1, X_s^0) : k = 1, \ldots, K; j = 1, \ldots, J; i = n_0 + 1, \ldots, N; s = 1, \ldots, n_0\}$. Since φ_{ijks} are not independent, standard methods for generalized linear models can not be applied directly. We consider three different assumptions on the correlation structure. First, as conforming to the ANOVA model (9.28), we assume that φ_{ijks} and $\varphi_{i'j'k's'}$ are correlated only when $i = i'$ or $s = s'$. Then φ_{ijks} are sparsely correlated as defined by Lumley (1998, 2005). In their notation, for each "observation" φ_{ijks}, we define the set $S_{ijks} = \{(i', j', k', s') : i' = i$ or $s' = s\}$, which contains the indices of all "observations" correlated to φ_{ijks}. It is easy to see that the number of "observations" in S_{ijks} is $M = KJ(N-1) = O(KJn_0 + KJn_1)$. Now consider a subset $\mathcal{T}$ of $\{(i, j, k, s) : k = 1, \ldots, K; j = 1, \ldots, J; i = n_0 + 1, \ldots, N; s = 1, \ldots, n_0\}$, which satisfies that for any two elements $(i', j', k', s') \in \mathcal{T}$ and $(i'', j'', k'', s'') \in \mathcal{T}$, $(i', j', k', s') \notin S_{i''j''k''s''}$ and $(i'', j'', k'', s'') \notin S_{i'j'k's'}$. Thus any two elements in $\mathcal{T}$ must have different i and s. Hence the maximum number of elements in $\mathcal{T}$ is $m = \min(n_0, n_1)$. Therefore $Mm = O(KJn_0n_1)$. Noticing that KJn_0n_1 is the number of "observations", we conclude that the condition of sparse correlation is satisfied.

This assumption can be relaxed to that φ_{ijks} and $\varphi_{i'j'k's'}$ are correlated only when $j = j'$ or $i = i'$ or $s = s'$; in this case, $S_{ijks} = \{(i', j', k', s') : j' = j$ or $i' = i$ or $s' = s\}$, $M = O(Kn_0n_1 + KJn_0 + KJn_1)$ and $m = \min(J, n_0, n_1)$. We can further relax the assumption to that φ_{ijks} and $\varphi_{i'j'k's'}$ are correlated only when $k = k'$ or $j = j'$ or $i = i'$ or $s = s'$; the corresponding $S_{ijks} = \{(i', j', k', s') : k' = k$ or $j' = j$ or $i' = i$ or $s' = s\}$, $M = O(Jn_0n_1 + Kn_0n_1 + KJn_0 + KJn_1)$ and $m = \min(K, J, n_0, n_1)$. Notice that under each of these conditions we always have $Mm = O(KJn_0n_1)$ and hence the data have a sparse correlation structure. To discriminate these assumptions, we call them Assumption I, II and III, respectively. Among the three assumptions, Assumption I is the strongest; it only allows correlations among two test results of the same subject and assumes that test results of two different subjects are not correlated, regardless of whether they are from the same test or are interpreted by the same reader. Assumption II is the second strongest; it allows possible correlations among two test results of the same subject and possible correlations among two test results of different subjects, interpreted by the same reader. Assumption III is the weakest assumption; it allows possible correlations among two test results of the same subject or two different subjects interpreted by the same reader.

Now consider the pseudo-likelihood

$$L = \prod_{k=1}^{K}\prod_{j=1}^{J}\prod_{s=1}^{n_0}\prod_{i=n_0+1}^{N} \{g(\beta'W_{ijks})\}^{\varphi_{ijks}} \{1 - g(\beta'W_{ijks})\}^{1-\varphi_{ijks}}, \quad (9.40)$$

where $W'_{ijks} = (Z'_k, Q'_j, (X^1_k)', (X^0_s)')$. Expression (9.40) is the likelihood when φ_{ijks} are independent. The log pseudo-likelihood equation is

$$U = \frac{\partial \log L}{\partial \beta'} = \sum_{k=1}^{K}\sum_{j=1}^{J}\sum_{s=1}^{n_0}\sum_{i=n_0+1}^{N} U_{ijks}(\beta) = 0, \quad (9.41)$$

where

$$U_{ijks}(\beta) = \left[\frac{\{\varphi_{ijks} - g(\beta'W_{ijks})\} g'(\beta'W_{ijks})}{g(\beta'W_{ijks}) \{1 - g(\beta'W_{ijks})\}} \right] W_{ijks},$$

$g'(\cdot)$ is the derivative of $g(\cdot)$. Let $\hat{\beta}$ be the solution to (9.41) that maximizes (9.40). By Theorem 7 of Lumley (2005), under some regularity conditions, as $m \to \infty$, $\hat{\beta}$ is consistent and asymptotically normal with variance consistently estimated by $C^{-1}B(C^{-1})'$ (Song and Zhou, 2005), where

$$C = \sum_{k=1}^{K}\sum_{j=1}^{J}\sum_{s=1}^{n_0}\sum_{i=n_0+1}^{N} \frac{\partial U_{ijks}(\hat{\beta})}{\partial \beta'},$$

$$B = \sum_{k=1}^{K}\sum_{j=1}^{J}\sum_{s=1}^{n_0}\sum_{i=n_0+1}^{N} \sum_{(i',j',k',s')\in S_{ijks}} U_{ijks}(\hat{\beta})U'_{i'j'k's'}(\hat{\beta}).$$

A consistent estimator for the AUCs can then be obtained by substituting $\hat{\beta}$ for β in (9.38). In practice, to utilize the asymptotic normality, m is required to be large. Under Assumption I, this corresponds to that both the number of diseased subjects and the number of non-diseased subjects are large. Assumption II further requires that the number of readers is large and Assumption III requires in addition that both the number of tests and the number of readers are large. Hence Assumption I is more reasonable in practice.

It is easy to see that the mixed-effects ANOVA model in Dorfman et al. (1992) is a special case of the proposed marginal model; that is,

$$\Pr\left(\varphi_{ijks} = 1 | Z_k, Q_j, X_k, X_s\right) = \phi(\beta_1' Z_k),$$

where $\phi(\cdot)$ is the distribution function for the standard normal, and

$$\beta_1 = \frac{(\mu_1 - \mu_0 + \alpha_{11} - \alpha_{10}, \ldots, \mu_1 - \mu_0 + \alpha_{I1} - \alpha_{I0})'}{\sum_{t=0}^{1} \left(\sigma_{Ct}^2 + \sigma_{\alpha Ct}^2 + \sigma_{RCt}^2 + \sigma_{\varepsilon t}^2\right)^{1/2}}.$$

The marginal model (9.39) can incorporate patient-level and reader-level covariates in (9.39). The asymptotic properties provide a sound and theoretical basis for statistical inference. Since the estimating equations (9.41) have the same form as the generalized estimating equations (GEE) with the independent working correlation structure, estimators can be obtained by standard statistical software such as SAS and R, although the standard errors need to be recomputed using the sandwich estimator described above. We have written the code for computing the standard errors under the logit and probit links using PROC IML in SAS, which can be easily extended to other links or converted to SPlus. The implementation of the marginal model approach includes three steps: i) derive the data set $\{\varphi_{ijks}, Z_i, Q_j, X_k, X_s\}$ from the original data; ii) obtain the estimates using PROC GENMOD or PROC LOGISTIC in SAS or function gee() or glm() in R; iii) compute the standard errors using self-coded functions based on the sandwich estimator and the output obtained from step ii). Song and Zhou (2005) have also conducted a simulation study to evaluate finite-sample properties of their marginal approach and compared the performance of the marginal approach with that of the DBM method. The simulation results show that that both the marginal and DBM method perform well under the null hypothesis that the accuracy of the tests are the same and that the marginal method outperforms the DBM method for inference on individual AUCs under an alternative hypothesis that the accuracy of the tests are not the same. SAS and R codes for implementing the marginal model approach, proposed by Song and Zhou (2005), are available at the web site for the book (http://faculty.washington.edu/azhou/books/diagnostic.html).

9.2.3 Analysis of the Interstitial Disease Example

In this section, we apply the above four methods to the interstitial disease example, as discussed in the beginning of Section 9.2.1.1. The results on the DBM, OR, and BWC methods were taken from Obuchowski et al. (2004).

The goal of the analysis is to test whether the diagnostic accuracies for the two resolution (high and median) chest images PACS are different. Under mixed-effects ANOVA model (9.27), the DBM method gives the estimated AUCs for the high and medium resolution chest images as $\widehat{\mu}_1 = 0.725$ and $\widehat{\mu}_2 =$

0.718, respectively. The 95% confidence interval for the difference between these two AUCs is $[-0.037, 0.051]$.

Next we apply the method of Obuchowski and Rockette (1995) to this data set. For each of 5 reader and two test combinations, we obtain a nonparametric estimate for the ROC curve area and its associated standard error. The OR gives the estimated AUCs of these two tests as 0.725 and 0.719, respectively. Using formula (9.25) we can also obtain the 95% confidence interval for the difference in the means of diagnostic accuracies over readers between any two tests. The resulting two-sided 95% confidence interval between the high and median resolution images is $[-0.043, 0.056]$.

Using the BWC's bootstrap method, we obtain that the estimated AUCs for the two resolutions of the chest images are 0.727 and 0.720, respectively. With the BWC's bootstrap method, the 95% confidence interval between the high and medium resolution images is $[-0.059, 0.071]$.

Using the marginal method, we obtain the estimated AUCs for the two resolutions of the chest images as 0.725 and 0.718, respectively. We also obtain the 95% confidence interval between the high and medium resolution images as $[-0.042, 0.055]$.

All four methods give similar point estimates for the AUCs of the high and medium resolution imaging techniques and similar 95% confidence intervals for the difference in the AUCS of these two imaging techniques.

9.2.4   Comparisons between MRMC Methods

Following Obuchowski et al. (2004), we compare and contrast the four MRMC methods - the DBM, the OR, the bootstrap, and the marginal method - in four key features: (1) accounting for the correlation in the estimates of test accuracy, (2) modeling test accuracy, (3) accounting for the variation in reader performance, and (4) adjusting for patient and reader characteristics (covariates).

The first major difference between the methods is how each method handles correlations among estimates of test accuracy. These correlations are from three types of correlation among original test results of subjects: correlations between different test results of the same patient, interpreted by the same reader; correlations between different test results of the same patient, interpreted by different readers; and correlations between test results of two different patients, interpreted by the same reader. Due to these types of correlations and since the estimates of test accuracy are functions of the original test results of subjects, the estimates of test accuracy for each test and each reader are also correlated. The DBM, OR, and the bootstrap methods incorporate correlations of the estimated test accuracy implicitly through interaction terms and correlated error terms on estimates of test accuracy. On the other hand, the marginal method directly incorporates correlations of original test results in estimation.

The second major difference between the methods is the level at which the different methods model test accuracy. The marginal method specifies a model for the confidence scores assigned by the readers to the images; both the DBM and bootstrap method define a model for a transformation of the observed confidence scores through jackknifed pseudovalues; the OR method directly models the summary measure of accuracy (e.g., the area under the ROC curve).

The third important difference is how the methods handle variation in reader performance via fixed or random effects. If the readers are selected from available readers at the institution where the study is performed, this sample of readers is often not generalizable to a broad population of radiologists. For these studies, the conclusions of the study should pertain to these particular readers only (so called "fixed effects"). However, if the selected readers represent a random sample of a well-defined population of readers so that the estimates of accuracy are generalizable to patients as well as readers at other institutions, the variation in reader performance can be treated as a source of variability and modeled by "random effects." The DBM, OR, and the bootstrap methods can be applied to either fixed effects or random effects situations; the marginal method is suitable to the fixed effects situation only.

The fourth important difference is whether the methods can handle patient or reader covariates, which affect the accuracy of diagnostic tests. For example, test accuracy may depend on a range of patient difficulties (because of the differences in tissue densities or disease characteristics) and a range of reader skill (because of training, experience, and natural aptitude). The DBM, OR, and the bootstrap methods can be extended to handle discrete patient-level covariates if there are enough patients in each covariate combination to permit calculation of the summary accuracy measure, but they cannot handle continuous covariates at the patient-level. Only the marginal method can adjust for both discrete and continuous covariates at the patient- and reader-level in the analysis.

9.3 ANALYSIS OF MULTIPLE TESTS DESIGNED TO LOCATE AND DIAGNOSE LESIONS

In Section 2.10 we discussed measuring the accuracy of diagnostic tests designed to locate lesions and characterize their significance. We pointed out that correct localization of the lesions must be part of the definition of sensitivity. We also pointed out the bias associated with patient-level metrics of diagnostic accuracy and suggested other metrics more applicable to these diagnostic tasks. In this section we briefly describe three methods commonly used to assess and compare the diagnostic accuracy of these tests in MRMC studies.

The first method is the location receiver operating characteristic (LROC) curve proposed by Starr et al. (1975). The second method is the free-response

ROC (FROC) approach originally proposed by Bunch and further developed by Chakraborty and others. The third one is based on regions of interest (ROI), originally proposed by Obuchowski et al. (2000).

9.3.1   LROC Approach

In the Location Receiver Operating Curve (LROC) experiment, the reader is asked to mark the location of one suspected abnormality and assign a confidence score to it. The marked place can be classified as a true positive (TP) or false positive (FP) finding depending on whether or not it contains an actual abnormality (Starr et al., 1975). The LROC curve has the same abscissa as the ROC curve, but has the true localization rate (TLR) (probability that a lesion is correctly localized and the rating of the lesion exceeds a threshold) as its ordinate. The area under the LROC curve provides a measure of a radiologist's ability to correctly localize a lesion on an abnormal image. Swensson (2000) proposed an elegant parametric model to estimate the LROC curve. His model is analogous to the binormal model in ROC analysis (Dorfman and Alf, 1969). Recently, Popescu (2007) proposed a nonparametric method to estimate the area under the LROC curve. The method is an extension of empirical AUC estimators. One limitation of the LROC curve is that it only allows for the presence of one true lesion per image.

9.3.2   FROC Approach

In the FROC "experiment", the reader is asked to mark the location of all suspected abnormalities and assign a confidence score to each. Every marked place can be classified as a true positive (TP) or false positive (FP) finding depending on whether or not it contains an actual abnormality (Chakraborty and Berbaum, 1989). The data are summarized in an FROC plot, where the y axis is the proportion of abnormalities that are detected and correctly located to within a specified distance, denoted by TMR, and the x axis is the mean number of false-positive findings generated per patient, denoted by FMN.

When Bunch et al. (1978) first introduced the FROC curve, they assumed that ratings were independent within the same image and proposed a parametric method for estimating the FROC curve parameters. Other parametric methods proposed by Chakraborty and Berbaum (1989) and Chakraborty and Berbaum (2004) assumed that ratings of a true mark (TM) and a false mark (FM) follow two different normal distributions with mean zero. Specifically, Chakraborty and Berbaum (1989) assumed independence on ratings from the same image and normal distributions for ratings of TM and FM, and then obtain the ML estimators for the FROC parameters. This ML method has been heavily criticized mainly because of the independence assumption. A more recent paper by Chakraborty (2006) used a jackknife technique at the level of images by deleting one image at a time to calculate the variance of the area under the FROC curve; this technique does not require the independence assumption.

Bandos et al. (2009) recently proposed an empirical estimator for the area under the FROC curve (FAUC), and obtained its variance based on a bootstrap procedure. One issue in estimating the FAUC is that unlike the area under the ROC curve, the area under the empirical FROC curve is generally not bounded by one; Bandos et al. (2009) address this issue.

Another complexity with the FROC curve is that the range of the FMN may vary from imaging system to system. This makes the comparison between two imaging systems almost impossible. For instance, if one FROC curve is on top of the other, but has a smaller FMN range, this may result in similar FAUCs of the two FROC curves. Chakraborty and Berbaum (2004) proposed an alternative FROC curve (AFROC), which maintains the same ordinate of the FROC curve, but changes the abscissa to be the probability of the maximum FM rating greater than a constant c. The main advantage of using the AFROC curve is that it essentially puts all systems on the same scale, allowing a fair comparison between imaging systems. Two summary measures of the AFROC curve are the probability of having a TM's rating greater than a FM rating on any image, and the probability of having a TM's rating greater than a FM rating on an abnormal image. Chakraborty (2006) introduced nonparametric methods to estimate these two measures, and used jackknife resampling methods to estimate the variances. Chakraborty (2006) also proposed a Jackknife alternative free-response receiver operating characteristic (JAFROC) curve method for measuring human observer performance in localization tasks.

9.3.3 ROI Approach

The ROI method was originally proposed to handle multiple anatomic locations from the same patient, where each location was scored separately by the reader (e.g. multiple artery segments each evaluated for their degree of stenosis, or breast quadrants from the same patient each scored for the probability of malignancy). The method, however, can be adapted for the case of characterizing readers' ability to correctly locate and diagnose lesions. As with the FROC experiment, each suspicious lesion is marked by the reader and assigned a confidence score for the probability of disease. Regions of interest (ROI) are defined a priori based on relevant clinical units. For example, in breast cancer each breast, or breast quadrant, could be considered an ROI. In screening for lung cancer, each lung or lung lobe might be considered an ROI. For colon cancer screening, the segments of the colon could be used as the ROIs. Each ROI with one or more true lesions (as defined by the gold standard) is used to estimate the reader's sensitivity. A true positive is defined as an ROI where the reader correctly located and diagnosed at least one of the lesions in the ROI. If the reader did not correctly locate any of the lesions in the ROI, then the ROI is considered a false negative. Similarly, each

ROI without a true lesion is used to estimate the reader's specificity. A true negative is defined as an ROI where the reader did not identify any lesions in the ROI; a false positive is an ROI where the reader identified one or more false lesions in the ROI. Treating the test result from each ROI as an observation, an ROC curve and its area can be estimated for each reader. Methods for estimating the variance and covariance of the ROC area from clustered data were described in Chapters 4 and 5. These methods can be used here to estimate the variance-covariance matrix of the readers' estimated ROC areas, where the clustered data is the multiple ROIs from the same patient. The ROC area estimates from each reader, along with the estimated variance-covariance matrix, can be inputted into OBUMRM2 to test hypotheses and construct confidence intervals for the readers' average performance and the difference in readers' average performance between modalities (Obuchowski, 2007).

In comparing the three methods, the FROC and ROI methods can be used when there are multiple lesions in the same patient, while the LROC method is limited to cases of a single lesion. Both the ROI method and recently proposed FROC extensions appropriately handle the correlation between lesions from the same patient. The ROI method uses the well-known ROC area as its summary measure, where the FROC method yields a less-known summary measure with an interpretation specific to the FROC experiment. The ROI method requires pre-defined ROIs and if these ROIs are not well defined, then estimation of sensitivity and specificity can be problematic. Furthermore, if multiple lesions exist often in the same ROI, then the ROI method has less power than the FROC method in detecting small differences between modalities.

CHAPTER 10

METHODS FOR CORRECTING VERIFICATION BIAS

In Chapters 4, 5, 8, and 9, we discussed the analytic methods for evaluating the accuracy of diagnostic tests. Those methods require that the condition status for each patient (present or absent) be determined independently of the patient's test result. The procedure that establishes the patient's condition status without an error is referred to as the gold standard. If a gold standard does not exist, we have a problem of imperfect gold standard bias, which we first described in Chapter 3 and will discuss in more detail in Chapter 11. In this chapter we assume a gold standard exists; however, some patients who underwent the test might not have their condition status verified by the gold standard. Usually the patients who did not have their condition status verified are not a random sample but rather are a selected group. For example, if the gold standard is invasive surgery, then patients with negative test results are less likely to receive the gold standard evaluation than patients with positive test results. Although this approach may be sensible and cost-effective in clinical practice, when it occurs in studies designed to evaluate the accuracy of diagnostic tests, the estimated accuracy of the tests may be biased. Considering as an example a test to diagnose coronary artery disease, Diamond (1991) pointed out that the diagnosis of coronary artery

Statistical Methods in Diagnostic Medicine,
Second Edition. By Xiao-Hua Zhou, Nancy A. Obuchowski, Donna K. McClish
Copyright © 2011 John Wiley & Sons, Inc.

disease is usually confirmed by coronary angiography. In clinical practice, however, only a small proportion of patients suspected of having coronary artery disease are actually referred for angiography. Those who are referred for angiography on clinical grounds usually have more abnormal clinical findings and more extreme test results than those not referred. As a result, patients who are referred are often not a representative sample of the target population that they represent, and this bias can cause a systematic over-estimation or under-estimation of the diagnostic accuracy of the test. This type of bias is called verification bias, as we described in Chapter 3. Diamond (1991) has humorously illustrated verification bias in a song, called "Accentuate the Positive" by Johnny Mercer, whose lyrics go like "You've got to accentuate the positive, Eliminate the negative, Latch on to the affirmative, Don't mess with Mister in-between."

Although verification bias can distort the estimated accuracy of a diagnostic test, many published studies on the accuracy of diagnostic tests fail to recognize verification bias. For example, Greenes and Begg (1985) reviewed 145 studies published between 1976 and 1980 and found that at least 26% of the articles had verification bias but failed to recognize it. Bates et al. (1993) reviewed 54 pediatric studies and found more than one third had verification bias. Philbrick et al. (1980) reviewed 33 studies on the accuracy of exercise tests for coronary disease and found that 31 might have had verification bias. Finally, Reid et al. (1995) looked at 112 studies published in the New England Journal of Medicine, the Journal of the American Medical Association, the British Medical Journal, and the Lancet between 1978 and 1993 and found 54% had verification bias.

In this chapter, we present methods for correcting verification bias in the analysis of accuracy data. In Section 10.1, we give five examples that will be used to illustrate the proposed verification bias models in later sections. In Section 10.2 we first describe the impact of verification bias on estimated accuracy of diagnostic tests. Then, in Section 10.3 we describe bias-correction methods for estimating sensitivity and specificity of a single diagnostic test, and in Section 10.4 we discuss bias-correction methods for comparing the sensitivity and specificity of two correlated tests. In Section 10.5 we discuss bias-correction methods for making inferences about the ROC curve and the area under it for a single ordinal-scale diagnostic test, and in Section 10.6, we present bias-correction methods for comparing the ROC curves and the areas under them of correlated ordinal-scale diagnostic tests. In Section 10.7, we describe bias-correction methods for estimating and comparing ROC curves of continuous-scale tests.

10.1   EXAMPLES

In this section we describe five diagnostic accuracy studies that have the problem of verification bias. The first four studies focus on diagnostic tests with ordinal-scale results, and the fifth study contains both continuous-scale and ordinal-scale tests.

10.1.1 Hepatic Scintigraph

A hepatic scintigraph is an imaging scan used in detecting liver disease. Drum and Chrisacopoulos (1972) conducted an experiment to determine the sensitivity and specificity of the hepatic scintigraph in detecting liver disease. There were 650 patients who participated in the study. Of the 429 patients who had positive hepatic scintigraph results, 263 (61%) were referred to undergo further disease verification by autopsy, biopsy, or surgical inspection. Of the 221 patients with negative hepatic scintigraph results, only 81 (37%) were referred to undergo the disease verification procedure by the liver pathology independent of the scintigraphic diagnosis. Hence, we have a potential problem of verification bias in estimation of the sensitivity and specificity of the hepatic scintigraph in detecting liver disease.

10.1.2 Screening Tests for Dementia Disorder Example

Alzheimer's disease is likely to be caused by a complex interaction of genetic and environmental influences. Hendrie et al. (1995) conducted an epidemiological study to investigate the role of environmental risk factors for development of dementia in two black populations from Indianapolis, USA, and Ibadan, Nigeria. The study used a two-stage design. In the first phase, subjects were selected and screened for dementia. The definitive diagnosis of dementia was established by a clinical assessment, which consisted of a neurological examination, a neuropsychological test battery, laboratory tests, CT scans, and a detailed interview with a relative of the subject. Because of time and cost restrictions, not all screened subjects could be assessed clinically, and in the second phase of the study, only a subset of the individuals screened in the first phase were selected for clinical assessment. Selection for clinical assessment was based on the score of the screening instruments and the age of a subject. Specifically, all subjects screened into the 'poor performance' category, 50% of the subjects screened into the 'intermediate performance' category, and 5% of the subjects screened into the 'good performance' group were invited for a clinical assessment. In order to have enough older subjects from the 'good performance' group, a stratified random sample was taken selecting 75% from those age 75 and older. Disease status was not ascertained for all subjects who were selected for disease verification because some subjects were unable to be clinically assessed, while others refused. Thus, whether a subject had a clinical diagnosis might depend on the screening test result as well as other factors, and the sampling fractions for the diagnosis were unknown and had to be estimated.

One of the goals of the study was to compare the accuracy of a new screening test (T_1) with that of a standard screening test (T_2). The new test was based on information from both a cognitive test given to the subject and a test given to someone who knew the subject (Hall et al., 1993). The standard test used results from the cognitive test only (Murden et al., 1991). Since not all subjects received the gold standard, we have a problem of verification bias in the comparison of the accuracy of these two screening tests.

10.1.3   Fever of Uncertain Origin

Gray et al. (1984) reported data from a study on the accuracy of computed tomography (CT) in differentiating focal from non-focal sources of sepsis among patients with fever of uncertain origin. The true disease status of each patient was obtained by the means of surgery, biopsy, or autopsy. In this study only some patients were verified by those disease verification procedures, depending on their CT results. Hence, this study had verification bias.

10.1.4   CT and MRI for Staging Pancreatic Cancer Example

Megibow et al. (1995) conducted a study on the relative accuracies of MRI and CT in the evaluation of pancreatic cancer. All patients had pancreatic cancer and were clinically judged to be candidates for surgical resection of the pancreatic gland. According to the design, all patients enrolled in the study were supposed to be examined with both MRI and CT before undergoing surgery. The MRI and CT examinations were then interpreted separately. A critical issue in this analysis was the presence or absence of vascular invasion. The radiologist's degree of suspicion about the presence of vascular invasion was grouped into a 3-point ordinal categorical scale. The gold standard on vascular invasion was established by a pathologist's examination of the patient's specimens obtained from surgery. All imaged patients were supposed to have surgery performed within three weeks of imaging; however, 39 of the 143 imaged patients didn't have surgery. The probability of having verified disease status ranged from 90% for a patient with both MRI and CT indicating non-invasion to 39% for a patient with both MRI and CT indicating invasion. Since the reasons for not having surgery might be related to the test results of MRI and CT, analysis using only disease verified cases might lead to biased results in comparing the relative accuracies of MRI and CT.

10.1.5   NACC MDS on Alzheimer Disease (AD)

The National Alzheimer's Coordinating Center (NACC) Minimum Data Set (MDS) contains subjects from 32 Alzheimer's Disease Centers (ADCs) throughout North America. Since 1984, these centers have conducted clinical and laboratory research on the causes and clinical course of Alzheimer's disease. Many patients at ADCs were referred or self-referred for evaluation of possible dementia; some were recruited specifically to participate in research. At enrollment, nearly all underwent clinical evaluation and neuropsychological testing. They were then followed over time with periodic clinical re-evaluation and cognitive testing. For patients who died, permission for brain autopsy was sought. The analytic sample was formed in several stages. One of the clinical questions was the assessment of diagnostic accuracy of the clinical diagnosis by clinicians and the mini-mental state examination (MMSE) in distinguishing AD from non-AD subjects (Koepsell et al., 1978). The gold standard ascertainment of AD is the diagnosis made by a pathologist, based on brain autopsy. Therefore, subjects who are still alive are missing the true disease status. We may get biased estimates for the accuracy of MMSE and clinical assessments in detecting AD if we only include subjects who have the gold standard.

10.2 IMPACT OF VERIFICATION BIAS

To illustrate how verification bias operates and affects the estimated accuracy of a test, we consider one real and one hypothetical example where verification bias can seriously bias the estimated diagnostic accuracy of tests.

Punglia et al. (2003) have nicely illustrated the impact of verification bias on estimation of the accuracy of the prostate-specific antigen (PSA) as a screening test in detecting prostate cancer. Although about 75 percent of U.S. men who are 50 years or older receive the PSA test to screen for prostate cancer, controversy still exists as to whether the traditional cut-point of 4.1 ng per millimeter for recommending prostate biopsy, the gold standard, should be lowered to improve the sensitivity of the test. One difficulty of estimating the accuracy of the PSA test is that many men who underwent the PSA-based screening for prostate cancer did not receive biopsy, particularly the men with negative PSA results. In the study sample given in Punglia et al. (2003), among the 6691 men who underwent the PSA test, only 705 received the prostate biopsy. To correct for verification bias, Punglia et al. (2003) have convincingly argued that the verification bias process is missing-at-random (MAR); that is, the decision to verify the prostate-cancer status of a man who receives a PSA test depends only on the results of the PSA test, the digital rectal examination, and other observed patient characteristics, including age, the presence or absence of a family history of prostate cancer. Under the MAR assumption, Punglia et al. (2003) applied the statistical method to be discussed in Sections 10.3.1 and   10.7 to their data set and concluded that adjusting for verification bias significantly increased the area under the ROC curve (AUC) of the PSA test, as compared with the estimated AUC based on only the verified cases. Specifically, in men 65 years or younger, the adjustment increased the AUC from 0.69, obtained using the verified cases only, to 0.86 (p-value < 0.001). In men 65 years or older, the adjustment increased the AUC from 0.62, obtained using the only verified cases, to 0.72 (p-value =0.008).

In our hypothetical example we want to estimate the sensitivity of a certain stress radiographic procedure in the diagnosis of coronary artery disease (Tavel et al., 1987). We use angiography as the gold standard for coronary artery disease. Assume that the actual sensitivity of the radiographic procedure (which we need to estimate) is 80%. Thus, 20% of all diseased patients will have false-negative test results. Suppose 500 patients with coronary artery disease undergo the stress test; 400 respond positively and 100 respond negatively. Since angiography is a risky and expensive procedure, instead of verifying all tested patients by angiography, only 75% of patients with a positive test undergo angiography, and 10% of patients with a negative test undergo angiography. Thus, among 400 patients who tested positive, 300 have angiography, and among 100 who tested negative, only 10 have angiography. Analysis using only those patients who have angiography would lead to the mistaken conclusion that the sensitivity of the stress test is 97% (300/310), a gross overestimation of the true sensitivity. Similarly, we can show an estimator of specificity using only verified cases is also biased.

10.3 A SINGLE BINARY-SCALE TEST

A patient who does not receive the gold standard verification can be regarded as missing the value of the true condition status. Thus, the framework of missing data can be used to handle the verification bias problem. If the probability of selecting a patient for disease verification depends only on the observed characteristics of the patient, we say the verification process is missing-at-random (MAR), a term first coined by Rubin for the analysis of missing data (Little and Rubin, 1987). Begg and Greenes (1983) refer to the MAR assumption as the assumption of conditional independence. In this section, we present bias correction methods for estimating the sensitivity and specificity first under the MAR assumption and then without the MAR assumption.

10.3.1 Correction Methods Under the MAR Assumption

Under the MAR assumption, without knowing the process of selecting a patient for disease verification, we can derive consistent estimators for sensitivity and specificity of a test. We first define the MAR assumption. Let V, T, and D be random variables representing verification status, the test result, and the condition status of a patient, respectively. Let $V = 1$ indicate a verified patient and $V = 0$ a non-verified patient; let $T = 1$ indicate a positive test result and $T = 0$ a negative test result; and let $D = 1$ indicate a patient with the condition, and $D = 0$ a patient without the condition. If the diagnostic test result is the only observed factor that affects the verification process, the MAR assumption for the verification mechanism is equivalent to

$$P(V = 1 \mid T, D) = P(V = 1 \mid T). \tag{10.1}$$

Table 10.1   Observed Data for a Single Binary Scale Test

		Diagnostic results	
		T=1	T=0
Verified	D=1	s_1 TP	s_0 FN
	D=0	r_1 FP	r_0 TN
Unverified		u_1	u_0
Total		m_1	m_0

In this case, the observed data may be displayed as in Table 10.1.

Next we derive the maximum likelihood estimators of sensitivity and specificity of the test, T. Denote

$$\phi_{1t} = P(T = t) \text{ and } \phi_{2t} = P(D = 1 \mid T = t), \tag{10.2}$$

where $t = 0, 1$. Let $\phi_1 = \phi_{11}$ and $\phi_2 = (\phi_{20}, \phi_{21})'$. Under the MAR assumption, the log-likelihood can be written as

$$l(\phi_1, \phi_2) = \sum_{t=0}^{1} m_t \log(\phi_{1t}) + \sum_{t=0}^{1} (s_t \log(\phi_{2t}) + r_t \log(1 - \phi_{2t})), \tag{10.3}$$

where $\phi_{10} = 1 - \phi_1$. Maximizing the above log-likelihood yields the following ML estimators for ϕ_1 and ϕ_2:

$$\hat{\phi}_1 = \frac{m_1}{N}, \text{ and } \hat{\phi}_{2t} = \frac{s_t}{s_t + r_t}, \tag{10.4}$$

where $N = m_0 + m_1$, the total number of patients in the sample. The asymptotic covariance matrix of the ML estimators, $\hat{\phi}_1$, $\hat{\phi}_{21}$, and $\hat{\phi}_{20}$, follows from its observed Fisher information matrix and has the following form:

$$\Sigma = \text{diag}(\frac{\phi_1^2(1 - \phi_1)^2}{m_1(1 - \phi_1)^2 + m_0\phi_1^2}, \frac{\phi_{21}^2(1 - \phi_{21})^2}{s_1(1 - \phi_{21})^2 + r_1\phi_{21}^2}, \frac{\phi_{20}^2(1 - \phi_{20})^2}{s_0(1 - \phi_{20})^2 + r_0\phi_{20}^2}).$$
$$\tag{10.5}$$

Since both the sensitivity (Se) and specificity (Sp) of T are functions of ϕ_1, ϕ_{20}, and ϕ_{21}, using the delta method we can derive the ML estimators of Se and Sp and their associated variances. Begg and Greenes (1983) derived the following ML estimators for the sensitivity and specificity:

$$\widehat{Se} = \frac{m_1 s_1/(N(s_1 + r_1))}{m_0 s_0/(N(s_0 + r_0)) + m_1 s_1/(N(s_1 + r_1))},$$

and

$$\widehat{Sp} = \frac{m_0 r_0/(N(s_0 + r_0))}{m_0 r_0/N(s_0 + r_0)) + m_1 r_1/(N(s_1 + r_1))},$$

and their respective consistent variance estimators are

$$\widehat{Var}(\widehat{Se}) = (\widehat{Se}(1 - \widehat{Se}))^2(\frac{N}{m_0 m_1} + \frac{r_1}{s_1(s_1 + r_1)} + \frac{r_0}{s_0(s_0 + r_0)}),$$

$$\widehat{Var}(\widehat{Sp}) = (\widehat{Sp}(1 - \widehat{Sp}))^2(\frac{N}{m_0 m_1} + \frac{s_1}{r_1(s_1 + r_1)} + \frac{s_0}{r_0(s_0 + r_0)}).$$

For a proof, see Zhou (1993).

Based on the asymptotic normality of

$$\frac{\widehat{Se} - Se}{\sqrt{\widehat{Var}(\widehat{Se})}} \text{ and } \frac{\widehat{Sp} - Sp}{\sqrt{\widehat{Var}(\widehat{Sp})}},$$

we construct $100(1 - \delta)\%$ confidence intervals for Se and Sp to be

$$\widehat{Se} \pm z_{1-\delta/2}\sqrt{\widehat{Var}(\widehat{Se})}$$

and

$$\widehat{Sp} \pm z_{1-\delta/2}\sqrt{\widehat{Var}(\widehat{Sp})},$$

respectively, where z_δ is the $100(1 - \delta)$th percentile of the standard normal distribution.

Instead of assuming normality of $\widehat{Se}$, we may believe a logit transformation of $\widehat{Se}$, $\log\left[\widehat{Se}/(1 - \widehat{Se})\right]$, is closer to a normal distribution with mean $\log\left[Se/(1 - Se)\right]$. Using the same method as the one for Se, we obtain a $100(1 - \delta)\%$ confidence interval for $\log\left[Se/(1 - Se)\right]$ as

$$\widehat{Se}/(1 - \widehat{Se}) \pm z_{1-\delta/2}\sqrt{\widehat{Var}(\log(\widehat{Se}/(1 - \widehat{Se})))},$$

where

$$\widehat{Var}(\log(\widehat{Se}/(1 - \widehat{Se}))) = \frac{N}{m_0 m_1} + \frac{r_1}{s_1(s_1 + r_1)} + \frac{r_0}{s_0(s_0 + r_0)}.$$

The resulting confidence interval for Se is

$$\left(\frac{\exp(\frac{\widehat{Se}}{1-\widehat{Se}} - z_{1-\delta/2}\sqrt{\widehat{Var}(\log\frac{\widehat{Se}}{1-\widehat{Se}})})}{1 + \exp(\frac{\widehat{Se}}{1-\widehat{Se}} - z_{1-\delta/2}\sqrt{\widehat{Var}(\log\frac{\widehat{Se}}{1-\widehat{Se}})})}\right.,$$

$$\left.\frac{\exp(\frac{\widehat{Se}}{1-\widehat{Se}} + z_{1-\delta/2}\sqrt{\widehat{Var}(\log\frac{\widehat{Se}}{1-\widehat{Se}})})}{1 + \exp(\frac{\widehat{Se}}{1-\widehat{Se}} + z_{1-\delta/2}\sqrt{\widehat{Var}(\log\frac{\widehat{Se}}{1-\widehat{Se}})})}\right). \tag{10.6}$$

The CI for Sp has the same expression as above for Se.

So far we have assumed the diagnostic test result is the only observed factor affecting the verification mechanism. If the verification mechanism depends not only on the test results but also on other observed covariates, the method described above can be easily extended. See Zhou (1998a) for more details.

10.3.1.1 Analysis of Hepatic Scintigraph Example In this section we apply
the verification bias correction method, described in Section 10.3.1 above, to
the hepatic scintigraph example, described in Section 10.1.1. Let T, D, and
V denote the test result, the true disease status, and the disease verification
status of a subject, respectively. We can then summarize the observed data
in Table 10.2.

Table 10.2 Hepatic Scintigraph Data

		Diagnostic results	
		T=1	T=0
V=1	D=1	231	27
	D=0	32	54
V=0		166	140
Total		429	221

If only the patients with verified condition status are used in the calculation, the biased estimate of sensitivity is 0.90 with a 95% confidence interval
of (0.86,0.93); and the biased estimate of specificity is 0.63 with the 95%
confidence interval of (0.53,0.73).

If the probability of verifying a patient depends only on the test results
of the hepatic imaging scan, the verification process is MAR. Using the correction method described above, the estimated sensitivity is reduced to 0.84
with a 95% confidence interval of (0.79,0.88), and the estimated specificity is
increased to 0.74 with a 95% confidence interval of (0.66,0.81).

10.3.2 Correction Methods Without the MAR Assumption

The validity of the above methods depends on the MAR assumption for the
verification mechanism. If the verification process depends on unobserved
variables that are related to the condition status, the verification process is not
MAR. This is most likely to occur when there is a long time lag between the
initial test and verification, when there are multiple investigators at various
institutions, when the patient population is very heterogeneous, or when the
disease process is not well understood (Baker, 1995; Begg and Greenes, 1983).
In this section, we discuss a general ML method for estimating sensitivity and
specificity without assuming that the verification mechanism is MAR (Zhou,
1993).

Without the MAR assumption, we need to model the verification process
to make inferences about the test's sensitivity and specificity. Let λ_{11} be the
conditional probability of selecting a patient for verification given that the
patient has a positive test result and has the condition, λ_{01} be the conditional
probability of selecting a patient for verification given a positive test result and
the absence of the condition, λ_{10} be the conditional probability of selecting

a patient for verification given a negative test result and the presence of the condition, and λ_{00} be the conditional probability of selection for verification a patient given a negative test result and the absence of the condition. Let ϕ_{1t} and ϕ_{2t} be defined by (10.2).

Based on the observed data given in Table 10.1, we may write the log-likelihood function as

$$
\begin{aligned}
l &= \sum_{t=0}^{1} m_t \log \phi_{1t} + s_t \log(\lambda_{1t}\phi_{2t}) + r_t \log(\lambda_{0t}(1 - \phi_{2t})) \\
&+ \sum_{t=0}^{1} u_t \log((1 - \lambda_{1t})\phi_{2t} + (1 - \lambda_{0t})(1 - \phi_{2t})).
\end{aligned}
$$

Set $e_t = \lambda_{1t}/\lambda_{0t}$. Then, the log-likelihood becomes

$$
\begin{aligned}
l &= \sum_{t=0}^{1} m_t \log \phi_{1t} + s_t \log(e_t\lambda_{0t}\phi_{2t}) + r_t \log(\lambda_{0t}(1 - \phi_{2t})) \\
&+ \sum_{t=0}^{1} u_t \log((1 - e_t\lambda_{0t})\phi_{2t} + (1 - \lambda_{0t})(1 - \phi_{2t})).
\end{aligned}
$$

Since there are only five degrees of freedom in the data, not all seven parameters $\phi_{11}, \phi_{20}, \phi_{21}, \lambda_{00}, \lambda_{01}, e_0$, and e_1 are estimable. If we can assume that two of them are known, the remaining five parameters may be estimable. Since parameters ϕ_{1t} and ϕ_{2t} determine the sensitivity and specificity and parameters e_k and λ_{0t} govern the verification process, a natural choice is to assume e_0 and e_1 are known. Here e_0 is the ratio of the probability of selecting a diseased subject with a negative test result to that of selecting a non-diseased subject with a negative test result; and e_1 is the ratio of the probability of selecting a diseased subject with a positive test result to that of selecting a non-diseased subject with a positive test result.

Under the assumption that e_0 and e_1 were known, Zhou (1993) showed that the resulting ML estimators for sensitivity and specificity are

$$
\widehat{Se}(e_0, e_1) = \frac{(s_1 m_1)/(s_1 + e_1 r_1)}{(s_1 m_1)/(s_1 + e_1 r_1) + (s_0 m_0)/(s_0 + e_0 r_0)} \tag{10.7}
$$

and

$$
\widehat{Sp}(e_0, e_1) = \frac{(e_0 r_0 m_0)/(s_0 + e_0 r_0)}{(e_1 r_1 m_1)/(s_1 + e_1 r_1) + (e_0 r_0 m_0)/(s_0 + e_0 r_0)}, \tag{10.8}
$$

respectively.

If $e_0 = e_1 = 1$, the verification process is MAR, and the ML estimators given above become the ones given in Section 2.3.1. In general, we cannot estimate e_0 and e_1 from the observed data. However, based on the observed data, we may find lower and upper bounds for e_0 and e_1. Recall that e_0 and

e_1 are ratios of two conditional probabilities: $e_1 = P(V = 1 \mid T = 1, D = 1)/P(V = 1 \mid T = 1, D = 0)$ and $e_0 = P(V = 1 \mid T = 0, D = 1)/P(V = 1 \mid T = 0, D = 0)$. Using the observed data, Zhou (1993) showed the ranges of possible values of e_0 and e_1 are as follows.

$$\frac{s_1}{s_1 + u_1} \le e_1 \le \frac{r_1 + u_1}{r_1}, \quad \frac{s_0}{s_0 + u_0} \le e_0 \le \frac{r_0 + u_0}{r_0}. \tag{10.9}$$

Using these bounds, we can study how sensitive the ML estimators of sensitivity and specificity derived under the MAR assumption are to the departure from the MAR assumption.

10.3.3 Analysis of Hepatic Scintigraph Example, Continued

Without the MAR assumption, we need to assume that the two ratios e_1 and e_0 are known in order to derive the ML estimators for sensitivity and specificity. Here, e_1 is the ratio of the probability of verifying a patient who has a positive hepatic scintigraph result and liver disease to that of verifying a patient who has a positive hepatic scintigraph result but does not have liver disease, and e_0 is the ratio of the probability of verifying a patient who has a negative hepatic scintigraph result and liver disease to that of verifying a patient who has a negative hepatic scintigraph result and does not have liver disease. For given values of e_1 and e_0, ML estimators for sensitivity and specificity are

$$\widehat{Se}(e_0, e_1) = \frac{1}{1 + 0.06(32e_1 + 231)/(54e_0 + 27)}$$

and

$$\widehat{Sp}(e_0, e_1) = \frac{1}{1 + 1.15(e_1(54e_0 + 27))/(e_0(32e_1 + 231))},$$

respectively. If $e_0 = e_1 = 1$, the verification process is MAR, and the resulting ML estimates are 84% and 74%, respectively. To study how sensitive the estimated sensitivity and specificity derived under the MAR assumption are to the departure from the MAR assumption, using formula (10.9), we obtain lower and upper bounds for e_1 and e_0,

$$0.58 \le e_1 \le 6.19, \quad 0.16 \le e_0 \le 3.59.$$

From these bounds, we can derive lower and upper bounds for the estimated sensitivity and specificity. Note that for a given e_0 both $\widehat{Se}(e_1, e_0)$ and $\widehat{Sp}(e_1, e_0)$ are decreasing functions of e_1, and for a given e_1 both $\widehat{Se}(e_1, e_0)$ and $\widehat{Sp}(e_1, e_0)$ are increasing functions of e_0. Thus,

$$0.68 \le \frac{1}{1 + 17.16/(54e_0 + 27)} \le \widehat{Se}(e_1, e_0) \le \frac{1}{1 + 14.95/(54e_0 + 27)} \le 0.95$$

and

$$0.37 \leq \frac{1}{1 + (54e_0 + 27)/216.73} \leq \widehat{Sp}(e_1, e_0) \leq \frac{1}{1 + (54e_0 + 27)/248.73} \leq 0.86.$$

Therefore, the ML estimators for sensitivity and specificity could vary from 0.68 to 0.95 and 0.37 to 0.86 respectively, depending on the values of e_0 and e_1. Figures 10.1 to 10.3 are plots of ML estimators for sensitivity and specificity for reasonable values of e_0 when $e_1 = 0.57$, $e_1 = 1.0$, and $e_1 = 1.72$, respectively, along with the Begg and Greenes (BG) estimators (Begg and Greenes, 1983).

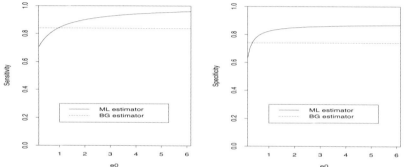

Figure 10.1   Estimates for Sensitivity and Specificity in the Hepatic Scintigraph Example When $e_1 = 0.57$

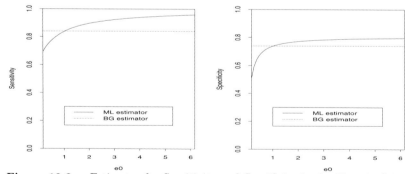

Figure 10.2   Estimates for Sensitivity and Specificity in the Hepatic Scintigraph Example When $e_1 = 1.0$

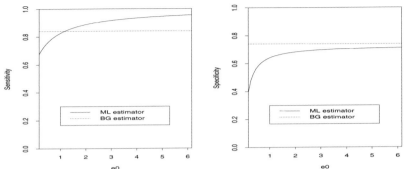

Figure 10.3 Estimates for Sensitivity and Specificity in the Hepatic Scintigraph Example When $e_1=1.72$

From Figure 10.1 to Figure 10.3 we conclude empirically that corrected estimators of the sensitivity and specificity derived under the MAR assumption are sensitive to the MAR assumption, and the ML estimator for sensitivity is less sensitive to the assumed value of e_1 than that for specificity.

10.4 CORRELATED BINARY-SCALE TESTS

If we are interested in assessing the relative accuracy of two binary diagnostic tests applied to the same set of subjects, we would compare the sensitivities and specificities of the two tests, respectively. In this section, like in Section 10.3, we also use the framework of missing data to correct for verification bias, and we assume the verification process is MAR. We first discuss bias correction methods when the probability of verification depends only on the results of two diagnostic tests. Then we extend the correction methods to the situation where the probability of verification depends not only on the results of the two diagnostic tests but also on other observed covariates.

Let T_1 and T_2 be binary results of two diagnostic tests from the same patient. We also let (Se_1, Sp_1) and (Se_2, Sp_2) denote the sensitivity and specificity pair for the first and second test, respectively.

10.4.1 ML Approach Without Any Covariates

We first assume that the probability of selecting a patient for condition status verification depends only on the diagnostic test results of the patient; that is,

$$P(V = 1 \mid T_1, T_2, D) = P(V = 1 \mid T_1, T_2). \tag{10.10}$$

This assumption implies the MAR assumption for the verification mechanism. Let

$$\varphi_{t\tilde{t}} = P(D = 1 \mid T_1 = t, T_2 = \tilde{t}), \quad \eta_{t\tilde{t}} = P(T_1 = t, T_2 = \tilde{t}), t, \tilde{t} = 0, 1,$$

where $\eta_{11} = 1 - \eta_{00} - \eta_{10} - \eta_{01}$. Let $\boldsymbol{\varphi} = (\varphi_{00}, \varphi_{01}, \varphi_{10}, \varphi_{11})$ and $\boldsymbol{\eta} = (\eta_{00}, \eta_{01}, \eta_{10})$. The respective sensitivities of the two diagnostic tests can be expressed as

$$Se_1 = (\sum_{\tilde{t}=0}^{1} \varphi_{1\tilde{t}}\eta_{1\tilde{t}})/p \text{ and } Se_2 = (\sum_{t=0}^{1} \varphi_{t1}\eta_{t1})/p, \tag{10.11}$$

and their specificities as

$$Sp_1 = (\sum_{\tilde{t}=0}^{1}(1-\varphi_{0\tilde{t}})\eta_{0\tilde{t}})/(1-p) \text{ and } Sp_2 = (\sum_{t=0}^{1}(1-\varphi_{t0})\eta_{t0})/(1-p), \tag{10.12}$$

where $p = \sum_{t=0}^{1}\sum_{\tilde{t}=0}^{1}\varphi_{t\tilde{t}}\eta_{t\tilde{t}}$. To find ML estimators for Se_i and Sp_i, where $i = 1, 2$, we need ML estimators for $\boldsymbol{\varphi}$ and $\boldsymbol{\eta}$.

Under the MAR assumption, valid likelihood-based inference can be made from the observed data without specifying a distribution for the verification mechanism (Little and Rubin, 1987). The observed data consist of the diagnostic test results and the true condition status for verified patients, and the diagnostic test results alone for unverified patients.

Table 10.3 summarizes the observed data with a total number of N $(=m_{11} + m_{10} + m_{01} + m_{00})$ patients in the study. For the observed data given in

Table 10.3   Observed Data for Two Paired Binary Scale Tests

		$T_1 = 1$		$T_1 = 0$	
		$T_2 = 1$	$T_2 = 0$	$T_2 = 1$	$T_2 = 0$
V=1	D=1	s_{11}	s_{10}	s_{01}	s_{00}
	D=0	r_{11}	r_{10}	r_{01}	r_{00}
V=0		u_{11}	u_{10}	u_{01}	u_{00}
Total		m_{11}	m_{10}	m_{01}	m_{00}

Table 10.3, the log-likelihood function is

$$l(\boldsymbol{\varphi}, \boldsymbol{\eta}) = \sum_{t,\tilde{t}=0}^{1} (s_{t\tilde{t}} \log \varphi_{t\tilde{t}} + r_{t\tilde{t}} \log(1 - \varphi_{t\tilde{t}})) + \sum_{t,\tilde{t}=0}^{1} m_{t\tilde{t}} \log \eta_{t\tilde{t}}. \tag{10.13}$$

Maximizing $l(\boldsymbol{\varphi}, \boldsymbol{\eta})$ with respect to $\boldsymbol{\varphi}$ and $\boldsymbol{\eta}$, we obtain the ML estimators of $\boldsymbol{\varphi}$ and $\boldsymbol{\eta}$. By substituting these ML estimators into (10.11), we obtain ML estimators for the sensitivities, $\widehat{Se}_1$ and $\widehat{Se}_2$. Using the delta method (Agresti, 1990), we derive their corresponding asymptotic covariance matrix. If the verification process is MAR, as defined by (10.10), the ML estimators for sensitivities and specificities of two diagnostic tests have the following forms:

$$\widehat{Se}_1 = \frac{\sum_{\tilde{t}=0}^{1} \frac{s_{1\tilde{t}}}{s_{1\tilde{t}}+r_{1\tilde{t}}} m_{1\tilde{t}}}{\sum_{t=0}^{1}\sum_{\tilde{t}=0}^{1} \frac{s_{t\tilde{t}}}{s_{t\tilde{t}}+r_{t\tilde{t}}} m_{t\tilde{t}}}, \quad \widehat{Se}_2 = \frac{\sum_{t=0}^{1} \frac{s_{t1}}{s_{t1}+r_{t1}} m_{t1}}{\sum_{t=0}^{1}\sum_{\tilde{t}=0}^{1} \frac{s_{t\tilde{t}}}{s_{t\tilde{t}}+r_{t\tilde{t}}} m_{t\tilde{t}}}; \tag{10.14}$$

and

$$\widehat{Sp}_1 = \frac{\sum_{\tilde{t}=0}^1 \frac{r_{0\tilde{t}}}{s_{0\tilde{t}}+r_{0\tilde{t}}} m_{0\tilde{t}}}{\sum_{t=0}^1 \sum_{\tilde{t}=0}^1 \frac{r_{t\tilde{t}}}{s_{t\tilde{t}}+r_{t\tilde{t}}} m_{t\tilde{t}}}, \quad \widehat{Sp}_2 = \frac{\sum_{t=0}^1 \frac{r_{t0}}{s_{i0}+r_{t0}} m_{t0}}{\sum_{t=0}^1 \sum_{\tilde{t}=0}^1 \frac{r_{t\tilde{t}}}{s_{t\tilde{t}}+r_{t\tilde{t}}} m_{t\tilde{t}}}. \tag{10.15}$$

For the ith and $\tilde{i}$th tests, the asymptotic covariance between $\widehat{Se}_i$ and $\widehat{Se}_{\tilde{i}}$ has the following explicit expression:

$$cov(\widehat{Se}_i, \widehat{Se}_{\tilde{i}}) = \sum_{t,\tilde{t}=0}^1 \frac{\varphi_{t\tilde{t}}^2(1-\varphi_{t\tilde{t}})^2}{s_{t\tilde{t}}(1-\varphi_{t\tilde{t}})^2 + r_{t\tilde{t}}\varphi_{t\tilde{t}}^2} \frac{\partial Se_i}{\partial \varphi_{t\tilde{t}}} \frac{\partial Se_{\tilde{i}}}{\partial \varphi_{t\tilde{t}}} + \sum_{(t,\tilde{t})\neq(1,1)} \frac{\eta_{t\tilde{t}}^2}{m_{t\tilde{t}}} \frac{\partial Se_i}{\partial \eta_{t\tilde{t}}} \frac{\partial Se_{\tilde{i}}}{\partial \eta_{t\tilde{t}}}$$

$$- \frac{1}{\sum_{t,\tilde{t}=0}^1 \frac{\eta_{t\tilde{t}}^2}{m_{t\tilde{t}}}} \left(\sum_{(t,\tilde{t})\neq(1,1)} \frac{\eta_{t\tilde{t}}^2}{m_{t\tilde{t}}} \frac{\partial Se_i}{\partial \eta_{t\tilde{t}}} \right) \left(\sum_{(t,\tilde{t})\neq(1,1)} \frac{\eta_{t\tilde{t}}^2}{m_{t\tilde{t}}} \frac{\partial Se_{\tilde{i}}}{\partial \eta_{t\tilde{t}}} \right), \tag{10.16}$$

and the asymptotic covariance between $\widehat{Sp}_i$ and $\widehat{Sp}_{\tilde{i}}$ has the following explicit expression:

$$cov(\widehat{Sp}_i, \widehat{Sp}_{\tilde{i}}) = \sum_{t,\tilde{t}=0}^1 \frac{\varphi_{t\tilde{t}}^2(1-\varphi_{t\tilde{t}})^2}{s_{t\tilde{t}}(1-\varphi_{t\tilde{t}})^2 + r_{t\tilde{t}}\varphi_{t\tilde{t}}^2} \frac{\partial Sp_i}{\partial \varphi_{t\tilde{t}}} \frac{\partial Sp_{\tilde{i}}}{\partial \varphi_{t\tilde{t}}} + \sum_{(t,\tilde{t})\neq(1,1)} \frac{\eta_{t\tilde{t}}^2}{m_{t\tilde{t}}} \frac{\partial Sp_i}{\partial \eta_{t\tilde{t}}} \frac{\partial Sp_{\tilde{i}}}{\partial \eta_{t\tilde{t}}}$$

$$- \frac{1}{\sum_{t,\tilde{t}=0}^1 \frac{\eta_{t\tilde{t}}^2}{m_{t\tilde{t}}}} \left(\sum_{(t,\tilde{t})\neq(1,1)} \frac{\eta_{t\tilde{t}}^2}{m_{t\tilde{t}}} \frac{\partial Sp_i}{\partial \eta_{t\tilde{t}}} \right) \left(\sum_{(t,\tilde{t})\neq(1,1)} \frac{\eta_{t\tilde{t}}^2}{m_{t\tilde{t}}} \frac{\partial Sp_{\tilde{i}}}{\partial \eta_{t\tilde{t}}} \right), \tag{10.17}$$

where $i, \tilde{i} = 1, 2$, and the partial derivatives of Se_i and Sp_i with respect to φ and η are given in Zhou (1998a).

Substituting unknown parameters in the variance-covariance matrix of Se_1 and Se_2 by their ML estimators, we derive the statistic,

$$\frac{\widehat{Se}_1 - \widehat{Se}_2 - (Se_1 - Se_2)}{\sqrt{\widehat{var}(\widehat{Se}_1) + \widehat{var}(\widehat{Se}_2) - 2\widehat{cov}(\widehat{Se}_1, \widehat{Se}_2)}},$$

which is approximately normally distributed when the total sample size N is large. Using this statistic, we may construct a confidence interval for the difference in sensitivities, $Se_1 - Se_2$, and perform a hypothesis test that H_0: $Se_1 = Se_2$. Similarly, we have the statistic,

$$\frac{\widehat{Sp}_1 - \widehat{Sp}_2 - (Sp_1 - Sp_2)}{\sqrt{\widehat{var}(\widehat{Sp}_1) + \widehat{var}(\widehat{Sp}_2) - 2\widehat{cov}(\widehat{Sp}_1, \widehat{Sp}_2)}},$$

for constructing a confidence interval and performing a hypothesis test about the difference in specificities of two diagnostic tests.

10.4.2   Analysis of Two Screening Tests for Dementia Disorder Example

To illustrate the method, we focus on the relative performance of the two tests for subjects 75 years or older in Indianapolis. Table 10.4 displays the resulting classification data for this group. Applying the bias correction method described above, we obtain the estimated sensitivities of the standard and new test as 0.725 and 0.795, respectively. Their corresponding standard error estimates are 0.105 and 0.089 with the estimated correlation of 0.492. The estimated difference in the sensitivities of the two tests is -0.070 with 95% confidence interval of $(-0.184, 0.043)$.

Table 10.4   Paired Screening Tests for Dementia Among 75 or Older Subjects in Indianapolis

		Test 1 negative		*Test 1 positive*	
		Test 2 negative	Test 2 positive	Test 2 negative	Test 2 positive
Verified	dementia	1	3	5	31
	non-dementia	55	19	10	25
Not verified		346	65	6	22
Total		402	87	21	78

Similarly, we obtain corrected estimates for the specificities of the two tests as 0.906 and 0.788, respectively. The corresponding variance estimates are 0.0003 and 0.0006 with the estimated correlation of 0.574. The estimated difference in the specificities of the two tests is 0.118 with 95% confidence interval, $(0.078, 0.157)$.

10.4.3   ML Approach With Covariates

If the probability of verification depends not only on the test results but also on other observed covariates X, we need to modify the above correction method. Let us assume that the vector of covariates X has G different covariate patterns and that its gth covariate pattern is denoted by the vector x_g, where $g = 1, \ldots, G$. If

$$P(V = 1 \mid T_1, T_2, X, D) = P(V = 1 \mid T_1, T_2, X), \qquad (10.18)$$

the MAR assumption on the verification process holds. We further assume that X is a random sample from a discrete space $(x_1, \ldots, x_G)$ with probabilities $\xi = (\xi_1, \ldots, \xi_G)$. Then we can summarize the observed data in Table 10.5.

Define

$$\varphi_{gt\tilde{t}} = P(D = 1 \mid T_1 = t, T_2 = \tilde{t}, X = x_g)$$

and

$$\eta_{gt\tilde{t}} = P(T_1 = t, T_2 = \tilde{t} \mid X = x_g).$$

Table 10.5   Observed Data for Two Paired Binary Scale Tests at the gth Covariate Pattern $(\mathbf{X} = \mathbf{x}_g)$

		$T_1 = 1$		$T_1 = 0$	
		$T_2 = 1$	$T_2 = 0$	$T_2 = 1$	$T_2 = 0$
$V=1$	D=1	s_{g11}	s_{g10}	s_{g01}	s_{g00}
	D=0	r_{g11}	r_{g10}	r_{g01}	r_{g00}
$V=0$		u_{g11}	u_{g10}	u_{g01}	u_{g00}
Total		m_{g11}	m_{g10}	m_{g01}	m_{g00}

Let N_g be the total number of patients with $X = x_g$. The contribution of a verified patient to the likelihood is

$$P(T_1, T_2, D, X) = P(D \mid T_1, T_2, X)P(T_1, T_2 \mid X)P(X),$$

and the likelihood contribution of an unverified case is $P(T_1, T_2, X) = P(T_1, T_2 \mid X)P(X)$. Thus, the likelihood of the observed data is the product of $P(D \mid T_1, T_2, X)$, $P(T_1, T_2 \mid X)$ and $P(X)$. The number of free parameters could grow uncontrollably as the number of covariates grows if we use unrestricted multinomial distributions. Thus we need to model the covariate effects. We model $P(D \mid T_1, T_2, X)$ by a logistic regression model and $P(T_1, T_2 \mid X)$ by a multinomial logit model (Agresti, 1990). For example, we can specify these models by the following forms:

$$\varphi_{gt\tilde{t}} = P(D = 1 \mid T_1 = t, T_2 = \tilde{t}, X = x_g)$$

$$= \frac{\exp(\beta_0 + \beta_1 t + \beta_2 \tilde{t} + \beta_3' x_g)}{1 + \exp(\beta_0 + \beta_1 t + \beta_2 \tilde{t} + \beta_3' x_g)}, \tag{10.19}$$

and

$$\eta_{gt\tilde{t}} = P(T_1 = t, T_2 = \tilde{t} \mid X = x_g)$$

$$= \frac{\exp(\alpha_{0t\tilde{t}} + \alpha_{1t\tilde{t}}' x_g)}{\sum_{h_1,h_2=0}^{1} \exp(\alpha_{0h_1h_2} + \alpha_{1h_1h_2}' x_g)}, \tag{10.20}$$

for $t, \tilde{t} = 0, 1$, where $\alpha_{011} = 0$ and $\alpha_{111} = 0$. Let $\beta = (\beta_0, \beta_1, \beta_2, \beta_3')'$, $\alpha = (\alpha_{000}, \alpha_{001}, \alpha_{010}, \alpha_{100}', \alpha_{101}', \alpha_{110}')'$, $\xi_g = P(\mathbf{X} = x_g)$, $\boldsymbol{\xi} = (\xi_1, \dots, \xi_{G-1})$, and $N = \sum_{g=1}^{G} N_g$. Then, the log-likelihood function is

$$l(\alpha, \beta, \xi) = \sum_{g=1}^{G} \sum_{t,\tilde{t}=0}^{1} m_{gt\tilde{t}} \log \eta_{gt\tilde{t}} + \sum_{g=1}^{G} \sum_{t,\tilde{t}=0}^{1} s_{gt\tilde{t}} \log \varphi_{gt\tilde{t}}$$

$$+ \sum_{g=1}^{G} \sum_{t,\tilde{t}=0}^{1} r_{gt\tilde{t}} \log(1 - \varphi_{gt\tilde{t}}) + \sum_{g=1}^{G} N_g \log \xi_g, \tag{10.21}$$

where $\xi_G = 1 - \xi_1 - \ldots - \xi_{G-1}$. We denote

$$l_1(\boldsymbol{\alpha}) = \sum_{g=1}^{G} \sum_{t,\tilde{t}=0}^{1} m_{gt\tilde{t}} \log \eta_{gt\tilde{t}},$$

$$l_2(\boldsymbol{\beta}) = \sum_{g=1}^{G} \sum_{t,\tilde{t}=0}^{1} \left\{ s_{gt\tilde{t}} \log \varphi_{gt\tilde{t}} + r_{gt\tilde{t}} \log(1 - \varphi_{gt\tilde{t}}) \right\},$$

and

$$l_3(\boldsymbol{\xi}) = \sum_{g=1}^{G} N_g \log \xi_g.$$

We can write $l(\boldsymbol{\alpha}, \boldsymbol{\beta}, \boldsymbol{\xi})$ as the sum of $l_1(\boldsymbol{\alpha})$, $l_2(\boldsymbol{\beta})$, and $l_3(\boldsymbol{\xi})$. Furthermore, we can consider $l_1(\boldsymbol{\alpha})$ as the log-likelihood function of all observations modeled by a multinomial logit model (the equation (10.20)), $l_2(\boldsymbol{\beta})$ as the log-likelihood function of verified cases modeled by a logistic regression model (the equation (10.19)), and $l_3(\boldsymbol{\xi})$ as the log-likelihood function for a multinomial distribution based on all observations. As the parameters $\boldsymbol{\alpha}$, $\boldsymbol{\beta}$, and $\boldsymbol{\xi}$ are distinct, their ML estimators $\hat{\boldsymbol{\alpha}}$, $\hat{\boldsymbol{\beta}}$, and $\hat{\boldsymbol{\xi}}$ can be obtained by maximizing l_1, l_2, and l_3 with respect to $\boldsymbol{\alpha}$, $\boldsymbol{\beta}$, and $\boldsymbol{\xi}$, respectively. The ML estimators $\hat{\boldsymbol{\alpha}}$ and $\hat{\boldsymbol{\beta}}$ and their corresponding observed Fisher information matrices I_1 and I_2 can be computed using any statistical software that can fit a logistic regression model and a multinomial logit model, such as SAS. The ML estimators for ξ_g are

$$\hat{\xi}_g = \frac{N_g}{N},$$

where $g = 1, \ldots, I$, and their corresponding observed Fisher information matrix is

$$I_3 = Diag(\frac{m_1}{\xi_1^2}, \ldots, \frac{m_{G-1}}{\xi_{G-1}^2}) + \frac{N_G}{\xi_G^2}(1, \ldots, 1)'(1, \ldots, 1).$$

Next we give the ML estimators $\widehat{Se}_i$ and $\widehat{Sp}_i$ for the sensitivity and specificity of the ith test and the asymptotic covariance matrix of the ML estimators of two sensitivities, as well as two specificities (Zhou, 1998a).

If the verification process is MAR, as defined by (10.18), the ML estimators for the sensitivities of the two diagnostic tests are

$$\widehat{Se}_1 = (\sum_{g=1}^{G} \sum_{\tilde{t}=0}^{1} \hat{\varphi}_{g1\tilde{t}} \hat{\eta}_{g1\tilde{t}} \hat{\xi}_g)/\hat{p} \text{ and } \widehat{Se}_2 = (\sum_{g=1}^{G} \sum_{t=0}^{1} \hat{\varphi}_{gt1} \hat{\eta}_{gt1} \hat{\xi}_g)/\hat{p}, \qquad (10.22)$$

respectively, and the ML estimators for their specificities are

$$\widehat{Sp}_1 = (\sum_{g=1}^{G} \sum_{\tilde{t}=0}^{1} (1 - \hat{\varphi}_{g0\tilde{t}}) \hat{\eta}_{g0\tilde{t}} \hat{\xi}_g)/(1 - \hat{p}),$$

$$\widehat{Sp}_2 = (\sum_{g=1}^{G}\sum_{t=0}^{1}(1 - \hat{\varphi}_{gt0})\hat{\eta}_{gt0}\hat{\xi}_g)/(1 - \hat{p}), \qquad (10.23)$$

respectively. The asymptotic variance-covariance matrix of $\widehat{Se}_1$ and $\widehat{Se}_2$ has the following form:

$$[\frac{\partial(Se_1, Se_2)}{\partial\alpha}]'I_1^{-1}(\alpha)[\frac{\partial(Se_1, Se_2)}{\partial\alpha}] + [\frac{\partial(Se_1, Se_2)}{\partial\beta}]'I_2^{-1}(\beta)[\frac{\partial(Se_1, Se_2)}{\partial\beta}]$$

$$+[\frac{\partial(Se_1, Se_2)}{\partial\boldsymbol{\xi}}]'I_3^{-1}(\boldsymbol{\xi})[\frac{\partial(Se_1, Se_2)}{\partial\boldsymbol{\xi}}], \qquad (10.24)$$

where the partial derivatives of Se_1, Se_2, Sp_1, and Sp_2 with respect to α, β, and $\boldsymbol{\xi}$ are given in Zhou (1998a).

10.4.4 Analysis of Two Screening Tests for Dementia Disorder Example, Continued

To illustrate the bias correction methods, we use the data from the Indianapolis site and define a positive result of a screening test as "poor performer" on the test. Table 10.6 displays the resulting classification data in Indianapolis.

Table 10.6 Data from the Alzheimer study: Entries are Numbers of Subjects

		Age $\geq$ 75			
		Test 1 negative		Test 1 positive	
		Test 2 negative	Test 2 positive	Test 2 negative	Test 2 positive
Verified	nondisease	55	19	10	25
	disease	1	3	5	31
Not verified		346	65	6	22
Total		402	87	21	78

		Age < 75			
		Test 1 negative		Test 1 positive	
		Test 2 negative	Test 2 positive	Test 2 negative	Test 2 positive
Verified	nondisease	34	6	19	10
	disease	0	0	0	7
Not verified		759	52	11	9
Total		793	58	30	26

In this data set, we have one covariate, x, that affects the probability of selecting a subject for disease verification; this covariate $x=1$ for a subject with 75 years or older, and $x=0$ otherwise. Using the SAS Proc Logistic procedure, we fitted the logistic regression model (10.19) to the verified cases, and using the SAS Proc Catmod procedure, we fitted the multinomial logit model (10.20) to all observations.

Let Se_1 and Se_2 be the sensitivities of the new screening test and the standard screening test. Using the methods discussed in Section 10.4.3, we calculate the ML estimates for the sensitivities of the new and standard screening tests as 0.59 and 0.58, respectively, and their corresponding variances are 0.0182 and 0.0148. The two-sided p-value for the test of the equality of the two sensitivities is 0.91, and the 95% confidence interval for $Se_1 - Se_2$ is $(-0.18, 0.20)$. Thus, we fail to reject the null hypothesis that the two sensitivities are equal.

Let Sp_1 and Sp_2 be the specificities of the new screening test and the standard screening test. We obtain the ML estimates for the specificities of the new and standard screening tests to be 0.9346 and 0.8858, respectively, with the corresponding variances being 0.000142 and 0.00009. Hence, the two-sided p-value for the equality of the two specificities is less than 0.00001, and the 95% confidence interval for $Sp_1 - Sp_2$ is $(0.036, 0.062)$. Therefore, we conclude that the specificity of the new screening test is higher than that of the standard screening test.

10.5 A SINGLE ORDINAL-SCALE TEST

In this section, we present bias correction methods for estimating the ROC curve and the area under the ROC curve. We focus on the verification bias problem when the verification process is MAR. See Zhou and Rodenberg (1997) for a discussion on the non-MAR verification process.

10.5.1 ML Approach Without Covariates

Let T be the ordinal scale test result; the definitions of random variables D and V are the same as those in Section 10.3.1. We can summarize the observed data as in Table 10.7. In this section we assume that the probability of verifying a patient depends only on the test result T; that is,

$$P(V = 1 \mid T, D) = P(V = 1 \mid T). \tag{10.25}$$

10.5.1.1 Estimation of ROC Curves For an ordinal scale test, by varying the definition of a positive test, we can calculate $K + 1$ pairs of true positive rates (TPR) and false positive rates (FPR) of the test. Specifically, if we define a positive test as the one with $T \geq t$, a corresponding pair of TPR and FPR are

$$TPR(t) = P(T \geq t \mid D = 1), \ FPR(t) = P(T \geq t \mid D = 0),$$

Table 10.7   Observed Data for a Single Ordinal Scale Test

		Diagnostic test results		
		T=1	...	T=K
Verified	D=1	s_1	...	s_K
	D=0	r_1	...	r_K
Unverified		u_1	...	u_K
Total		m_1	...	m_K

respectively, for $t = 1, \ldots, K + 1$. Using the trapezoidal rule (Bamber, 1975), we produce an empirical ROC curve by connecting the coordinates, $(FPR(t), TPR(t))$ (see Chapter 4 for details). Since $TPR(1) = FPR(1) = 1$ and $TPR(K + 1) = FPR(K + 1) = 0$, to provide an unbiased estimator of an empirical ROC curve we need to find unbiased estimators for $(FPR(t), TPR(t))$, $t = 2, \ldots, K$. Define $\phi_{1t} = P(T = t)$ and $\phi_{2t} = P(D = 1 \mid T = t)$, where $t = 1, \ldots, K$. Then, $\phi_{1K} = 1 - \phi_{11} - \ldots - \phi_{1(K-1)}$. Denote $\boldsymbol{\phi}_1 = (\phi_{11}, \ldots, \phi_{1(K-1)})$ and $\boldsymbol{\phi}_2 = (\phi_{21}, \ldots, \phi_{2K})$. Under the assumption that the verification mechanism is MAR, valid likelihood-based inferences on ϕ_{1t} and ϕ_{2t} can be made based on observed data without specifying a distribution for the verification mechanism. The log-likelihood function based on the observed data is

$$l(\boldsymbol{\phi}_1, \boldsymbol{\phi}_2) = \sum_{t=1}^{K} m_t log(\phi_{1t}) + \sum_{t=1}^{K} (s_t log(\phi_{2t}) + r_t log(1 - \phi_{2t})). \quad (10.26)$$

Let $l_1(\boldsymbol{\phi}_1) = \sum_{t=1}^{K} m_t log(\phi_{1t})$ and $l_2(\boldsymbol{\phi}_2) = \sum_{t=1}^{K} (s_t log(\phi_{2t}) + r_t log(1 - \phi_{2t}))$. We can write $l(\boldsymbol{\phi}_1, \boldsymbol{\phi}_2)$ as the sum of $l_1(\boldsymbol{\phi}_1)$ and $l_2(\boldsymbol{\phi}_2)$. Since $\boldsymbol{\phi}_1$ and $\boldsymbol{\phi}_2$ are distinct parameters and both l_1 and l_2 are the log-likelihood functions for multinomial distributions, the ML estimators for $\boldsymbol{\phi}_1$ and $\boldsymbol{\phi}_2$ are

$$\hat{\phi}_{1t} = \frac{m_t}{N}, t = 1, \ldots, K - 1, \hat{\phi}_{2t} = \frac{s_t}{s_t + r_t}, t = 1, \ldots, K; \quad (10.27)$$

and the observed Fisher information matrix on $(\boldsymbol{\phi}_1, \boldsymbol{\phi}_2)$ is

$$\text{diag}(I_1(\boldsymbol{\phi}_1), I_2(\boldsymbol{\phi}_2)), \quad (10.28)$$

where $I_1(\boldsymbol{\phi}_1)$ and $I_2(\boldsymbol{\phi}_2)$ are the observed Fisher information matrices on the log-likelihood $l_1(\boldsymbol{\phi}_1)$ and $l_1(\boldsymbol{\phi}_2)$, respectively.

Next, we derive the ML estimators for the empirical ROC curve. Note that the coordinates of the empirical ROC curve can be written as functions of $\boldsymbol{\phi}_1$ and $\boldsymbol{\phi}_2$,

$$TPR(t) = \frac{\sum_{\tilde{t}=t}^{K} \phi_{1\tilde{t}} \phi_{2\tilde{t}}}{\sum_{\tilde{t}=1}^{K} \phi_{1\tilde{t}} \phi_{2\tilde{t}}} \text{ and } FPR(t) = \frac{\sum_{\tilde{t}=t}^{K} \phi_{1\tilde{t}}(1 - \phi_{2\tilde{t}})}{\sum_{\tilde{t}=1}^{K} \phi_{1\tilde{t}}(1 - \phi_{2\tilde{t}})}.$$

We summarize the ML estimators of $TPR(t)$ and $FPR(t)$ and the associated covariance matrix below. Under the MAR assumption, defined by (10.25), for $2 \leq t \leq K$ the ML estimators of $TPR(t)$ and $FPR(t)$ are defined as follows:

$$\widehat{TPR}(t) = \frac{\sum_{\tilde{t}=t}^{K} \frac{m_{\tilde{t}}}{N} \frac{s_{\tilde{t}}}{s_{\tilde{t}}+r_{\tilde{t}}}}{\sum_{\tilde{t}=1}^{K} \frac{m_{\tilde{t}}}{N} \frac{s_{\tilde{t}}}{s_{\tilde{t}}+r_{\tilde{t}}}} \text{ and } \widehat{FPR}(t) = \frac{\sum_{\tilde{t}=t}^{K} \frac{m_{\tilde{t}}}{N} \frac{r_{\tilde{t}}}{s_{\tilde{t}}+r_{\tilde{t}}}}{\sum_{\tilde{t}=1}^{K} \frac{m_{\tilde{t}}}{N} \frac{r_{\tilde{t}}}{s_{\tilde{t}}+r_{\tilde{t}}}}. \quad (10.29)$$

Their asymptotic variance-covariance matrix has the following form:

$$var(\widehat{TPR}(t)) = \sum_{\tilde{t}=1}^{K} \frac{\phi_{2\tilde{t}}^2(1-\phi_{2\tilde{t}})^2}{s_{\tilde{t}}(1-\phi_{2\tilde{t}})^2 + r_{\tilde{t}}\phi_{2\tilde{t}}^2} \left(\frac{\partial TPR(t)}{\partial \phi_{2\tilde{t}}}\right)^2 + \sum_{\tilde{t}=1}^{K-1} \frac{\phi_{1\tilde{t}}^2}{m_{\tilde{t}}} \left(\frac{\partial TPR(t)}{\partial \phi_{2\tilde{t}}}\right)^2$$

$$- \frac{1}{\sum_{\tilde{t}=1}^{K} \frac{\phi_{1\tilde{t}}^2}{m_{\tilde{t}}}} \left(\sum_{\tilde{t}=1}^{K-1} \frac{\phi_{1\tilde{t}}^2}{m_{\tilde{t}}} \frac{\partial TPR(t)}{\partial \phi_{2\tilde{t}}}\right)^2,$$

$$var(\widehat{FPR}(t)) = \sum_{\tilde{t}=1}^{K} \frac{\phi_{2\tilde{t}}^2(1-\phi_{2\tilde{t}})^2}{s_{\tilde{t}}(1-\phi_{2\tilde{t}})^2 + r_{\tilde{t}}\phi_{2\tilde{t}}^2} \left(\frac{\partial FPR(t)}{\partial \phi_{2\tilde{t}}}\right)^2 + \sum_{\tilde{t}=1}^{K-1} \frac{\phi_{1\tilde{t}}^2}{m_{\tilde{t}}} \left(\frac{\partial FPR(t)}{\partial \phi_{2\tilde{t}}}\right)^2$$

$$- \frac{1}{\sum_{\tilde{t}=1}^{K} \frac{\phi_{1\tilde{t}}^2}{m_{\tilde{t}}}} \left(\sum_{\tilde{t}=1}^{K-1} \frac{\phi_{1\tilde{t}}^2}{m_{\tilde{t}}} \frac{\partial FPR(t)}{\partial \phi_{2\tilde{t}}}\right)^2,$$

and

$$cov(\widehat{TPR}(t), \widehat{FPR}(t)) = \sum_{\tilde{t}=1}^{K} \frac{\phi_{2\tilde{t}}^2(1-\phi_{2\tilde{t}})^2}{s_{\tilde{t}}(1-\phi_{2\tilde{t}})^2 + r_{\tilde{t}}\phi_{2\tilde{t}}^2} \frac{\partial TPR(t)}{\partial \phi_{2\tilde{t}}} \frac{\partial FPR(t)}{\partial \phi_{2\tilde{t}}}$$

$$+ \sum_{\tilde{t}=1}^{K-1} \frac{\phi_{1\tilde{t}}^2}{m_{\tilde{t}}} \frac{\partial TPR(t)}{\partial \phi_{2\tilde{t}}} \frac{\partial FPR(t)}{\partial \phi_{2\tilde{t}}}$$

$$- \frac{1}{\sum_{\tilde{t}=1}^{K} \frac{\phi_{1\tilde{t}}^2}{m_{\tilde{t}}}} \left(\sum_{\tilde{t}=1}^{K-1} \frac{\phi_{1\tilde{t}}^2}{m_{\tilde{t}}} \frac{\partial TPR(t)}{\partial \phi_{2\tilde{t}}}\right) \left(\sum_{\tilde{t}=1}^{K-1} \frac{\phi_{1\tilde{t}}^2}{m_{\tilde{t}}} \frac{\partial FPR(t)}{\partial \phi_{2\tilde{t}}}\right),$$

where the partial derivatives of $TPR(t)$ and $FPR(t)$ with respect to $\phi_{1\tilde{t}}$ and $\phi_{2\tilde{t}}$ are given in Zhou (1998a).

In the preceding paragraph, we discussed the correction methods for estimating an empirical ROC curve. Next, we consider correction methods for estimating a smooth ROC curve. In Chapter 4, we discussed how to estimate a smooth ROC curve when all patients are verified. Under the most commonly used binormal model, in Chapter 4 we showed that the ROC curve of the test is a plot of $1 - \Phi(c)$ versus $1 - \Phi(bc - a)$, where $\Phi(\cdot)$ is the cumulative distribution function of the standard normal random variable, $a = (\mu_1 - \mu_0)/\sigma_1$, and $b = \sigma_0/\sigma_1$. Or, the ROC curve is defined by

$$ROC(\text{FPR}) = \Phi(b\Phi^{-1}(\text{FPR}) - a),$$

where FPR is the false positive rate ranging from 0 to 1 as the corresponding implicit cut-off point varies from $-\infty$ to $+\infty$. Hence, under the binormal model, an ROC curve is determined by two parameters, a and b, which may be estimated using the maximum likelihood method. In the absence of verification bias, Dorfman and Alf (1969) developed the method of scoring to compute the ML estimates of a and b, as discussed in Chapter 4. In the presence of verification bias, Gray et al. (1984) developed a modified scoring algorithm to compute the ML estimates of a and b.

Next we discuss Gray's approach in more detail. Let $p_d = P(D = d)$ and $\pi_{td} = P(T = t \mid D = d)$. We can write π_{td} as functions of the parameters of an ROC curve:

$$\pi_{t0} = \Phi(c_{t-1}) - \Phi(c_t) \text{ and } \pi_{t1} = \Phi(bc_{t-1} - a) - \Phi(bc_t - a),$$

where c_t is a cut-off point, as defined in Chapter 4, $t = 1, \ldots, K$. Notice that the probability of having $T = t$ and $D = d$ for a verified patient is $p_d \pi_{td}$ and that the probability of having $T = t$ for an unverified patient is $\sum_{d=0}^{1} p_d \pi_{td}$, a mixture of two distributions. Hence, under the MAR assumption, as defined by (10.25), the log-likelihood for the observed data, given in Table 10.7, is

$$\sum_{t=1}^{K} \sum_{d=0}^{1} z_{td} \log p_d \pi_{td} + \sum_{t=1}^{K} u_t \log(p_1 \pi_{t1} + p_0 \pi_{t0}). \tag{10.30}$$

Gray et al. (1984) developed a modified scoring algorithm to compute the ML estimates $\hat{a}$ and $\hat{b}$ of a and b by maximizing (10.30), and they also provided the covariance of $\hat{a}$ and $\hat{b}$ using the inverse of the expected Fisher information matrix. The resulting smooth ROC curve is given by

$$ROC(\text{FPR}) = \Phi(\hat{b}\Phi^{-1}(\text{FPR}) - \hat{a}),$$

where FPR is the false positive rate ranging from 0 to 1.

10.5.1.2 Estimation of ROC Curve Areas

We first observe that the area under the empirical ROC curve is a function of the parameters ϕ_1 and ϕ_2,

$$A = \frac{\sum_{t=1}^{K-1} \sum_{\tilde{t}=t+1}^{K}(1 - \phi_{2t})\phi_{1t}\phi_{2\tilde{t}}\phi_{1\tilde{t}} + (1/2)\sum_{t=1}^{K}(1 - \phi_{2t})\phi_{2t}\phi_{1t}^2}{\sum_{t=1}^{K}(1 - \phi_{2t})\phi_{1k}\sum_{\tilde{t}=1}^{K}\phi_{2\tilde{t}}\phi_{1\tilde{t}}}. \tag{10.31}$$

Substituting for unknown parameters in (10.31) by their ML estimates, defined by (10.27), we obtain the following ML estimator of the empirical AUC:

$$\hat{A} = \frac{\sum_{t=1}^{K-1} \sum_{\tilde{t}=t+1}^{K} \frac{r_t m_t}{s_t + r_t} \frac{s_{\tilde{t}} m_{\tilde{t}}}{s_{\tilde{t}} + r_{\tilde{t}}} + (1/2)\sum_{t=1}^{K} \frac{s_t r_t m_t^2}{(s_t + r_t)^2}}{\sum_{t=1}^{K} \frac{r_t m_t}{s_t + r_t} \sum_{\tilde{t}=1}^{K} \frac{s_{\tilde{t}} m_{\tilde{t}}}{s_{\tilde{t}} + r_{\tilde{t}}}}. \tag{10.32}$$

Then, using the delta method we obtain the corresponding variance of the estimated AUC:

$$var(\hat{A}) = \sum_{t=1}^{K} \frac{\phi_{2t}^2(1 - \phi_{2t})^2}{s_t(1 - \phi_{2t})^2 + r_t\phi_{2t}^2}\left(\frac{\partial A}{\partial \phi_{2t}}\right)^2 + \sum_{t=1}^{K-1} \frac{\phi_{1t}^2}{m_t}\left(\frac{\partial A}{\partial \phi_{1t}}\right)^2 -$$

$$\frac{1}{\sum_{t=1}^{K} \frac{\phi_{1t}^2}{m_t}} \left(\sum_{t=1}^{K-1} \frac{\phi_{1t}^2}{m_t} \frac{\partial A}{\partial \phi_{1t}} \right)^2.$$

Here

$$\frac{\partial A}{\partial \phi_{1t}} = \frac{\frac{\partial B_1}{\partial \phi_{1t}} + (1/2)\frac{\partial B_2}{\partial \phi_{1t}}}{w(1-w)} - A \times \frac{1-2w}{w(1-w)}(\phi_{2t} - \phi_{2K}),$$

and

$$\frac{\partial A}{\partial \phi_{2\tilde{t}}} = \frac{\frac{\partial B_1}{\partial \phi_{2\tilde{t}}} + (1/2)\frac{\partial B_2}{\partial \phi_{2\tilde{t}}}}{w(1-w)} - A \times \frac{1-2w}{w(1-w)}\phi_{1\tilde{t}},$$

where

$$w = \sum_{t=1}^{K} \phi_{1t}\phi_{2t},$$

$$B_1(\phi) = \sum_{t=1}^{K-1} \sum_{\tilde{t}=t+1}^{K} (1-\phi_{2t})\phi_{1t}\phi_{2\tilde{t}}\phi_{1\tilde{t}}, \quad B_2(\phi) = \sum_{t=1}^{K}(1-\phi_{2t})\phi_{2t}\phi_{1t}^2,$$

and the partial derivatives of $B_1(\phi)$ and $B_2(\phi)$ with respect to ϕ_{1t} and $\phi_{2\tilde{t}}$ are given in Zhou (1998a)

For a smooth ROC curve based on a binormal model, the ML estimator for the area under the ROC curve is

$$\hat{A} = \Phi\left(\frac{\hat{a}}{\sqrt{1+\hat{b}^2}}\right),$$

where $\hat{a}$ and $\hat{b}$ are the ML estimators of a and b, obtained using Gray's modified scoring algorithm. Let $var(\hat{a})$, $cov(\hat{a}, \hat{b})$, and $var(\hat{b})$ be the asymptotic variance-covariance matrix of the ML estimators $\hat{a}$ and $\hat{b}$ obtained using the expected Fisher information. Then, the asymptotic variance of $\hat{A}$ is

$$(\phi(\frac{a}{\sqrt{1+b^2}}))^2[(1+b^2)^{-1}var(\hat{a}) - 2ab(1+b^2)^{-2}cov(\hat{a},\hat{b}) + (ab)^2(1+b^2)^{-3}var(\hat{b})].$$

The Fortran program, written by R. Gray, is available at the web site (http://faculty.washington.edu/azhou/books/diagnostic.html).

10.5.2   Analysis of Fever of Uncertain Origin Example

Gray et al. (1984) reported data from a study on the accuracy of computed tomography in differentiating focal from nonfocal sources of sepsis among patients with fever of uncertain origin. In this study, only some patients were verified, depending on their CT results. Hence, this study had verification bias. Table 10.8 displays the data.

If we use only the verified cases, the estimates of a and b are 1.44 and 1.93, respectively. The resulting empirical and smooth ROC curves are displayed in

Table 10.8   CT Data of 53 Patients with Fever of Uncertain Origin

		T=1	T=2	T=3	T=4	T=5
V=1	D=1	7	7	2	3	37
	D=0	8	0	1	1	4
V=0		40	11	3	5	12
Total		55	18	6	9	53

Figure 10.4. The area under the smooth ROC curve is 0.75 with the standard deviation of 0.108. If we assume that the probability of verification depends only on the result of CT, using all the cases, the ML estimates of a and b are 1.80 and 1.75, respectively. We display the corrected empirical and smooth ROC curves in Figure 10.4. The area under the corrected smooth ROC curve is 0.81 with standard deviation of 0.07.

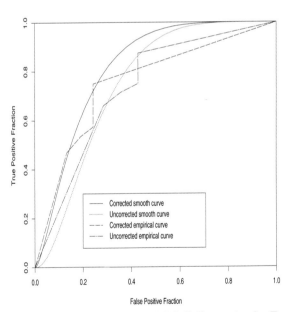

Figure 10.4   Uncorrected and Corrected ROC Curves in the Fever of Uncertain Origin Example

10.5.3 ML Approach With Covariates

If the probability of verifying a patient depends not only on the test results but also on some observed covariates, we need to modify the correction methods discussed in Section 10.5.1. Let X be the vector of observed covariates that may affect the verification process and the accuracy of the test. Assume that X has G distinct combinations, and x_g represents the values of the covariates for the gth combination. The observed data with $X = x_g$ form a contingency table, displayed in Table 10.9. The MAR assumption becomes

Table 10.9   Observed Data for a Single Ordinal Scale Test at the gth Covariate Pattern $(\mathbf{X} = \mathbf{x}_g)$

		T=1	T=2	...	T=K
V=1	D=1	z_{11g}	z_{21g}	$\cdots$	z_{K1g}
	D=0	z_{10g}	z_{20g}	$\cdots$	z_{K0g}
V=0		u_{1g}	u_{2g}	$\cdots$	u_{Kg}
Total		m_{1g}	m_{2g}	$\cdots$	m_{Kg}

$$P(V = 1 \mid T, X, D) = P(V = 1 \mid T, X). \tag{10.33}$$

10.5.3.1 Estimation of ROC Curves   We first discuss a non-parametric approach for estimating the empirical ROC curve. Define $\phi_{1tg} = P(T = t \mid X = x_g)$, $\phi_{2tg} = P(D = 1 \mid T = t, \mathbf{X} = \mathbf{x}_g)$, and $p_{dg} = P(D = d \mid X = x_g)$. For the subpopulation with $X = x_g$, the empirical ROC curve is a plot of $TPR_g(t) = P(T \geq t \mid D = 1, X = x_g)$ against $FPR_g(t) = P(T \geq t \mid D = 0, X = x_g)$, for $t = 1, \ldots, K$. For the whole population, the empirical ROC curve is a plot of $TPR(t) = P(T \geq t \mid D = 1)$ against $FPR(t) = P(T \geq t \mid D = 0)$, for $t = 1, \ldots, K + 1$. Observe that

$$TPR_g(t) = \frac{\sum_{\tilde{t}=t}^{K} \phi_{1\tilde{t}g}\phi_{2\tilde{t}g}}{\sum_{\tilde{t}=1}^{K} \phi_{1\tilde{t}g}\phi_{2\tilde{t}g}}, \; FPR_g(t) = \frac{\sum_{\tilde{t}=t}^{K} \phi_{1\tilde{t}g}(1 - \phi_{2\tilde{t}g})}{\sum_{\tilde{t}=1}^{K} \phi_{1\tilde{t}g}(1 - \phi_{2\tilde{t}g})},$$

$$TPR(t) = \frac{\sum_{g=1}^{G} \sum_{\tilde{t}=t}^{K} \phi_{1\tilde{t}g}\phi_{2\tilde{t}g}\xi_g}{\sum_{g=1}^{G} \sum_{\tilde{t}=1}^{K} \phi_{1\tilde{t}g}\phi_{2\tilde{t}g}\xi_g},$$

and

$$FPR(t) = \frac{\sum_{g=1}^{G} \sum_{\tilde{t}=t}^{K} \phi_{1\tilde{t}g}(1 - \phi_{2\tilde{t}g})\xi_g}{\sum_{g=1}^{G} \sum_{\tilde{t}=1}^{K} \phi_{1\tilde{t}g}(1 - \phi_{2\tilde{t}g})\xi_g}. \tag{10.34}$$

Hence, to estimate the empirical ROC curve, we need to estimate ϕ_{1tg}, ϕ_{2tg}, and ξ_g. Under the MAR assumption, the log-likelihood for the observed data given in Table 10.9 is

$$\sum_{g=1}^{G}\sum_{t=1}^{K} m_{tg} \log(\phi_{1tg}) + \sum_{g=1}^{G}\sum_{t=1}^{K}(z_{t1g}\log(\phi_{2tg}) + z_{t0g}\log(1-\phi_{2tg})).$$

Maximizing the above log-likelihood yields the following ML estimators for ϕ_{1tg} and ϕ_{2tg}:

$$\hat{\phi}_{1tg} = \frac{m_{tg}}{N_g} \text{ and } \hat{\phi}_{2tg} = \frac{z_{t1g}}{z_{t1g}+z_{t0g}},$$

where $N_g = \sum_{t=1}^{K} m_{tg}$. By substituting unknown parameters in (10.34) with their ML estimators, we obtain the ML estimators for the subpopulation-specific and overall ROC curves. Their variance estimators can be found in Zhou (1996b).

Next, we discuss the correction method for estimating smooth ROC curves. Using Rodenberg and Zhou's approach (Rodenberg, 1996; Rodenberg and Zhou, 2000), we model the effects of the covariates $\mathbf{X} = \mathbf{x}_g$ on the distribution of the results by ordinal regression with a probit link (McCullagh, 1980; Tosteson and Begg, 1988)

$$\sum_{\tilde{t} \le t} \pi_{\tilde{t}dg} = \Phi\left(\frac{c_t - (\beta_D d + \beta_X' x_g)}{\exp(\alpha_D d + \alpha_X' x_g)}\right), \text{ for } t = 1, \ldots, K-1,$$

where $\pi_{\tilde{t}dg} = P(T = \tilde{t} \mid D = d, X = x_g)$, and c_t's are cut-off points of a latent continuous variable T^*, as defined in Chapter 4. Denote $\boldsymbol{\alpha} = (\alpha_D, \alpha_X)$, $\boldsymbol{\beta} = (\beta_D, \beta_X)$, and $c = (c_1, \ldots, c_{K-1})$. To emphasize the dependence of π_{ldg} on $\boldsymbol{\alpha}$, $\boldsymbol{\beta}$, and c, we write $\pi_{tdg} = \pi_{tdg}(\boldsymbol{\alpha}, \boldsymbol{\beta}, c)$. Hence, under the MAR assumption, defined by (10.33), the log-likelihood is

$$\sum_{t=1}^{K}\sum_{d=0}^{1}\sum_{g=1}^{G} z_{tdg}\log(p_{dg}\pi_{tdg}(\boldsymbol{\alpha},\boldsymbol{\beta},c))$$

$$+\sum_{t=1}^{K}\sum_{g=1}^{G} u_{tg}\log(p_{1g}\pi_{t1g}(\boldsymbol{\alpha},\boldsymbol{\beta},c) + p_{0g}\pi_{t0g}(\boldsymbol{\alpha},\boldsymbol{\beta},c)),$$

where $p_{dg} = P(D = d \mid \mathbf{X} = \mathbf{x}_g)$, the prevalence of condition in the gth subgroup of patients with $\mathbf{X} = \mathbf{x}_g$.

The above log-likelihood, based on the observed data, has a complicated form, involving mixture distributions. Let w_{dtg} be the number of unverified patients with $T = t$ and $X = x_g$ whose condition status is d ($D = d$). Because of selective verification, one does not observe w_{tdg}, but instead one observes $u_{tg} = w_{t0g} + w_{t1g}$. However, if all subjects had been verified, a much simpler complete-data log-likelihood could be written as

$$\sum_{g=1}^{G}\sum_{t=1}^{K}\sum_{d=0}^{1}\{z_{tdg}+w_{tdg}\}\log(p_{dg}) + \sum_{g=1}^{G}\sum_{t=1}^{K}\sum_{d=0}^{1}\{z_{tdg}+w_{tdg}\}\log(\pi_{tdg}(\boldsymbol{\alpha},\boldsymbol{\beta},c)).$$

These two separate sums suggest that p_{dg} and π_{tdg} can be maximized separately. The EM algorithm can be used here with a maximization step for an ordinal regression model of $\pi_{tdg}(\boldsymbol{\alpha}, \boldsymbol{\beta}, c)$ with w_{tdg} assumed known; a computer program PLUM, developed by McCullagh (1980), already exists for such a task. The expectation step finds new estimates of w_{kdg} given the current values of $\boldsymbol{\alpha}$, $\boldsymbol{\beta}$, c, and p, $\boldsymbol{\alpha}^{(m)}$, $\boldsymbol{\beta}^{(m)}$, $c^{(m)}$, and $p^{(m)}$, using

$$E(w_{tg} \mid \boldsymbol{\alpha} = \boldsymbol{\alpha}^{(m)}, \boldsymbol{\beta} = \boldsymbol{\beta}^{(m)}, p = p^{(m)}) = u_{tg} \frac{p_{dg}^{(m)} \; \pi_{tdg}(\boldsymbol{\alpha}^{(m)}, \boldsymbol{\beta}^{(m)}, c^{(m)})}{\sum_{d=0}^{1} p_{dg}^{(m)} \; \pi_{tdg}(\boldsymbol{\alpha}^{(m)}, \boldsymbol{\beta}^{(m)}, c^{(m)})}.$$

This iterative process is continued until the relative change in successive ML estimates is small. The convergent values are the ML estimates of the parameters. Their asymptotic covariance matrix is given by the inverse of the expected information matrix, defined by the equation (10.35).

Once we have the ML estimates $\hat{\boldsymbol{\alpha}}$, $\hat{\boldsymbol{\beta}}$, and $\hat{c}$ and their associated covariance matrix estimate, V, we can estimate the smooth ROC curves for the different covariate levels. For the subpopulation with $X = x_g$, the ROC curve is the plot

$$1 - \Phi\left(\frac{c - L_{0,g}}{S_{0,g}}\right)$$

against

$$1 - \Phi\left(\frac{c - L_{1,g}}{S_{1,g}}\right)$$

for $-\infty < c < \infty$, where

$$L_{d,g} = \beta_D d + \boldsymbol{\beta}_X' x_g, \text{ and } S_{d,g} = \exp(\alpha_D d + \boldsymbol{\alpha}_X' x_g).$$

Letting $z = (c - L_{0,g})/S_{0,g}$, we obtain the ROC curve for patients with $X = x_g$ as follows:

$$1 - \Phi(z) \quad \text{versus} \quad 1 - \Phi\left(\frac{S_{0,g}}{S_{1,g}} z - \frac{L_{1,g} - L_{0,g}}{S_{1,g}}\right). \tag{10.35}$$

Denoting $b_g = S_{0,g}/S_{1,g}$ and $a_g = (L_{1,g} - L_{0,g})/S_{1,g}$, we can express the ROC curve using the notation given in the standard parametric ROC curve literature,

$$1 - \Phi(z) \quad \text{versus} \quad 1 - \Phi\left(b_g z - a_g\right) \tag{10.36}$$

for $-\infty < z < \infty$.

10.5.3.2 Estimation of ROC Curve Areas

To estimate the area under the empirical ROC curve using the trapezoidal rule, we first observe that the empirical ROC area is a function of the parameters ϕ_1 and ϕ_2,

$$A = \frac{\sum_{t=1}^{K-1} \sum_{\tilde{t}=t+1}^{K} \sum_{g=1}^{G} (1 - \phi_{2tg}) \phi_{1\tilde{t}g} \xi_g \sum_{g=1}^{G} \phi_{2tg} \phi_{1\tilde{t}g} \xi_g}{\sum_{t=1}^{K} \sum_{g=1}^{G} (1 - \phi_{2tg}) \phi_{1tg} \xi_g \sum_{t=1}^{K} \sum_{g=1}^{G} \phi_{2tg} \phi_{1tg} \xi_g}$$

$$+ \frac{1}{2} \frac{\sum_{t=1}^{K} \sum_{g=1}^{G} (1 - \phi_{2tg}) \phi_{1tg} \xi_g \sum_{g=1}^{G} \phi_{2tg} \phi_{1tg} \xi_g}{\sum_{t=1}^{K} \sum_{g=1}^{G} (1 - \phi_{2tg}) \phi_{1tg} \xi_g \sum_{t=1}^{K} \sum_{g=1}^{G} \phi_{2tg} \phi_{1tg} \xi_g}. \tag{10.37}$$

Substituting for unknown parameters in (10.37) by their ML estimates, we obtain the following non-parametric estimator of A:

$$\hat{A} = \frac{\sum_{t=1}^{K-1} \sum_{\tilde{t}=t+1}^{K} \sum_{g=1}^{G} \frac{z_{t0g} m_{tg}}{z_{t1g} + z_{t0g}} \sum_{g=1}^{G} \frac{z_{t1g} m_{tg}}{z_{t1g} + z_{t0g}}}{\sum_{t=1}^{K} \sum_{g=1}^{G} \frac{z_{t0g} m_{tg}}{z_{t1g} + z_{t0g}} \sum_{t=1}^{K} \sum_{g=1}^{G} \frac{z_{t1g} m_{tg}}{z_{t1g} + z_{t0g}}}$$

$$+ \frac{1}{2} \frac{\sum_{t=1}^{K} \sum_{g=1}^{G} \frac{z_{t0g} m_{tg}}{z_{t1g} + z_{t0g}} \sum_{g=1}^{G} \frac{z_{t1g} m_{tg}}{z_{t1g} + z_{t0g}}}{\sum_{t=1}^{K} \sum_{g=1}^{G} \frac{z_{t0g} m_{tg}}{z_{t1g} + z_{t0g}} \sum_{t=1}^{K} \sum_{g=1}^{G} \frac{z_{t1g} m_{tg}}{z_{t1g} + z_{t0g}}}, \tag{10.38}$$

where z_{t0g}, z_{t1g}, and m_{tg} are defined in Table 10.9. The corresponding variance estimator can be obtained by either the jackknife method or the information method as described in Zhou (1996b).

With a binormal assumption, the area under the smooth ROC curve for patients with $X = x_g$ is given by

$$A_g = \Phi \left(\frac{a_g}{\sqrt{1 + b_g}} \right). \tag{10.39}$$

By substituting $\hat{a}_i$ and $\hat{b}_i$ into equation (10.39), we obtain the following ML estimate for the ROC area for patients with $X = x_g$:

$$\hat{A}_g = \Phi \left(\frac{\hat{a}_g}{\sqrt{1 + \hat{b}_g}} \right).$$

We can use the delta method to estimate the variance of $\hat{A}_g, g = 1, 2, \ldots, G$. See Rodenberg and Zhou (2000) for a formula for this variance.

10.5.4 Analysis of New Screening Test for Dementia Disorder

In Section 10.1.2, we described a study of dementia disorders. One of the goals of the study was to assess how the accuracy of the new screening test was affected by the study site and the age of a subject. To illustrate the methods the project leaders were asked to further classify the 'poor performers' group into two subgroups, 'poor performers' and 'very poor performers.' The classification data on the new screening test result are given in Table 10.10. Let two binary variables X_1 and X_2 indicate the site of the study and the age group

Table 10.10 New Screening Test for Dementia Disorder Data

Study Site	Age Group			New Screening Test 1	2	3	4
Ibadan	65 − 74	V=1	D=1	0	0	4	3
Ibadan	65 − 74		D=0	35	49	62	12
Ibadan	65 − 74	V=0		1558	54	12	4
Ibadan	75+	V=1	D=1	2	2	8	9
Ibadan	75+		D=0	75	46	87	29
Ibadan	75+	V=0		350	44	28	21
Indianapolis	65 − 74	V=1	D=1	0	0	3	7
Indianapolis	65 − 74		D=0	27	34	40	12
Indianapolis	65 − 74	V=0		1106	43	30	5
Indianapolis	75+	V=1	D=1	1	5	20	29
Indianapolis	75+		D=0	71	39	54	9
Indianapolis	75+	V=0		578	46	39	14

of a subject, respectively: (1) $X_1 = 0$ for subjects in Ibadan, and $X_1 = 1$ for subjects in Indianapolis; (2) $X_2 = 0$ for subjects with age less than 75, and $X_2 = 1$ for subjects with age greater than or equal to 75. Using the likelihood ratio test, Rodenberg and Zhou (2000) have derived a best model as follows:

$$\Phi^{-1}(T \leq t \mid D, X_1, X_2) = \frac{c_t - (\beta_1 D + \beta_2 X_1 + \beta_3 X_2 + \beta_4(X_1 * X_2))}{\alpha_1 D + \alpha_2(X_1 * X_2) + \alpha_3(D * X_2)}$$

$$- \frac{(\beta_5(D * X_2) + \beta_6(X_1 * X_2 * D))}{\alpha_1 D + \alpha_2(X_1 * X_2) + \alpha_3(D * X_2)}.$$

Figure 10.5 illustrates the fitted ROC curves and empirical (TPF,FPF) estimates, where the empirical estimates are obtained by applying the nonparametric method, described in Section 10.5.1, to the subgroups stratified by site and age group. From this figure, we conclude that the estimated ROC curves for Indianapolis and Ibadan's young subjects are the same, but the estimated ROC curves for Indianapolis and Ibadan's older subjects are different. We now consider the less stringent question of whether the discriminatory ability of the test, measured by the area under the curve, depends on age and site. Table 10.11 reports the estimated areas under the ROC curves and their standard errors under the best model. Because the same ROC curve is fit for the two sites in the young age group, the area estimates for these two subgroups are identical. Table 10.12 compares various area estimates and tests the hypothesis that the two values are the same.

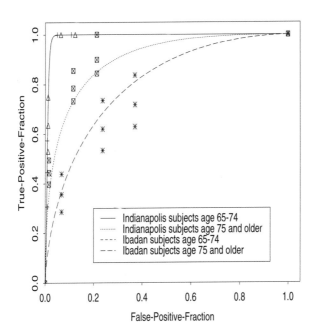

Figure 10.5   ROC Curves and Empirical (FPF,TPF) Estimates for the Dementia Screening Test by Site and Age Group under the Best Model

Table 10.11   Area under the ROC Curve of the Ordinal Scale Screening Test

Subgroup	Estimate(Standard Error)
Ibadan 65 − 74	0.990 (0.003)
Ibadan 75+	0.782 (0.074)
Indianapolis 65 − 74	0.990 (0.003)
Indianapolis 75+	0.914 (0.036)
Indianapolis Combined	0.944 (0.024)
Ibadan Combined	0.885 (0.046)

Table 10.12 P-Values for the Null Hypothesis That There Are No Differences in ROC Areas

Comparison			p-value
Indianapolis 75+	vs.	Ibadan 75+	0.056
Indianapolis 75+	vs.	Indianapolis 65 − 74	0.037
Ibadan 75+	vs.	Ibadan, 65 − 74	0.005
Indianapolis	vs.	Ibadan	0.154

From the results in Tables 10.12 and 10.11, we conclude the screening test performs better in the younger age group than in the older age group for both sites. There is a moderate indication that for subjects age 75 and above, the screening test is more accurate for Indianapolis subjects than it is for Ibadan subjects. If we consider the overall performance of the screening instrument within a site, however, no statistically significant difference exists between the two sites.

10.6 CORRELATED ORDINAL-SCALE TESTS

When we have two ordinal scale tests, we would be interested in comparing the relative ROC curves of the two tests and their corresponding areas under the ROC curves. Let T_1 and T_2 be the ordinal scale results of two diagnostic tests from the same patients. Let T_1 and T_2 range from 1 to K_1 and from 1 to K_2, respectively. Let X be a vector of observed discrete covariates that may affect the probability of disease verification and that has G different covariate patterns. Let the definitions of random variables D and V be the same as those defined in Section 10.3.1. We display the observed data with the ith covariate pattern, $X = x_g$, in Table 10.13.

In this section, we assume that the probability of selecting a patient for condition status verification depends only on the diagnostic test results of the patient and the observed covariates X; that is,

$$P(V = 1 \mid T_1, T_2, D, X) = P(V = 1 \mid T_1, T_2, X). \tag{10.40}$$

If the verification process is non-MAR, see Zhou and Castelluccio (2003) for a more detailed discussion on a bias correction method.

One main difficulty in analyzing such data is the dependence between T_1 and T_2 because both the tests are performed on the same patients. In this section we discuss two methods for handling such correlations. One is based

Table 10.13   Observed Data for Paired Ordinal Scale Tests at the gth
Covariate Pattern

		$T_1 = 1$			...	$T_1 = K_1$			
		$T_2 = 1$	...	$T_2 = K_2$	...	$T_2 = 1$	...	$T_2 = K_2$
$V = 1$	$D = 1$	s_{g11}	...	s_{g1K_2}	...	s_{gK_11}	...	$s_{gK_1K_2}$
	$D = 0$	r_{g11}	...	r_{g1K_2}	...	r_{gK_11}	...	$r_{gK_1K_2}$
$V = 0$		u_{g11}	...	u_{g1K_2}	...	u_{gK_11}	...	$u_{gK_1K_2}$
Total		m_{g11}	...	m_{g1K_2}	...	m_{gK_11}	...	$m_{gK_1K_2}$

on the idea of weighted generalized estimating equations (GEE) (Toledano
and Gatsonis, 1999; Zheng et al., 2005), and the other is based on a likelihood
approach (Zhou, 1998b).

10.6.1   Weighted Estimating Equation Approaches for Latent Smooth ROC Curves

In this section, we discuss three forms of weighted estimating equations based
on imputation and inverse probability weighting for correcting for verification
bias in estimation of the covariate-specific smooth ROC curves of an ordinal-
scale test.

The first approach is inverse probability weighting (IPW), proposed by
Toledano and Gatsonis (1999), where each verified observation is weighted
by the inverse of the probability of getting disease verification. The second
approach is mean score imputation (MSI), where the missing disease statuses
for unverified cases are imputed. The validity of the IPW method requires that
both the models for the test results and verification be correctly specified, and
the validity of the MSI method requires both the models for the test results
and disease status be correctly specified. The strong dependence of these
two methods on two correctly specified models may limit their applications in
practice (Liu and Zhou, 2011b). The third method is a doubly robust method,
whose validity requires either a correctly specified model for disease status or
a correctly specified model for the verification in addition to the correct model
for the test outcomes (Zheng et al., 2005).

10.6.1.1   The IPW approach   Toledano and Gatsonis (1999) proposed an inverse probability weighting (IPW) approach to correct for verification bias.
Since this approach is an extension of the GEE approach, as discussed in Section 8.3.1, to the problem of verification bias, it retains the semi-parametric
feature of the GEE approach in the sense that we only need to specify the
first two moments of T_1 and T_2, respectively, and a "working covariance" for
T_1 and T_2 without a full specification of the joint distribution of T_1 and T_2

(Robins et al., 1994), where the "working covariance" does not have to be the true covariance matrix of T_1 and T_2.

Let T_{ki} be the result of the ith test on the kth patient, and let D_k and X_k be the condition status and the covariate value of the kth patient, where $i = 1, 2$, and $k = 1, \ldots, N$. Let us denote the indicator variable $Y_{kit} \equiv I(T_{ki} \leq t)$ for $t = 1, \cdots, K - 1$. We then assume the following location-scale model for the cumulative indicator Y_{kit}:

$$E\left(T_{kit} | D_{ki}, X_{ki}\right) = \mu_{kit} = \Pr(T_{ki} \leq t | D_{ki}, X_{ki}) = \Phi\left[\frac{c_t - \nu(D_{ki}, X_{ki})}{\sigma(D_{ki}, X_{ki})}\right],$$

where Φ is the standard normal cumulative distribution function, and

$$\nu(D_{ki}, X_{ki}) = \beta_1' X_{ki} + \beta_2 D_{ki} + \beta_3' X_{ki} D_{ki}.$$

In our application we assume the scale parameter only depends on disease status, $\sigma(D_{ki}, \boldsymbol{X}_{ki}) = \exp(\alpha D_{ki})$, but this can be generalized to include other covariates. Let $\boldsymbol{B} \equiv (c_1, \cdots, c_{K-1}, \beta_1', \beta_2, \beta_3', \alpha)'$ be all the unknown parameters. For a given covariates value $\boldsymbol{X} = x$, the ROC curve can be derived as

$$ROC_x(p) = \Phi\left(a + b\Phi^{-1}(p)\right),$$

with $a = e^{-\alpha}(\beta_2 + \beta_3' x)$ and $b = e^{-\alpha}$. The corresponding area under the ROC curve is given by $AUC = \Phi\left(\frac{a}{\sqrt{1+b^2}}\right)$.

To describe the IPW approach, we first need to fit the following parametric logistic regression model for the verification model:

$$\pi_{ki} \equiv \Pr(V_{ki} = 1 | T_{ki}, \boldsymbol{X}_{ki}) = \frac{\exp(\zeta' Z_{ki})}{1 + \exp(\zeta' Z_{ki})},$$

where $Z_{ki} = \left[1, T_{ki}, \boldsymbol{X}_{ki}'\right]'$. The estimating function for ζ can be written as $U_{vki}(\zeta) \equiv Z_{ki}(V_{ki} - \pi_{ki})$.

Then, the IPW approach estimates the parameters, $\boldsymbol{B}$ and ζ, using the following IPW estimating equations:

$$U_{IPW}(\boldsymbol{B}, \zeta) = \sum_{k=1}^{N} \sum_{i=1}^{C_k} \left[\begin{array}{c} \frac{V_{ki}}{\pi_{ki}} U_{oki}\left(\boldsymbol{B}; T_{ki}, \boldsymbol{X}_{ki}, D_{ki}\right) \\ U_{vki}(\zeta; V_{ki}, T_{ki}, \boldsymbol{X}_{ki}) \end{array}\right],$$

where

$$U_{oki}(\boldsymbol{B}) = \frac{\partial \boldsymbol{\mu}_{ki}}{\partial \boldsymbol{B}'} \boldsymbol{V}_{ki}^{-1}(\boldsymbol{Y}_{ki} - \boldsymbol{\mu}_{ki}), \tag{10.41}$$

with $\boldsymbol{\mu}_{ki}$ and $\boldsymbol{Y}_{ki}$ being vectors with $K-1$ elements: $\boldsymbol{\mu}_{ki} = [\mu_{ki1}, \cdots, \mu_{ki(K-1)}]'$ and $\boldsymbol{Y}_{ki} = [Y_{ki1}, \cdots, Y_{ki(K-1)}]'$. Here $\boldsymbol{V}_{ki}$ is a working covariance matrix of $\boldsymbol{Y}_{ki}$. Toledano and Gatsonis (1999) showed that the resulting estimator, $\hat{\boldsymbol{B}}$ of $\boldsymbol{B}$, is consistent regardless of whether the working covariance matrix, $\boldsymbol{V}_{ki}$, is the true covariance matrix of $\boldsymbol{Y}_{ki}$, under the assumption that the verification process is MAR. They have also derived the asymptotic distribution and variance-covariance matrix of the resulting estimator, $\hat{\boldsymbol{B}}$.

10.6.1.2 The MSI approach The MSI method imputes the missing disease status, D_{ki}, of an unverified case, $V_{ki} = 0$, by the expected value of D_{ki}, given the observed data, V_{ki}, Y_{ki}, and X_{ki}, $E(D_{ki} \mid V_{ki} = 0, Y_{ki}, X_{ki})$. We use two ways to model this conditional expectation. We first model $D_{ki} \mid X_{ki}$ by the following logistic regression:

$$\rho_{ki} \equiv \Pr(D_{ki} = 1 \mid X_{ki}) = \frac{\exp(\gamma_1' X_{ki}^*)}{1 + \exp(\gamma_1' X_{ki}^*)}, \tag{10.42}$$

where $X_{ki}^* = [1, X_{ki}]$. Let $U_{ki}^{(1)} \equiv X_{ki}^*(D_{ki} - \rho_{ki})$ be the estimating functions for α_1. Then

$$
\begin{aligned}
w_{kid}(B, \gamma_1) &= \Pr(D_{ki} = d \mid T_{ki}, X_{ki}) \\
&= \frac{P(T_{ki} \mid X_{ki}, D_{ki} = d)p(D_{ki} = d \mid X_{ki})}{\sum_{d=0}^{1} P(T_{ki} \mid X_{ki}, D_{ki} = d)P(D_{ki} = d \mid X_{ki})}.
\end{aligned}
$$

We can then estimate parameters, B and γ_1, by solving the following estimating functions:

$$U_{IB}^{(1)}(B, \gamma_1) = \sum_{k=1}^{N} \sum_{i=1}^{C_k} \left[\begin{array}{c} V_{ki}U_{oki}(B; T_{ki}, X_{ki}, D_{ki}) \\ V_{ki}U_{ki}^{(1)}(\gamma_1; D_{ki}, X_{ki}) \end{array} \right]$$

$$+ \sum_{k=1}^{N} \sum_{i=1}^{C_k} \left[\begin{array}{c} (1 - V_{ki}) \sum_{d=0}^{1} w_{kid}(B, \gamma_1)U_{oki}(B; T_{ki}, X_{ki}, D_{ki} = d)) \\ (1 - V_{ki}) \sum_{d=0}^{1} w_{kid}(B, \gamma_1)U_{ki}^{(1)}(\gamma_1; D_{ki} = d, X_{ki})) \end{array} \right].$$

Here we use an EM-type algorithm to estimate the conditional expectation $E[D_{ki} \mid T_{ki}, X_{ki}]$ from $D_{ki} \mid X_{ki}$ and $T_{ki} \mid D_{ki}, X_{ki}$. This approach is valid if the model for $D_{ki} \mid X_{ki}$ is correctly specified. We refer to this estimator as the MSI1 estimator.

The second approach directly models $D_{ki} \mid T_{ki}, X_{ki}$ by the following logistic regression:

$$\rho_{ki}^{(2)} \equiv \Pr(D_{ki} = 1 \mid T_{ki}, X_{ki}) = \frac{\exp(\gamma_2' Z_{ki})}{1 + \exp(\gamma_2' Z_{ki})}, \tag{10.43}$$

where $Z_{ki} = \left[1, T_{ki}, X_{ki}'\right]'$. Let us denote $U_{ki}^{(2)} \equiv V_{ki}Z_{ki}(D_{ki} - \rho_{ki}^{(2)})$. We then estimate the parameters, B and γ_2, by solving the following estimating functions:

$$
\begin{aligned}
U_{IB}^{(2)}(B, \gamma_2) &= \sum_{k=1}^{N} \sum_{i=1}^{C_k} \left[\begin{array}{c} V_{ki}U_{oki}(B; T_{ki}, X_{ki}, D_{ki}) \\ U_{ki}^{(2)}(\gamma_2; D_{ki}, T_{ki}, X_{ki}) \end{array} \right] \\
&+ \sum_{k=1}^{N} \sum_{i=1}^{C_k} \left[\begin{array}{c} (1 - V_{ki})\rho_{ki}^{(2)}U_{oki}(B; T_{ki}, X_{ki}, D_{ki} = 1)) \\ 0 \end{array} \right] \\
&+ \sum_{k=1}^{N} \sum_{i=1}^{C_k} \left[\begin{array}{c} (1 - V_{ki})\left(1 - \rho_{ki}^{(2)}\right)U_{oki}(B; T_{ki}, X_{ki}, D_{ki} = 0)) \\ 0 \end{array} \right].
\end{aligned}
$$

This approach is valid if the model for $D_{ki}|T_{ki}, \boldsymbol{X}_{ki}$ is correctly specified. We refer to this estimator as the MSI2 estimator.

10.6.1.3 The doubly robust approach The third method is a doubly robust (DR) method, whose validity requires either a correctly specified model for disease status or a correctly specified model for the verification in addition to the correct model for the test outcomes. The DR estimator makes use of both $[V|\boldsymbol{X}, T]$ and $[D|X, T]$ in estimating the model for $[T|X, D]$. Similar to the MSI1 and MSI2 estimators, there are two forms of DR estimators: one models $[D|X]$ first and uses an EM-type algorithm to obtain $[D|X, T]$, the other directly models $[D|X, T]$. We refer to them as DR1 and DR2 estimators. The corresponding estimating functions are

$$U_{DR}^{(1)}(\boldsymbol{B}, \gamma_1, \zeta)$$

$$= \sum_{k=1}^{N} \sum_{i=1}^{C_k} \left[\begin{array}{c} \frac{V_{ki}}{\pi_{ki}} U_{oki}(\boldsymbol{B}; T_{ki}, X_{ki}, D_{ki}) \\ \frac{V_{ki}}{\pi_{ki}} U_{ki}^{(1)}(\gamma_1; D_{ki}, X_{ki}) \\ U_{vki}(\zeta; V_{ki}, T_{ki}, X_{ki}) \end{array} \right]$$

$$+ \sum_{k=1}^{N} \sum_{i=1}^{C_k} \left[\begin{array}{c} (1 - \frac{V_{ki}}{\pi_{ki}}) \sum_{d=0}^{1} w_{kid}(\boldsymbol{B}, \gamma_1) U_{oki}(\boldsymbol{B}; T_{ki}, X_{ki}, D_{ki} = d)) \\ (1 - \frac{V_{ki}}{\pi_{ki}}) \sum_{d=0}^{1} w_{kid}(\boldsymbol{B}, \gamma_1) U_{ki}^{(1)}(\gamma_1; D_{ki} = d, X_{ki})) \\ 0 \end{array} \right],$$

and

$$U_{DR}^{(2)}(\boldsymbol{B}, \gamma_2, \zeta) =$$

$$\sum_{k=1}^{N} \sum_{i=1}^{C_k} \left[\begin{array}{c} \frac{V_{ki}}{\pi_{ki}} U_{oki}(\boldsymbol{B}; T_{ki}, X_{ki}, D_{ki}) + (1 - \frac{V_{ki}}{\pi_{ki}}) \rho_{ki}^{(2)} U_{oki}(\boldsymbol{B}; T_{ki}, X_{ki}, D_{ki} = 1) \\ U_{ki}^{(2)}(\gamma_2; D_{ki}, T_{ki}, X_{ki}) \\ U_{vki}(\zeta; V_{ki}, T_{ki}, X_{ki}) \end{array} \right]$$

$$+ \sum_{k=1}^{N} \sum_{i=1}^{C_k} \left[\begin{array}{c} \left(1 - \frac{V_{ki}}{\pi_{ki}}\right) \left(1 - \rho_{ki}^{(2)}\right) U_{oki}(\boldsymbol{B}; T_{ki}, X_{ki}, D_{ki} = 0) \\ 0 \\ 0 \end{array} \right]$$

The DR estimator requires either $[D \mid X, T]$ or $[V \mid X, T]$ is correctly specified but not necessarily both.

The variance estimator for the estimated parameters has the sandwich form

$$\frac{1}{n} \left[E \frac{\partial U_i}{\partial \boldsymbol{B}} \right]^{-1} cov(U_i) \left[E \frac{\partial U_i}{\partial \boldsymbol{B}} \right]^{-1}.$$

The information matrix $E \frac{\partial U_i}{\partial \boldsymbol{B}}$ is estimated by the sample mean of the derivative of the estimating functions, while $cov(U_i)$ is estimated by the sample covariance matrix.

10.6.1.4 Analysis of the clinical diagnosis in the NACC MDS Example

To illustrate the methods discussed in the above section, we apply them to the NACC MDS example by assessing the accuracy of the clinical diagnosis of AD, which has four categories, ranging from definitely not AD to definitely AD. In our analysis, we use a total of 20,299 deceased patients. The gold standard verification for AD comes from brain autopsy. Since the main reason for missing the gold standard is that the patients or their families opted not to have the brain autopsy, the MAR assumption is likely to hold. Table 10.14 displays the test results versus disease status.

Covariates include age (continuous variable), gender (1 for male and 0 for female), race (1 for white and 0 for non-white), marital status (1 for married and 0 otherwise), stroke (1 for patients who had stroke and 0 otherwise), Parkinson's disease (1 for patients with Parkinson's disease and 0 otherwise), and depression status (1 for patients with depression and 0 otherwise).

We use the following verification model in the analysis:

$$\text{logit}(\pi_k) = \zeta_0 + \zeta_1 T_k + \zeta_2' X_k, \tag{10.44}$$

where T_k is the test result for the kth patient, and X_k includes all the patient covariates above. The disease models corresponding to the methods in equations (10.42) and (10.43) are specified, respectively, as follows:

$$\text{logit}(\rho_k) = \gamma_{10} + \gamma_{11}' X_k,$$

and

$$\text{logit}(\rho_k) = \gamma_{20} + \gamma_{21} T_k + \gamma_{22}' X_k,$$

Table 10.14   The Clinical Assessment (T) Data in the NACC MDS Example

	$T = 1$	$T = 2$	$T = 3$	$T = 4$
$D = 0$	859	509	176	426
$D = 1$	530	425	613	2957
$D = NA$	1994	1748	2108	7954

where X_k includes all the patient covariates above. The R code for implementing this analysis can be found at the web site (http://faculty.washington.edu/azhou/books/diagnostic.html).

The estimated location-scale parameters are shown in Table 10.15, where the DR1, DR2, IPW, MSI1, and the complete-case (CC) analysis estimates are displayed. It is worth noting that the MSI2 estimating equations, using the quasi-Newton algorithm, does not converge in this example.

The DR1, DR2 and IPW estimates generally agree with each other, implying that the verification model is approximately correct. The IB1 estimates are a bit different from the DR and IPW estimates. Hence the disease model $D|X$ may not be correctly specified. Perhaps there are some other unobserved covariates or interactions affecting the disease probability. The CC estimates are very different from the DR and IPW estimates; this result indicates that the MCAR assumption is too strong, noting the validity of the CC analysis method requires the MCAR assumption.

We also display three estimated covariate-specific ROC curves in Figure 10.6, corresponding to (a) a 70 years old non-white female without Parkinson's disease, stroke or depression; (b) a 60 years old non-white female with stroke and without Parkinson's disease or depression; and (c) a 60 years old white male with Parkinson's disease, stroke and depression, respectively. We also examine the goodness of fit for the DR estimators. The only continuous variable, age, is dichotomized at the threshold 70 years old. We calculate the observed and expected cell count for the contingency table generated by test result, disease status and covariates. As the number of cells is large ($4 \times 2^8 = 1024$), the contingency table is very sparse and we are not able to perform the formal χ^2 test. Instead, we could visualize the goodness of fit for the proposed method in Figure 10.7, which is a plot of the expected versus observed cell counts in log scale. We can see that the points are scattered around the diagonal line, and hence conclude that the DR method fist the data reasonably well.

Table 10.15 The Estimated Location and Scale Parameters with the Associated Standard Errors for the NACC MDS Clinical Diagnosis Data under the MAR Verification Assumption

		DR1	DR2	IPW	MSI1	CC
Location	Cutoff 1	-0.220 (0.11)	-0.234 (0.12)	-0.098 (0.15)	0.004 (0.09)	0.104 (0.14)
	Cutoff 2	0.314 (0.11)	0.300 (0.13)	0.392 (0.15)	0.572 (0.10)	0.666 (0.14)
	Cutoff 3	0.776 (0.12)	0.761 (0.13)	0.783 (0.15)	1.072 (0.10)	1.080 (0.14)
	Age	0.082 (0.02)	0.084 (0.03)	0.030 (0.03)	-0.008 (0.02)	-0.012 (0.02)
	Gender	-0.064 (0.05)	-0.093 (0.06)	-0.004 (0.06)	-0.020 (0.05)	0.010 (0.06)
	Race	-0.092 (0.11)	-0.104 (0.13)	-0.084 (0.15)	0.040 (0.09)	0.038 (0.14)
	Married	0.165 (0.06)	0.169 (0.06)	0.220 (0.07)	0.238 (0.05)	0.243 (0.06)
	Stroke	0.139 (0.06)	0.201 (0.07)	0.097 (0.08)	0.339 (0.05)	0.111 (0.07)
	Parkinson	0.361 (0.08)	0.460 (0.09)	0.341 (0.10)	0.318 (0.07)	0.349 (0.09)
	Depression	-0.044 (0.06)	-0.069 (0.07)	0.046 (0.08)	0.095 (0.05)	0.094 (0.07)
	D	1.562 (0.16)	1.536 (0.17)	1.670 (0.19)	2.018 (0.14)	1.905 (0.19)
	D × *Age*	-0.101 (0.03)	-0.103 (0.04)	-0.067 (0.04)	0.048 (0.03)	-0.020 (0.03)
	D × *Gender*	-0.077 (0.07)	-0.042 (0.07)	-0.061 (0.08)	-0.142 (0.06)	-0.106 (0.07)
	D × *Race*	-0.121 (0.14)	-0.098 (0.17)	-0.200 (0.17)	-0.331 (0.10)	-0.351 (0.17)
	D × *Married*	-0.058 (0.07)	-0.065 (0.08)	-0.118 (0.08)	-0.146 (0.06)	-0.052 (0.08)
	D × *Stroke*	-0.480 (0.08)	-0.569 (0.10)	-0.402 (0.10)	-0.812 (0.07)	-0.467 (0.09)
	D × *Parkinson*	-0.825 (0.107)	-0.963 (0.13)	-0.825 (0.12)	-0.805 (0.11)	-0.889 (0.12)
	D × *Depression*	-0.162 (0.08)	-0.130 (0.09)	-0.172 (0.09)	-0.391 (0.07)	-0.215 (0.09)
Scale	*D*	0.033 (0.04)	0.031 (0.04)	0.051 (0.046)	0.113 (0.05)	0.156 (0.04)

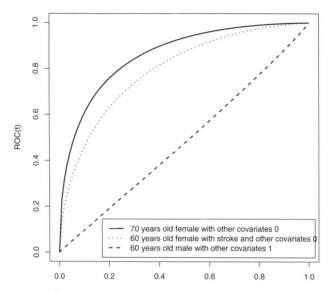

Figure 10.6   NACC Example: Several Estimated Covariate-specific ROC Curves

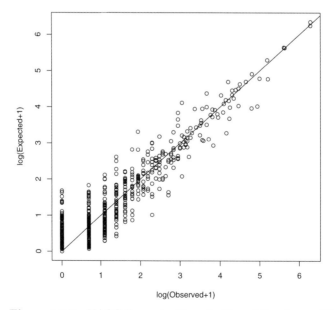

Figure 10.7   NACC Example: Examination of Goodness of Fit

10.6.2 Likelihood-Based Approach for ROC Areas

If one is interested in comparing the areas under the ROC curves, an approach simpler than the weighted GEE method is available (Zhou, 1998b). This approach is an extension of the previous method for a single ROC curve.

To derive this approach, we need the following notation. For the observed data given as in Table 10.13, we define the following parameters:

$$\phi_{2gt\tilde{t}} = P(D = 1 \mid T_1 = t, T_2 = \tilde{t}, \mathbf{X} = \mathbf{x}_g), \phi_{1gt\tilde{t}} = P(T_1 = t, T_2 = \tilde{t} \mid \mathbf{X} = \mathbf{x}_g),$$

and

$$\xi_g = P(\mathbf{X} = \mathbf{x}_g).$$

We can write the area under the ROC curves of the two diagnostic tests, A_1 and A_2 as a function of $\phi_{2gt\tilde{t}}$, $\phi_{1gt\tilde{t}}$, and ξ_g. After we obtain the ML estimates for $\phi_{1gt\tilde{t}}$, $\phi_{2gt\tilde{t}}$, and ξ_g, we then calculate the ML estimates for A_1 and A_2 and their covariance matrix.

Under the MAR assumption, defined by (10.40), the contribution of a verified patient to the likelihood is $P(T_1, T_2, D, \mathbf{X}) = P(D \mid T_1, T_2, \mathbf{X})P(T_1, T_2 \mid \mathbf{X})P(\mathbf{X})$, and the likelihood contribution of an unverified case is $P(T_1, T_2, \mathbf{X}) = P(T_1, T_2 \mid \mathbf{X})P(X)$. Because the number of free parameters can grow uncontrollably as the number of covariates grows, we need to model the joint probability $P(T_1, T_2, D \mid \mathbf{X})$. One may model effects of T_1, T_2, and X on D by a logistic regression model:

$$\phi_{2gt\tilde{t}} = \frac{\exp(\beta_{1t} + \beta_{2\tilde{t}} + \beta_3'\mathbf{x}_g)}{1 + \exp(\beta_{1t} + \beta_{2\tilde{t}} + \beta_3'\mathbf{x}_g)}, \tag{10.45}$$

where $\beta_{1K_1} = 0$ and $\beta_{2K_2} = 0$. We model the effects of X on T_1 and T_2 by the following multinomial logit regression:

$$\phi_{1gt\tilde{t}} = P(T_1 = t, T_2 = \tilde{t} \mid \mathbf{X} = \mathbf{x}_g) = \frac{\exp(\alpha_{t\tilde{t}}'\mathbf{x}_g)}{\sum_{h_1=1}^{K_1} \sum_{h_2=1}^{K_2} \exp(\alpha_{h_1 h_2}'\mathbf{x}_g)}, \tag{10.46}$$

where $\alpha_{K_1 K_2} = 0$. Denote $\beta = (\beta_{11}, \ldots, \beta_{1(K_1-1)}, \beta_{21}, \ldots, \beta_{2(K_2-1)}, \beta_3')$, $\alpha = (\alpha_{11}, \ldots, \alpha_{K_1(K_2-1)})'$, $\xi_g = P(\mathbf{X} = \mathbf{x}_g)$, $\xi = (\xi_1, \ldots, \xi_{G-1})$, $N_g = \sum_{t=1}^{K_1} \sum_{\tilde{t}=1}^{K_2} m_{gt\tilde{t}}$, and $N = \sum_{g=1}^{G} N_g$.

To emphasize the dependence of $\phi_{1gt\tilde{t}}$ on α and the dependence of $\phi_{2gt\tilde{t}}$ on β, one may write $\phi_{1gt\tilde{t}} = \phi_{1gt\tilde{t}}(\alpha)$ and $\phi_{2gt\tilde{t}} = \phi_{2gt\tilde{t}}(\beta)$. Under the MAR assumption, a valid log-likelihood function is

$$l(\alpha, \beta, \xi) = \sum_{g=1}^{G} \sum_{t=1}^{K_1} \sum_{\tilde{t}=1}^{K_2} m_{gt\tilde{t}} \log \frac{\exp(\alpha_{t\tilde{t}}'\mathbf{x}_g)}{\sum_{h_1,h_2=1}^{K} \exp(\alpha_{h_1 h_2}'\mathbf{x}_g)} + \sum_{g=1}^{G} N_g \log \xi_g$$

$$+ \sum_{g=1}^{G} \sum_{t=1}^{K_1} \sum_{\tilde{t}=1}^{K_2} s_{gt\tilde{t}} \log \frac{\exp(\beta_{1t} + \beta_{2\tilde{t}} + \beta_3'\mathbf{x}_g)}{1 + \exp(\beta_{1t} + \beta_{2\tilde{t}} + \beta_3'\mathbf{x}_g)}$$

$$+ \sum_{g=1}^{G} \sum_{t=1}^{K_1} \sum_{\tilde{t}=1}^{K_2} r_{gt\tilde{t}} \log \frac{1}{1 + \exp(\beta_{1t} + \beta_{2\tilde{t}} + \beta_3' \mathbf{x}_g)}, \qquad (10.47)$$

where $\xi_G = 1 - \xi_1 - \ldots - \xi_{G-1}$. Let

$$l_1(\boldsymbol{\alpha}) = \sum_{g=1}^{G} \sum_{t=1}^{K_1} \sum_{\tilde{t}=1}^{K_2} m_{gt\tilde{t}} \log \frac{\exp(\alpha_{t\tilde{t}}' \mathbf{x}_g)}{\sum_{h_1,h_2=1}^{K} \exp(\alpha_{h_1 h_2}' \mathbf{x}_g)}, \qquad (10.48)$$

$$l_2(\boldsymbol{\beta}) = \sum_{g=1}^{G} \sum_{t=1}^{K_1} \sum_{\tilde{t}=1}^{K_2} s_{gt\tilde{t}} \log \frac{\exp(\beta_{1t} + \beta_{2\tilde{t}} + \beta_3' \mathbf{x}_g)}{1 + \exp(\beta_{1t} + \beta_{2\tilde{t}} + \beta_3' \mathbf{x}_g)}$$

$$+ \sum_{g=1}^{G} \sum_{t=1}^{K_1} \sum_{\tilde{t}=1}^{K_2} r_{gt\tilde{t}} \log \frac{1}{1 + \exp(\beta_{1t} + \beta_{2\tilde{t}} + \beta_3' \mathbf{x}_g)}, \qquad (10.49)$$

and

$$l_3(\xi) = \sum_{g=1}^{G} N_g \log \xi_g. \qquad (10.50)$$

Then $l(\boldsymbol{\alpha}, \boldsymbol{\beta}, \boldsymbol{\xi})$ may be written as the sum of $l_1(\boldsymbol{\alpha})$, $l_2(\boldsymbol{\beta})$, and $l_3(\boldsymbol{\xi})$. Here, $l_1(\boldsymbol{\alpha})$, $l_2(\boldsymbol{\beta})$, and $l_3(\boldsymbol{\xi})$ may be considered as the log likelihood function of all cases modeled by the multinomial logit model defined by (10.46), the log likelihood function of verified cases modeled by the logistic regression model defined by (10.45), and the log likelihood function for a multinomial distribution based on all cases, respectively. Since the parameters $\boldsymbol{\alpha}$, $\boldsymbol{\beta}$, and $\boldsymbol{\xi}$ are distinct, their ML estimators, $\hat{\boldsymbol{\alpha}}$, $\hat{\boldsymbol{\beta}}$, and $\hat{\boldsymbol{\xi}}$, may be obtained by maximizing l_1, l_2, and l_3 with respect to $\boldsymbol{\alpha}$, $\boldsymbol{\beta}$, and $\boldsymbol{\xi}$, separately. The observed Fisher information for $(\boldsymbol{\alpha}, \boldsymbol{\beta}, \boldsymbol{\xi})$ is

$$diag(I_1(\boldsymbol{\alpha}), I_2(\boldsymbol{\beta}), I_3(\boldsymbol{\xi})), \qquad (10.51)$$

where I_1, I_2, and I_3 are the observed Fisher information matrices on the log-likelihood functions $l_1(\boldsymbol{\alpha})$, $l_2(\boldsymbol{\beta})$, and $l_3(\boldsymbol{\xi})$, respectively. Maximizing $l_1(\boldsymbol{\alpha})$ with respect to $\boldsymbol{\alpha}$ and $l_2(\boldsymbol{\beta})$ with respect to $\boldsymbol{\beta}$ yields ML estimators $\hat{\boldsymbol{\alpha}}$ and $\hat{\boldsymbol{\beta}}$, respectively. Since $\xi_G = 1 - \ldots - \xi_{G-1}$, maximizing $l_3(\boldsymbol{\xi})$ with respect to ξ_g yields ML estimators of ξ_g:

$$\hat{\xi}_g = \frac{N_g}{N},$$

$g = 1, \ldots, G - 1$.

Zhou (1998b) derived the ML estimators of A_1 and A_2 and their covariance matrix, under the MAR assumption on the verification process defined by (10.40). He showed that the ML estimator for the ith test, A_i, has the following form:

$$\hat{A}_i = \frac{1}{\hat{\gamma}(1 - \hat{\gamma})} \sum_{t=1}^{K_i - 1} \hat{\phi}_{i1}^*(t) \sum_{\tilde{t}=t+1}^{K_i} \hat{\phi}_{i2}^*(\tilde{t}),$$

where

$$\hat{\gamma} = \sum_{g=1}^{G}\sum_{t=1}^{K_1}\sum_{\tilde{t}=1}^{K_2}\phi_{2gt\tilde{t}}(\hat{\boldsymbol{\beta}})\phi_{1gt\tilde{t}}(\hat{\boldsymbol{\alpha}})\hat{\xi}_g,$$

$$\hat{\phi}_{11}^*(t) = \sum_{g=1}^{G}\sum_{\tilde{t}=1}^{K_2}(1-\phi_{2gt\tilde{t}}(\hat{\boldsymbol{\beta}}))\phi_{1gt\tilde{t}}(\hat{\boldsymbol{\alpha}})\hat{\xi}_g, \quad \hat{\phi}_{12}^*(t) = \sum_{g=1}^{G}\sum_{\tilde{t}=1}^{K_2}\phi_{2gt\tilde{t}}(\hat{\boldsymbol{\beta}})\phi_{1gt\tilde{t}}(\hat{\boldsymbol{\alpha}})\hat{\xi}_g,$$

and

$$\hat{\phi}_{21}^*(\tilde{t}) = \sum_{g=1}^{G}\sum_{t=1}^{K_1}(1-\phi_{2gt\tilde{t}}(\hat{\boldsymbol{\beta}}))\phi_{1gt\tilde{t}}(\hat{\boldsymbol{\alpha}})\hat{\xi}_g, \quad \hat{\phi}_{22}^*(\tilde{t}) = \sum_{g=1}^{G}\sum_{t=1}^{K_1}\phi_{2gt\tilde{t}}(\hat{\boldsymbol{\beta}})\phi_{1gt\tilde{t}}(\hat{\boldsymbol{\alpha}})\hat{\xi}_g.$$

The corresponding covariance matrix of $\hat{A}_1$ and $\hat{A}_2$ is

$$[\frac{\partial(A_1, A_2)}{\partial\alpha}]'I_1^{-1}(\alpha)\frac{\partial(A_1, A_2)}{\partial\alpha} + [\frac{\partial(A_1, A_2)}{\partial\beta}]'I_2^{-1}(\beta)\frac{\partial(A_1, A_2)}{\partial\beta}$$

$$+[\frac{\partial(A_1, A_2)}{\partial\xi}]'I_3^{-1}(\xi)\frac{\partial(A_1, A_2)}{\partial\xi},$$

where the partial derivatives, $\partial(A_1, A_2)/\partial\alpha$, $\partial(A_1, A_2)/\partial\beta$, and $\partial(A_1, A_2)/\partial\xi$, are given in Zhou (1998b). For a proof, see Zhou (1998b).

Assuming the normality of $\hat{A}_1 - \hat{A}_2$, one can then perform hypothesis tests and construct confidence intervals about $A_1 - A_2$. The main strength of this approach is that it does not require a model for the verification process under the MAR assumption, and its main weakness is that it can only be used to estimate the areas under ROC curves, but not ROC curves themselves.

10.6.3 Analysis of CT and MRI for Staging Pancreatic Cancer

We illustrate the use of the method described in Section 10.6.2 using data from a study designed to assess the relative accuracies of MRI and CT in the evaluation of the extent of pancreatic cancer (Megibow et al., 1995). All study patients had pancreatic cancer and were clinically judged to be candidates for surgical resection of the pancreatic gland. According to the design, all patients enrolled in the study would be examined with both MRI and CT before undergoing surgery. The MRI and CT examinations were interpreted separately. A critical issue in a patient's prognosis was the presence or absence of vascular invasion. We grouped the radiologist's degree of suspicion about the presence of vascular invasion into a 3-point ordinal categorical scale. The gold standard on vascular invasion was pathologic analysis of the patient's specimens obtained from surgery. All imaged patients were supposed to have surgery performed within three weeks of imaging. However, 39 of the 143 imaged patients didn't have surgery, and thus were missing verified diseased status. Let T_1 and T_2 denote the results of MRI and CT examinations of a patient, respectively, and let X denote the gender of a patient. If a patient is male, then $X = 1$; otherwise, $X = 0$. One patient was excluded from the analysis because the patient was missing the gender code. Table 10.16 gives the resulting classification data.

Since the reasons for not having surgery might be related to the results of MRI and CT, analysis using only disease verified cases might lead to biased results in comparing the relative accuracies of MRI and CT. Let A_1 and A_2 denote the areas under the ROC curves of MRI and CT, respectively. The null and alternative hypotheses of interest are

$$H_0 : A_1 = A_2 \text{ vs } H_1 : A_1 \neq A_2.$$

Assuming the probability of verifying a patient depends only on the results of MRI and CT and the gender of a patient, using the SAS PROC LOGISTIC procedure. We fitted the logistic regression model (10.19) to the verified cases, and using the SAS PROC CATMOD procedure. we fitted the multinomial logit model (10.20) to all observations. Then, the p-value of our two-sided test is 0.69, and the 95% confidence interval for $A_1 - A_2$ is $(-0.12, 0.17)$. Therefore, we cannot conclude that the areas under the ROC curves of MRI and CT are different.

10.7 CONTINUOUS-SCALE TESTS

When the response of a test is continuous, Alonzo and Pepe (2005) proposed several methods for correcting for verification bias in estimation of a single ROC curve when the verification process is MAR. He et al. (2009) proposed a non-parametric estimator of the area under the ROC curve under the MAR verification process. Liu and Zhou (2011b) proposed several verification bias corrected semi-parametric regression methods, including a doubly robust method, for estimating covariate-specific ROC curves when the verification process is MAR.

Rotnitzky et al. (2006) studied estimation of the area under the ROC curve under a non-MAR verification process. They developed a doubly robust estimator of the area under the ROC curve under a non-MAR verification model. Their non-MAR verification bias model assumes the non-MAR parameter (the log odds ratio of verification for diseased versus non-diseased individuals) is known. Fluss et al. (2009) applied the same methodology as in Rotnitzky et al. (2006) to construct the doubly robust estimators for sensitivity and specificity of the test at each cutoff point.

In practice, specifying the non-MAR parameter can be challenging because there is usually little prior information about the magnitude of the non-MAR parameter. Liu and Zhou (2011a) proposed a likelihood approach to estimate the ROC curve and its area under a parametric model for the non-MAR verification process and a parametric model for the disease regression model. In the next three subsections, we introduce these methods in detail.

Table 10.16   MRI and CT Data in Staging Pancreatic Cancer Example

Female (X=0)

	$T_1 = 1$			$T_1 = 2$			$T_1 = 3$		
	$T_2 = 1$	$T_2 = 2$	$T_2 = 3$	$T_2 = 1$	$T_2 = 2$	$T_2 = 3$	$T_2 = 1$	$T_2 = 2$	$T_2 = 3$
$V=1$ D=0	3	3	4	1	1	1	1	1	0
D=1	5	2	1	1	2	5	4	2	4
$V=0$	3	0	2	3	0	3	0	1	10
Total	11	5	7	5	3	9	5	4	14

Male (X=1)

	$T_1 = 1$			$T_1 = 2$			$T_1 = 3$		
	$T_2 = 1$	$T_2 = 2$	$T_2 = 3$	$T_2 = 1$	$T_2 = 2$	$T_2 = 3$	$T_2 = 1$	$T_2 = 2$	$T_2 = 3$
$V=1$ D=0	7	2	4	3	0	1	4	0	1
D=1	12	3	8	2	0	3	4	0	7
$V=0$	0	0	2	1	2	2	0	1	9
Total	19	5	14	6	2	6	8	1	17

10.7.1 Estimation of ROC Curves and Their Areas Under the MAR Assumption

In this section, we describe verification bias methods for estimating the ROC curve and their areas when the verification process can be assumed to be MAR. Here we assume the following MAR assumption:

$$P(V = 1 \mid T, D, X) = P(V = 1 \mid T, X).$$

For a cutoff point c defining a positive test, we can write $P(T \geq c, D = 1)$ and $P(T < c, D = 0)$ as the following expressions, respectively:

$$P(T \geq c, D = 1) = \int \int I_{[t \geq c]} P(D = 1 \mid T = t, X = x) P(T = t, X = x) dx dt,$$

$$P(T < c, D = 0) = \int \int I_{[t < c]} P(D = 0 \mid T = t, X = x) P(T = t, X = x) dx dt,$$

$$(10.52)$$

respectively. We can also write $P(D = 1)$ as follows:

$$P(D = 1) = \int \int P(D = 1 \mid T = t, X = x) P(T = t, X = x) dx dt.$$

From the above expressions, we can see that to consistently estimate the sensitivity and specificity of the test at a cutoff point, c, we need to consistently estimate $P(D = 1 \mid T = t, X = x)$.

Let $(T_i, D_i, V_i = 1, X_i), i = 1, \ldots, n$ denote observed data of verified subjects and $(T_i, V_i = 0, X_i), i = 1, \ldots, n$ denote observed data of unverified subjects. Under the MAR assumption, we can consistently estimate $P(D = 1 \mid T = t, X = x)$, based on a regression model (e.g. a logistic regression model), using only verified subjects, $(T_i, D_i, V_i = 1, X_i), i = 1, \ldots, n$; we denote the resulting estimator by $\widehat{\rho}_i$. Under the MAR assumption, $\widehat{\rho}_i$ is a consistent estimator if the assumed model for $P(D_i = 1 \mid T_i, X_i)$ is correct. If we use the empirical estimator for $P(T = t, X = x)$, based on the observed data, $(T_i, X_i), i = 1, \ldots, n$, Alonzo and Pepe (2005) proposed the following consistent full imputation (FI) estimators for $Se(c)$ and $Sp(c)$:

$$\widehat{Se}_{FI}(c) = \frac{\sum_{i=1}^{n} I_{[T_i \geq c]} \widehat{\rho}_i}{\sum_{i=1}^{n} \widehat{\rho}_i}, \quad \widehat{Sp}_{FI}(c) = \frac{\sum_{i=1}^{n} I_{[T_i < c]} (1 - \widehat{\rho}_i)}{\sum_{i=1}^{n} (1 - \widehat{\rho}_i)}.$$

Alonzo and Pepe (2005) also proposed a mean score imputation (MSI) based estimator, by only imputing disease status for unverified subjects and still using the observed disease status for verified subjects. The MSI-based estimators for sensitivity and specificity are defined as follows:

$$\widehat{Se}_{MSI}(c) = \frac{\sum_{i=1}^{n} I_{[T_i \geq c]} [V_i D_i + (1 - V_i) \widehat{\rho}_i]}{\sum_{i=1}^{n} [V_i D_i + (1 - V_i) \widehat{\rho}_i]},$$

$$\widehat{Sp}_{MSI}(c) = \frac{\sum_{i=1}^{n} I_{[T_i < c]}[V_i(1 - D_i) + (1 - V_i)(1 - \widehat{\rho}_i)]}{\sum_{i=1}^{n} [V_i(1 - D_i) + (1 - V_i)(1 - \widehat{\rho}_i)]}.$$

Alonzo and Pepe (2005) also proposed the third estimators for sensitivity and specificity using the idea of semiparametric efficient (SPE) inverse probability weighted estimation proposed by Robins and his colleagues. Let $\pi_i = P(V_i = 1 | T_i, X_i)$ and $\widehat{\pi}_i$ be its consistent estimator. These SPE estimators are defined as follows:

$$\widehat{Se}_{SPE}(c) = \frac{\sum_{i=1}^{n} I_{[T_i \geq c]}[V_i D_i + (\widehat{\pi}_i - V_i)\widehat{\rho}_i]/\widehat{\pi}_i}{\sum_{i=1}^{n} [V_i D_i + (\widehat{\pi}_i - V_i)\widehat{\rho}_i]/\widehat{\pi}_i},$$

$$\widehat{Sp}_{MSI}(c) = \frac{\sum_{i=1}^{n} I_{[T_i < c]}[V_i(1 - D_i) + (\widehat{\pi}_i - V_i)(1 - \widehat{\rho}_i)]/\widehat{\pi}_i}{\sum_{i=1}^{n} [V_i(1 - D_i) + (\widehat{\pi}_i - V_i)(1 - \widehat{\rho}_i)]/\widehat{\pi}_i}.$$

He et al. (2009) proposed a direct non-parametric estimator of the area under the ROC curve under the MAR verification process. Their method is based on the following equality under the MAR assumption:

$$E(\frac{V_i V_j}{\pi_i \pi_j} I_{[T_i > T_j]} I_{[D_i > D_j]}) = E(I_{[T_i > T_j]} I_{[D_i > D_j]})$$

$$= P(D_i = 1, D_j = 0)P(T_i > T_j \mid D_i = 1, D_j = 0).$$

Note that the last quantity above is the area under the ROC curve, AUC. Hence, a consistent estimator of the AUC is given as follows:

$$\widehat{AUC} = \frac{\sum_{i=1}^{n} \sum_{j=1}^{n} \widehat{\pi}_i^{-1} \widehat{\pi}_j^{-1} V_i V_j I_{[T_i > T_j]} I_{[D_i > D_j]}}{\sum_{i=1}^{n} \sum_{j=1}^{n} \widehat{\pi}_i^{-1} \widehat{\pi}_j^{-1} V_i V_j I_{[D_i > D_j]}}.$$

We may use the bootstrap method to estimate the variance of the estimated AUC, $\widehat{AUC}$.

10.7.1.1 Covariate-specific ROC curves and areas under the MAR assumption

In the previous section we discussed the bias correction procedures for ROC curves and areas under them. In practice, the patient covariates may be associated with the test result and hence may affect the classification accuracy. In this case, investigators are often more interested in the covariate-specific ROC curve. In this section, we introduce a regression model for assessing the covariate-specific ROC curve, adjusting for verification bias, proposed by Liu and Zhou (2011b).

We assume a location and scale model for T_i:

$$T_i = \mu_i(X_i, D_i; \beta) + \sigma_i(X_i, D_i; \gamma) \times \epsilon_i(D_i), \tag{10.53}$$

where $\mu_i(X_i, D_i; \beta)$ and $\sigma_i(X_i, D_i; \gamma)$ is the mean and standard deviation for T_i, respectively. We may use μ_i and σ_i as abbreviations. Let G_0 and G_1 be the unknown distribution functions of $\epsilon_i(0)$ and $\epsilon_i(1)$, respectively, with mean 0 and variance 1.

We can show that the covariate specific sensitivity and false positive rate of the test at a cutoff point c have the following forms:

$$Se_x(c) = \Pr(T \geq c|\, D = 1) = 1 - G_1 \left(\frac{c - \mu(x, 1; \beta)}{\sigma(x, 1; \gamma)} \right),$$

$$1 - Sp_x(c) = \Pr(T \geq c|\, D = 0) = 1 - G_0 \left(\frac{c - \mu(x, 0; \beta)}{\sigma(x, 0; \gamma)} \right).$$

Hence, we can express the ROC curve in the following form:

$$ROC_x(t) = 1 - G_1 \left[\frac{\sigma(x, 0; \gamma)}{\sigma(x, 1; \gamma)} G_0^{-1}(1 - t) + \frac{\mu(x, 0; \beta) - \mu(x, 1; \beta)}{\sigma(x, 1; \gamma)} \right].$$

Here we call G_1 and G_0^{-1} the link function and the baseline functions of the ROC curve, respectively. Allowing the link and baseline to remain unspecified gives more flexibility for the ROC curve.

In the ROC curve expression, the unknown quantities to be estimated are finite dimensional parameters β and γ, and infinite dimensional curves G_0^{-1} and G_1. When the gold standard is observed for each subject, the estimation of β and γ is easily obtained by the following estimating functions:

$$U_1 \equiv \sum_i U_{1i} \equiv \sum_i \left(\frac{\partial \mu_i}{\partial \beta} \right)' \frac{(T_i - \mu_i)}{\sigma_i^2},$$

$$U_2 \equiv \sum_i U_{2i} \equiv \sum_i \left(\frac{\partial \sigma_i^2}{\partial \beta} \right)' \frac{(T_i - \mu_i)^2 - \sigma_i^2}{\text{var}\left[(T_i - \mu_i)^2 \right]}.$$

Substituting the unknown μ_i and σ_i in the model (10.53) by the estimated $\hat{\beta}$ and $\hat{\gamma}$, we obtain the fitted residuals as $\hat{\epsilon}_i(D_i) = \frac{(T_i - \hat{\mu}_i)}{\hat{\sigma}_i}$. For each fixed s, the two distribution functions, G_1 and G_0, can then be estimated by the following kernel smoothing estimators:

$$U_3(s) \equiv \sum_i U_{3i}(s) \equiv \sum_i D_i \left[K \left(\frac{s - \hat{\epsilon}_i(D_i)}{h} \right) - G_1(s) \right],$$

$$U_4(s) \equiv \sum_i U_{4i}(s) \equiv \sum_i (1 - D_i) \left[K \left(\frac{s - \hat{\epsilon}_i(D_i)}{h} \right) - G_0(s) \right],$$

where $K(\cdot)$ is some distribution function, such as the standard normal distribution Φ, and h is the bandwidth. In order to estimate the $1 - t$ quantile of G_0, $G_0^{-1}(1 - t)$, we solve the following estimating function for every fixed t:

$$U_5(t) \equiv \sum_i U_{5i}(t) \equiv \sum_i (1 - D_i) \left[K \left(\frac{G_0^{-1}(1 - t) - \hat{\epsilon}_i(0)}{h} \right) + t - 1 \right].$$

Although t may take an infinite number of values between 0 and 1, we may just need to set finite grid points to get a good approximation for the smooth ROC curve. In practice, we may choose $t = 0.01, 0.02, \cdots, 0.99$ with linear extrapolation between the adjacent grid points. The estimated $\hat{G}_0$ and $\hat{G}_1$ have the same $\sqrt{n}$-consistency as the empirical distribution function, as long as the bandwidth is sufficiently small (Nadaraya, 1964).

As the gold standard is only available for a portion of the subjects, we need to reweight the estimating equations. Let $\rho_i = \Pr(D_i = 1|T_i, X_i) = \Pr(D_i = 1|T_i, X_i, V_i = 1)$ be the disease probability, and $\pi_i = \Pr(V_i = 1|T_i, X_i)$ be the verification probability. Under the missing at random assumption, ρ_i and π_i can be estimated, for example, using logistic regression. We then construct the weighted estimating equations with the estimated $\hat{\rho}_i$ and $\hat{\pi}_i$. Three types of estimating methods are considered: doubly robust (DR), inverse probability weighting (IPW), and imputation based (IB) approach. Let

$$S_k^{DR} = \sum_i S_{ki}^{DR} = \sum_i \left\{ \frac{V_i}{\hat{\pi}_i} U_{ki} + \left(1 - \frac{V_i}{\hat{\pi}_i} \right) E_{D_i|T_i, X_i} U_{ki} \right\}, \tag{10.54}$$

$$S_k^{IPW} = \sum_i S_{ki}^{IPW} \equiv \sum_i \frac{V_i}{\hat{\pi}_i} U_{ki}, \tag{10.55}$$

$$S_k^{IB} = \sum_i S_{ki}^{IB} = \sum_i \left\{ V_i U_{ki} + (1 - V_i) E_{D_i|T_i, X_i} U_{ki} \right\}, \tag{10.56}$$

for $k = 1, 2, 3, 4, 5$. We abbreviate the superscript and use S_k to denote the general weighted estimating functions in the text below. The conditional expectation $E_{D_i|T_i, X_i}$ can be written as weighted summations, as D_i takes the value of 0 or 1. For example,

$$
\begin{aligned}
E_{D_i|T_i, X_i} U_{1i} &= \sum_{d=0}^{1} \Pr(D_i = d| T_i, X_i) \left(\frac{\partial \mu_i(X_i, d; \beta)}{\partial \beta} \right)' \frac{(T_i - \mu_i(X_i, d; \beta))}{\sigma_i^2(X_i, d; \gamma)} \\
&= (1 - \rho_i) \left(\frac{\partial \mu_i(X_i, 0; \beta)}{\partial \beta} \right)' \frac{(T_i - \mu_i(X_i, 0; \beta))}{\sigma_i^2(X_i, 0; \gamma)} \\
&\quad + \rho_i \left(\frac{\partial \mu_i(X_i, 1; \beta)}{\partial \beta} \right)' \frac{(T_i - \mu_i(X_i, 1; \beta))}{\sigma_i^2(X_i, 1; \gamma)}.
\end{aligned}
$$

The DR estimating functions (10.54) enjoy the "doubly robust" property: as long as either $\hat{\rho}_i$ or $\hat{\pi}_i$ is consistently estimated, the DR estimator is consistent; the IPW estimating equations (10.55) require that the verification probability, π_i, be consistently estimated; the MSI estimating equations (10.56) require that the disease probability, ρ_i, be consistently estimated.

Let $B_1(\alpha_1) = \sum_i B_{1i}(\alpha_1)$ and $B_2(\alpha_2) = \sum_i B_{2i}(\alpha_2)$ be the estimating functions for modeling ρ and π, respectively. Let $\theta_1 = \begin{pmatrix} \beta \\ \gamma \end{pmatrix}$, the location and scale parameters, and $\hat{\theta}_1$ be its estimate. Let $U_{12,i} = \begin{pmatrix} U_{1i} \\ U_{2i} \end{pmatrix}$ and $S_{12,i} = \begin{pmatrix} S_{1i} \\ S_{2i} \end{pmatrix}$. Define $I = -\frac{\partial}{\partial \theta'_1} ES_{12,i}$, $J_1 = -\frac{\partial}{\partial \alpha'_1} ES_{12,i}$, $J_2 = -\frac{\partial}{\partial \alpha'_2} ES_{12,i}$, $K_1 = -\frac{\partial}{\partial \alpha'_1} EB_{1i}$, $K_2 = -\frac{\partial}{\partial \alpha'_2} EB_{2i}$. Let $Q_i = U_{12,i} - J_1 K_1^{-1} B_{1i} - J_2 K_2^{-1} B_{2i}$.

Under the standard regularity conditions stated in Liu and Zhou (2011b), we can show that

$$\sqrt{n}\left(\hat{\theta}_1 - \theta_1\right) \xrightarrow{d} N(0, \Omega_1),$$

where

$$\Omega_1 = I^{-1} \mathrm{var}(Q_i) I^{-1}.$$

Our primary interest is not only to estimate the location and scale model, but also to construct the covariate-specific ROC curve. With the estimated $\hat{\beta}$, $\hat{\gamma}$, $\hat{G}_0^{-1}$ and $\hat{G}_1$, we could estimate the covariate-specific ROC curve as follows:

$$\widehat{ROC}_x(t) = 1 - \hat{G}_1 \left[\frac{\sigma(x,0;\hat{\gamma})}{\sigma(x,1;\hat{\gamma})} \hat{G}_0^{-1}(1-t) + \frac{\mu(x,0;\hat{\beta}) - \mu(x,1;\hat{\beta})}{\sigma(x,1;\hat{\gamma})} \right].$$

We can show that $\widehat{ROC}_x(t)$ is consistent and asymptotically normally distributed. That is, for any $t \in (0,1)$,

$$\sqrt{n}\left(\widehat{ROC}_x(t) - ROC_x(t)\right) \xrightarrow{d} N(0, \Omega_2)$$

where the expression of Ω_2 is given in Liu and Zhou (2011b).

10.7.1.2 Analysis of NACC MDS Example with the MMSE test
We apply the proposed method in Section 10.7.1.1 to the NACC MDS data set. We included a total of 17,403 deceased patients for our analysis. The Mini Mental State Examination (MMSE) is an instrument that assesses cognitive impairment. The MMSE score ranges from 0 to 30, with lower scores indicating more severe impairment. Our goal is to evaluate the diagnostic accuracy of the MMSE test in discriminating Alzheimer's disease (AD) from non-AD. The gold standard ascertainment of AD, based on brain autopsy, is only available for about 31% of the cohort. The missingness may be due to the patients' or their family's decision. We believe that their decision may be associated with patient's demographic characteristics (such as age, gender, race, etc.), but is unlikely to be correlated with true AD status. So the MAR assumption seems to be reasonable here. Other covariates extracted from the database include age (continuous variable indicating age at the MMSE test), gender (binary variable with 1 indicating male), race (binary variable with 1 indicating non-white), marital status (binary variable with 1 indicating married), clinical diagnosis of AD (binary variable with 1 indicating clinical diagnosis of AD), stroke (binary variable with 1 indicating having had stroke), Parkinson's disease (binary variable with 1 indicating presence of the disease), and

depression (binary variable with 1 indicating presence of the disease). Figure 10.8 displays the distribution of the MMSE scores among all the patients and among subgroups stratified by verification and disease status. The distribution of the test result seems to be irregular, so it is difficult to justify any parametric distribution. The test distributions for the cases and controls are very different too.

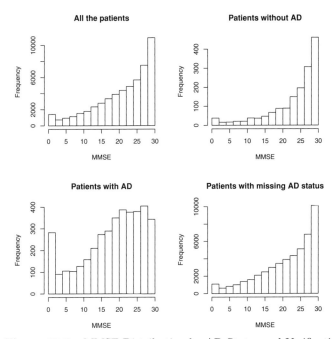

Figure 10.8 MMSE Distribution by AD Status and Verification

We transform the MMSE score using $\tilde{T} = (30 - T)/5$ so that a diseased subject tends to have a larger test result than a non-diseased subject, and transform the age using $age_1 = (age - 70)/10$. All the aforementioned covariates, as well as the MMSE score are included in the verification model. The disease model also includes the quadratic term of the test score, as well as interaction terms between the test and the covariates.

We use the following regression model for $\tilde{T}_i$:

$$\tilde{T}_i = \beta_0 + \beta_1 D_i + \beta_2' X_i + \beta_3' D_i X_i + exp((\gamma_0 + \gamma_1 D_i)/2) \times \epsilon_i,$$

where $E(\epsilon_i) = 0$ and $Var(\epsilon_i) = 1$. We report the estimates for β and γ, using the DR, IPW and MSI methods, in Table 10.17.

The results from the three methods generally agree with each other. The DR method identifies main effects of race, clinical AD, and true disease status to be significant, indicating that these variables affect the magnitude of the MMSE score. Only the $race \times D$ interaction is significant.

Table 10.17   The Estimated Location and Scale Parameters with the
Associated Standard Errors for the MMSE Test Using the NACC MDS Data

	DR	IPW	MSI
	Location parameter estimates and SEs in parentheses		
Intercept	**1.394 (0.125)**	**1.452 (0.199)**	**1.408 (0.131)**
Age	-0.064 (0.039)	**-0.114 (0.051)**	-0.054 (0.032)
Gender	-0.049 (0.079)	0.046 (0.096)	-0.028 (0.074)
Race	**-0.303 (0.131)**	**-0.525 (0.203)**	**-0.304 (0.128)**
Marital status	0.083 (0.086)	**0.219 (0.102)**	0.031 (0.076)
Clinical AD	**1.120 (0.077)**	**1.160 (0.097)**	**1.128 (0.070)**
Stroke	0.129 (0.095)	0.100 (0.125)	0.129 (0.083)
Parkinson's	0.186 (0.138)	0.228 (0.153)	**0.292 (0.124)**
Depression	-0.007 (0.108)	0.144 (0.156)	-0.006 (0.083)
D	**0.984 (0.167)**	**1.090 (0.250)**	**0.982 (0.170)**
$D \times Age$	0.049 (0.052)	0.085 (0.063)	0.035 (0.041)
$D \times Gender$	-0.146 (0.099)	-0.065 (0.119)	**-0.180 (0.090)**
$D \times Race$	**-0.322 (0.158)**	-0.339 (0.240)	**-0.330 (0.152)**
$D \times Marital\ status$	0.039 (0.108)	-0.090 (0.127)	0.110 (0.094)
$D \times Clinical\ AD$	-0.150 (0.106)	-0.154 (0.127)	-0.166 (0.095)
$D \times Stroke$	-0.124 (0.120)	-0.082 (0.156)	-0.115 (0.105)
$D \times Parkinson's$	0.074 (0.172)	0.012 (0.190)	-0.058 (0.155)
$D \times Depression$	-0.225 (0.135)	-0.119 (0.180)	-0.153 (0.102)
	Scale parameter estimates and SEs in parentheses		
Intercept	**0.301 (0.024)**	**0.391 (0.028)**	**0.310 (0.022)**
D	**0.120 (0.027)**	**0.149 (0.031)**	**0.109 (0.025)**

We take the bandwidth to be 0.02 in estimating the covariate-specific ROC curves. In Figure 10.9, we show the DR estimates of the two specific ROC curves: one for 70-year-old non-white female with other covariate values being 0, the other for 60-year-old white male with depression and other covariate values being 0. The 95% CI's are also plotted. The results show that the

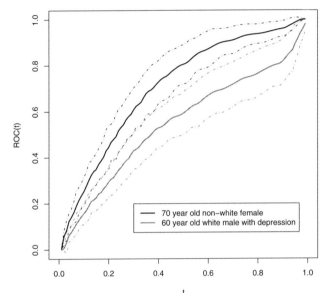

Figure 10.9   The Covariate-Specific ROC Curves

classification ability of the MMSE test could differ substantially for different covariate groups.

10.7.2   Estimation of ROC Curves and Areas under a Non-MAR Process

The proposed methods above assume that the verification bias is MAR. However, disease verification may also depend on some unobserved covariates related to the disease, and hence the MAR assumption may not hold, which is known as the non-MAR verification mechanism. When we have the non-MAR missing data mechanism, the observed likelihood involves the verification mechanism given by a selection model.

We assume the following selection model for the verification mechanism:

$$Pr(V_i = 1 | D_i, T_i, X_i) = \text{expit}(h(T_i, X_i; \boldsymbol{\beta}) + \alpha D_i), \tag{10.57}$$

where $\text{expit}(x) \equiv \frac{\exp(x)}{1+\exp(x)}$, and α is the non-MAR parameter. For simplicity, we take $h(T_i, X_i; \boldsymbol{\beta}) = \beta_0 + \beta_1 T_i + \boldsymbol{\beta}' X_i$, which is a natural consideration in practice. This can be easily extended to allow for interactions between T_i and X_i. If $\alpha = 0$, the missing mechanism is MAR; otherwise, it is non-MAR. Note that the link function in (10.57) could also be Φ (standard normal cdf) for a probit model. We allow the link functions to be either expit or Φ in the next section, but we only use expit here for the purpose of easy interpretation. It follows from (10.57) that

$$\frac{\Pr(D = 1 \mid V = 1, T, X)}{\Pr(D = 1 \mid V = 0, T, X)}$$

$$= \frac{\Pr(V = 1 \mid D = 1, T, X)\Pr(D = 1 \mid T, X)/\Pr(V = 1 \mid T, X)}{\Pr(V = 0 \mid D = 1, T, X)\Pr(D = 1 \mid T, X)/\Pr(V = 0 \mid T, X)}$$

$$= \frac{\Pr(V = 0 \mid T, X)}{\Pr(V = 1 \mid T, X)} \exp(\beta_0 + \beta_1 T + \beta_2' X + \alpha). \tag{10.58}$$

Similarly, we can obtain the following equation:

$$\frac{\Pr(D = 0 \mid V = 1, T, X)}{\Pr(D = 0 \mid V = 0, T, X)} = \exp(\beta_0 + \beta_1 T + \beta_2' X)\frac{\Pr(V = 0 \mid T, X)}{\Pr(V = 1 \mid T, X)}. \tag{10.59}$$

From (10.58) and (10.59), we have

$$\frac{\Pr(D = 1 \mid V = 1, T, X)/\Pr(D = 0 \mid V = 1, T, X)}{\Pr(D = 1 \mid V = 0, T, X)/\Pr(D = 0 \mid V = 0, T, X)} = \exp(\alpha). \tag{10.60}$$

The original interpretation of α based on the selection model is the log odds ratio of verification for a diseased subject versus a non-diseased subject. According to (10.60), α can also be interpreted as the log odds ratio of having the disease for a verified case as compared to an unverified case with the same test result and covariates, as long as (10.57) holds. Then $\Pr(D = 1 \mid V = 0, T, X)$ can be solved from (10.60) as a function of $\Pr(D = 1 \mid V = 1, T, X)$,

$$\Pr(D = 1 \mid V = 0, T, X)$$

$$= \frac{\Pr(D = 1 \mid V = 1, T, X)}{\exp(\alpha) + \Pr(D = 1 \mid V = 1, T, X)(1 - \exp(\alpha))}. \tag{10.61}$$

As Rotnitzky et al. (2006) argued, the observed data are governed by $\Pr(D = 1 \mid V = 1, T, X)$, $\Pr(V = 1 \mid T, X)$, and $f(T, X)$. Hence if we changed α in (10.61) and kept $\Pr(D = 1 \mid V = 1, T, X)$ the same, we would get a different disease probability for the unverified sample, while the observed (marginal) distribution still remains the same. Intuitively, since the disease model is restricted in the verified sample, $\Pr(D = 1 \mid V = 0, T, X)$ could be any structure. They proposed to specify α and developed the doubly robust estimate for the area under the ROC curve; that is, they showed that their AUC estimator is consistent if either $\Pr(V = 1 \mid D, T, X)$ or $\Pr(D = 1 \mid V = 1, T, X)$ has a correctly specified parametric form. Although the doubly robust property is desirable, it depends on the correct specification of the log odds ratio, α. It is quite a strong assumption to set α as known, and specifying α correctly could be challenging in practice.

In order to make α estimable, we need to assume a disease model for the whole sample,

$$\Pr(D_i = 1 | T_i, X_i) = \text{expit}(m(T_i, X_i; \boldsymbol{\gamma})). \tag{10.62}$$

For simplicity, we take $m(T_i, X_i; \boldsymbol{\gamma}) = \gamma_0 + \gamma_1 T_i + X_i' \boldsymbol{\gamma}_2$. The doubly robust property also has to be sacrificed as a cost of estimating α. Intuitively in this case, if we fix $\Pr(D = 1 | V = 1, T, X)$ and change α in (10.61), $\Pr(D = 1 | V = 0, T, X)$ will be changed and (10.62) may no longer hold in general. In other words, the restriction of (10.62) does provide some information in estimating α.

Let $\boldsymbol{\beta} = (\beta_0, \beta_1, \boldsymbol{\beta}_2')'$ and $\boldsymbol{\gamma} = (\gamma_0, \gamma_1, \boldsymbol{\gamma}_2')'$. Let $\pi_{di} = \Pr(V_i = 1 | D_i = d, T_i, X_i)$, given by the selection model (10.57), and $\rho_i = \Pr(D_i = 1 | T_i, X_i)$, given by the disease model (10.62). The log likelihood could be written as follows:

$$l(\alpha, \boldsymbol{\beta}, \boldsymbol{\gamma}) = \sum_i \{ D_i V_i \left(\log \pi_{1i} \rho_i \right) + (1 - D_i) V_i \left(\log \pi_{0i} (1 - \rho_i) \right)$$

$$+ (1 - V_i) \log \left(1 - \pi_{1i} \rho_i - \pi_{0i} (1 - \rho_i) \right) \},$$

which has the same form as the multinomial likelihood. The three cells are given by $DV = 1$, $(1 - D)V = 1$, and $V = 0$, with the corresponding cell probabilities $\pi_{1i} \rho_i$, $\pi_{0i} (1 - \rho_i)$ and $1 - \pi_{1i} \rho_i - \pi_{0i} (1 - \rho_i)$, respectively. If the expit link is used for the selection and disease model, then the score equations for α, $\boldsymbol{\beta}$ and $\boldsymbol{\gamma}$ are given as follows:

$$0 = \sum_i \left[D_i V_i (1 - \pi_{1i}) - \frac{(1 - V_i) \rho_i \pi_{1i} (1 - \pi_{1i})}{1 - \pi_{1i} \rho_i - \pi_{0i} (1 - \rho_i)} \right],$$

$$0 = \sum_i \begin{pmatrix} 1 \\ T_i \\ X_i \end{pmatrix} \{ D_i V_i (1 - \pi_{1i}) + (1 - D_i) V_i (1 - \pi_{0i})$$

$$- \frac{(1 - V_i)(\rho_i \pi_{1i}(1 - \pi_{1i}) + (1 - \rho_i)\pi_{0i}(1 - \pi_{0i}))}{1 - \pi_{1i} \rho_i - \pi_{0i}(1 - \rho_i)} \},$$

$$0 = \sum_i \begin{pmatrix} 1 \\ T_i \\ X_i \end{pmatrix} \left[V_i (D_i - \rho_i) - \frac{(1 - V_i)(\pi_{1i} - \pi_{0i})\rho_i(1 - \rho_i)}{1 - \pi_{1i} \rho_i - \pi_{0i} (1 - \rho_i)} \right].$$

The model parameters could be estimated by solving the above score equations using the Newton-Raphson algorithm, or as suggested by previous literature, using an EM algorithm to facilitate the calculation.

As mentioned above, the likelihood function takes the form of the multinomial distribution, and the cell probabilities are determined by the disease and verification models. Although one could employ the Hosmer-Lemeshow test to assess the goodness of fit, we do not recommend any formal test for the goodness of fit. The non-MAR verification model itself could not be tested nonparametrically from the data set, and hence the usefulness of the goodness of fit test is in doubt. Instead, the disease and verification models should be based on scientific considerations, which may come from exogenous or prior knowledge about the disease and the sampling scheme.

After we have calculated the estimates for π_i and ρ_i, $\hat{\pi}_i$ and $\hat{\rho}_i$, we can then obtain estimates for the empirical ROC curve and the AUC using a similar approach as in Alonzo and Pepe (2005). Specifically, we propose four types of empirical ROC curve estimates using $\hat{\pi}_i$ and $\hat{\rho}_i$.

The first approach is full imputation (FI), where D_i in the estimating functions for complete data are replaced by $\hat{\rho}_i$. In other words, all the disease statuses are imputed by the estimated ones, no matter whether they are observed or missing. The FI estimators for $Se(s)$, $Sp(s)$, and the AUC are given as follows:

$$\widehat{Se}_{FI}(s) = \frac{\sum_i I(T_i \geq s)\hat{\rho}_i}{\sum_i \hat{\rho}_i}, \quad \widehat{Sp}_{FI}(s) = \frac{\sum_i I(T_i < s)(1 - \hat{\rho}_i)}{\sum_i (1 - \hat{\rho}_i)},$$

$$\hat{\nu}_{FI} = \left\{\sum_{i \neq j} I_{ij}\hat{\rho}_i(1 - \hat{\rho}_j)\right\} \bigg/ \left\{\sum_{i \neq j} \hat{\rho}_i(1 - \hat{\rho}_j)\right\}.$$

Denote $\rho_{0i} \equiv \Pr(D = 1 | V = 0, T, X)$ to be the disease probability given the disease status is missing. Its estimated version can be expressed as

$$\hat{\rho}_{0i} = \frac{(1 - \hat{\pi}_{1i})\hat{\rho}_i}{(1 - \hat{\pi}_{1i})\hat{\rho}_i + (1 - \hat{\pi}_{0i})(1 - \hat{\rho}_i)},$$

where $\hat{\pi}_{1i} \equiv \widehat{\Pr}(V_i = 1 | D_i = 1, T_i, X_i)$ and $\hat{\pi}_{0i} \equiv \widehat{\Pr}(V_i = 1 | D_i = 0, T_i, X_i)$. The second approach is mean score imputation (MSI), where only the missing D_i's are replaced by $\hat{\rho}_{0i}$. Let $D_{MSI,i} = V_i D_i + (1 - V_i)\rho_{0i}$ and $\hat{D}_{MSI,i}$ be the estimated version with ρ_{0i} replaced by $\hat{\rho}_{0i}$. The estimated $Se(s)$, $Sp(s)$, and the AUC are then given as follows:

$$\widehat{Se}_{MSI}(s) = \frac{\sum_i I(T_i \geq s)\hat{D}_{MSI,i}}{\sum_i \hat{D}_{MSI,i}},$$

$$\widehat{Sp}_{MSI}(s) = \frac{\sum_i I(T_i < s)(1 - \hat{D}_{MSI,i})}{\sum_i (1 - \hat{D}_{MSI,i})},$$

$$\hat{\nu}_{MSI} = \left\{\sum_{i \neq j} I_{ij}\hat{D}_{MSI,i}(1 - \hat{D}_{MSI,j})\right\} \bigg/ \left\{\sum_{i \neq j} \hat{D}_{MSI,i}(1 - \hat{D}_{MSI,j})\right\}.$$

The third approach is inverse probability weighting (IPW). Each observation is weighted by the probability of getting disease verification. The corresponding estimates of $TPR(s)$, $FPR(s)$ and the AUC are:

$$\widehat{Se}_{IPW}(s) = \frac{\sum_i I(T_i \geq s) V_i D_i / \hat{\pi}_i}{\sum_i V_i D_i / \hat{\pi}_i},$$

$$\widehat{Sp}_{IPW}(s) = \frac{\sum_i I(T_i < s) V_i(1 - D_i)/ \hat{\pi}_i}{\sum_i V_i(1 - D_i)/ \hat{\pi}_i},$$

$$\hat{\nu}_{IPW} = \left\{ \sum_{i \neq j} I_{ij} \frac{V_i V_j D_i(1 - D_j)}{\hat{\pi}_i \hat{\pi}_j} \right\} \bigg/ \left\{ \sum_{i \neq j} \frac{V_i V_j D_i(1 - D_j)}{\hat{\pi}_i \hat{\pi}_j} \right\}.$$

The fourth approach is the pseudo doubly robust estimate (PDR). Let $D_{PDR,i} \equiv V_i D_i / \pi_i + (1 - V_i / \pi_i)\rho_{0i}$. The estimated $\hat{D}_{PDR,i}$ have π_i and ρ_{0i} replaced by $\hat{\pi}_i$ and $\hat{\rho}_{0i}$. The estimated $Se(s)$, $Sp(s)$ and AUC are then given as follows:

$$\widehat{Se}_{PDR}(s) = \frac{\sum_i I(T_i \geq s)\hat{D}_{PDR,i}}{\sum_i \hat{D}_{PDR,i}},$$

$$\widehat{Sp}_{PDR}(s) = \frac{\sum_i I(T_i < s)(1 - \hat{D}_{PDR,i})}{\sum_i(1 - \hat{D}_{PDR,i})},$$

$$\hat{\nu}_{PDR} = \left\{ \sum_{i \neq j} I_{ij} \hat{D}_{PDR,i}(1 - \hat{D}_{PDR,i}) \right\} \bigg/ \left\{ \sum_{i \neq j} \hat{D}_{PDR,i}(1 - \hat{D}_{PDR,i}) \right\}.$$

The functional form of the PDR estimate is the same as that in Rotnitzky, Faraggi, and Schisterman (2006). However, it does not have the doubly robust property in general, as the two probabilities $\hat{\pi}_i$ and $\hat{\rho}_i$ are estimated together from the likelihood function, and correct specification of both the verification model and the disease model is required.

The empirical ROC curves using the FI and MSI methods are monotonic, because $\hat{\rho}_i$ and $\hat{D}_{MSI,i}$ are both between 0 and 1. The IPW estimate of the ROC curve is also monotonic, because $V_i D_i / \hat{\pi}_i$ and $V_i(1 - D_i)/ \hat{\pi}_i$ are both positive. However, the PDR estimate of the ROC curve may be nonmonotonic, as $\hat{D}_{PDR,i}$ could be outside the $[0, 1]$ interval. One can use isotonic regression techniques for a correction as suggested by Fluss et al. (2009).

Liu and Zhou (2011a) have shown that $D_{MSI,i}$ and $D_{PDR,i}$ are both unbiased estimators of ρ_i and that the FI, MSI, IPW, and PDR estimators of $Se(s)$, $Sp(s)$ and AUC are all consistent.

10.7.2.1 Analysis of NACC MDS Example with the MMSE under a non-MAR model
In Section 10.7.1.2, we analyzed the accuracy of the MMSE test under the MAR assumption. In this section, we re-analyze this data set under a parametric non-MAR model for the verification process. In the previous analysis, we restricted the sample to those patients who had died during the study to make the MAR assumption feasible. Here we also include the alive

patients, and the resulting sample has a total of 53,063 patients with about 11% verification proportion.

We choose the following selection model for this non-MAR verification process:

$$\Pr(V = 1 | D, T, X) = \text{expit}(\beta_0 + X'\beta_1 + \beta_2 T + \alpha D),$$

and the following model for the probability of the disease:

$$\Pr(D = 1 | T, X) = \text{expit}(\gamma_0 + X'\gamma_1 + \gamma_2 T),$$

where X was the vector of all the aforementioned covariates. In the above models, we use a linear transformation on age and test result by considering $(age - 70)/10$ and $(30 - T)/15$, just for the convenience of reporting their coefficients. The estimated parameters and their standard errors are given in Table 10.18.

Table 10.18   Estimated Model Parameters and Their Standard Errors for the MMSE Data under a Non-MAR Verification Model. (Significant Coefficients are in Bold Font.)

	Verification model	Disease model
Intercept	**-4.527 (0.089)**	**-1.101 (0.252)**
age	**0.086 (0.017)**	**0.134 (0.034)**
gender	**0.587 (0.037)**	**-0.468 (0.075)**
race	**1.696 (0.070)**	-0.025 (0.175)
marital status	**-0.195 (0.035)**	0.129 (0.080)
clinical AD diagnosis	0.079 (0.083)	**1.881 (0.070)**
stroke	**0.305 (0.043)**	-0.100 (0.095)
Parkinson's disease	**0.641 (0.058)**	0.234 (0.122)
depression	**-0.202 (0.044)**	0.110 (0.099)
T	**0.203 (0.040)**	**0.784 (0.071)**
D	**0.718 (0.178)**	-

We find that all variables except clinical AD status are significant in the selection model. The non-MAR parameter is estimated to be 0.718, indicating that the odds ratio of verification for the diseased versus the non-diseased is 2.05 (95% CI: 1.45, 2.91). The disease model identifies some significant risk factors such as age, gender, clinical AD diagnosis, as well as the test result. In fact, our main interest here is not on the risk factors, but on the predicted individual verification probability and disease probability. Hence we just keep the predetermined model that is scientifically plausible, rather than considering any model selection.

We can also try different predictors in the models, but it seems that the non-MAR parameter does not change much. For example, when deleting the race variable in the disease model, α is estimated to be 0.721 (95% CI: 0.375, 1.067); when adding the interaction between T and gender, $\hat{\alpha} = 0.696$

(95% CI: 0.331, 1.060); when adding the interaction between age and gender, $\hat{\alpha} = 0.759$ (95% CI: 0.418, 1.100). Here we just report the models with main effects of the covariates, and calculate the AUC thereafter. Figure 10.10 shows the estimated ROC curves using the FI, MSI, IPW and PDR methods.

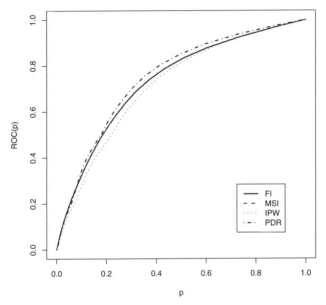

Figure 10.10   Estimated ROC Curve Using FI, MSI, IPW and PDR Approaches Under the Non-ignorable Verification

We can see that the FI and MSI estimates of the ROC curve virtually overlap with each other. The IPW curve is a little lower than the FI curve, and the PDR curve is slightly higher than the FI curve. As for the AUC, the FI estimate for the AUC is 0.7350 (95% CI: 0.7215, 0.7484); the MSI estimate for the AUC is 0.7355 (95% CI: 0.7243, 0.7468); the IPW estimate for the AUC is 0.7164 (95% CI: 0.6983, 0.7344); the PDR estimate for the AUC is 0.7514 (95% CI: 0.7340, 0.7688). Similar to the simulation studies, FI and MSI estimates have narrower confidence intervals than the IPW and PDR estimates. The reason why IPW estimates are not as precise as the FI and MSI estimates may be due to the low verification probability. With only about 10% verification, the inverse of selection probability would be large for many subjects, so as to make the IPW estimates less stable and precise.

CHAPTER 11

METHODS FOR CORRECTING IMPERFECT GOLD STANDARD BIAS

In the previous chapters, we assume that the gold standard for establishing the true disease status of a subject exists. However, for many disease conditions, it is difficult or impossible to establish a definitive diagnosis of the disease. A perfect gold standard may not exist or may be too expensive or impractical to administer. For example, in Case Study 3 on the accuracy of MRA for detecting carotid artery plaque, described in Chapter 1, the gold standard is catheter angiography, which is not a perfect test, and radiologists often disagree in their interpretations of its findings.

Similarly, the diagnosis of Alzheimer's disease cannot be definitive until a patient has died and a neuropathological examination is performed. Even the "definitive" diagnosis of a well-defined condition, such as an infection by a known agent, requires culture of the organism or other detection methods, any of which may be subject to laboratory and other errors. Consequently, in many diagnostic accuracy studies, an imperfect standard is used to evaluate the test. When an imperfect gold standard is used as if it were a gold standard or if no gold standard is available, the accuracy of the test is often either underestimated or overestimated. This type of bias is called imperfect gold standard bias, as we described in Chapter 3.

Statistical Methods in Diagnostic Medicine,
Second Edition. By Xiao-Hua Zhou, Nancy A. Obuchowski, Donna K. McClish
Copyright © 2011 John Wiley & Sons, Inc.

Valenstein (1990) reported sensitivity and specificity of a new latex immunoagglutination assay for detecting *Clostridium difficile*-associated diarrhea from six studies. These studies used the stool cytotoxicity test as a gold standard. Since the cytotoxicity test has been shown to give positive results in some asymptomatic patients and negative results in some patients with compatible clinical histories and biopsy proven pseudomembranous colitis, the cytotoxicity test is almost certainly an imperfect gold standard. The six studies reported that the new latex immunoassay test had an overall sensitivity of 81% and specificity of 94%. However, using a clinical definition of *C. difficile*-associated diarrhea as the gold standard, the sensitivity and specificity were 90% and 97%, respectively.

In the absence of a gold standard, one may just be interested in assessing agreement between a new test and an imperfect gold standard, which is often reported as a Kappa statistic (Kraemer et al., 2004). However, agreement data on two tests will not tell us the accuracy of the tests – if two tests agree, they can both be either correct or wrong.

In this chapter we present methods for correcting imperfect gold standard bias in the analysis of accuracy data in the absence of any gold standard or when an imperfect gold standard is used.

In Section 11.1, we introduce six real-world examples, which all have the problem of an imperfect gold standard. In Section 11.2 we discuss the effects of imperfect gold standard bias on the estimated accuracy of diagnostic tests. Then, in Section 11.3 we describe bias-correction methods for estimating the sensitivity and specificity of a single diagnostic test against an imperfect gold standard in one single population, and in Section 11.4 we extend these correction methods to G populations. In Section 11.5 we discuss bias-correction methods when I ($I > 2$) tests are applied to a single population, and in Section 11.6, we present bias-correction methods for estimating sensitivities and specificities of I tests when they are applied to G populations. In Section 11.7 we present bias-correction methods for estimating the ROC curves of tests when multiple ordinal-scale tests are applied to sample patients in the absence of any reference standard. In Section 11.8, we discuss bias-correction methods for estimating ROC curves of continuous-scale tests when they are applied to the same subjects and no reference standard is used.

11.1   EXAMPLES

In this section, we describe six diagnostic accuracy studies that have the problem of imperfect gold standard bias. The first four studies focus on binary-scale diagnostic tests; the fifth study focuses on ordinal-scale tests; and the sixth study contains both continuous-scale and ordinal-scale tests. In the first two studies, an imperfect gold standard is used, and in the last four studies, no gold standard is available.

11.1.1 Binary Stool Test for Strongyloides Infection

Gyorkos et al. (1990) reported a study on the effectiveness of a screening and treatment program for intestinal parasite infections among newly arrived Southeast Asian refugees in Canada between July 1982 and February 1983. One goal of the study was to assess the accuracy of a binary-scale stool examination test in detecting Strongyloides infection among the Cambodian refugees. The serology test was used as a gold standard in the study. However, using a separate coprologic test, which is known to be better than serology, as the "gold standard," the sensitivity and specificity of the serotogic test, were 95% and specificity 29%, respectively, and its positive and negative predictive values were 30% and 95%, respectively. Hence, the serology test, used as the "gold standard" in this study, is not perfect.

11.1.2 Binary Tine Test for Tuberculosis

Hui and Walter (1980) provided data on the accuracy of a new binary-scale skin Tine test in detecting tuberculosis against the binary-scale reference standard, the Mantoux skin test. For each study subject, both were applied to the subject's forearm. The presence of an induration larger than a fixed size after 48 hours of administering a skin test constitutes a positive result. Both tests were applied to a southern U.S. school district population and the Missouri State Sanatorium population. Pouchot et al. (1997) have shown that the Mantoux skin test, the reference standard, itself has many potential sources of error and variability, such as standardization of the tuberculin reagent, the meaning of the test results, and the reading of the test. Hence, estimation of diagnostic accuracy of the Tine skin test, using the Mantoux skin test as a gold standard, is subject to imperfect gold standard bias.

11.1.3 Binary-Scale X-rays for Pleural Thickening

Irwig et al. (1979) conducted a study on the accuracy of chest X-rays in detecting the presence of pleural thickening. One goal of this study was to estimate the sensitivities and specificities of the three radiologists in interpreting X-rays in the absence of any reference standard. Three experienced radiologists independently evaluated the chest X-rays of 1692 male workers in South African asbestos mines for the presence/absence of pleural thickening according to the ILO U/C International Classification of Radiographs of pneumoconioses. Their responses, based on the chest X-rays, are binary. In this study, no reference standard was used.

11.1.4 Bioassays for HIV

Alvord et al. (1988) studied the sensitivity and specificity of four conventional bioassays for detecting HIV infection without the use of any reference standard: an enzyme-linked immunosorbent assay (ELISA) and three radioim-munoassay (RIA) tests utilizing recombinant antigen ag1, p24, and gp120, denoted by RIA1, RIA2, and RIA3, respectively. In this study, serum samples of each patient were tested by the four tests. One goal of this study was to estimate the sensitivity and specificity of the four binary tests in the absence of a gold standard.

11.1.5 Ordinal-Scale Evaluation by Pathologists for Detecting Carcinoma in Situ of the Uterine Cervix

Holmquist et al. (1967) studied variability in detection of carcinoma in situ of the uterine cervix among seven study pathologists. During the period July 1, 1964 through June 30, 1965, the seven study pathologists at Louisiana State University Medical Center independently evaluated and classified lesions on each of the 118 randomly ordered slides into a five category ordinal-scale result, ranging from 1 (negative) to 5 (invasive carcinoma). In this study, there was a clinical definition of carcinoma in situ of the uterine cervix. However, due to technological limitations, diagnosis based on the clinical definition was not available. The original data were given in Landis and Koch (1977), who assessed variability in detection of carcinoma among the seven readers using Kappa agreement measures. However, the agreement information cannot be translated into the accuracy information. For example, while the seven readers might agree on the disease status of a patient, they all could be wrong. We would be interested in estimating the ROC curves and associated areas of the seven pathologists in the absence of a reference standard.

11.1.6 Ordinal-Scale and Continuous-Scale MRA for Carotid Artery Stenosis

As described as Case Study 3 in Chapter 1, Masaryk et al. (2007) reported a study on the accuracy of Magnetic Resonance Angiography (MRA) for detecting carotid artery plaque. Each patient in the study first underwent an MRA, then a conventional catheter angiogram. Four radiologists from three institutions independently interpreted the conventional catheter angiograms, and the same four radiologists independently interpreted the MRA images. The conventional catheter angiograms were used as a gold standard to define a significant stenosis requiring surgical intervention as stenosis that blocked 60-99 percent of the carotid vessel.

Using an MRA, the radiologists were asked to grade their confidence that a significant stenosis was present using a 5-point scale as well as to indicate the percent of stenosis present (a number between 0 and 100). Since the "gold standard" for this study, catheter angiography, is not a perfect test, we need to correct for the imperfect gold standard bias in estimating the accuracy of the MRA.

11.2   IMPACT OF IMPERFECT GOLD STANDARD BIAS

To illustrate how imperfect gold standard bias operates and affects the estimated accuracy of a test, we consider two hypothetical examples. The first example shows how the true sensitivity and specificity of a new test may be underestimated, and the second example shows how the true sensitivity and specificity of a new test may be overestimated. In the first example, the new test is evaluated against an imperfect gold standard that has sensitivity of 90% and specificity of 70%. Assume that the new test and imperfect gold standard are conditionally independent given the condition status and that the actual sensitivity and specificity of the new test (which we need to estimate) are 80% and 60%, respectively. The conditional independence assumption (CIA) means that classification errors made by the new test and imperfect gold standard occur independently, given the true disease status. Suppose the study population consists of 100 patients with the condition and 100 patients without the condition. Since the imperfect standard has a sensitivity of 90% and a specificity of 70%, of all study patients with the condition, 90 respond positively and 10 respond negatively to the imperfect standard; of all study patients without the condition, 30 respond positively and 70 respond negatively to the imperfect standard. Given that the sensitivity of the new test is 80%, when it is applied to the 90 patients with the condition who have a positive test on the imperfect gold standard, 72 respond p̲   ̱ ̰ ̱ᵗᵒ ᵗʰᵉ new test and the remaining 18 respond negatively. Since the sᵖ test is 60%, when it is applied to the 30 patients withou are wrongly diagnosed as positive by the imperfect gold positive result to the new test and the other 18 have a ᵣ larly, in the 70 patients without the condition who have ₐ imperfect gold standard, 28 respond positively to the nᵢ 42 respond negatively. Of the 10 patients with the cond diagnosed as negative by the imperfect gold standard to the new test and the other 2 respond negatively. Table 11.1 ₛᵤₘₘ the cross-classification results of the new test and imperfect gold standard. Using the imperfect gold test as a "gold standard", the estimated sensitivity and specificity of the new test would be 70% ($84/120$) and 55% ($44/80$), respectively, considerably less than its true sensitivity and specificity.

The second example uses an imperfect gold standard with a sensitivity of 90% and a specificity of 90%. The new test and reference standard are conditionally dependent given the condition status, which means that they have a tendency to make misdiagnoses in the same patients. We assume that 10% of patients with the condition produce negative results with both the new test and the imperfect gold standard, that none of the patients with the condition yield a positive result with the new test and a negative result with the imperfect gold standard, and that 10% of patients with the condition yield negative results with the new test and positive results with the imperfect gold standard. Similarly, for patients without the condition, we assume that 10%

[handwritten margin note: are most conditionally dependent or independent]

Table 11.1   Results of a New Test (T) and an Imperfect Gold Standard (R) with Known Sensitivity of 90% and Specificity of 70%

| Reference test | Diagnostic results | | Total |
	T=1	T=0	
R=1	84	36	120
R=0	36	44	80
Total	120	80	200

of them produce positive results with both the new test and imperfect gold standard, that none of them yield a negative result with the new test and a positive result with the imperfect gold standard, and that 10% of them yield positive results with the new test and negative results with the imperfect gold standard. Table 11.2 summarizes the joint probability of the test and imperfect reference standard given the true condition status. The actual sensitivity

Table 11.2   Conditional Joint Probability of a New Test (T) and an Imperfect Gold Standard (R) Given the Condition Status (D)

| Reference test | $D=1$ | | $D=0$ | |
	T=1	T=0	T=1	T=0
R=1	0.8	0.1	0.1	0.0
R=0	0.0	0.1	0.1	0.8

and specificity of the new test (which we need to estimate) is 80% and 80%, respectively. Suppose the study population consists of 100 patients with the condition and 100 patients without the condition. Using similar reasoning as in the first example, we get the cross-classification results of the new test and imperfect gold standard, summarized in Table 11.3. Using the imperfect

Table 11.3   Classification of Results by T and R Based on the Conditional Joint Probability Given in Table (11.2)

| Reference test | Diagnostic results | | Total |
	T=1	T=0	
R=1	90	10	100
R=0	10	90	100
Total	100	100	200

gold test as a "gold standard", the estimated sensitivity and specificity of the new test would be 90% (90/100) and 90% (90/100), respectively, considerably higher than its true sensitivity and specificity.

In general, if a test and an imperfect gold standard are conditionally independent, the test's sensitivity and specificity are underestimated. When a test and an imperfect gold standard are conditionally dependent, the estimated sensitivity and specificity of the test against the imperfect standard can be biased in either direction. The direction of the bias is determined by the degree to which the test and standard tend to missclassify the same patients. When this tendency is slight, the accuracy of the test is generally underestimated; when the tendency is strong, the accuracy of the test is generally overestimated (Valenstein, 1990; Vacek, 1985; Torrance-Rynard and Walter, 1997).

11.3 ONE SINGLE BINARY TEST IN A SINGLE POPULATION

When we are interested in assessing the accuracy of a single binary test against an imperfect gold standard, we run into a model non-identifiability problem, which occurs when different sets of parameter values correspond to the one same distribution of observed data. Model identification is a necessary condition for many nice asymptotic properties associated with model-based parameter estimators, such as root-n-consistency.

To overcome estimation problem of a non-identified model, frequentist methods impose additional constraints on the parameters in the model, and Bayesian methods assume a proper prior distribution and make inferences on parameters, based on the posterior distribution. In order to obtain useful parameter estimates, the Bayesian methods need to elicit an informative prior on at least as many parameters as would be constrained when using the frequentist method (Dendukuri and Joseph, 2001).

In this section, we discuss the issue of model identifiability and both the frequentist and Bayesian methods for estimating the accuracy of a single binary test with an imperfect gold standard. Let $D = 1$ indicate a patient with the condition, and $D = 0$ a patient without the condition. Let T and R represent results of a new diagnostic test and an imperfect gold standard, respectively, where $T = 1$ indicates a positive test result, and $T = 0$ a negative test result; similarly, $R = 1$ indicates a positive result from the imperfect gold standard, and $R = 0$ a negative result from the imperfect gold standard. The observed data may be displayed as in Table 11.4.

If we denote $p_{tr} = P(T = t, R = r)$, the observed data may be modeled by a multinomial distribution with cell probabilities, p_{tr}, where $t, r = 0, 1$.

Let $Se(T)$ and $Sp(T)$ denote the true sensitivity and specificity of a new test, and let $Se(R)$ and $Sp(R)$ be the sensitivity and specificity of an imperfect gold standard. That is,

$$Se(T) = P(T = 1 \mid D = 1),\ Sp(T) = P(T = 0 \mid D = 0),$$

$$Se(R) = P(R = 1 \mid D = 1),\ Sp(R) = P(R = 0 \mid D = 0).$$

Table 11.4   A General Data Structure For a Single Test and Imperfect Gold Standard

Reference test	Diagnostic results	
	T=1	T=0
R=1	s_{11}	s_{10}
R=0	s_{01}	s_{00}
Total	n_1	n_0

Let $\pi = P(D = 1)$ denote the prevalence, and define conditional models for T and R, given D, as follows:

$$\eta_{0,tr} = P(T = t, R = r \mid D = 0), \eta_{1,tr} = P(T = t, R = r \mid D = 1).$$

Hence, the model parameters include π, $\eta_{0,tr}$, and $\eta_{1,tr}$, where $t, r = 0, 1$.

11.3.1   Conditions for Model Identifiability

Note the following relationship between p_{tr} and the model parameters:

$$p_{tr} = \pi\eta_{0,tr} + (1 - \pi)\eta_{1,tr}, \tag{11.1}$$

where $(t, r) = (1, 1), (1, 0), (0, 1)$. Since $\sum_{t,r=0} p_{tr} = 1$, we stack p_{tr}'s, except p_{00} into a single q-dimensional vector $p = (p_{11}, p_{10}, p_{01})'$, where $q = 3$. We stack $\eta_{0,tr}$'s, $\eta_{1,tr}$'s, and π into a r-dimensional vector,

$$\theta = (\eta_{1,11}, \eta_{1,10}, \eta_{1,01}, \eta_{1,00}, \eta_{0,11}, \eta_{0,10}, \eta_{0,01}, \eta_{0,00}, \pi)',$$

where $r = 9$. Here θ is the vector of model parameters. Based on (11.1), the model specifies a mapping F from $\mathcal{R}^q$ to $\mathcal{R}^r$ such that

$$p = F(\theta). \tag{11.2}$$

The model is identifiable if F is invertible; that is, the model is identifiable if we can determine a unique θ for a given p. Let us define $J(\theta)$ as the $q \times r$ Jacobian matrix of the mapping function F at θ; that is, $J(\theta) = \partial F(\theta)/\partial\theta$. If the Jacobian matrix $J(\theta)$ has a full column rank for all θ, the model (11.1) is identifiable. If not, the model (11.1) is not identifiable.

One necessary condition for the model (11.1) being identifiable is that the number of parameters in the model is less than or equal to the degrees of freedom. However, even when the number of parameters is less than or equal to the degrees of freedom, the model (11.1) is not automatically identifiable. To show that a model like (11.1) is identifiable, we need to show that the Jacobian matrix $J(\theta)$ has full column rank.

Applying the above principle to our case, we conclude that the model (11.1) is not identifiable. To reduce the number of unknown parameters, we usually make the conditional independence assumption (CIA) of the errors between the new test and the imperfect gold standard; that is,

$$P(R, T \mid D) = P(R \mid D)P(T \mid D). \tag{11.3}$$

The CIA means that the test and standard are not prone to misdiagnose the same patients.

Under the CIA, the equation (11.1) becomes the following equations:

$$p_{11} = \pi Se(T)Se(R) + (1 - \pi)(1 - Sp(T))(1 - Sp(R)),$$

$$p_{10} = \pi Se(T)(1 - Se(R)) + (1 - \pi)(1 - Sp(T))Sp(R),$$

$$p_{01} = \pi(1 - Se(T))Se(R) + (1 - \pi)Sp(T)(1 - Sp(R)). \tag{11.4}$$

Even with the CIA, the system of equations (11.4) still has 5 parameters with only three equations. Hence, these five parameters are still not identifiable. We need to further assume two of these parameters are known to obtain an identifiable model. Since the parameters of interest are the sensitivity and specificity of the new test, T, we usually consider three common cases to derive an identifiable model: (1) the sensitivity and specificity of the imperfect gold standard, $Se(R)$ and $Sp(R)$, are known; (2) the sensitivities of both the new test and reference standard are 100%; (3) the specificities of both the new test and reference standard are 100%. Under these additional assumptions, we can show that the Jacobian matrix $J(\theta)$ has a full column rank.

11.3.2 The Frequentist-Based ML Method Under an Identifiable Model

In this section, we derive the ML estimators for the sensitivity and specificity of the new test under the conditional independence assumption and the assumption that $Se(R)$ and $Sp(R)$ are known. Under these two assumptions, the likelihood, based on the observed data, is given as follows:

$$L = \{Se(R)Se(T)\pi + (1 - Sp(R))(1 - Sp(T))(1 - \pi)\}^{s_{11}}$$

$$\times \{Se(R)(1 - Se(T))\pi + (1 - Sp(R))Sp(T)(1 - \pi)\}^{s_{10}}$$

$$\times \{(1 - Se(R))Se(T)\pi + Sp(R)(1 - Sp(T))(1 - \pi)\}^{s_{01}}$$

$$\times \{(1 - Se(R))(1 - Se(T))\pi + Sp(R)Sp(T)(1 - \pi)\}^{s_{00}}. \tag{11.5}$$

By maximizing the above likelihood function with respect to $Se(T)$, $Sp(T)$, and π, we obtain the ML estimators of the sensitivity and specificity of the new test as well as the disease prevalence rate as follows:

$$\widehat{Se}(T) = \frac{Sp(R)(s_{11} + s_{01}) - s_{01}}{NSp(R) - (s_{01} + s_{00})}, \widehat{Sp}(T) = \frac{Se(R)(s_{10} + s_{00}) - s_{10}}{NSe(R) - (s_{11} + s_{10})},$$

$$\widehat{\pi} = \frac{NSp(R) - (s_{01} + s_{00})}{N},$$

respectively, where N is the total number of study patients.

11.3.3   Bayesian Methods Under a Non-Identifiable Model

Instead of imposing constraints on parameters, we may use a Bayesian approach to estimation of sensitivity and specificity of the tests by first imposing a prior distribution for all unknown parameters (Johnson and Gastwirth, 1991; Joseph et al., 1995). In the Bayesian method, the uncertainty about each parameter in θ is summarized in a prior distribution, which is utilized to differentiate between the numerous possible solutions to the system of equations (11.1) for the non-identifiable model.

Although Bayesian inferences based on the posterior distribution can provide useful estimates for the sensitivity and specificity of the new test and the imperfect gold standard if a proper prior is correctly specified, the resulting estimates can be greatly affected by a change in the prior distribution, regardless of how large the sample size is. In addition, Dendukuri and Joseph (2001) pointed out that to obtain useful Bayesian inferences, one needs to specify informative priors on at least as many parameters as one would need to put constraints on when using the frequentist approach.

Next, we discuss how to apply a Bayesian approach to estimation of sensitivity and specificity of the tests under the conditional independence assumption (CIA) and then describe a Bayesian approach without the CIA. Under the CIA, from (11.5) we see that we have five parameters: $Se(R)$, $Se(T)$, $Sp(R)$, $Sp(T)$, and π. We assume independent conjugate beta priors for knowledge of these parameters:

$$Se(R) \sim beta(\alpha_{R1}, \beta_{R1}), Sp(R) \sim beta(\alpha_{R2}, \beta_{R2}),$$

$$Se(T) \sim beta(\alpha_{T1}, \beta_{T1}), Sp(T) \sim beta(\alpha_{T2}, \beta_{T2}), \pi \sim beta(\alpha_{\pi}, \beta_{\pi}),$$

where $beta(\alpha, \beta)$ denotes a beta distribution with the following density function:

$$f(x) = \begin{cases} \frac{\Gamma(\alpha)\Gamma(\beta)}{\Gamma(\alpha+\beta)} x^{\alpha-1}(1-x)^{\beta-1} & \text{if } 0 \leq x \leq 1 \\ 0 & \text{otherwise} \end{cases},$$

with $\Gamma(\cdot)$ being the gamma function. Then, the joint posterior density distribution is proportional to

$$Se(R)^{\alpha_{R1}-1}(1 - Se(R))^{\beta_{R1}-1} Sp(R)^{\alpha_{R2}-1}(1 - Sp(R))^{\beta_{R2}-1}$$
$$\times Se(T)^{\alpha_{T1}-1}(1 - Se(T))^{\beta_{T1}-1} Sp(T)^{\alpha_{T2}-1}(1 - Sp(T))^{\beta_{T2}-1}$$
$$\times \pi^{\alpha_{\pi}-1}(1 - \pi)^{\beta_{\pi}} L(\theta), \qquad (11.6)$$

where $L(\theta)$ is defined by (11.5). Since the likelihood function $L(\theta)$ has a complicated form, involving mixture structures, it is difficult to compute this posterior distribution directly. To compute this posterior distribution, Joseph et al. (1995) used the method of augmented data with a Gibbs sampler (Tanner, 1993). To see why this augmented data approach allows us to easily compute this posterior distribution, we define Y_{jk} to be the unobserved number of patients with the condition out of the observed cell value s_{jk} in the 2x2 data of Table 11.4. Then, the number of patients without the condition out of the observed cell value s_{jk} is $s_{jk} - Y_{jk}$. Denote $\mathbf{s} = (s_{jk}, j, k = 0, 1)$ and $Y = (Y_{jk}, j, k = 0, 1)$. Then, the likelihood function of the augmented data $(\mathbf{s}, Y)$ has a very simple form,

$$(Se(R))^{Y_{11}+Y_{10}} (1 - Se(R))^{Y_{01}+Y_{00}} (Se(T))^{Y_{11}+Y_{01}} (1 - Se(T))^{Y_{10}+Y_{00}}$$
$$\times (Sp(R))^{s_{00}-Y_{00}+s_{01}-Y_{01}} (1 - Sp(R))^{s_{11}-Y_{11}+s_{10}-Y_{10}}$$
$$\times (Sp(T))^{s_{00}-Y_{00}+s_{10}-Y_{10}} (1 - Sp(T))^{s_{11}-Y_{11}+s_{01}-Y_{01}}$$
$$\times (\pi)^{Y_{00}+Y_{01}+Y_{10}+Y_{11}} (1 - \pi)^{n-Y_{00}-Y_{01}-Y_{10}-Y_{11}}. \quad (11.7)$$

With a conjugate beta prior distribution for θ, the corresponding posterior distribution of θ, given the augmented data, also has a simple form and is proportional to

$$(Se(R))^{Y_{11}+Y_{10}+\alpha_{R1}-1} (1 - Se(R))^{Y_{01}+Y_{00}+\beta_{R1}-1}$$

$$\times (Se(T))^{Y_{11}+Y_{01}+\alpha_{T1}-1} (1 - Se(T))^{Y_{10}+Y_{00}+\beta_{T1}-1}$$

$$\times (Sp(R))^{s_{00}-Y_{00}+s_{01}-Y_{01}+\alpha_{R2}-1} (1 - Sp(R))^{s_{11}-Y_{11}+s_{10}-Y_{10}+\beta_{R2}-1}$$

$$\times (Sp(T))^{s_{00}-Y_{00}+s_{10}-Y_{10}+\alpha_{T2}-1} (1 - Sp(T))^{s_{11}-Y_{11}+s_{01}-Y_{01}+\beta_{T2}-1}$$

$$\times (\pi)^{Y_{00}+Y_{01}+Y_{10}+Y_{11}+\alpha_p-1} (1 - \pi)^{n-Y_{00}-Y_{01}-Y_{10}-Y_{11}+\beta_p-1}. \quad (11.8)$$

From (11.8), a Gibbs sampler allows us to generate a random sample from the posterior distribution of any parameter of interest, such as the sensitivity of T. See Joseph et al. (1995) for more detail on this Gibbs sampling method.

Without the CIA, Jones et al. (2010) proposed a Bayesian method that takes into account the possible dependence between test and imperfect gold standard, conditional on the disease status. They proposed two methods - the fixed effects and random effects models - to account for the conditional dependence between T and R. Let us denote the covariance between T and S among the diseased and nondiseased subjects by $covs_{12}$ and $covc_{12}$, respectively. Vacek (1985) has shown that the conditional joint probabilities of T and R, given D, can be expressed in the following forms:

$$\eta_{1,11} = Se(T)Se(R) + covs_{12}, \eta_{1,10} = Se(T)(1 - Se(R)) - covs_{12},$$

$$\eta_{1,01} = (1 - Se(T))Se(R) - covs_{12}, \eta_{1,00} = (1 - Se(T))(1 - Se(R)) + covs_{12},$$

$$\eta_{0,11} = (1 - Sp(T))(1 - Sp(R)) - covc_{12}, \eta_{0,10} = (1 - Sp(T))(1 - Se(R)) - covc_{12},$$

$$\eta_{0,01} = (1 - Se(T))Se(R) - covc_{12}, \eta_{0,00} = (1 - Se(T))(1 - Se(R)) + covc_{12}.$$

Without assuming the CIA, under the fixed effects model, we have now a vector of seven unknown parameters, $Se(T)$, $Sp(T)$, $Se(R)$, $Se(T)$, $covs_{12}$, $covc_{12}$, π, denoted by θ. Dendukuri and Joseph (2001) proposed the use of the same prior for $Se(T)$, $Sp(T)$, $Se(R)$, $Se(T)$, and π as in Joseph et al. (1995)

under the CIA. For additional parameters, $covs_{12}$ and $covc_{12}$, Dendukuri and Joseph (2001) used the following generalized beta prior distributions:

$$covs_{12} \sim genbeta(\alpha_{covs_{12}}, \beta_{covs_{12}}),$$

where $0 \leq covs_{12} \leq min(Se(T), Se(R)) - Se(T)Se(R)$ and

$$covc_{12} \sim genbeta(\alpha_{covc_{12}}, \beta_{covc_{12}}),$$

where $0 \leq covc_{12} \leq min(Sp(T), Sp(R)) - Sp(T)Sp(R)$. Using the same Gibbs sampling algorithm as the one for the CIA, described above, we can obtain the marginal posterior distribution of each parameter.

The second way to model the conditional dependence of T and R, given D, uses a random effect model, which assumes there is a latent variable ξ such that conditional on D and ξ, T and R are independent. Specifically, the random effects model assumes that

$$P(T, R \mid D, \xi) = P(T \mid D, \xi)P(R \mid D, \xi),$$

$$P(T = 1 \mid D = d, \xi) = \Phi(a_{1d} + b_{1d}\xi), P(R = 1 \mid D = d, \xi) = \Phi(a_{2d} + b_{2d}\xi),$$

$$\xi \sim N(0, 1).$$

Under the random effects model for the conditional dependence of T and R, given D, the vector of parameters is $\theta = (\pi, a_{10}, b_{10}, a_{20}, b_{20}, a_{11}, b_{11}, a_{21}, b_{21})'$. Dendukuri and Joseph (2001) proposed the following prior for θ: a beta prior distribution for π; a bivariate normal distribution for (a_{jd}, b_{jd}) with mean (A_{jd}, B_{jd}) and diagonal variance-covariance matrix $\begin{pmatrix} \sigma_{ajd}^2 & 0 \\ 0 & \sigma_{bjd}^2 \end{pmatrix}$, where $d = 0, 1$ and $j = 1, 2$. As in the case of the fixed-effects model, Dendukuri and Joseph (2001) used a Gibbs sampler to obtain samples from the marginal posterior distribution of θ. BUGS code for implementing these Bayesian methods can be found at the website for the book (http://faculty.washington.edu/azhou/books/diagnostic.html).

11.3.4   Analysis of Strongyloides Infection Example

In this section, we illustrate the application of the Bayesian methods, described in Section 11.3.2, in the study of the accuracy of stool examination in detecting Strongyloides infection among Cambodian refugees, described in Section 11.1.1. Table 11.5 displays the results of stool examination and serology test in 162 Cambodian refugees.

Joseph et al. (1995) used a Bayesian approach to estimate sensitivities and specificities of both stool examination and serology tests under the CIA. To apply the Bayesian analysis, one first needs to assign a prior distribution for all parameters, which include the sensitivity and specificity of each test, as well as the prevalence of Strongyloides infection. Joseph et al. (1995) chose a prior

Table 11.5   Results by Stool Examination (T) and Serologic Test (R) for Strongyloides Infection

Reference test	Diagnostic results		Total
	T=1	T=0	
R=1	38	87	125
R=0	2	35	37
Total	40	122	162

distribution by first determining equal-tailed 95 percent probability intervals for sensitivity and specificity of each test from a review of published literature and clinical opinion. They then matched the mean and the standard deviation of the beta distribution with the center of the range and one quarter of the total range, respectively. These two requirements gave unique values of α and β parameters in a beta distribution. Since very little was known about the prevalence of Strongyloids infection among the Cambodian refugees, Joseph et al. (1995) used a uniform prior over the range [0,1], which was equivalent to a beta distribution with $\alpha = \beta = 1$. We summarize this process of choosing a prior in Table 11.6.

Table 11.6   Results by Stool Examination (T) and Serologic test (R) For Strongyloides Infection

	Serology test			Stool examination		
	Range (%)	α	β	Range (%)	α	β
Sensitivity	65-95	21.96	5.49	5-45	4.44	13.31
Specificity	35-100	4.1	1.76	90-100	71.25	3.75
	Range		α		β	
Prevalence	0-100		1		1	

Applying the Bayesian method with the prior distribution given in Table 11.6, Joseph et al. (1995) obtained the posterior distribution of the parameters, which in turn gave us the median estimates for each parameter and its corresponding 95% credible interval. These results, along with the chosen priors, are summarized in Table 11.7. The results show that the stool examination has a low sensitivity and a high specificity.

Without the CIA, Joseph et al. (1995) applied the Bayesian method with a fixed-effects model for the conditional dependence, as discussed in Section 11.3.3, to the data set. The results are reported in Table 11.8.

The estimated values for the sensitivity and specificity of the stool examination under the assumed conditional dependence model are similar to those derived under the conditional independence model. However, the specificity

Table 11.7   Marginal Prior and Posterior Medians and Equal-tailed 95% Credible Intervals in Strongyloides Infection Example Under the CIA

Test	Parameter	Prior information		Posterior results	
	Prevalence	0.50	0.03-0.98	0.76	0.52-0.91
Stool examination	$S_e(T)$	0.24	0.07-0.47	0.31	0.22-0.44
	$S_p(T)$	0.95	0.89-0.99	0.96	0.91-0.99
Serology test	$S_e(R)$	0.81	0.63-0.92	0.89	0.80-0.95
	$S_p(R)$	0.72	0.31-0.96	0.67	0.36-0.95

Table 11.8   Marginal Prior and Posterior Medians and Equal-tailed 95% Credible Intervals in Strongyloides Infection Example Under a Conditional Dependence Model

Test	Parameter	Prior information		Posterior results	
	Prevalence	0.50	0.03-0.98	0.78	0.63-0.89
Stool examination	$S_e(T)$	0.24	0.07-0.47	0.34	0.25-0.44
	$S_p(T)$	0.95	0.89-0.99	0.92	0.78-0.98
Serology test	$S_e(R)$	0.81	0.63-0.92	0.91	0.81-0.97
	$S_p(R)$	0.72	0.31-0.96	0.81	0.56-0.96

of the serology test, the imperfect reference standard, has a higher estimate under the conditional dependence model than the one derived under the conditional independence model.

11.4   ONE SINGLE BINARY TEST IN G POPULATIONS

In this section, we discuss imperfect gold standard bias correction methods when both the new test and reference test are applied to each individual from G populations $(G \geq 2)$.

Let X be the subpopulation indicator ($X = g$ corresponds to Population g). Let $Se(1, g)$ and $Sp(1, g)$ be the sensitivity and specificity of the new test in the gth population, and let $Se(2, g)$ and $Sp(2, g)$ be the sensitivity and specificity of the reference test in the gth population. Let π_g be the prevalence of the condition in the gth population and $\xi_g = P(X = g)$. We define conditional models for T and R, given D and X as follows:

$$\eta_{0,tr,g} = P(T = t, R = r \mid D = 1, X = g),$$

and

$$\eta_{1,tr,g} = P(T = t, R = r \mid D = 0, X = g).$$

Hence, the model parameters include π, $\eta_{0,tr,g}$, $\eta_{1,tr,g}$, π_g, and ξ_g, where $(t,r) = (0,1), (1,0), (1,1)$, and $g = 1, \ldots, G$. Let $p_{tr,g} = P(T = t, R = r, X = g)$. Note that there is a relationship between $p_{tr,g}$ and the model parameters,

$$p_{tr,g} = (\pi_g \eta_{0,tr,g} + (1 - \pi_g)\eta_{1,tr,g})\xi_g. \tag{11.9}$$

Similar to Section 11.3.1, we stack probabilities of observing T, R, and X, $p_{tr,g}$'s, except $p_{00,0}$, into a single q-dimensional vector p, where $q = 4G$. We also stack the corresponding model parameters, $\eta_{0,tr,g}$'s and $\eta_{1,tr,g}$'s, π_g, and ξ_g, where $(t,r) \neq (0,1)$ and $g \neq 0$, into a r-dimensional vector θ, where $r = 6G$. Let F be the mapping from $\mathcal{R}^q$ to $\mathcal{R}^r$ such that

$$p = F(\theta). \tag{11.10}$$

As in Section 11.3.1, the model (11.9) is identifiable if the Jacobian matrix of $F(\theta)$ has a full column rank for all θ.

11.4.1   Estimation Methods

To make model (11.10) identifiable, we often assume the conditional independence assumption (CIA). Under the CIA,

$$P(T, R \mid D, X) = P(T \mid D, X)P(R \mid D, X), \tag{11.11}$$

the log-likelihood function has the following form:

$$l = \sum_{g=1}^{G} N_g \log \xi_g + \sum_{g=1}^{G} \sum_{k=1}^{N_g} \log[\prod_{i=1}^{2}(Se(i,g))^{t_{ikg}}(1 - Se(i,g))^{1-t_{ikg}}\pi_g$$

$$+ \prod_{i=1}^{2}(1 - Sp(i,g))^{t_{ikg}}(Sp(i,g))^{1-t_{ikg}}(1 - \pi_g)], \tag{11.12}$$

where π_g is the prevalence of the condition in the gth population and $\xi_g = P(X = g)$. The data provide $4G - 1$ degrees of freedom for $6G - 1$ parameters. Therefore, not all parameters are estimable. To reduce the number of unknown parameters, Hui and Walter (1980) assumed that the error rate for each test was the same in each population ($Se(i,g) = Se(i)$ and $Sp(i,g) = Sp(i)$). With this assumption, the log-likelihood (11.12) becomes

$$l = \sum_{g=1}^{G} N_g \log \xi_g + \sum_{g=1}^{G} \sum_{k=1}^{N_g} \log[\prod_{i=1}^{2}(Se(i))^{t_{ikg}}(1 - Se(i))^{1-t_{ikg}}\pi_g +$$

$$\prod_{i=1}^{2}(1 - Sp(i))^{t_{ikg}}(Sp(i))^{1-t_{ikg}}(1 - \pi_g)]. \tag{11.13}$$

The log-likelihood (11.13) contains $2G + 3$ parameters, which is equal to the degrees of freedom when $G = 2$ and is less than the degrees of freedom when $G > 2$. Even when the number of parameters does not exceed the degrees of freedom, the log-likelihood (11.13) does not have a unique ML solution because both $(\widehat{\pi}_g, \widehat{Se}(i), \widehat{Sp}(i))$ and $(1-\widehat{\pi}_g, 1-\widehat{Se}(i), 1-\widehat{Sp}(i))$ are ML estimates. To obtain the unique ML estimates, Hui and Walter (1980) introduced the following constraint:

$$Sp(i) + Se(i) > 1.$$

Under this constraint and when $G = 2$, Hui and Walter (1980) derived closed-form expressions for the unique ML estimates of the prevalence rates and the error rates of both tests, and they also derived variances for the ML estimators, based on the expected information matrix.

The validity of Hui and Walter's estimators relies on two critical assumptions: (1) availability of two populations with equal test accuracy and different prevalences, and (2) the conditional independence of tests given the condition status. When either of these two assumptions is violated, Hui and Walter's estimators are biased. Sinclair (1989) showed Hui and Walter's procedure can either underestimate or overestimate test error rates, depending on the magnitudes of the true error rates. Vacek (1985) showed that if the test errors are not independent and equal in both subpopulations, Hui and Walter's procedure can substantially underestimate the test error rates. When $G > 2$, it may be difficult to derive a closed-form expression for the ML estimators from (11.13). Alternatively, iterative numerical algorithms are often used. Two such algorithms are the weighted least squares algorithm and the EM algorithm. The method of weighted least squares (WLS) obtains estimates by minimizing the objective function, which is equal to the weighted sum of squares between the observed frequencies and their expected values, with the weights equal to the inverse of the expected cell frequencies. Sinclair (1989) showed the resulting WLS estimates are equivalent to ML estimates.

Let $Se^{(m)}(i)$, $Sp^{(m)}(i)$, $\pi_g^{(m)}$, and $\xi^{(m)}$ be current values of parameters $Se(i)$, $Sp(i)$, π_g, and ξ after m iterations in the EM algorithm. The next iteration estimates are given by

$$Se^{(m+1)}(i) = \frac{\sum_{g=1}^{G} \sum_{k=1}^{N_g} t_{ikg} q_{kg}^{(m)}}{\sum_{g=1}^{G} \sum_{k=1}^{N_g} q_{kg}^{(m)}},$$

$$Sp^{(m+1)}(i) = \frac{\sum_{g=1}^{G} \sum_{k=1}^{N_g} (1 - t_{ikg})(1 - q_{kg}^{(m)})}{\sum_{g=1}^{G} \sum_{k=1}^{N_g} (1 - q_{kg}^{(m)})},$$

$$\pi_g^{(m+1)} = \frac{\sum_{k=1}^{N_g} q_{kg}^{(m)}}{N_g}, \xi^{(m+1)} = \frac{N_g}{\sum_{g=1}^{G} N_g}. \tag{11.14}$$

Here

$$q_{kg}^{(m)} = \frac{A}{A + B}, \tag{11.15}$$

where

$$A = \prod_{i=1}^{2} (Se^{(m)}(i))^{t_{ikg}} (1 - Se^{(m)}(i))^{1-t_{ikg}} \pi_g^{(m)},$$

and

$$B = \prod_{i=1}^{2} (1 - Sp^{(m)}(i))^{t_{ikg}} (Sp^{(m)}(i))^{1-t_{ikg}} (1 - \pi_g^{(m)}).$$

We iterate this process until the estimates converge. The convergent values $\widehat{Se}(i)$, $\widehat{Sp}(i)$, and $\widehat{\pi}_g$ are ML estimates for $Se(i)$, $Sp(i)$, and π_g.

The output of the EM algorithm does not provide a direct estimate for the asymptotic covariance matrix of $\widehat{Se}$, $\widehat{Sp}$, and $\widehat{\pi}$. One way of estimating this covariance matrix is to first compute the expected Fisher information matrix using the log-likelihood function, given by (11.12). Then, its inverse provides an estimate for the covariance matrix of the ML estimates (Little and Rubin, 1987).

We next describe a Bayesian method to estimate sensitivities and specificities of the new test and reference test under the same assumptions as the ones for the ML-based method. The sampled data from the gth population can be represented by $y_g = (y_{11g}, y_{10g}, y_{01g}, y_{00g})$, where y_{11g} (y_{00g}) is the number of sample subjects from the gth population who have positive (negative) results on both the new and reference tests, and y_{10g} (y_{01g}) is the number of subjects sampled from the gth population who have positive (negative) results on the new test but negative (positive) results on the reference test. Let $p_{tr|g} = P(T = t, R = r \mid X = g)$. We assume that the observed data from the G populations follow G independent multinomial distributions:

$$y_g \sim \text{multinomial}(n_g, (p_{11|g}, p_{10|g}, p_{01|g}, p_{00|g})), g = 1, \ldots, G, \qquad (11.16)$$

where $n_g = y_{11,g} + y_{10,g} + y_{01,g} + y_{00,g}$. Under the CIA, we have the following model

$$p_{11|g} = \pi_g Se(1)Se(2) + (1 - \pi_g)(1 - Sp(1))(1 - Sp(2)),$$

$$p_{12|g} = \pi_g Se(1)(1 - Se(2)) + (1 - \pi_g)(1 - Sp(1))Sp(2),$$

$$p_{21|g} = \pi_g(1 - Se(1))Se(2) + (1 - \pi_g)Sp(1)(1 - Sp(2)),$$

$$p_{22|g} = \pi_g(1 - Se(1))(1 - Se(2)) + (1 - \pi_g)Sp(1)Sp(2). \qquad (11.17)$$

In the model (11.17), we have $4+G$ parameters, denoted by θ. To complete the Bayesian specification, we need to assume beta prior distributions for θ. To allow possible zero disease prevalence in the gth population, Branscum et al. (2005) assumed π_g had a mixture of point mass at zero with a probability $1 - \pi_{g0}$ and a continuous beta distribution, $beta(a_{\pi g}, b_{\pi g})$, with probability π_{g0}. The independent beta prior distributions for two sensitivities and two specificities are given as follows:

$$Se(1) \sim beta(a_{Se1}, b_{Se1}), Se(2) \sim beta(a_{Se1}, b_{Se2}),$$

$$Sp(1) \sim beta(a_{Sp1}, b_{Sp1}), Sp(2) \sim beta(a_{Sp1}, b_{Sp2}).$$

Then the MCMC method can be used to obtain samples from the posterior distributions for the parameters of interest.

Without assuming the conditional independence assumption, like in Section 11.3.3, we can also use a Bayesian approach under either an identifiable or non-identifiable model to estimate sensitivities and specificities of the tests, as proposed by Joseph et al. (1995); Dendukuri and Joseph (2001). This Bayesian estimation method has been implemented in WinBUGS by Branscum et al. (2005), whose BUGS code can found at the website (http://faculty.washington.edu/azhou/books/diagnostic.html).

11.4.2 Tuberculosis Example

Hui and Walter (1980) provided data on the accuracy of a new Tine test in detecting tuberculosis against the reference standard, the Mantoux test. Both tests were applied to a southern U.S. school district population and the Missouri State Sanatorium population. Table 11.9 displays the test results.

Table 11.9 Results of Mantoux and Tine Tests for Tuberculosis in Two Populations

Mantoux test	Population 1 Tine test		Population 2 Tine test	
	Positive	Negative	Positive	Negative
Positive	14	4	887	31
Negative	9	528	37	367
Total	23	532	924	398

Under the CIA and the assumption that the sensitivities and specificities of the Tine test and the reference test are the same in the two populations and that the prevalences of tuberculosis are different in the two populations, we obtain the ML estimates of the sensitivity and specificity of the Tine test with associated 95% confidence intervals. We report the results in Table 11.10.

We also apply the Bayesian methods, outlined in Branscum et al. (2005), to this data set. We first apply the Bayesian method under the CIA to the data set and report the resulting posterior distribution results in Table 11.11. We then apply another Bayesian analysis to the data set without assuming conditional independence and instead assuming a conditional dependence model, as described in Section 11.4.1 and report the results in Table 11.12. From these results, we see that under the CIA, both ML and Bayesian estimates of the sensitivities and specificities of the Mantoux and Tine test have very similar high values. Under the specified conditional dependence model, the

Table 11.10   Parameter Estimates of Mantoux and Tine Tests for
Tuberculosis in Two populations Using the ML Approach Under the CIA

Test	Parameter	Estimates	95% Confidence Interval
	Prevalence 1	0.027	(0.016, 0.045)
	Prevalence 2	0.717	(0.691, 0.741)
Mantoux test	$S_e(T)$	0.966	(0.950, 0.977)
	$S_p(T)$	0.993	(0.980, 0.998)
Tine test	$S_e(R)$	0.969	(0.954, 0.979)
	$S_p(R)$	0.984	(0.968, 0.992)

Table 11.11   Bayesian Results for the Accuracy of Mantoux and Tine Tests
Under the CIA

Test	Parameter	Prior information Modal value	Posterior results Median	95% C.I.
	Prevalence 1	0.03	0.029	(0.016, 0.044)
	Prevalence 2	0.30	0.714	(0.689, 0.714)
Mantoux test	$S_e(T)$	0.55	0.965	(0.950, 0.978)
	$S_p(T)$	0.98	0.991	(0.992, 0.998)
Tine test	$S_e(R)$	0.90	0.968	(0.955, 0.980)
	$S_p(R)$	0.85	0.980	(0.967, 0.990)

Table 11.12   Bayesian Estimates of the Accuracy of Mantoux and Tine Tests
for Tuberculosis Assuming a Conditional Dependence Model

Test	Parameter	Prior information Modal value	Posterior results Median	95% C.I.
Mantoux test	$S_e(T)$	0.83	0.882	(0.773, 0.953)
	$S_p(T)$	0.90	0.976	(0.955, 0.992)
Tine test	$S_e(R)$	0.70	0.886	(0.777, 0.959)
	$S_p(R)$	0.85	0.969	(0.946, 0.986)

estimated sensitivities and specificities are lower than those obtained under the CIA.

11.5   MULTIPLE BINARY TESTS IN ONE SINGLE POPULATION

In this section, we consider correction methods for estimating sensitivities and specificities of multiple tests simultaneously applied to a random sample from a single population without a gold standard. Let T_{ik} denote the result of the ith test for the kth patient, where $k = 1, \ldots, N$, and $i = 1, \ldots, I$ $(I > 2)$. Let D_k denote the condition status for the kth patient. Define $Se(i)$ and $Sp(i)$ to be the sensitivity and specificity of the ith test, respectively, $i = 1, \ldots, I$. That is,

$$Se(i) = P(T_{ik} = 1 \mid D_k = 1), \text{ and } Sp(i) = P(T_{ik} = 0 \mid D_k = 0).$$

Let t_{ik} be the observed value of T_{ik}; $t_{ik} = 1$ if the kth patient yields a positive result on the ith test, and $t_{ik} = 0$ otherwise. Denote $\mathbf{t}_k = (t_{1k}, \ldots, t_{Ik})'$. The observed data consist of $\mathbf{t}_1, \ldots, \mathbf{t}_N$. We are interested in estimating the sensitivities and specificities of I tests. We first discuss bias correction methods when I tests are conditionally independent given the condition status.

As in Section 11.3 for one test, non-identifiability of a model is an issue for estimation of the accuracy of I tests. We first discuss how to check whether a model is identifiable and then discuss estimation methods for sensitivities and specificities of I tests under an identifiable and non-identifiable model.

11.5.1   Checking for Model Identifiability

In this section, we discuss how to check whether a given model is identifiable. Let us define $p_{t_1,\ldots,t_I} = P(T_1 = t_1, \ldots, T_I = t_I)$, $\eta_{1,t_1\ldots,t_I} = P(T_1 = t_1, \ldots, T_I = t_I \mid D = 1)$, and $\eta_{0,t_1\ldots t_I} = P(T_1 = t_1, \ldots, T_I = t_I \mid D = 0)$. Then, we obtain the following relationship between p_{tr} and the model parameters, $\eta_{0,t_1\ldots t_I}$, $\eta_{1,t_1\ldots t_I}$, and π:

$$p_{t_1\ldots t_I} = \pi \eta_{0,t_1\ldots t_I} + (1 - \pi)\eta_{1,t_1\ldots t_I}, \tag{11.18}$$

where $(t_1, \ldots, t_I) \neq (0, \ldots, 0)$, and $t_1, \ldots, t_I = 0, 1$.

We stack $p_{t_1\ldots t_I}$'s, except $p_{0\ldots 0}$, into a single q-dimensional vector $p = (p_{1\ldots 1}, \ldots, p_{0\ldots 01})'$, where $q = 2^I - 1$ and $\eta_{0,tr}$'s and $\eta_{1,tr}$'s, π into a r-dimensional vector $\theta = (\eta_{1,1\ldots 1}, \ldots, \eta_{1,0\ldots 1}, \eta_{0,1\ldots 1}, \ldots, \eta_{0,0\ldots 01}, \pi)'$, where $r = 2^{I+1} - 1$. Note that θ is the vector of model parameters. Based on (11.18), the model specifies a mapping F from $\mathcal{R}^q$ to $\mathcal{R}^r$ such that

$$p = F(\theta). \tag{11.19}$$

Let $J(\theta)$ be the Jacobian matrix of the transformation $F(\theta)$; that is, $J(\theta) = \frac{\partial F(\theta)}{\partial \theta}$, a $q \times r$ matrix. If the column rank of $J(\theta)$ is full for all θ, the model is globally identifiable. Global identifiability is hard to achieve for a diagnostic testing model. If $J(\theta)$ is full column rank at $\theta = \theta_0$, the model is locally identifiable at $\theta = \theta_0$.

Since $q < r$ in model (11.18), model (11.18) is not identifiable without further assumptions. One common assumption is the CIA of the errors among I tests; that is,

$$P(T_1, \ldots, T_I \mid D) = P(T_1 \mid D) \ldots P(T_I \mid D). \qquad (11.20)$$

Under the CIA, the number of parameters in model (11.18) is $2I + 1$. Hence, the degrees of freedom from the data are greater than the number of parameters if $I \geq 3$; that is, $q \geq r$. When $q > r$, to show $J(\theta)$ has a full column rank, we can use singular value decomposition. If all eigenvalues of $J'(\theta)J(\theta)$, a $r \times r$ matrix, are nonzero, $J(\theta)$ has full column rank. If $q = r$, we can compute its determinant. Computation of eigenvalues and determinant of a squared matrix may be performed using symbolic algebra software, such as *Mathematica* or *Matlab*. If the determinant is not zero for all θ, $J(\theta)$ has full column rank. We next illustrate how to check for identifiability under the CIA when $I = 3$. When $I = 3$, the Jacobian matrix is a 7×7 matrix, and its determinant is given as follows:

$$\mid J(\theta) \mid = \pi^3 (\pi-1)^3 (Se(1)+Sp(1)-1)^2 (Se(2)+Sp(2)-1)^2 (Se(3)+Sp(3)-1)^3.$$

For a proof, see Jones et al. (2010). From this expression, we see that there are five points in the parameter space that make the determinant zero. Hence, excluding them from the parameter space leads to local identifiability of the model. Therefore, we conclude that in the region in which $0 < \pi < 1$ and $Se(i) + Sp(i) > 1$, for $i = 1, 2, 3$, model (11.18) under the CIA is locally identifiable.

11.5.2 ML Estimates under the CIA

Under the CIA, we may write the log-likelihood function of the observed data as

$$l = \sum_{i=1}^{I} \sum_{k=1}^{N} \log[Se(i)^{t_{ik}}(1 - Se(i))^{1-t_{ik}}\pi + Sp(i)^{1-t_{ik}}(1 - Sp(i))^{t_{ik}}(1 - \pi)].$$

$$(11.21)$$

This likelihood function has $2K + 1$ parameters, and the observed data can provide $K^2 - 1$ degrees of freedom. Thus, when $K \geq 3$, all parameters are estimable. It is worth noting that this likelihood function has a complicated form, involving mixture structures. To maximize this likelihood function, we can employ an iterative numerical algorithm, such as the Newton-Raphson or Fisher scoring algorithm.

Alternatively we may use the EM algorithm to find ML estimates for $Se(i)$, $Sp(i)$, and p, $i = 1, \ldots, I$ in (11.21). We next summarize this EM algorithm.

Let $Se^{(m)}(i)$, $Sp^{(m)}(i)$ and $\pi^{(m)}$ be current values of parameters $Se(i)$, $Sp(i)$, and π after m iterations in the EM algorithm. The next iteration estimates are

$$Se^{(m+1)}(i) = \frac{\sum_{k=1}^{N} t_{ik} q_k^{(m)}}{\sum_{k=1}^{N} q_k^{(m)}}, \quad Sp^{(m+1)}(i) = \frac{\sum_{k=1}^{N} (1 - t_{ik})(1 - q_k^{(m)})}{\sum_{k=1}^{N} (1 - q_k^{(m)})},$$

and

$$\pi^{(m+1)} = \frac{\sum_{k=1}^{N} q_k^{(m)}}{N}. \tag{11.22}$$

Here

$$q_k^{(m)} = \frac{A_2}{A_2 + B_2}, \tag{11.23}$$

where

$$A_2 = \prod_{i=1}^{I} (Se^{(m)}(i))^{t_{ik}} (1 - Se^{(m)}(i))^{1-t_{ik}} (\pi^{(m)}),$$

and

$$B_2 = \prod_{i=1}^{I} (1 - Sp^{(m)}(i))^{t_{ik}} (Sp^{(m)}(i))^{1-t_{ik}} (1 - \pi^{(m)}).$$

We iterate this process until the estimates converge. The convergent values $\widehat{Se}(i)$, $\widehat{Sp}(i)$, and $\hat{p}$ are the ML estimates for $Se(i)$, $Sp(i)$, and p, $k = 1, \ldots, K$. Their asymptotic covariance matrix can be estimated from the expected Fisher information of the observed data log-likelihood function, given by (11.21).

All iteratively numerical algorithms, including the EM, Newton-Raphson, and Fisher scoring algorithms, require a suitable starting value for each parameter. One way of choosing initial estimates is to use the majority rule among the tests. We will discuss this approach in more detail in the pleural thickening example given in Section 11.5.3. Regardless of how one chooses initial estimates, in practice, it is advisable to repeat the algorithm for several different sets of initial estimates to check whether the global maximum of interest is achieved (Dawid and Skene, 1979; Walter and Irwig, 1988).

11.5.3   Assessment of Pleural Thickening Example

We report the analysis of the pleural thickening example, described in Section 11.1.3, using the ML method. Table 11.13 presents the result of cross-classification of three radiologists on the presence of pleural thickening for 1692 males. Under the CIA, Walter and Irwig (1988) used the EM algorithm to compute the ML estimates of the parameters in the likelihood function (11.21) with initial estimates based on the majority opinion among the radiologists. For example, the initial estimate of prevalence of pleural thickening was the proportion of subjects with at least two positive X-ray assessments. Similarly, the initial estimate of sensitivity for each radiologist was calculated

Table 11.13   Assessments of Pleural Thickening by Three Radiologists

Reader 1	Reader 2	Reader 3	Observed Frequency
0	0	0	1513
0	0	1	21
0	1	0	59
0	1	1	11
1	0	0	23
1	0	1	19
1	1	0	12
1	1	1	34

1=positive result (pleural thickening present)
0=negative result (pleural thickening absent)

by the proportion of subjects rated as positive by this radiologist among all subjects rated positive by at least two radiologists. Table 11.14 reports the initial estimates and the ML estimates and their associated standard deviations. From the second and third rows of Table 11.14, we see that Readers 1

Table 11.14   ML Parameter Estimates for the Pleural Thickening Example

	Sensitivity		
	Reader 1	Reader 2	Reader 3
Initial estimates	0.855	0.750	0.842
ML estimates	0.765	0.644	0.749
Standard Deviation	0.112	0.171	0.119
	Specificity		
Initial estimates	0.986	0.963	0.987
ML estimates	0.989	0.965	0.990
Standard Deviation	0.004	0.005	0.003

and 3 have very similar sensitivity and specificity, which are higher than the sensitivity and specificity of Reader 2. The estimated standard deviations of the sensitivities are much larger than those of the specificities, which reflects the low prevalence of the condition.

11.5.4   ML Approaches Under Identifiable Conditional Dependence Models

In an earlier section, Section 11.5.2, we made the conditional independence assumption in parameter estimation. While the conditional independence assumption usually simplifies the statistical problem, various authors have pointed out that the CIA may not be reasonable in many applications (Vacek, 1985; Torrance-Rynard and Walter, 1997; Goetghebeur et al., 2000; Uebersax, 1999). For example, when there is a spectrum of severity of the condition, the most severe cases are unlikely to be missed by any test, whereas the least severe cases are more likely to be negative on more than one test.

In this section, we discuss available correction methods without assuming the CIA. These methods allow conditional dependence between tests by treating the true condition status as a latent variable with two classes. Even though the use of more than two latent classes of the condition status may improve the goodness of fit of a latent model (Rindskopf and Rindskopf, 1986), it is difficult to define the sensitivity and specificity of a diagnostic test with more than two latent classes. Here, we discuss latent models with two latent classes of the true condition status. Three general models are available for incorporating the dependencies among tests: (1) a random effects latent class model (Qu et al., 1996), (2) a latent class joint cell probability log-linear model (Espeland et al., 1989), and (3) a marginal latent class model (Yang and Becker, 1997).

In a random effects latent two class model, we allow the I test results of the same patient to be dependent, even after conditioning on the true disease status, but these test results become independent conditional on the true disease status and additional random effects due to some unobserved patient characteristics. Let $T_{k1}, \ldots, T_{kI}$ be the results of I tests for the kth patient. Let D_k be the true condition status of the kth patient and U_k denote a one-dimensional random effect due to the kth patient. Qu et al. (1996) proposed a random effects latent two class model, defined by

$$P(T_{k1}, \ldots, T_{kI} \mid D_k, U_k) = P(T_{k1} \mid D_k, U_k) \ldots P(T_{kI} \mid D_k, U_k),$$

$$P(T_{ki} = 1 \mid D_k = d, U_k = u) = \Phi(\zeta_{id} + v_{id}u), \qquad (11.24)$$

where U_k has the standard normal distribution and is independent of D_k, and $\Phi(\cdot)$ is the cumulative distribution of the standard normal variate. They called this model the 2LCR. By integrating out the random effect u in (11.24), we obtain the sensitivity and specificity of the kth test:

$$Se(i) = \int_{-\infty}^{+\infty} \Phi(\zeta_{i1} + v_{i1}u)d\Phi(u) = \Phi\left(\frac{\zeta_{i1}}{\sqrt{1 + v_{i1}^2}}\right),$$

$$Sp(i) = 1 - \int_{-\infty}^{+\infty} \Phi(\zeta_{i0} + v_{i0}u)d\Phi(u) = 1 - \Phi\left(\frac{\zeta_{i0}}{\sqrt{1 + v_{i0}^2}}\right)$$

$$= \Phi\left(\frac{-\zeta_{i0}}{\sqrt{1 + v_{i0}^2}}\right). \qquad (11.25)$$

Next, we discuss maximum likelihood (ML) estimation for the 2LCR model. Under (11.24), we may write the likelihood function of the observed data as

$$L = \prod_{k=1}^{N} \left\{ \int_{-\infty}^{+\infty} \left[\prod_{i=1}^{I} (\Phi(\zeta_{i1} + v_{i1}u))^{t_{ik}} (1 - \Phi(\zeta_{i1} + v_{i1}u))^{1-t_{ik}} \right] \pi_1 d\Phi(u) \right.$$

$$+ \int_{-\infty}^{+\infty} [\prod_{i=1}^{I} (\Phi(\zeta_{i0} + v_{i0}u))^{t_{ik}} (1 - \Phi(\zeta_{i0} + v_{i0}u))^{1-t_{ik}}] \pi_0 d\Phi(u)\}, \qquad (11.26)$$

where $\pi_d = P(D = d)$. We can employ an iterative numerical algorithm, such as the Newton-Raphson or Fisher scoring algorithm, to directly maximize this likelihood function to obtain ML estimates. However, since this likelihood function has a very complicated form, involving both one-dimensional integral and mixture structures, a better alternative is the EM algorithm which exploits the simple structure of the likelihood function when the condition status D is known. By approximating an integral in (11.26) by the Gauss-Hermite quadrature over a finite number of mass points $(u_1, \ldots, u_J)$, Qu et al. (1996) identified the likelihood function (11.26) as one of a finite mixture model. By applying the EM algorithm developed by Jansen (1993) for a finite mixture model, they obtained the ML estimates. Specifically, using the Gauss-Hermite quadrature over a finite number of mass points $(u_1, \ldots, u_J)$, one can approximate (11.26) by

$$L_2 = \prod_{k=1}^{N} \sum_{j=1}^{J} \sum_{d=0}^{1} \pi_d w_j g_{dj}(\mathbf{t}_k), \qquad (11.27)$$

where

$$g_{dj}(\mathbf{t}_k) = \prod_{i=1}^{I} \Phi(\zeta_{id} + v_{id}u_j)^{t_{ik}} (1 - \Phi(\zeta_{id} + v_{id}u_j))^{1-t_{ik}},$$

and $w_j = \phi(u_j)$ with $\phi(\cdot)$ being the density function of the standard normal distribution. Observe that the likelihood function, defined by (11.27), is also the likelihood of a finite mixture model with mixing proportions $\pi_d w_j$ and $2J$ component distributions $g_{dj}(t_k)$ $(d = 0, 1; j = 1, \ldots, J)$. Applying an EM algorithm for a finite mixture distribution (Jansen, 1993), one can obtain the ML estimates.

Estimation in a 2LCR model involves computation of the one-dimensional integral in (11.26). To avoid such an integral computation, one can use two alternative approaches. The first approach allows conditional dependence among tests through a log-linear model of the joint cell probabilities defined by the cross-classification of the K tests and D with interactions between tests (Espeland et al., 1989). Let $\eta_{t_1 \ldots t_I d}$ be the joint cell probability of a patient with $T_1 = t_1, \ldots, T_I = t_I$, and $D = d$. Then, a latent log-linear model is of the form

$$\log \eta_{d,t_1 \ldots t_I} = E\mathbf{b}, \qquad (11.28)$$

where E is the model matrix and $\mathbf{b}$ is a vector of parameters.

The CIA is equivalent to the latent log-linear model without any interaction between two tests within latent classes,

$$\log \eta_{d,t_1 \ldots t_4} = \lambda_d + \sum_{k=1}^{4} \lambda_{t_k d}.$$

A conditional dependence model is defined by allowing interaction terms between two tests within latent classes. For example, a latent log-linear model,

$$\log \eta_{d,t_1 \dots t_4} = \lambda_d + \sum_{k=1}^{4} \lambda_{t_k d} + \psi_{t_2 t_3 d}, \tag{11.29}$$

allows the diagnostic tests 2 and 3 to be dependent on each other even after conditioning on the true condition status. Espeland et al. (1989) used a Fisher scoring algorithm to obtain ML estimates of the parameters and their variances. A drawback of this approach is that with the addition of interactions between tests, the main effects in a latent log-linear model for individual tests will no longer have direct interpretations in terms of sensitivity and specificity. For example, in the latent log-linear model defined by (11.29), the parameters $\lambda_{t_2 d}$ and $\lambda_{t_3 d}$ do not have direct interpretations in terms of sensitivity and specificity. To correct for this drawback, Yang and Becker (1997) proposed to model the joint cell probabilities through a marginal model and a model for bivariate marginal associations between tests within a latent class. The constraints are that all higher than two-order associations within a latent class are assumed to be zero. For example, we may use a marginal logit to model the ith test,

$$\log \frac{P(T_i = 0 \mid D = d)}{P(T_i = 1 \mid D = d)} = \alpha_{id}, \tag{11.30}$$

where $i = 1, \dots, I$, and we specify the association between two tests within the same latent class by a log-odds ratio model,

$$\log \frac{P(T_i = 0, T_{\tilde{i}} = 0 \mid D = d)P(T_i = 1, T_{\tilde{i}} = 1 \mid D = d)}{P(T_i = 0, T_{\tilde{i}} = 1 \mid D = d)P(T_i = 1, T_{\tilde{i}} = 0 \mid D = d)} = \psi_{i\tilde{i}d}, \tag{11.31}$$

where $1 \leq i \neq \tilde{i} \leq I$.

Let $\boldsymbol{\theta}$ denote the vector of all unknown parameters, α_{id}, and $\psi_{i\tilde{i}d}$, and let $\boldsymbol{\Psi}$ be the vector of joint cell probabilities within the latent classes; that is

$$\boldsymbol{\Psi} = (P(T_1 = t_1, \dots, T_I = t_I \mid D = d), t_1, \dots, t_I = 0, 1; d = 0, 1).$$

A latent class marginal model relates $\boldsymbol{\Psi}$ to the vector of parameters $\boldsymbol{\theta}$ by the following model,

$$\mathbf{C} \log(\mathbf{B}\boldsymbol{\Psi}) = \mathbf{Z}\boldsymbol{\theta}, \tag{11.32}$$

where the matrix B contains ones and zeros for mapping $\boldsymbol{\Psi}$ into the marginal probabilities with the latent classes, and $\mathbf{C}$ is the known matrix that forms the required logits, log-odds ratios and log-odds ratio contrasts. When $I = 4$, Yang and Becker (1997) gave the expressions for B and $\mathbf{C}$.

One major advantage of this marginal model over a joint log-linear model is that sensitivity and specificity of a test can be directly obtained from its marginal parameters. Under Model (11.30), we see the sensitivity and specificity of the ith test are

$$Se(i) = \frac{1}{1 + \exp(\alpha_{i1})} \text{ and } Sp(i) = \frac{\exp(\alpha_{i0})}{1 + \exp(\alpha_{i0})}.$$

Yang and Becker (1997) used a modified gradient EM algorithm to obtain the ML estimates of the model parameters. The EM is recommended for latent class models because if D were known, the kernel of the complete-data log-likelihood would have a simple form,

$$\sum y^*_{t1...t_I} \log(\eta_{d,t_1...t_I}),$$

where $y^*_{t1...t_I d}$ is the unobserved cell count with $T_1 = t_1, \ldots, T_I = t_I, D = d$. The maximization step in the EM algorithm assumes that the joint cell probabilities for the complete-data satisfy the latent class model, defined by (11.30) and (11.31) and the constraints that all interactions higher than two-way among tests within a latent class are zero. Because of the constraint on the association parameters, the Lagrangian multiplier method has to be used in conjunction with the EM algorithm, which makes its computation more complicated than Espeland's method.

We can assess the goodness of fit of a latent class model using formal tests and graphical methods. While formal goodness of fit tests give an indication of overall fit, graphical methods can describe patterns of any lack of fit. Standard goodness-of-fit methods assess the fit of a model by comparing the expected cell counts under the assumed model against the observed frequencies. However, since we do not observe D, we cannot directly assess the fit of the latent model for the contingency table formed by $T_1, \ldots, T_I$, and D. But, we may indirectly assess its fit by comparing the observed frequencies in a collapsed table over D formed by $T_1, \ldots, T_I$. A lack of fit in the collapsed table also indicates a lack of fit of a latent model. Of course, a good fit in the latter table does not guarantee a good fit in the former table. The two best known goodness-of-fit tests are Pearson's test and the likelihood ratio test. For large sample sizes, both tests have the same chi-square distribution under the null hypothesis and the assumption that the assumed latent model is identifiable. However, since the proposed latent class model here is a restricted one, as defined by Goodman (1974), further research is needed to assess the validity of this identifiability assumption.

Let $n_{t_1...t_I}$ and $\hat{n}_{t_1...t_I}$ be the observed count and the estimated count under the assumed latent model at the cell with $T_1 = t_1, \ldots, T_I = t_I$. A standardized residual for cell $(t_1, \ldots, t_I)$ is defined by

$$e^{(1)}_{t_1...t_I} = \frac{n_{t_1...t_I} - \hat{n}_{t_1...t_I}}{\widehat{SD}_{t_1...t_I}},$$

where $\widehat{SD}_{t_1...t_I}$ is the estimated standard deviation of $\hat{n}_{t_1...t_I}$. A plot of $e^{(1)}_{t_1...t_I}$, for $t_1, \ldots, t_I = 0, 1$, can reveal any lack of fit in cells formed by $T_1, \ldots, T_I$.

Since higher-than-second-order dependencies are less likely to occur in practice, a lack-of-fit plot may start with pairwise dependencies. Let $n_{t_i t_{\bar{i}}}$ and $\hat{n}_{t_i t_{\bar{i}}}$ be the observed and the estimated counts under the assumed model in the cell formed by two tests, $T_i = t_i, T_{\bar{i}} = t_{\bar{i}}$. We define a standardized residual for cell $(t_i, t_{\bar{i}})$ by

$$e_{t_i t_{\bar{i}}}^{(2)} = \frac{n_{t_1 t_{\bar{i}}} - \hat{n}_{t_i t_{\bar{i}}}}{\widehat{SD}_{t_i t_{\bar{i}}}},$$

where $\widehat{SD}_{t_i t_{\bar{i}}}$ is the estimated standard deviation of $\hat{n}_{t_i t_{\bar{i}}}$. A plot of $e_{t_i t_{\bar{i}}}^{(2)}$'s can reveal any lack of fit in cells formed by two tests. See Agresti (1990) for more details.

Instead of cell counts, Qu et al. (1996) proposed calculating the residuals of the observed and expected pairwise correlations. Let $corr_{i\bar{i}}^{(0)}$ be the observed Pearson's correlation coefficient between T_i and $T_{\bar{i}}$ and $corr_{i\bar{i}}^{(E)}$ be the estimated Pearson's correlation coefficient between T_i and $T_{\bar{i}}$ from the assumed latent model. Qu et al. (1996) defined residuals as

$$e_{i\bar{i}}^{(3)} = corr_{i\bar{i}}^{(0)} - corr_{i\bar{i}}^{(E)}.$$

This simple residual may have limited usefulness because the variance of $corr_{i\bar{i}}^{(0)}$ may not be constant. See Agresti (1990) for more details. Further research is needed to assess the asymptotic distribution of the three types of residuals discussed here.

11.5.5   Bioassays for HIV Example

Alvord et al. (1988) studied sensitivity and specificity of four conventional bioassays for detecting HIV infection without the use of a gold standard: an enzyme-linked immunosorbent assay (ELISA) and three radioimmunoassay (RIA) tests utilizing recombinant antigen ag1, p24, and gp120, denoted by RIA1, RIA2, and RIA3, respectively. In this study, serum samples of each patient were tested by the four tests; the data are summarized in Table 11.15. Using the computer program of Qu et al. (1996), written in Gauss, we fitted a two class latent model with conditional independence and found the likelihood ratio chi-square deviance was 16.23 with a p-value of 0.06. To explore the pattern of lack of fit, we first plotted the residuals of cell counts in the contingency table formed by four observed tests (see Figure 11.1). From this plot, we see evidence of lack of fit in four cells, which are related to two tests, RIA_3 and RIA_2. To confirm this observation, we also plot the correlation residuals, displayed in Figure 11.2, where we see that the correlation residual between the tests RIA_3 and RIA_2 is positively large. Both plots suggest that RIA_3 and RIA_2 may not be conditionally independent. This suspicion is consistent with the clinical fact that the RIA_3 and RIA_2 tests are so close biochemically. Thus, Qu et al. (1996) re-fitted a two class latent random

Table 11.15   Results of the Accuracy of Four HIV Tests

RIA1	RIA2	RIA3	ELISA	Observed Frequency
0	0	0	0	170
0	0	0	1	15
0	0	1	0	0
0	0	1	1	0
0	1	0	0	6
0	1	0	1	0
0	1	1	0	0
0	1	1	1	0
1	0	0	0	4
1	0	0	1	17
1	0	1	0	0
1	0	1	1	83
1	1	0	0	1
1	1	0	1	4
1	1	1	0	0
1	1	1	1	128

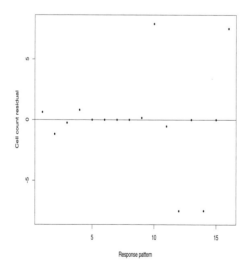

Figure 11.1   Cell count Residuals Under the CIA Model in the HIV Example

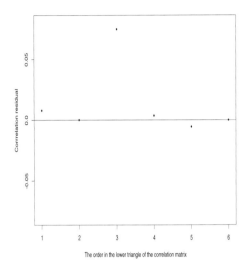

Figure 11.2   Pairwise Correlation Residuals Under the CIA Model in the HIV Example

effects model,

$$P(T_{ik} = 1 \mid D_k = d, U_k = u) = \Phi(\zeta_{kd} + \upsilon_{kd}u), \qquad (11.33)$$

where $b_{21} = b_{31} = b$ and $\upsilon_{kd} = 0$ if $(k, d) = (2, 1), (3, 1)$. This 2LCR model fits the data much better than the CIA model, with a deviance of 3.056 and a corresponding p-value of 0.93. Both the cell count residual plot (Figure 11.3) and correlation residual plot (Figure 11.4) confirm the good fit of the model to the contingency table formed by RIA_1, RIA_2, RIA_3, and ELISA.

Table 11.16 displays the ML estimates for sensitivity and specificity for the four tests and their corresponding 95% confidence intervals under the CIA model and the 2LCR model. Note that when the estimated sensitivity or specificity is 1.00, the computer program given in Qu et al. (1996) has a problem calculating the standard errors. This problem is related to the sparseness of the observed data. In these situations when the standard errors are not obtainable, their program sets the estimates for the standard errors to zero.

Yang and Becker (1997) re-analyzed the HIV data using latent class marginal models with no three and four-factor associations within latent classes. That is,

$$\log \frac{P(T_{ik} = 0 \mid D_k = d)}{P(T_{ik} = 1 \mid D_k = d)} = \alpha_{id},$$

$$\log \frac{P(T_{ik} = 0, T_{\tilde{i}k} = 0 \mid D_k = d)P(T_{ik} = 1, T_{\tilde{i}k} = 1 \mid D_k = d)}{P(T_{ik} = 0, T_{\tilde{i}k} = 1 \mid D_k = d)P(T_{ik} = 1, T_{\tilde{i}k} = 0 \mid D_k = d)} = \psi_{\tilde{i}id},$$

$$(11.34)$$

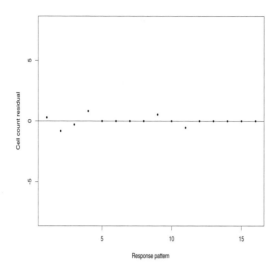

Figure 11.3   Cell Count Residuals Under the 2LCR Model in the HIV Example

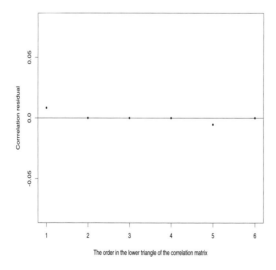

Figure 11.4   Pairwise Correlation Residuals Under the 2LCR Model in the HIV Example

Table 11.16   ML Estimates and the 95% Confidence Intervals for Sensitivity and Specificity of the Four HIV Tests Using a Random Effect Model

		Diagnostic test		
Model	RIA1	RIA2	RIA3	ELISA
		Sensitivity		
The CIA model	1.00 (*)	0.57 (0.51,0.64)	0.92 (0.88,0.95)	1.00 (*)
The 2LCR model	1.00 (*)	0.57 (0.51,0.63)	0.91 (0.87,0.95)	1.00 (*)
		Specificity		
The CIA model	0.97 (0.94,0.99)	0.96 (0.94,0.99)	1.00 (*)	0.92 (0.88,0.96)
The 2LCR model	0.97 (0.95,0.99)	0.96 (0.94,0.99)	1.00 (*)	0.92 (0.88,0.96)

*: the program fails to calculate the SE, resulting in no confidence interval

for $1 \leq i < \tilde{i} \leq 4$, where there is no three-way or four-way interactions within latent classes. Because of the sparseness of the observed data, they added the constant 0.1 to each cell frequency to provide greater computational stability. Yang and Beck first consider two models, called Models I and II, which are equivalent to the CIA and 2LCR models used in Qu et al. (1996). Model I is defined by (11.34) when $\psi_{i\tilde{i}d} = 0$ for all $i, \tilde{i}, d$, and Model II is defined by (11.34) when $\psi_{i\tilde{i}d} = 0$ if $(i, \tilde{i}) \neq (2, 3)$. Table 11.17 displays the ML estimates of sensitivities and specificities for the four tests with corresponding 95% confidence intervals.

Table 11.17   ML Estimates for Sensitivity and Specificity of the Four HIV Tests, with 95% Confidence Intervals, Using Marginal Log-linear Models

		Diagnostic test		
Model	ELISA	RIA1	RIA2	RIA3
		Sensitivity		
Model I	1.00 (0.91,1.00)	0.57 (0.51,0.63)	0.91 (0.87, 0.94)	1.00 (0.91,1.00)
Model II	1.00 (0.90,1.00)	0.57 (0.51,0.63)	0.91 (0.87,0.94)	1.00 (0.92,1.00)
Model III	1.00 (0.91,1.00)	0.57 (0.51,0.63)	0.91 (0.87,0.94)	1.00 (0.92,1.00)
Model IV	0.95 (0.90,0.98)	0.61 (0.54,0.67)	0.92 (0.86,0.95)	0.95 (0.89,0.97)
		Specificity		
Model I	0.97 (0.93,0.99)	0.96 (0.93,0.98)	1.00 (0.92,1.00)	0.92 (0.87,0.95)
Model II	0.97 (0.93,0.99)	0.96 (0.93,0.98)	1.00 (0.92,1.00)	0.92 (0.87,0.95)
Model III	0.97 (0.93,0.99)	0.96 (0.92,0.98)	1.00 (0.92,1.00)	0.92 (0.87,0.95)
Model IV	0.91 (0.84,0.95)	1.00 (0.00,1.00)	1.00 (0.50,1.00)	0.85 (0.78,0.90)

From this table, we see that Models I, II, and III give almost identical results and that even though Model IV gives a slightly different result, it also gives the very high level of uncertainty for the specificities of RIA2 and RIA3.

11.5.6   Bayesian Methods Under Conditional Dependence Models

Without the CIA, model (11.18) is non-identifiable. As in Section 11.3.3 for a single test, when the model is non-identifiable, we can use a Bayesian method to estimate sensitivities and specificities of I tests with the help of an informative prior distribution. To complete a Bayesian inference on $Se(i)$ and $Sp(i)$, where $i = 1, \ldots, I$, we need to model two joint conditional distributions, $P(T_1, \ldots, T_I \mid D = 1)$ and $P(T_1, \ldots, T_I \mid D = 0)$.

When $I \geq 3$, it is not easy to model the above joint conditional distributions using a fixed effects model, as done in Section 11.3.3 when $I = 2$. Here we choose to use a random effects model for $P(T_1, \ldots, T_I \mid D = 1)$ and $P(T_1, \ldots, T_I \mid D = 0)$. We assume that there exists a latent variable ξ such that conditional on D and ξ, $T_1, \ldots, T_I$ are independent; that is,

$$P(T_1, \ldots, T_I \mid D, \xi) = P(T_1 \mid D, \xi) \ldots P(T_I \mid D, \xi),$$

$$P(T_i = 1 \mid D = d, \xi) = \Phi(a_{id} + b_{id}\xi), \text{ and } \xi \sim N(0, 1).$$

Under the random effects model for the conditional dependence of $T_1, \ldots, T_I$, given D, the vector of parameters is $\theta = (\pi, a_{id}, b_{id}, i = 1, \ldots, d = 0, 1)'$. We choose a beta prior distribution for π and independent bivariate normal prior distributions for (a_{id}, b_{id})'s with mean (A_{id}, B_{id}) and diagonal variance-covariance matrix, $\begin{pmatrix} \sigma_{aid}^2 & 0 \\ 0 & \sigma_{bid}^2 \end{pmatrix}$, where $d = 0, 1$ and $i = 1, \ldots, I$. A Gibbs sampler can be used to obtain samples from the marginal posterior distribution of θ.

11.5.7   Analysis of the MRA for Carotid Stenosis Example

We analyze Case Study 3, described in Chapter one, which investigated the accuracy of MRA for detection of significant carotid stenosis in patients who had suffered TIA or stroke. Here we are interested in assessing the accuracy of the first three radiologists, who indicated the percent of stenosis present in the left of the carotid arteries. We dichotomize a radiologist's response into a binary response: 1 if the percent of stenosis is ≥ 60 and 0 otherwise. There is no gold standard for the diagnosis of a significant carotid stenosis. Table 11.18 summarizes the data.

We use the Bayesian methods discussed in Section 11.5.6 to assess the diagnostic accuracy of the two binary-scale tests in the absence of a gold standard under a conditional dependence model. Table 11.19 displays the results. From the results in Table 11.19 we see that Reader 3 has both the highest estimated sensitivity and specificity among the three readers, and

Table 11.18   Assessments of Left Carotid Artery Stenosis by Three Radiologists

Reader 1	Reader 2	Reader 3	Observed Frequency
0	0	0	62
0	0	1	4
0	1	0	7
0	1	1	5
1	0	0	1
1	0	1	1
1	1	0	5
1	1	1	78

1=positive result (% of stenosis ≥ 60)
0=negative result (% of stenosis < 60)

Table 11.19   Parameter Estimates of Left Carotid Artery Stenosis Data

Test	Parameter	Prior information Modal value	Posterior results Median	95% C.I.
	Prevalence	0.70	0.497	(0.421, 0.574)
Reader 1	$S_e(T)$	0.75	0.898	(0.822, 0.958)
	$S_p(T)$	0.90	0.912	(0.846, 0.965)
Reader 2	$S_e(R)$	0.75	0.818	(0.729, 0.894)
	$S_p(R)$	0.90	0.953	(0.899, 0.989)
Reader 3	$S_e(T)$	0.90	0.932	(0.861, 0.983)
	$S_p(T)$	0.98	0.977	(0.951, 0.994)

Reader 1 has the worst estimated specificity, while Reader 2 has the worst estimated sensitivity.

11.6 MULTIPLE BINARY TESTS IN G POPULATIONS

In this section we introduce bias correction methods when I different tests with binary outcomes are applied to the same individuals in G populations when no reference standard is used. Let T_i be the result of the ith test for a patient, where $i = 1, \ldots, I$, and $g = 1, \ldots, G$, and let D and X denote the condition status and the population indicator for the patient. Here $X_k = g$ if the patient is from the gth population. Let $Se(i, g)$ and $Sp(i, g)$ be the sensitivity and specificity of the ith test in the gth population. That is,

$$Se(i, g) = P(T_i = 1 \mid D = 1, X = g), Sp(i, g) = P(T_i = 0 \mid D = 0, X = g).$$

Let $\pi_g = P(D = 1 \mid X = g)$ be the prevalence of the condition in the gth population. Denote **Se** as a vector with components $Se(i, g)$, $i = 1, \ldots, I$; $g = 1, \ldots, G$. Denote **Sp** as a vector with components $Sp(i, g)$, $i = 1, \ldots, I$; $g = 1, \ldots, G$. Denote **p** as a vector with components $\widehat{\pi}_g$, $g = 1, \ldots, G$. Let t_{ikg} be the observed value of T_i for the kth sampled patient from the gth population, where $k = 1, \ldots, N_g$, and N_g be the number of patients sampled from the gth population. The observed data consist of $t_{ikg}, i = 1, \ldots, I$, $k = 1, \ldots, N_g$, and $g = 1, \ldots, G$.

11.6.1 ML Approaches Under the CIA

If conditional independence holds, then

$$P(T_1 \ldots T_I \mid D, X) = P(T_1 \mid D, X) \ldots P(T_I \mid D, X), \tag{11.35}$$

can be assumed between the tests, and we can put the log-likelihood in the following general expression:

$$l = \sum_{g=1}^{G} \sum_{k=1}^{N_g} \log[\widehat{\pi}_g \prod_{i=1}^{I} (Se(i, g)^{t_{ikg}} (1 - Se(i, g))^{1 - t_{ikg}})$$

$$+ \sum_{g=1}^{G} \sum_{k=1}^{N_g} (1 - \widehat{\pi}_g) \prod_{i=1}^{I} ((1 - Sp(i, g))^{t_{ikg}} (Sp(i, g))^{1 - t_{ikg}})]. \tag{11.36}$$

For any given values of I and G in such designs, the data provide $G(2^I - 1)$ degrees of freedom for $G(2I + 1) - 1$ parameters if the prevalence and test error rates vary with the populations. Hence, if $2^{(I-1)} \geq I + 1$, then all parameters in (11.36) are estimable. Walter and Irwig (1988) presented many specific examples from the literature with various combinations of K and G.

They also covered some special irregular designs, including different schemes of sequential testing.

To find ML estimators of the parameters we can use an iterative numerical algorithm, such as Fisher scoring, to directly maximize the likelihood function in (11.36). A more computationally efficient approach is to use the EM algorithm, just as in Section 11.4, because the likelihood function would have a much simpler form than the observed-data log-likelihood function if the true condition status had been known for each patient. We summarize this EM algorithm below. Let $Se^{(m)}(i,g)$, $Sp^{(m)}(i,g)$, and $\pi_g^{(m)}$ be current values of parameters $Se(i,g)$, $Sp(i,g)$, and π_g after m iterations. The next iteration estimators of the parameters have the following explicit solutions.

$$Se^{(m+1)}(i,g) = \frac{\sum_{k=1}^{N_g} t_{ikg} q_{kg}^{(m)}}{\sum_{k=1}^{N_g} q_{kg}^{(m)}}, Sp^{(m+1)}(i,g) = \frac{\sum_{k=1}^{N_g} (1 - t_{ikg})(1 - q_{kg}^{(m)})}{\sum_{k=1}^{N_g} (1 - q_{kg}^{(m)})},$$

$$\pi_g^{(m+1)} = \frac{\sum_{k=1}^{N_g} q_{kg}^{(m)}}{N_g}. \tag{11.37}$$

Here

$$q_{kg}^{(m)} = \frac{A_3}{A_3 + B_3}, \tag{11.38}$$

where

$$A_3 = \prod_{i=1}^{I} (Se^{(m)}(i,g))^{t_{ikg}} (1 - Se^{(m)}(i,g))^{1-t_{ikg}} (\pi^{(m)}),$$

and

$$B_3 = \prod_{i=1}^{I} [(1 - Sp^{(m)}(i,g))^{t_{ikg}} (Sp^{(m)}(i,g))^{1-t_{ikg}}](1 - \widehat{\pi}_g^{(m)}).$$

We iterate this process until the estimates converge. The convergent values are the ML estimates.

11.6.2   ML Approach Without the CIA Assumption

Instead of assuming conditional independence among tests, we can allow possible conditional dependence between tests by using the three types of models discussed in Section 11.5.4. For example, using a random effects model, we assume there exists a random variable U such that

$$P(T_1 \ldots T_I \mid D, X, U) = P(T_1 \mid D, X, U) \ldots P(T_I \mid D, X, U). \tag{11.39}$$

We model the conditional marginal distribution T_i given D, X, and U by the following probit model:

$$P(T_i = 1 \mid D = d, X = x, U = u) = \Phi(\zeta_{id} + v_{id} u + c_{id} x). \tag{11.40}$$

Under this model, we can use the same EM algorithm as described in Section 11.5.4 to find the ML estimates of the parameters (Qu et al., 1996). As pointed in Section 11.5.4, the issue of parameter identifiability in a random effects latent class model remains an unresolved problem. The requirement that the number of non-redundant parameters in the model should be less than or equal to the number of independent observations is a necessary condition for identifying latent class models, but it is not sufficient.

11.7 MULTIPLE ORDINAL-SCALE TESTS IN ONE SINGLE POPULATION

In this section, we discuss methods for estimating ROC curves of multiple ordinal-scale tests in the absence of a gold standard. We first describe a non-parametric method for estimating the ROC curves of ordinal-scale tests under the conditional independence assumption (CIA). Then, we introduce two parametric methods for estimating the ROC curves without the CIA, in the absence of a gold standard.

11.7.1   Non-Parametric Estimation of ROC Curves Under the CIA

Due to the issue of non-identifiability, Zhou et al. (2005) proposed a non-parametric maximum likelihood (ML) method for estimation of ROC curves and their areas for ordinal-scale tests under the CIA in the absence of a gold standard when the number of tests is greater than 2. Let $T_1, \cdots, T_I$ be responses from I diagnostic tests for a particular patient, ranging from 1 to J, and let D denote the unknown disease status of the patient, where $D = 1$ if the patient is diseased and $D = 0$ if the patient is non-diseased. To compute a discrete ROC curve from the ordinal data, by varying the threshold for a positive test we obtain $I + 1$ pairs of true positive rates (TPR) and false positive rates (FPR). Specifically, for the ith test, if we define a positive test as one with $T_i \geq j$, the corresponding pair of TPR and FPR are given by

$$TPR_i(j) = P(T_i \geq j \mid D = 1), \ FPR_i(j) = P(T_i \geq j \mid D = 0),$$

respectively, for $j = 1, \cdots, J + 1$. Here, $TPR_i(1) = FPR_i(1) = 1$, and $TPR_i(J + 1) = FPR_i(J + 1) = 0$. A discrete ROC curve is defined as a discrete function of $(FPR_i(j), TPR_i(j))$, $j = 1, \cdots, J + 1$. By connecting coordinates with straight lines, we obtain the non-parametric ROC curve. Using the trapezoidal rule for integration, we can obtain the area under the non-parametric ROC curve of the ith test as follows:

$$A_i = \sum_{j=1}^{J-1} \left[P(T_i = j \mid D = 0) \sum_{l=j+1}^{J} P(T_i = l \mid D = 1) \right]$$

$$+\frac{1}{2}\sum_{j=1}^{J}P(T_i = j \mid D = 0)P(T_i = j \mid D = 1).$$

Let $\phi_{0ij} = P(T_i = j \mid D = 0)$ and $\phi_{1ij} = P(T_i = j \mid D = 1)$. Then, the ROC curve and its area are functions of ϕ_{0ij} and ϕ_{1ij} in the following form:

$$FPR_i(j) = \sum_{l=j}^{J}\phi_{0il}, \; TPR_i(j) = \sum_{l=j}^{J}\phi_{1il}, \qquad (11.41)$$

and

$$A_i = \sum_{j=1}^{J-1}\left[\phi_{0ij}\sum_{l=j+1}^{J}\phi_{1il}\right] + \frac{1}{2}\sum_{j=1}^{J}\phi_{0ij}\phi_{1ij}. \qquad (11.42)$$

We next introduce a ML method for ϕ_{0ij} and ϕ_{1ij}. Let y_{ijk} be a binary variable such that $y_{ijk} = 1$ if the response of the ith test is j for the kth patient and $y_{ijk} = 0$ otherwise, where $k = 1, \cdots, N$, $j = 1, \cdots, J$, and $i = 1, \cdots, I$. Let $\mathbf{y}_k = (y_{11k}, \cdots, y_{IKk})$ denote the vector of all binary test results for kth patient. Let D_k denote the disease status of the kth patient, where $D_k = 1$ if the kth patient is diseased and $D_k = 0$ if the kth patient is not diseased. Let $g_d(\mathbf{y}_k) = P(\mathbf{y}_k \mid D_k = d)$ denote the conditional probability of the kth patient's test score vector $\mathbf{y}_i$ given the disease status $D_k = d$. Let us denote $\mathbf{y} = (\mathbf{y}_1, \ldots, \mathbf{y}_N)$, the observed data.

Under the CIA of the K tests, we obtain that

$$g_d(\mathbf{y}_k) = \prod_{j=1}^{J}\prod_{i=1}^{I}[\phi_{dij}]^{y_{ijk}}. \qquad (11.43)$$

Let $\boldsymbol{\phi}_0 = (\phi_{011}, \cdots, \phi_{0IJ})$, $\boldsymbol{\phi}_1 = (\phi_{111}, \cdots, \phi_{1IJ})$, and $\pi_d = P(D_i = d)$.

We next describe the EM algorithm for finding the maximum likelihood estimators for ϕ_0 and ϕ_1, subject to the normalizing conditions $\sum_{j=1}^{J}\phi_{dij} = 1$, where $d = 0, 1$ and $i = 1, \cdots, I$. Let $\theta = (p_1, \phi_0, \phi_1)$. We can show that the complete-data log-likelihood is given by the following form:

$$l_c(\theta) = \sum_{k=1}^{N}[D_k \log \pi_1 g_1(\mathbf{y}_k) + (1 - D_k) \log \pi_0 g_0(\mathbf{y}_k)].$$

Let $\theta^{(t)}$ denote the estimate of θ after the tth iteration of the EM algorithm. The next iteration value of θ is obtained after the following E and M steps:

- **E step**: The E step computes the conditional expectation of $l_c(\theta)$ given the observed data $\mathbf{y}$ and current parameter estimates $\theta = \theta^{(t)}$,

$$E(l_c(\theta) \mid \mathbf{y}, \theta = \theta^{(t)}) = \sum_{k=1}^{N}\sum_{d=0}^{1}P(D_k = d \mid \mathbf{y}_k, \theta^{(t)}) \log \pi_d g_d(\mathbf{y}_k).$$

If we write

$$q_{kd}^{(t)} = P(D_k = d \mid \mathbf{y}_k, \pi_1^{(t)}, \phi_0^{(t)}, \phi_1^{(t)}),$$

and

$$g_d^{(t)}(\mathbf{y}_i) = \prod_{j=1}^{J} \prod_{i=1}^{I} [\phi_{dij}^{(t)}]^{y_{ijk}},$$

we can show that

$$q_{kd}^{(t)} = \frac{\pi_d^{(t)} g_d^{(t)}(\mathbf{y}_k)}{\pi_0^{(t)} g_0^{(t)}(\mathbf{y}_k) + \pi_1^{(t)} g_1^{(t)}(\mathbf{y}_k)}, \tag{11.44}$$

and

$$E(l_c(\theta) \mid \mathbf{y}, \theta = \theta^{(t)}) = \sum_{k=1}^{N} \sum_{d=0}^{1} q_{kd}^{(t)} \log g_d(\mathbf{y}_k). \tag{11.45}$$

- **M step**: The M step finds the updated estimate $\theta^{(t+1)}$ for θ by maximizing $E(l_c(\theta) \mid \mathbf{y}, \theta = \theta^{(t)})$ in (11.45) with respect to θ. We can show that $\theta^{(t+1)}$ has the following explicit expression:

$$\pi_1^{(t+1)} = \frac{1}{N} \sum_{k=1}^{N} q_{k1}^{(t)}, \tag{11.46}$$

and

$$\phi_{dij}^{(t+1)} = \frac{\sum_{k=1}^{N} q_{kd}^{(t)} y_{ijk}}{\sum_{k=1}^{N} q_{kd}^{(t)}}. \tag{11.47}$$

Let us denote the convergent values of the EM algorithm by $\hat{\pi}_0$, $\hat{\pi}_1$, $\hat{\phi}_{0ij}$, and $\hat{\phi}_{1ij}$, which are ML estimates of π_0, π_1, ϕ_{0ij}, and ϕ_{1ij}. We obtain the estimated covariance matrix for θ using the Fisher information matrix. See Zhou et al. (2005) for the detailed expression.

11.7.2 Estimation of ROC Curves Under Some Conditional Dependence Models

If we assume that an ordinal-scale test result is a categorization of a latent continuous scale random variable with a parametric distribution, we do not need to make the conditional independence assumption (CIA) and produce a smooth ROC curve, just like in Chapter 4. Henkelman et al. (1990) proposed a maximum likelihood estimation method for the ROC curves of five-point rating scale tests using a multivariate normal mixture latent model. The assumption of a multivariate normal distribution for multivariate latent variables may be too strong in practice. In addition, in a published commentary on this paper, Begg and Metz (1990) pointed out three serious potential limitations to this method and called for further research into its properties before they could recommend it for general use. Albert (2007) proposed a random effects model for conditional correlations and a marginal parametric probit model for the cumulative distribution of an ordinal-scale test. Next we describe this method in more detail.

Following the method of Qu et al. (1996), Albert (2007) used a random effects model to represent conditional correlations among test results of kth subject, $T_{1k}, \ldots, T_{Ik}$, given D_k, where $k = 1, \ldots, N$. He assumed that there exist two normally distributed random effects, ξ_{dk}, for $d = 0, 1$, such that $T_{1k}, \ldots, T_{Ik}$ are independent, given both $D_k = d$ and ξ_{dk}; that is,

$$P(T_{1k}, \ldots, T_{Ik} \mid D_k = d, \xi_{dk}) = P(T_{1k} \mid D_k = d, \xi_{kd}) \ldots P(T_{Ik} \mid D_k = d, \xi_{kd}),$$

$$\xi_{dk} \sim N(0, \sigma_d^2).$$

Here ξ_{dk} is assumed to follow a normal distribution with mean zero and variance σ_d^2. Albert (2007) assumed the following distributions for the random effects, ξ_{dk}, conditional on $D_k = d$. Conditional on $D_k = 1$,

$$\xi_{1k} = \begin{cases} +\infty & \text{with probability } \eta_0 \\ N(0, \sigma_0^2) & \text{with probability } 1 - \eta_0 \end{cases}$$

Conditional on $D_k = 0$,

$$\xi_{0k} = \begin{cases} -\infty & \text{with probability } \eta_1 \\ N(0, \sigma_1^2) & \text{with probability } 1 - \eta_1. \end{cases}$$

If $\eta_0 = \eta_1 = 0$, the above random effects model is the most commonly used Gaussian random effects (GRE) model. If $\sigma_1 = \sigma_0 = 0$, the above random effects model is a finite mixture (FM) of the normal model (Uebersax, 1999; Albert, 2007). In this section, we discuss estimation methods under the most commonly used GRE model for the conditional dependence.

Albert (2007) proposed the following model for the conditional distribution of T_{ik} given $D_k = d$ and ξ_{dk}:

$$\Phi^{-1}(P(T_{ik} \leq j \mid D_k = d, \xi_{dk})) = C_{d,j,i} + \xi_{dk}.$$

This model allows test-specific cutoff points and has a vector of parameters, $\boldsymbol{\theta}' = (\pi, C_{d,j,i}, \sigma_d, d = 0, 1, j = 1, \ldots, J - 1, i = 1, \ldots, I)$. Albert (2007) then proposed to directly maximize the observed data log-likelihood to find the maximum likelihood estimate of $\boldsymbol{\theta}$. A bootstrap method was suggested to find the variance of the result estimator of $\boldsymbol{\theta}$.

11.7.3   Analysis of Ordinal-Scale Tests for Detecting Carcinoma in Situ of the Uterine Cervix

Under the conditional independence assumption, we applied the EM algorithm, discussed in Section 11.7.1 to the data set to obtain the empirical

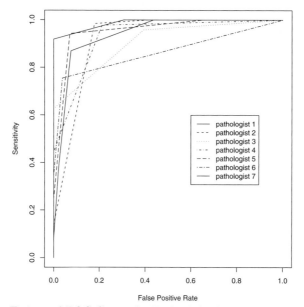

Figure 11.5   Estimated ROC Curves for Each of the Seven Pathologists Based on Non-parametric Model

ROC curves and their areas under the curves for the seven pathologists. We summarize the estimated non-parametric ROC curves of the seven pathologists in Figure 11.5. The corresponding areas under the ROC curves are 0.94, 0.92, 0.90, 0.93, 0.95, 0.87, and 0.98, respectively. The estimated prevalence is 0.61.

Without the CIA, we applied the ML-based method with the GRE conditional dependence model, discussed in Section 11.7.2, to the data set. We obtained the estimated AUCs of the seven pathologists as follows: 0.87, 0.83, 0.89, 0.99, 0.86, 0.79, and 0.95, respectively. Using the Akaike information criterion (AIC), Albert (2007) showed the conditional dependence GRE model has a smaller AIC than that obtained under the CIA model, suggesting that the conditional GRE model may fit the data better than the CIA model.

11.8   MULTIPLE-SCALE TESTS IN ONE SINGLE POPULATION

When tests yield results on a continuous scale, Henkelman et al. (1990) proposed a maximum likelihood method for estimating ROC curves of two or more tests applied to the same patients in the absence of the gold standard test, by assuming multivariate normal distributions for test results of a diseased and non-diseased subject. Choi et al. (2006) proposed a Bayesian method for estimating and comparing ROC curves of two continuous-scale tests in the absence of a gold standard by assuming the joint distribution of two test results of a patient is a mixture of two bivariate normal distributions.

In the case of two tests, both methods assume that unobserved test results of a diseased subject, X_1 and X_2, follow a bivariate normal distribution

$$\mathbf{X} = \begin{bmatrix} X_1 \\ X_2 \end{bmatrix} \sim N_2(\boldsymbol{\mu}_1, \boldsymbol{\Sigma}_1),$$

and that unobserved test results of a non-diseased subject, Y_1 and Y_2, also follow a bivariate normal distribution

$$\mathbf{Y} = \begin{bmatrix} Y_1 \\ Y_2 \end{bmatrix} \sim N_2(\boldsymbol{\mu}_0, \boldsymbol{\Sigma}_0).$$

Here

$$\boldsymbol{\mu}_1 = \begin{bmatrix} \mu_{11} \\ \mu_{21} \end{bmatrix}, \ \boldsymbol{\Sigma}_1 = \begin{bmatrix} \sigma_{11}^2 & \rho_1 \\ \rho_1 & \sigma_{21}^2 \end{bmatrix}, \ \boldsymbol{\mu}_0 = \begin{bmatrix} \mu_{10} \\ \mu_{20} \end{bmatrix} \text{ and } \boldsymbol{\Sigma}_0 = \begin{bmatrix} \sigma_{10}^2 & \rho_0 \\ \rho_0 & \sigma_{20}^2 \end{bmatrix}.$$

The vector of parameters in this setting is given by

$$\boldsymbol{\theta}' = (\pi, \mu_{11}, \mu_{21}, \mu_{10}, \mu_{20}, \sigma_{11}^2, \sigma_{21}^2, \sigma_{10}^2, \sigma_{20}^2, \rho_1, \rho_0),$$

where $\pi = P(D = 1)$. It is worth noting that under this model, the conditional independence assumption is a special case with $\rho_1 = \rho_0 = 0$.

Under the bivariate normal distribution assumption, the ROC curve of the diagnostic test j is given by $R_j(t) = 1 - \Phi(b_j \Phi^{-1}(1 - t) - a_j)$, where $a_j = (\mu_{j1} - \mu_{j0})/\sigma_{j1}$ and $b_j = \sigma_{j0}/\sigma_{j1}$, and the corresponding area under the ROC curve is $A_j = \Phi(\frac{a_j}{\sqrt{1+b_j^2}})$, for $j = 1, 2$, where $\Phi(\cdot)$ is the standard normal distribution function.

Since there is no gold standard, both $\mathbf{X}$ and $\mathbf{Y}$ are missing, Hsieh et al. (2009) proposed the use of the EM algorithm to obtain the ML estimate of $\boldsymbol{\theta}$ and the bootstrap method for the construction of an ML-based interval for $\Delta = A_1 - A_2$. Next we describe this EM algorithm for finding the ML estimate of $\boldsymbol{\theta}$ by treating D_i's as missing.

Let D_k and t_{ik} denote the unknown true disease status of the kth subject and the test result of the ith test applied to the kth patient, where $i = 1, 2$, and $k = 1, \ldots, N$. Let $\mathbf{t}_k = (t_{1k}, t_{2k})'$, $\mathbf{t}' = (\mathbf{t}'_1, \ldots, \mathbf{t}'_N)$, and $\mathbf{D} = (D_1, \ldots, D_N)$. If $\mathbf{D}$ had been observed, then the complete data log-likelihood function would be given as follows:

$$l^c(\boldsymbol{\theta}|\mathbf{t}, \mathbf{D}) = \sum_{k=1}^{N} [D_k \log(\pi f_{\mathbf{X}}(\mathbf{t}_k)) + (1 - D_k) \log((1 - \pi) f_{\mathbf{Y}}(\mathbf{t}_k))],$$

where $f_{\mathbf{X}}(\mathbf{t})$ is the density function of the bivariate normal distribution, $N_2(\boldsymbol{\mu}_1, \boldsymbol{\Sigma}_1)$, and $f_{\mathbf{Y}}(\mathbf{t})$ is the density function of the bivariate normal distribution, $N_2(\boldsymbol{\mu}_0, \boldsymbol{\Sigma}_0)$. Let $\boldsymbol{\theta}^{(m)}$ denote the estimate of $\boldsymbol{\theta}$ after the mth iteration of the EM algorithm. We can use the following E-step and M-step to obtain an updated estimate of $\boldsymbol{\theta}$, $\boldsymbol{\theta}^{(m+1)}$.

• E-step: Computes the following conditional expectation of $l^c(\boldsymbol{\theta})$ under the observed data $\mathbf{t}$ and the current parameter estimate, $\boldsymbol{\theta} = \boldsymbol{\theta}^{(m)}$:

$$E(l^c(\boldsymbol{\theta})|\mathbf{t}, \boldsymbol{\theta} = \boldsymbol{\theta}^m) = \sum_{k=1}^{N} z_{k1}^{(m)} \log(\pi) f_{\mathbf{X}}(\mathbf{t}_k) + z_{k0}^{(m)} \log(1 - \pi) f_{\mathbf{Y}}(\mathbf{t}_k),$$

where

$$z_{kd}^{(m)} = P(D_k = d \mid \mathbf{t}_k, \boldsymbol{\theta}^{(m)}).$$

Hsieh et al. (2009) showed the following explicit expressions for $z_{kd}^{(m)}$, $d = 0, 1$:

$$z_{k1}^{(m)} = \frac{\pi^{(m)} f_{\mathbf{X}}^{(m)}(\mathbf{t}_k)}{\pi^{(m)} f_{\mathbf{X}}^{(m)}(\mathbf{t}_k) + (1 - \pi^{(m)}) f_{\mathbf{Y}}^{(m)}(\mathbf{t}_k)}, \qquad (11.48)$$

and

$$z_{k0}^{(m)} = \frac{(1 - p)^{(m)} f_{\mathbf{Y}}^{(m)}(\mathbf{t}_k)}{\pi^{(m)} f_{\mathbf{X}}^{(m)}(\mathbf{t}_k) + (1 - \pi^{(m)}) f_{\mathbf{Y}}^{(m)}(\mathbf{t}_k)}. \qquad (11.49)$$

• M-step: Finds the updated estimate $\boldsymbol{\theta}^{(m+1)}$ for $\boldsymbol{\theta}$ by maximizing $E(l^c(\boldsymbol{\theta})|\mathbf{t}, \boldsymbol{\theta} = \boldsymbol{\theta}^m)$ with respect to $\boldsymbol{\theta}$. See Hsieh et al. (2009) for detailed expressions for the elements of $\boldsymbol{\theta}^{(m+1)}$.

The convergent value of $\boldsymbol{\theta}^{(m+1)}$ in the EM algorithm is the ML estimate of $\boldsymbol{\theta}$. Finally, inserting the ML estimate of $\boldsymbol{\theta}$ into the expressions for the ROC curves of the two tests and $\Delta = A_1 - A_2$, we obtain the ML estimates for the ROC curves of the two tests, $\widehat{R}_1(t)$ and $\widehat{R}_2(t)$, and their difference, $\widehat{\Delta}$.

To get a confidence interval for Δ, we need to find a variance estimate for $\widehat{\Delta}$. Due to the complicated variance form of $\widehat{\Delta}$, Hsieh et al. (2009) proposed a bootstrap method to obtain its variance estimate. We summarize their bootstrap procedure for constructing an equal-tailed $100(1 - \alpha)\%$ confidence interval for $\Delta = A_1 - A_2$ as follows.

Step 1: Choose an initial value for $\boldsymbol{\theta}$.

Step 2: Utilize the EM algorithm to obtain $\boldsymbol{\theta}$ and then $\widehat{\Delta}$, using the original observed data, $\mathbf{t} = (\mathbf{t}_1, \mathbf{t}_2, \ldots, \mathbf{t}_N)$.

Step 3: Obtain B bootstrap samples, by sampling from the original observed data, $\mathbf{t}$, without replacement, such that each bootstrap sample has a size N.

Step 4: Apply the EM algorithm to each bootstrap sample to obtain an estimate $\Delta = A_1 - A_2$. Then, based on these B bootstrap estimates of Δ, we can obtain the sample variance estimate for the variance of $\widehat{\Delta}$, denoted by $\widehat{var}(\widehat{\Delta}_{boot})$.

Step 5: Use the resulting $\widehat{\Delta}$ in Step 2 and $\widehat{var}(\widehat{\Delta}_{boot})$ in Step 4 to construct $(1 - \alpha)100\%$ confidence interval for Δ as follows:

$$(\widehat{\Delta} - z_{1-\alpha/2}\sqrt{\widehat{var}(\widehat{\Delta}_{boot})}, \widehat{\Delta} + z_{1-\alpha/2}\sqrt{\widehat{var}(\widehat{\Delta}_{boot})}).$$

Instead of using the ML-based inferences for the ROC curves of the two tests and their areas, Choi et al. (2006) proposed a Bayesian method. To complete their Bayesian inferences on the ROC curves and their areas, Choi et al. (2006) chose the following independent prior distributions for components in $\boldsymbol{\theta}$: $N(0, 1000)$ for μ_{jD} and $\mu_{j\bar{D}}$, $\Gamma(0.001, 0.001)$ for $1/\sigma_{jD}^2$ and $1/\sigma_{j\bar{D}}^2$, and $Uniform(-1, 1)$ for ρ_D and $\rho_{\bar{D}}$. This Bayesian method has been implemented in WinBUGS by Choi et al. (2006). The computer programs for the methods in Hsieh et al. (2009) and Choi et al. (2006) can be found at the web site (http://faculty.washington.edu/azhou/books/diagnostic.html).

The multivariate normal assumption in the above methods may be too strong in practice. Without assuming any parametric models for the joint distributions of I test results of a diseased and non-diseased subject, Hall and Zhou (2003) investigated identifiability of a non-parametric model and showed that under the conditional independence assumption and some mild regularity conditions, the problem is nonparametrically identifiable when the number of tests is greater than or equal to 3. Under the identifiable setting, they then proposed $\sqrt{n}$ consistent nonparametric estimators of univariate marginal distributions and the mixing proportion. We next describe their results briefly.

Let $F(.)$ denote the joint distribution of the I test results, $(T_{1k}, \ldots, T_{Ik})$, and G_{id} denote the conditional marginal distribution of T_{ik} conditional on $D_i = d$. Under the conditional independence assumption of $T_{1k}, \ldots, T_{Ik}$, conditional on D_i, we have

$$F(x) = \pi \prod_{i=1}^{I} G_{i1}(x_i) + (1 - \pi) \prod_{i=1}^{I} G_{i0}(x_i). \qquad (11.50)$$

Hall and Zhou (2003) considered non-parametric estimation of the above model (11.50). The vector of parameters in model (11.50) can be represented by

$$Q = (\pi, G_{11}, \ldots, G_{I1}, G_{10}, \ldots, G_{I0}).$$

Hall and Zhou (2003) showed that when $I = 1, 2$ neither π nor G_{id} is identifiable nonparametrically. However, for $I \geq 3$ and under mild regularity conditions, model (11.50) can determine Q uniquely, up to the dichotomy obtained by interchanging the two products on the right-hand side of (11.50). They then proceeded to consistently estimate all the components of Q using purely nonparametric methods. Since the ROC curve of the ith test is a function of G_{i0} and G_{i1}, we can also obtain a consistent estimator for the ROC curve of the ith test. The conditional independence assumption plays a crucial role in parametric identifiability nonparametrically. Hall and Zhou (2003) showed that the commonly used random effects conditional dependence model for multiple tests in the absence of a gold standard is not identifiable if one takes a nonparametric view of the mixture estimation problem.

11.8.1 Re-Analysis of the Accuracy of Continuous-Scale MRA for Detection of Significant Carotid Stenosis

In this section, we illustrate the methods described in Section 11.8 by applying them to the MRA test example, which was analyzed in Section 11.5.7, as the binary-scale tests. We estimated the accuracy of the binary-scale MRA tests, interpreted by three radiologists. Here we are interested in assessing the accuracy of the continuous-scale MRA tests, interpreted by the first two radiologists. Using the EM algorithm proposed by Hsieh et al. (2009) and described in Section 11.8, we obtained the 95% confidence interval for the difference between areas under the ROC curves of the first and second radiologists as $[0.0125, 0.0819]$ and the estimated disease prevalence of 0.38. However, when we applied the BUGS code for the Bayesian method, given in Choi et al. (2006), it failed to converge. Based on the ML results, we conclude that the accuracy of the MRA test differs between two radiologists.

CHAPTER 12

STATISTICAL ANALYSIS FOR META-ANALYSIS

Separate clinical studies, using patients from distinct populations, are often conducted to estimate the accuracy of the same diagnostic test. In combining the information statistically from the various studies, we hope to arrive at a better estimate of the true accuracy of the test. In doing so, we need to address questions such as: Why do the reported accuracy measures differ from study to study? Do the differences simply reflect within-study variation (experimental error)? Or do the differences also represent between-study variation - differences in design and execution of the study or differences in the characteristics of the patients enrolled? Different analysis methods are appropriate, depending on the assumptions that we wish to make regarding this variation.

In Chapter 7, we introduced meta-analysis of studies assessing the accuracy of diagnostic tests, described design issues, and presented simple methods of analysis. In this chapter, we develop more complex methods of analyzing data for meta-analytic studies. In Section 12.1, we discuss how to combine estimates of either sensitivity or specificity if data are binary, incorporating random effects. In Section 12.2, we discuss combining accuracy measures for interval or continuous data across studies that present single sensitivity and

Statistical Methods in Diagnostic Medicine,
Second Edition. By Xiao-Hua Zhou, Nancy A. Obuchowski, Donna K. McClish
Copyright © 2011 John Wiley & Sons, Inc.

specificity pairs. This discussion includes methods to specifically incorporate random effects (and, possibly, covariates) for comparing sensitivity and specificity and estimating summary ROC (SROC) curves. In Section 12.3 we present random-effects methods for combining accuracy measures across studies when they are presented as areas under the ROC curves.

12.1 BINARY-SCALE DATA

If the data are truly binary-scale, and only a single sensitivity or specificity is of interest, an average value can be used as a meta-analysis summary measure. As mentioned in Chapter 7, the assumption that any observed variation in accuracy is solely due to sampling error within studies is unrealistic. A more appropriate assumption is that there are true differences in accuracy between studies. The most common method to model between-study variation in meta-analysis uses random effects (DerSimonian and Laird, 1986). If we let η_i represent the true logit of sensitivity (TPR) of the i-th study, where the logit is ln[sensitivity/(1-sensitivity)], a random effects model assumes that true sensitivities vary across studies following a normal distribution

$$\eta_i \sim N(\eta, \sigma_\eta^2), \qquad (12.1)$$

where between-study variation is represented by σ_η^2. The within-study variation is usually modeled as an approximate normal distribution for the logit

$$\widehat{\eta}_i | \eta_i \sim N(\eta_i, \ \frac{1}{s_{1i}} + \frac{1}{s_{0i}}), \qquad (12.2)$$

where the variance of the logit of TPR in the i-th study is estimated as $1/s_{1i} + 1/s_{0i}$ (using notation from Chapter 4). Similarly, for the logit of the false positive rate ξ_i,

$$\xi_i \sim N(\xi, \sigma_\xi^2), \widehat{\xi}_i | \xi_i \sim N(\xi_i, \ \frac{1}{r_{0i}} + \frac{1}{r_{1i}}). \qquad (12.3)$$

This model is a linear random effects model and can be estimated using standard likelihood procedures with Linear Mixed Model software such as PROC MIXED in SAS (for SAS code see, for example, van Houwelingen et al. (2002)).

Hamza et al. (2008) pointed out that the method of DerSimonian and Laird (1986) could yield biased results when applied to proportions, because their method approximated the (true) binomial likelihood of the proportion within-study by the normal likelihood. This is particularly problematic if the sample size is small or if the proportion is close to 0 or 1. In addition, the normal approximation ignores the correlation between the mean and the variance. They suggested that a more appropriate approach was to directly use the exact binomial distribution of the number of true and false positives to represent the within-study variance. In other words, if s_{1i} is the observed number of true positives out of n_{1i} with the condition, we assume that s_{1i} follows a binomial distribution.

$$s_{1i} \sim B(n_{1i}, v_i), \tag{12.4}$$

where

$$v_i = 1/(1 + e^{-\eta_i}). \tag{12.5}$$

This is then a generalized linear mixed model (GLMM) which can be estimated with programs such as SAS's NLMIXED procedure or GLIMMIX. Hamza et al. (2008) performed simulations which showed that the exact (binomial) approach produced unbiased estimates of η as well as the between-study variance, whereas the approximate (normal) method was biased, particularly when individual studies were small and the median proportion was high. Also, when between study variation was large, the approximate method underestimated the logit of the sensitivity. Hamza et al. (2008) provided SAS code for estimation using both the approximate normal (PROC MIXED) and exact binomial (PROC NLMIXED) models.

12.1.1   Random Effects Model: Meta-analysis of Ultrasound for PAD

We consider again the meta-analysis analyzed in Chapter 7, section 7.5.2.1. That meta-analysis (DeVries et al., 1996), looked at diagnostic accuracy of duplex ultrasonography (US) with and without golor guidance, for use in the diagnosis of stenosis of 50-99% or occlusion. In Chapter 7 we saw that the mean sensitivity for regular duplex ultrasonography (i.e., without color guidance) was 0.84, with a standard error of 0.0257 (95% CI: 0.798,0.889). Using the random effects model (as in equations (12.1) and (12.2)), which is an approximate method (assuming normality of the logit of sensitivity), the estimate of the logit from SAS PROC MIXED is 1.5704, with confidence interval (1.2465, 1.8943). Transforming back to sensitivity units, the estimate of sensitivity is 0.838 with 95% CI: 0.777, 0.869. Between study variability is estimated as 0.1265. The exact method, which uses the binomial distribution of the true positive rate, (see Equations (12.4) and (12.5)) gives estimates of the logit of sensitivity of 1.6424 and 95% CI: 1.3008,1.9840 (from SAS PROC NLMIXED). Transformed to sensitivity units, the estimated sensitivity is 0.828 with 95% CI: 0.786, 0.879. The estimated between study variance is 0.1367. A test of significance of the between study variance in the exact method indicates that between study variance is not significantly different from zero (p=0.2649). Thus it should not be surprising that the width of the confidence intervals for the simple arithmetic mean, approximate and exact random effect models do not differ much.

12.2 ORDINAL- OR CONTINUOUS-SCALE DATA

As described in Chapter 7, Section 7.5, studies of diagnostic tests often only report a single sensitivity and specificity pair, even if the diagnostic test can produce results in several ordinal classes or is continuous. The appropriate model for summarizing the accuracy of the diagnostic test depends on the assumptions made. The most restrictive is to assume that all studies use the same decision threshold and have the same level of accuracy (i.e., ability to discriminate those with and without the condition of interest). A somewhat more realistic assumption is that the accuracy of the diagnostic test is the same across studies, but that the decision threshold varies between studies. That is, the sensitivity, specificity pairs from different studies actually lie on the same ROC curve, but at different locations along the curve (fixed effect). This model, popularized by Littenberg and Moses (1993) and Moses et al. (1993) was presented in Chapter 7

$$B_i = \phi_0 + \phi_1 S_i + e_i.$$

As described in Chapter 7, various fixed effect methods of estimation have been suggested. As also summarized there, many issues with these estimation methods exist, including 1) S_i is measured with error, 2) the correlation between S and B is ignored, 3) between study variation is ignored and 4) having to add a small amount such as 0.5 to cells to enable estimation of within-study errors when there are zero cells.

12.2.1 Random Effects Model

While covariates may be included in the above model to try to explain differences between levels of accuracy in studies as a function of specific patient or study characteristics or levels of quality, there may still be unmeasured or unexplained variation remaining between studies. The simplest refinement to the standard SROC method is the random intercept (RI) model, which is just a random effects model (Hamza et al., 2008)

$$B_i = \phi_{0i} + \phi_1 S_i + \epsilon_i, \tag{12.6}$$

where between study variability is captured through assuming random effect intercept.

$$\phi_{0i} \sim N(\phi, \sigma_{\phi_0}^2). \tag{12.7}$$

The within-study variation of $\widehat{B}_i$, the log of the odds ratio, is estimated as

$$\widehat{\sigma}_{B_i}^2 = \frac{1}{s_{1i}} + \frac{1}{s_{0i}} + \frac{1}{r_{1i}} + \frac{1}{r_{0i}}. \tag{12.8}$$

If any of the denominators are zero, the logits and variances are estimated by adding 0.5 to all cells. This model can also include covariates. Estimation can be accomplished with a linear mixed model program such as PROC MIXED in SAS. This method solves the problem in the original SROC model of ignoring between- study variability. But other problems such as measurement error in $\widehat{S}$, the correlation between B and S, as well as the necessity of adding 0.5 to cells if any are zero, remain.

12.2.2 Bivariate Approach

Reitsma et al. (2005), Arends et al. (2008) and others suggested a multivariate extension of the methods of DerSimonian and Laird (1986) and Hamza et al. (2008), by dealing with sensitivity and specificity simultaneously. These methods will avoid the issue of regression with errors in independent variables (S), and will directly model the correlation between sensitivity and specificity.

Let $\xi_i = \text{logit}(FPR_i)$ and $\eta_i = \text{logit}(TPR_i)$ be the true population parameters for each study. Between study variability can be modeled by assuming a bivariate normal model for (ξ_i, η_i),

$$(\xi_i, \eta_i) \sim N\left(\begin{pmatrix}\xi \\ \eta\end{pmatrix}, \begin{pmatrix}\sigma_\xi^2 & \sigma_{\xi\eta} \\ \sigma_{\xi\eta} & \sigma_\eta^2\end{pmatrix}\right). \tag{12.9}$$

This model implies that the standard univariate random-effects models apply for both ξ and η. It also allows for correlation between the two logits. In terms of the SROC regression line $B = \phi_0 + \phi_1 S$, the parameters ϕ_0 and ϕ_1 can be estimated from the model parameters as

$$\phi_1 = \frac{\sigma_\eta^2 - \sigma_\xi^2}{\sigma_\eta^2 + \sigma_\xi^2 + 2\sigma_{\eta\xi}} \text{ and } \phi_0 = \eta - \xi - \phi_1(\eta + \xi), \tag{12.10}$$

with the residual variance

$$\sigma_{D|S}^2 = \sigma_\eta^2 + \sigma_\xi^2 - 2\sigma_{\eta\xi} - \frac{(\sigma_\eta^2 - \sigma_\xi^2)^2}{\sigma_\eta^2 + \sigma_\xi^2 + 2\sigma_{\eta\xi}}. \tag{12.11}$$

The within-study variability has been modeled in one of two ways. Reitsma et al. (2005) and Arends et al. (2008) use the so called normal-normal (NN) approach that approximates the within-study variability as normal:

$$\widehat{\xi}_i|\xi \sim N(\xi_i, \frac{1}{r_{1i}} + \frac{1}{r_{0i}}), \tag{12.12}$$

$$\widehat{\eta}_i|\eta \sim N(\eta_i, \frac{1}{s_{1i}} + \frac{1}{s_{0i}}). \tag{12.13}$$

With the normal assumption for within study variation, these equations together specify a linear random effects or general linear mixed model (GLMM). The parameters can be estimated using restricted maximum likelihood such as with PROC MIXED in SAS. But this procedure in SAS will not provide estimates and standard errors of user defined functions of these parameters, which may be needed to specify the SROC curve. These can be estimated by "hand", though. An alternative is to use other procedures such as PROC NLMIXED which will provide estimates and SEs of user defined parameters.

This normal-normal method still suffers from two problems. First, the normality assumption is approximate, assuming large samples. In addition, if any of true positive or false positives are zero, then the add-hoc correction of adding 0.5 will be necessary to fit the model. These latter two problems can be avoided with the binomial-normal (BN) model. Extending the method in the univariate case by Hamza et al. (2008), others such as Arends et al. (2008), Chu and Cole (2006) and Hamza et al. (2008), suggested the error specification be modeled directly as binomial.

$$\widehat{\xi_i} \sim Binomial(\frac{1}{1 + e^{-\xi_i}}, n_{0i}), \tag{12.14}$$

$$\widehat{\eta_i} \sim Binomial(\frac{1}{1 + e^{-\eta_i}}, n_{1i}). \tag{12.15}$$

This is now a generalized linear mixed model, and can be estimated using software such as SAS PROC NLMIXED (Arends et al. (2008), Reitsma et al. (2005), Hamza et al. (2008) all provide SAS code to accomplish the analysis).

One advantage of directly modeling sensitivity and specificity (or false positive rate), as compared to the random intercept model is that it is possible to investigate whether covariates individually influence specificity, sensitivity or both.

Chu and Cole (2006) as well as Riley et al. (2007) in small simulations, showed that the BN model gave unbiased estimates of parameters, while the NN model did not. Hamza et al. (2008) did extensive simulations to compare the slope, intercept and variance of the regression model resulting from the three models (RI, NN, and BN) in terms of the bias, MSE and coverage probabilities. They also found that the BN model gave unbiased estimates of both the intercept and slope parameters, with reasonable coverage probabilities, while the random intercept (RI) and NN models often did not. Yet, when within-study sample sizes were large, differences were likely not practically important. That could be important, as analysis, particularly of the random effects model, may be simpler. In fact, surprisingly, the random intercepts model often outperformed the normal-normal model.

12.2.2.1 Simultaneous Summary of Sensitivity and Specificity: Meta-analysis of Ultrasound for PAD   Looking again at the ultrasound meta-analysis of DeVries et al. (1996), we can apply the three random effects models to simultaneously estimate sensitivity and specificity, as well as estimate the SROC curve. Using the RI model, as proposed by Hamza et al. (2008), to the data from studies of regular duplex ultrasonography, we estimate the SROC curve as $B = 4.5439 + 0.1419S$. The test of $\phi_1 = 0$ has p-value 0.6125.

Applying the normal-normal (NN) model, the estimates of false positive rate and sensitivity for regular duplex ultrasonography are 0.0496, 0.828, while for color guided ultrasonography are 0.0317 and 0.9028. Modeling modality as a covariate, the test comparing the two modalities is significant for sensitivity ($p = 0.0120$) but not for false positive rate ($p = 0.2503$).

Following the methodology of Hamza et al. (2008) for the bivariate random effects approach assuming the binomial distribution for within-study variability, we use the NLMIXED procedure to estimate the parameter of the SROC curve. For the regular duplex ultrasonography, the estimate of the intercept is 4.2983, and the slope is -0.29. This is similar to the results of the fixed effects model in Chapter 7, where the weighted least squares result was intercept= 4.19, slope= -0.25. The estimates for color guided ultrasonography in the random effects model were intercept= 5.66; slope= -0.30, while the fixed effects estimates were intercept= 5.45, slope= -0.25 (see Table 7.3 of Chapter 7).

12.2.3 Binary Regression Model

Rutter and Gatsonis (1995) proposed a binary regression model with maximum likelihood (ML) estimation that can account for errors in both $\widehat{FPR}_i$ and $\widehat{Se}_i$. The regression model was motivated by an ordinal regression model for indirect ROC regression, as discussed in Chapter 8. To introduce their method, we need different notation. Let T_{ki} and D_{ki} be the binary test results and the true condition status of the kth patient in the ith study, where $i = 1, \cdots, G$ and $k = 1, \cdots, N_i$. Here $T_{ki} = 1$ for a positive test result and 0 otherwise; $D_{ki} = 0.5$ when the kth patient in the ith study has the condition, and -0.5 otherwise; and N_i is the number of patients in the ith study. It is worth noting that patient-level data $-(T_{ki}, D_{ki})$, $k = 1, \cdots, N_i-$ in the ith study can be constructed easily from the 2×2 table, summarizing agreement between the binary test result and the gold standard. Rutter and Gatsonis (1995) assume the following binary regression model for T_{ki}:

$$\text{logit} P(T_{ki} = 1 | D_{ki}) = \frac{c_i - \beta D_{ki}}{e^{\alpha D_{ki}}}, \tag{12.16}$$

where c_i is a threshold specific to the ith study. This binary regression model is a special case of an ordinal regression model proposed by McCullagh (1980).

From this model, the SROC curve of a diagnostic test has the form,

$$SROC(FPR) = \text{logit}^{-1}[\text{logit}(FPR)e^{-\alpha} - \beta e^{-\alpha/2}],$$

where logit^{-1} is the inverse function $\text{logit}^{-1}(y) = e^y/(1 + e^y)$.

It is worth noting that when the location and scale parameters (α and β) are assumed constant across studies as above (a common assumption needed to be able to fit the model), that the binary regression model and the linear regression model of Moses et al. (1993) are equivalent, with

$$\phi_0 = \frac{-2\beta e^{-\alpha/2}}{1 + e^{-\alpha}}, \phi_1 = \frac{e^{-\alpha} - 1}{e^{-\alpha} + 1}. \tag{12.17}$$

The binary regression method assures that ϕ_1 is between -1 and 1, avoiding estimating implausible SROC curves.

We can use the ML method to estimate the parameters in model equation (12.16). Assuming that the test responses from the different studies are independent and that within the same study binary test responses are Bernoulli random variables, the log-likelihood function is given as follows:

$$l = \sum_{i=1}^{G} \sum_{k=1}^{N_i} \left[(\text{logit})^{-1} \left(\frac{c_i - \beta D_{ki}}{exp(\alpha D_{ki})} \right) \right]^{T_{ki}} \left[1 - (\text{logit})^{-1} \left(\frac{c_i - \beta D_{ki}}{exp(\alpha D_{ki})} \right) \right]^{1 - T_{ki}}.$$

The binary regression model equation (12.16) can also be extended to accommodate study-specific covariates. Let $Z_{i1}, \cdots, Z_{iM}$ be the values of M study-level covariates for the ith study. Then the extended binary regression model is defined by

$$\text{logit}[P(T_{ki} = 1 | D_{ki}, Z_i) = \frac{c_i - [\beta D_{ki} + \eta_1 Z_{i1} D_{ki} + \ldots + \eta_M Z_{iM} D_{ki}]}{e^{\alpha D_{ki}}}. \tag{12.18}$$

In this model, interactions between the disease status and the study-level covariates are included as location parameters. As noted by Rutter and Gatsonis (1995), it is not possible to also include study-level covariates as scale parameters, because of unidentifiability issues. Rutter and Gatsonis (1995) called this model the accuracy model. Under this model, the SROC curve of the test in a study with a vector of study-level covariates $Z = (Z_1, \ldots, Z_M)'$ has the following form:

$$SROC(FPR)_Z = \text{logit}^{-1}[\text{logit}(FPR)e^{-\alpha} - (\beta + \eta_1 Z_1 + \ldots + \eta_M Z_M)e^{-\alpha/2}].$$

The ML method can also be used to estimate the parameters $\alpha, \beta, \eta_1, \cdots, \eta_M$.

Maximizing the preceding log-likelihood function with respect to c_i, β and α, as well as the η's in the accuracy model, we can obtain the corresponding ML estimates (MLEs). Noting the relationship between binary regression model equation (12.16) and an ordinal regression model proposed by McCullagh (1980), Rutter and Gatsonis (1995) originally proposed using PLUM, an existing computer program developed by McCullagh for fitting model equation (12.16) to obtain the MLEs for the location and scale parameters β and α. Binary regression models such as this can also be fit with standard software such as SAS using PROC NLMIXED. Gatsonis and Paliwal (2006) provide SAS code that can be used to fit the binary regression model.

12.2.3.1 Binary Regression: Meta-analysis of Ultrasound for PAD   To illustrate use of the binary regression model proposed by Rutter and Gatsonis (1995), we apply it to the meta-analysis of the eight studies that used regular duplex US. Let $T_{ki} = 1$ if the kth patient in the ith study has a positive test result, and 0 otherwise, $D_{ki} = 0.5$ if the kth patient in the ith study has the condition, and -0.05 otherwise, and $Z_i = (Z_{i1}, \ldots, Z_{i7})$ be a vector of study-indicator variables for the ith study, where $Z_{ij} = 1$ if $i = j$ and 0 otherwise. We fit the binary regression model

$$\text{logit}(P(T_{ki}) = 1|D_{ki}, Z_{ki}) = \frac{c - \beta D_{ki} - \gamma' Z_i}{e^{\alpha D_{ki}}}.$$

Using PROC NLMIXED, we obtain that the parameter estimates as $\widehat{\beta} = -4.5201$, $se(\widehat{\beta}) = 0.297$, $\widehat{\alpha} = 1.0327$, and $se(\widehat{\alpha}) = 0.698$. Therefore, the estimated SROC curve for regular duplex ultrasonography in the diagnosis of stenosis of 50-99% or occlusion, in logit units as in the equation (12.6), is given by

$$B = 3.98 - 0.478S.$$

This can be compared to the results in Chapter 7, where the estimates using weighted least squares were $\widehat{\phi}_0 = 4.19$ and $\widehat{\phi}_1 = -0.25$.

12.2.4 Hierarchical SROC (HSROC) Curve

Because a fixed-effects model can incorporate between-study variability in only a limited way by the inclusion of study-level covariates, Rutter and Gatsonis (2001) proposed a hierarchical regression model that could account for between study variation in estimated sensitivity and specificity pairs more completely than a fixed-effects regression model. The proposed hierarchical model first accounts for within-study variation by a binary regression model as defined by the equation (12.16), with its own study-level positivity and location parameters. It then accounts for between-study variation by assuming that study-level positivity and location parameters are normally distributed with a mean that depends on a linear function of study-level covariates. More specifically, Rutter and Gatsonis (2001) proposed the following 3-level hierarchical regression model in the case of a single study-level covariate Z.

- Level I: The following ordinal regression model with a logit link is assumed for T_{ki}:

$$\text{logit}[P(T_{ki} = 1|D_{ki})] = \frac{c_i - \beta_i D_{ki}}{e^{\alpha D_{ki}}}. \tag{12.19}$$

Here, both the positivity parameter c_i and the location parameter β_i are allowed to vary across studies, but the scale parameter α remains constant across studies.

- Level II: The location parameter β_i and the threshold c_i are assumed to follow normal distributions, with means that depend on the study-level covariates Z_i :

$$c_i|(\gamma_0, \gamma_1, Z_i, \sigma_c^2) \sim N(\gamma_0 + \gamma_1 Z_i, \sigma_c^2),$$
$$\beta_i|(\lambda_0, \lambda_1, Z_i, \sigma_\beta^2) \sim N(\lambda_0 + \lambda_1 Z_i, \sigma_\beta^2). \tag{12.20}$$

Here, c_i and β_i are assumed to be conditionally independent, given γ_0, γ_1, Z_i, σ_c^2 and σ_β^2.

- Level III: The hyperparameters γ_0, γ_1, λ_0, λ_1, σ_c^2, σ_β^2 and α are assumed to have the following known distributions:

$$\gamma_0 \sim Uniform[\mu_{\gamma01}, \mu_{\gamma02}], \gamma_1 \sim Uniform[\mu_{\gamma11}, \mu_{\gamma12}],$$
$$\lambda_0 \sim Uniform[\mu_{\lambda01}, \mu_{\lambda02}], \lambda_1 \sim Uniform[\mu_{\lambda11}, \mu_{\lambda12}],$$
$$\sigma_c^2 \sim \Gamma^{-1}(\xi_1, \xi_2), \sigma_\beta^2 \sim \Gamma^{-1}(\xi_{\beta_1}, \xi_{\beta_2}), \alpha \sim Uniform[\mu_{\alpha_1}, \mu_{\alpha_2}],$$

where the notation $Uniform[a, b]$ refers to a uniform distribution over the interval $[a, b]$ and the notation $\Gamma^{-1}(a, b)$ refers to an inverse gamma distribution with parameters a and b. Here, $\mu_{\gamma01}$, $\mu_{\gamma02}$, $\mu_{\gamma11}$, $\mu_{\gamma12}$, ξ_1, ξ_2, $\mu_{\lambda01}$, $\mu_{\lambda02}$, $\mu_{\lambda11}$, $\mu_{\lambda12}$, ξ_{β_1}, and ξ_{β_2} are known constants and are chosen to reflect possible ranges. See Rutter and Gatsonis (2001) for a detailed discussion on the choice of prior ranges and related sensitivity analysis for chosen prior ranges.

As is standard in Bayesian inference, Rutter and Gatsonis (2001) based their inferences about quantities of interest on the posterior distributions of model parameters. Point estimates are given by the model or the expected value of the posterior distribution, and the highest posterior-density sets of intervals are used in place of confidence intervals (CIs) in the most frequent inferences (Gelman et al., 1995). Because there are no closed-form expressions for the posterior distributions, Rutter and Gatsonis (2001) estimated posterior quantities by simulating observations from the posterior distributions using Markov Chain Monte Carlo (MCMC) simulation, implemented by BUGS (Spiegelhalter et al., 1996), a publicly available software for MCMC sampling. Rutter and Gatsonis (2001) defined the SROC curve for the test as follows:

$$SROC(FPR) = logit^{-1}[logit(FPR)e^{-E(\alpha)} + E(\lambda_0 + \lambda_1 Z_i)e^{-E(\alpha)/2}.$$

This SROC curve is sometimes referred to as a hierarchical SROC curve, or HSROC curve.

Note that level III is only needed when a full Bayesian method is used to estimate the model. Macaskill (2004) suggested a likelihood based approximation which uses nonlinear mixed models. More specifically, she suggested using SAS PROC NLMIXED (she provided SAS code for the procedure). The procedure uses maximum likelihood to fit the model, with Adaptive Gaussian quadrature to maximize the marginal likelihood. Likelihood ratio tests can be used to assess significance of individual parameters or sets of parameters by comparing $-2\times$loglikelihood values for models with and without the parameters of interest. Empirical Bayes estimates of random effects are available using the PREDICT command in NLMIXED.

A clear advantage of the likelihood based approximation is the relative simplicity of implementation with the SAS software. A possible disadvantage is that with NLMIXED the random effects are assumed normal. While step II above shows a normal distribution, distributions other than normal could be chosen for c_i and β_i.

Habord et al. (2007) showed that the HSROC model and the bivariate normal (BN) model are equivalent (just different parameterizations) when study-level covariates are not included. The BN model has an advantage over the HSROC model in that it can accommodate covariates that effect sensitivity alone, specificity alone or both. On the other hand, the HSROC model allows covariates that modify the accuracy in terms of the odds ratio, the threshold parameter or both. When the model has the same covariates effecting both accuracy and threshold parameter, the HSROC model is equivalent of the BN model that has these covariates affecting both sensitivity and specificity. For an HSROC model that includes model. Estimation method effects whether results will agree in practice. If the same program such as SAS NLMIXED is used for both models, the results will agree, but if the Bayesian Markov chain Monte-Carlo method is used for estimation, results may differ.

12.2.5 Other Methods

Sometimes studies will present more than 1 sensitivity, specificity pair, or data corresponding to multiple thresholds. If sufficient data thresholds are presented, an ROC curve can be constructed and the area estimated. Methods for this are in the next section. If interest is in constructing a summary ROC curve, previous methods for single thresholds need to be extended. Hamza et al. (2009) took studies with more than one sensitivity/specificity pair and combined them. Dukic and Gatsonic (2003) also took studies with more than one threshold (but the number of thresholds could vary) and presented methods to combine them using both non-Bayesian and Bayesian methods. We do not present the details here. Kester and Buntinx (2000) presented a method to produce a pooled ROC curve, when each study provided data for a complete ROC curve. Their method was based on using sums and differences of logits, similar to Moses et al. (1993) except that entire ROC curves were used to estimate ROC curve parameters for each study.

12.3 ROC CURVE AREA

If the results of a diagnostic test are ordinal or continuous, and if the investigator reports the results with such measures as the ROC curve area or partial area, then different methods can be used to summarize these findings over studies. Fixed effects methods were described in Chapter 7, Section 7.5.3. When differences between ROC curves are not completely attributable to within-study variability, other methods must be considered. Zhou (1996a) suggested using an empirical Bayes (EB) method, which provided a simple way to express study-level heterogeneity through a two-stage model. In the first stage of the EB method, it is assumed that the area under the ROC curve for individual studies is conditionally independent, given the true ROC curve area, whereas in the second stage, it is assumed that the unobserved true ROC curve areas for individual studies are a random sample from a distribution, with a mean A and a variance τ^2 - the between-study variability. More specifically, we have

- Stage I
$$E(\widehat{A}_i | A_i) = A_i \text{ and } Var(\widehat{A}_i | A_i) = V_i. \tag{12.21}$$

- Stage II
$$E(\widehat{A}_i) = A \text{ and } Var(\widehat{A}_i) = \tau^2. \tag{12.22}$$

Thus we have that

$$E(\widehat{A}_i) = A \text{ and } Var(\widehat{A}_i) = V_i + \tau^2. \tag{12.23}$$

We can estimate A_i and V_i by using either parametric or nonparametric methods. To estimate the parameters A and τ^2, we use the theory of generalized estimating functions (Godambe, 1991). The estimating functions are

$$U_1(A, \tau^2) = \sum_{i=1}^{G} \frac{\widehat{A}_i - A}{V_i + \tau^2} = 0, \tag{12.24}$$

and

$$U_2(A, \tau^2) = \sum_{i=1}^{G} \frac{(\widehat{A}_i - A)^2}{(V_i + \tau^2)^2} - \sum_{i=1}^{G} \frac{1}{V_i + \tau^2} = 0. \tag{12.25}$$

The solution to these two equations provides estimates of A and τ^2. These estimators, $\widehat{A}$ and $\widehat{\tau}^2$, can be shown to be consistent estimators of A and τ and have an asymptotically joint normal distribution with a 0 mean and the following variances:

$$Var(\widehat{A}) = \left(\sum_{i=1}^{G} \frac{1}{V_i + \tau^2} \right)^{-1}, \tag{12.26}$$

and

$$Var(\widehat{\tau}^2) = \left(\sum_{i=1}^{G} \frac{1}{V_i + \tau^2} \right)^{-2} \sum_{i=1}^{G} \frac{(\widehat{A}_i - \widehat{A})^4 - (V_i + \widehat{\tau}^2)^2}{(V_i + \widehat{\tau}^2)^4}, \tag{12.27}$$

respectively. For a proof of this result, see Zhou (1996a).

Zhou (1996a) suggested two possible computational approaches. The first consists of the following four steps:

1. Choose an initial value of τ^2; call it $\widehat{\tau}_0^2$.

2. Estimate A as

$$\widehat{A}(\widehat{\tau}_0^2) = \sum_{i=1}^{G} \frac{\widehat{A}_i}{V_i + \widehat{\tau}_0^2} \Bigg/ \sum_{i=1}^{G} \frac{1}{V_i + \widehat{\tau}_0^2}. \tag{12.28}$$

3. Find an updated estimate of τ^2 by solving

$$\sum_{i=1}^{G} \frac{[\widehat{A}_i - \widehat{A}(\widehat{\tau}_0^2)]^2}{V_i + \tau^2} - \sum_{i=1}^{G} \frac{1}{V_i + \tau^2} = 0. \tag{12.29}$$

4. Continue this process until convergence occurs.

The second approach uses existing statistical packages. It relies on the fact that if the marginal distribution of $\widehat{A}_i$ is normal, with a mean A and a variance $V_i + \tau^2$, then the score functions for A and τ^2 from the normal random variables will be identical to equations (12.24, 12.25). Thus these equations can be solved with software designed specifically for this task, such as the LE program in BMDP statistical software package.

Note that if parameter $\tau^2 = 0$, the true areas under the ROC curves for individual studies are the same - that is, the studies are homogeneous and the methods of the previous section would be appropriate.

Hellmich et al. (1999) review other ML and moments methods for estimating these parameters and their variances. The authors also suggested a fully Bayesian approach to this meta-analysis of the ROC curve area, noting that the 2-stage approach does not account for the uncertainty in the estimates of A and τ^2. Thus they add a third stage to the analysis:

- Stage III

$$A|\tau^2 \sim F(A) \text{ and } \tau^2 \sim G(\tau^2), \tag{12.30}$$

where F and G are prior distributions that can be either informative or non-informative. The noninformative priors that the authors suggested include a vague normal prior, $N(0, 10^4)$, for F, and a gamma or Pareto distribution for G. Specifically, if $\log(\tau^2)$ has a uniform prior on $(-\infty, +\infty)$, then τ^2 is chosen to have a $\Gamma(0.001, 0.001)$ distribution. If τ has a locally uniform prior on $(0, 10)$, then τ^2 is chosen to have a Pareto $(0.5, 0.01)$ distribution.

There are no closed-form analytic solutions for the marginal of the joint prior densities or posterior predictive densities. Instead, techniques such as Gibbs sampling can be used and implemented with computer programs such as BUGS (Spiegelhalter et al., 1996).

12.3.1 Empirical Bayes Method: Meta-analysis of DST

We revisit the example, first presented in Chapter 7, Section 7.5.3.1 regarding the dexamethasone suppression test (DST) to assess pituitary-adrenal dysregulation. The article, by Mossman and Somoza (1989), presented the area under the curve of 7 studies of the accuracy of DST. In Chapter 7, we saw that a test of heterogeneity rejected the null hypothesis of a single underlying common area for the 7 studies. Thus the individual ROC curve areas from the 7 studies are subject to both within- and between-study variation. The EB method would then be more appropriate than the fixed effect method. For the EB method, using the LE program in BMDP, we obtain the estimates for A and τ^2 of $\widehat{A} = 0.77$ and $\widehat{\tau}^2 = 0.0051$. Using the equation (12.26) and the standard errors provided in Table 7.4 we can estimate the variance of $\widehat{A}$ as

$$\widehat{Var}(\widehat{A}) = \left(\frac{1}{0.057^2 + 0.0051} + \frac{1}{0.025^2 + 0.0051} + \cdots + \frac{1}{0.038^2 + 0.0051} \right)^{-1}$$

$$= 0.00103.$$

The variance of $\widehat{\tau}^2$ can be calculated as 0.00227. The fully Bayesian method with various noninformative priors gives an estimate of the population area of 0.769 to 0.771. Estimates for τ^2 are more variable; the means range from 0.00828 to 0.0203, whereas the medians of the posterior distributions range from 0.00561 to 0.0123. As estimated by the fully Bayesian method, the standard errors of area $\widehat{A}$ range from 0.0412 to 0.0600. This range is larger than that for the EB method - which is not surprising, for the fully Bayesian method attempts to capture more of the variability.

Previously, by the fixed effects methods, we found an estimate of the average value of the area for the 7 studies was 0.781 with variance 0.0001825. This area estimate is larger than any of the Bayesian estimates (EB or fully Bayesian), which were highly consistent. With the fixed-effects method, the standard error of the area estimates, at 0.0135, was considerably smaller than that for any of the Bayesian methods. This was to be expected, for the Bayesian methods incorporate both between-study and within-study variation, whereas the fixed-effects methods essentially assume that between-study variation is 0.

APPENDIX A

CASE STUDIES AND CHAPTER 8 DATA

1. Parathyroid Disease Data for Case Study 1:

Parathyroid glands are small endocrine glands usually located in the neck or upper chest that produce a hormone which controls the body's calcium levels. Most people have four parathyroid glands. In the most common form of parathyroid disease, one of these glands grows into a benign tumor, called a parathyroid adenoma, that produces excess amounts of parathyroid hormone. In a less common condition, called parathyroid hyperplasia, all four parathyroid glands become enlarged and secrete excess parathyroid hormone. In both conditions, a patient's serum calcium levels become elevated, and the patient experiences loss of energy, depression, kidney stones, and headaches. Surgical removal of the offending parathyroid lesion is considered curative in most cases.

Single photon emission computed tomography (SPECT) using the radio-pharmaceutical Tc-99m sestamibi is a nuclear medicine imaging test used to detect and localize parathyroid lesions prior to surgical intervention.

Table A.1 summarizes the SPECT accuracy data. There are 97 rows corresponding to the test results for 97 parathyroid glands.

Statistical Methods in Diagnostic Medicine,
Second Edition. By Xiao-Hua Zhou, Nancy A. Obuchowski, Donna K. McClish
Copyright © 2011 John Wiley & Sons, Inc.

Table A.1 Parathyroid Disease Data for Case Study 1

101	1	6	6	5	pos
102	1	4	5	5	pos
102	2	1	1	1	pos
102	3	1	1	1	pos
102	4	1	1	1	pos
103	1	6	7	5	pos
103	2	1	1	1	pos
104	1	7	7	5	pos
105	1	6	6	5	pos
106	1	5	5	4	pos
106	2	4	3	1	neg
107	1	5	4	1	pos
107	2	5	5	1	neg
107	3	5	1	1	neg
107	4	5	1	1	neg
108	1	7	7	5	pos
109	1	3	3	2	neg
110	1	7	7	4	pos
111	1	7	7	3	neg
111	2	1	5	5	pos
112	1	7	7	5	pos
113	1	5	5	5	pos
113	2	3	2	1	neg
114	1	6	6	5	pos
115	1	7	7	4	pos
115	2	1	1	1	pos
115	3	1	1	1	pos
116	1	5	6	5	pos
117	1	4	5	5	pos
118	1	7	7	5	pos
201	1	3	5	5	pos
201	2	3	5	1	neg
201	3	3	5	1	neg
202	1	6	6	5	pos
203	1	7	7	5	pos
204	1	3	3	1	neg
205	1	5	5	5	pos
205	2	4	5	1	neg
206	1	5	5	5	pos
207	1	5	6	5	pos
207	2	1	1	1	pos
208	1	5	6	5	pos
209	1	7	7	5	neg
210	1	7	7	5	pos

210	2	1	1	1	neg
211	1	1	1	1	neg
212	1	3	5	4	pos
213	1	5	5	5	pos
213	2	6	6	1	neg
214	1	1	3	1	pos
214	2	1	3	1	neg
214	3	1	3	1	neg
215	1	1	5	1	pos
215	2	5	5	1	neg
215	3	1	5	1	neg
301	1	7	7	5	pos
302	1	7	7	5	pos
303	1	4	5	5	pos
303	2	4	3	1	neg
304	1	5	6	4	pos
304	2	4	4	1	neg
305	1	4	5	5	pos
306	1	5	6	5	pos
307	1	6	7	5	pos
307	2	2	1	1	neg
308	1	1	5	5	pos
309	1	5	7	5	pos
310	1	6	7	5	pos
311	1	3	4	5	pos
311	2	5	6	3	neg
312	1	6	6	4	pos
312	2	5	1	1	pos
313	1	7	7	5	pos
314	1	1	1	3	pos
315	1	5	5	4	pos
315	2	1	1	1	pos
316	1	5	6	3	pos
317	1	5	6	5	pos
317	2	1	1	2	pos
318	1	5	4	4	pos
319	1	7	7	5	pos
320	1	7	7	5	pos
321	1	4	4	1	pos
321	2	4	4	1	neg
321	3	7	7	1	neg
322	1	3	4	1	pos
322	2	1	1	1	pos
322	3	1	1	1	pos
323	1	4	5	1	pos
323	2	4	4	1	pos

323	3	1	4	1	neg
323	4	1	4	1	neg
324	1	7	7	5	pos
325	1	5	6	5	pos
326	1	7	7	5	pos
327	1	6	6	4	pos
328	1	7	7	5	pos

1st column is the patient's study ID number

2nd column is the gland number (varies from 1 to 4 glands per patient)

3rd column is the test result for SPECT with no attenuation

4th column is the test result for SPECT with attenuation

5th column is the test result for SPECT/CT

6th column is the surgical results (pos=positive for disease; neg=negative for disease)

2. Colon Cancer Detection Data for Case Study 2

The data are presented in three tables:

1. Table A.2: The readers' detection of the polyps (sensitivity data).

2. Table A.3: The readers' false detections (the number of false positives per patient) which is described in chapter 2.

3. Table A.4: The readers' highest score assigned to each of the 8 colon segments (ROC data).

Table A.2 lists the 7 readers' results for 39 colon polyps >5mm in 25 patients. Each row represents a polyp (39 total rows). A score of zero indicates that the reader did not detect the polyp; a score of one indicates that the reader did detect the polyp.

Table A.3 lists the 7 readers' total number of false positives without CAD and the additional number of false positives with CAD for each of the 30 patients. Each row represents a patient (30 total rows). Note that the total number of false positives with CAD equals the sum of the total number of false positives without CAD and the additional number of false positives with CAD.

Table A.4 lists the 7 readers' score for each colon segment. Each row represents a colon segment; each patient had 8 segments evaluated (240 total rows). The third column is the reference standard diagnosis ("truth") for the segment, where F=no polyp exists in the segment, and T=one or more polyps are present in the segment.

Table A.2   Sensitivity Data for Case Study 2

1	0	1	1	1	0	1	1	1	1	1	1	1	1	1
2	1	1	1	1	1	1	1	1	0	1	1	1	1	1
2	1	1	1	1	1	1	1	1	1	1	1	1	1	1
3	1	1	1	1	1	1	1	1	1	1	1	1	1	1
3	1	1	1	1	1	1	1	1	1	1	1	1	1	1
4	0	1	1	1	1	1	0	1	1	1	1	1	1	1
5	1	1	1	1	1	1	1	1	0	1	1	1	1	1
5	1	1	1	1	1	1	1	1	1	1	1	1	1	1
6	1	1	1	1	1	1	1	1	1	1	1	1	1	1
6	1	1	1	1	1	1	1	1	1	1	1	1	1	1
7	1	1	1	1	1	1	1	1	1	1	1	1	1	1
8	1	1	1	1	1	1	1	1	1	1	1	1	1	1
9	0	1	1	1	1	1	1	1	0	1	0	1	1	1
10	1	1	1	1	1	1	1	1	1	1	1	1	1	1
11	1	1	1	1	1	1	1	1	1	1	1	1	1	1
11	1	1	1	1	1	1	1	1	1	1	1	1	1	1
12	0	0	1	1	1	1	1	1	1	1	1	1	1	1
13	1	1	1	1	0	1	1	1	1	1	1	1	0	1
13	0	0	0	0	0	0	0	0	1	1	0	0	1	1
13	0	1	0	1	1	1	1	1	1	1	1	1	1	1
14	1	1	1	1	1	1	1	1	0	1	0	1	1	1
14	1	1	1	1	0	0	1	1	1	1	1	1	1	1
15	1	1	1	1	1	1	1	1	1	1	1	1	1	1
16	1	1	1	1	1	1	1	1	1	1	1	1	1	1
17	1	1	1	1	1	1	1	1	1	1	1	1	1	1
18	0	1	1	1	1	1	1	1	0	1	1	1	0	1
18	1	1	1	1	1	1	1	1	1	1	1	1	1	1
19	1	1	1	1	1	1	1	1	1	1	1	1	1	1
19	0	0	1	1	1	1	0	0	1	1	1	1	1	1
20	0	0	0	0	0	0	1	1	0	0	1	1	0	0
20	0	0	0	0	1	1	1	1	0	0	1	1	0	0
21	1	1	1	1	1	1	1	1	1	1	1	1	1	1
22	1	1	1	1	0	1	1	1	1	1	1	1	1	1
22	1	1	1	1	0	1	1	1	1	1	1	1	1	1
23	0	1	1	1	1	1	1	1	0	1	1	1	1	1
23	1	1	1	1	1	1	1	1	1	1	1	1	0	1
24	1	1	0	1	0	1	1	1	0	1	1	1	1	1
24	1	1	1	1	1	1	1	1	0	1	1	1	1	1
25	0	0	0	0	0	0	0	0	0	0	0	0	0	0

1st column=patient id

2nd, 4th, 6th, 8th, 10nd, 12th, 14th and 16th columns are readers' 1-7 true detections without CAD

3rd, 5th, 7th, 9th, 11nd, 13th, 15th and 17th columns are readers' 1-7 true detections with CAD

Table A.3   # False Positives per Patient for Case Study 2

1	0	0	3	0	1	0	2	0	2	0	0	0	0	0
2	2	0	2	0	2	1	3	1	4	0	1	1	0	0
3	0	0	1	0	0	0	0	0	1	0	0	0	0	0
4	2	0	2	0	0	1	0	1	0	1	0	0	0	0
5	0	0	0	0	1	0	1	0	0	0	0	0	0	0
6	0	0	0	0	0	1	0	0	0	0	0	0	0	0
7	0	0	0	0	4	2	0	1	1	0	1	0	0	1
8	0	0	1	0	4	0	1	0	3	0	1	0	1	0
9	0	0	0	0	0	0	0	0	0	0	0	0	0	0
10	2	1	2	0	3	3	0	2	3	2	1	0	1	0
11	0	0	0	0	0	0	0	0	0	0	0	0	0	1
12	1	0	1	0	2	1	0	1	2	3	1	0	4	1
13	0	0	0	0	1	0	1	0	0	0	0	0	0	0
14	0	1	0	0	1	2	1	0	0	0	1	0	0	0
15	0	0	0	0	0	0	0	0	0	0	0	0	0	0
16	1	0	1	0	0	1	1	1	0	0	0	0	2	2
17	0	0	0	0	1	0	0	0	1	0	2	0	2	0
18	0	0	0	0	0	0	1	0	1	1	1	0	0	0
19	1	1	0	0	1	1	1	1	1	1	1	0	1	0
20	0	0	0	0	0	0	0	0	1	0	0	0	0	0
21	0	0	2	1	4	0	1	0	2	1	2	0	1	0
22	0	0	0	0	1	1	0	0	0	0	0	0	0	0
23	0	0	2	0	1	0	2	0	3	0	2	0	0	0
24	0	0	2	0	1	0	1	0	0	0	0	0	0	0
25	2	0	0	1	0	1	0	1	1	0	0	0	1	0
26	0	0	0	0	2	0	2	0	0	0	0	0	0	0
27	0	0	2	0	1	0	0	0	0	0	0	0	1	0
28	0	1	1	0	2	1	0	0	3	3	1	2	1	0
29	0	0	0	0	1	1	0	1	1	1	0	0	0	1
30	1	0	0	0	1	0	0	0	0	0	0	0	1	0

1st column=patient id
2nd, 4th, 6th, 8th, 10th, 12th, 14th and 16th columns are readers' 1-7 true detections without CAD
3rd, 5th, 7th, 9th, 11th, 13th, 15th and 17th columns are readers' 1-7 true detections with CAD

Table A.4   ROC Data for Case Study 2

1	S1	F	0	0	0	0	0	0	0	0	0	0	0	0	0	0
1	S2	F	0	0	0	0	0	0	0	0	0	0	0	0	0	0
1	S3	F	0	0	0	0	0	0	0	0	0	0	0	0	0	0
1	S4	F	0	3	0	0	0	0	0	0	3	0	0	0	0	0
1	S5	F	0	3	0	5	0	0	0	0	3	0	5	0	0	0
1	S6	F	0	0	5	0	5	0	0	0	0	5	0	5	0	0
1	S7	F	0	0	0	5	0	0	0	0	0	0	5	0	0	0
1	S8	F	0	0	0	0	0	0	0	0	0	0	0	0	0	0
2	S1	F	0	0	0	5	0	0	0	0	0	0	5	0	0	0
2	S2	F	4	0	0	5	3	5	0	4	0	0	5	3	5	0
2	S3	F	0	0	0	0	0	0	0	0	0	0	0	0	0	0
2	S4	F	0	4	0	5	5	0	0	0	4	0	5	5	0	0
2	S5	F	5	0	5	0	0	0	0	5	0	5	0	0	0	0
2	S6	T	5	4	5	5	4	3	0	0	0	0	0	3	0	0
2	S7	F	0	4	0	0	4	0	0	0	4	0	0	4	0	0
2	S8	F	0	0	5	5	0	0	0	0	0	5	0	0	0	0
3	S1	F	0	0	0	0	0	0	0	0	0	0	0	0	0	0
3	S2	F	0	0	3	0	4	4	5	0	0	3	0	4	4	0
3	S3	F	0	0	0	0	0	0	0	0	0	0	0	0	0	0
3	S4	T	4	5	5	0	4	5	5	4	5	5	0	4	5	5
3	S5	F	0	0	0	0	0	0	0	0	0	0	0	0	0	0
3	S6	F	0	0	0	0	0	0	0	0	0	0	0	0	0	0
3	S7	F	0	0	0	0	0	0	0	0	0	0	0	0	0	0
3	S8	T	5	5	5	5	5	5	5	5	5	5	3	5	5	5
4	S1	F	0	0	0	0	0	0	0	0	0	0	0	0	0	0
4	S2	F	0	0	0	0	0	0	0	0	0	0	0	0	0	0
4	S3	F	0	0	0	0	0	0	0	0	0	0	0	0	0	0
4	S4	F	0	0	0	0	0	0	0	0	0	0	0	0	0	0
4	S5	F	4	0	0	0	0	0	0	4	0	0	0	0	0	0
4	S6	F	0	0	0	0	0	0	0	0	0	0	0	0	0	0
4	S7	T	5	5	5	5	4	5	5	5	5	5	5	4	5	5
4	S8	F	0	0	0	0	0	0	0	0	0	0	0	0	0	0
5	S1	F	0	0	3	5	0	0	0	0	0	3	5	0	0	0
5	S2	F	0	0	0	0	0	0	0	0	0	0	0	0	0	0
5	S3	F	0	0	0	0	0	0	0	0	0	0	0	0	0	0
5	S4	F	0	0	0	0	0	0	0	0	0	0	0	0	0	0
5	S5	F	0	0	0	0	0	0	0	0	0	0	0	0	0	0
5	S6	F	0	0	0	0	0	0	0	0	0	0	0	0	0	0
5	S7	F	0	0	0	0	0	0	0	0	0	0	0	0	0	0
5	S8	F	0	0	0	0	0	0	0	0	0	0	0	0	0	0
6	S1	T	4	5	5	5	0	5	0	4	5	5	5	0	5	0
6	S2	F	0	0	0	0	0	0	0	0	0	0	0	0	0	0
6	S3	F	0	0	0	0	0	0	0	0	0	0	0	0	0	0
6	S4	F	0	0	4	0	0	0	0	0	0	0	0	0	0	0

6	S5	F	0	0	0	0	0	0	0	0	0	0	0	0	0	0
6	S6	F	0	0	0	0	0	0	0	0	0	0	0	0	0	0
6	S7	F	0	0	0	0	0	0	0	0	0	0	0	0	0	0
6	S8	F	0	0	0	0	0	0	0	0	0	0	0	0	0	0
7	S1	F	0	0	5	0	0	0	0	0	0	5	0	0	0	0
7	S2	F	0	0	0	5	0	0	3	0	0	0	0	0	0	0
7	S3	T	5	5	5	0	5	5	5	5	5	5	0	5	5	0
7	S4	F	0	0	0	0	0	0	0	0	0	0	0	0	0	0
7	S5	F	0	0	0	0	0	0	0	0	0	0	0	0	0	0
7	S6	T	4	5	5	5	5	5	5	4	5	5	5	4	5	5
7	S7	F	0	0	5	0	5	5	0	0	0	5	0	5	5	0
7	S8	F	0	0	0	0	0	0	0	0	0	0	0	0	0	0
8	S1	F	0	5	0	0	0	3	0	0	5	0	0	0	3	0
8	S2	F	0	0	0	0	0	0	4	0	0	0	0	0	0	4
8	S3	F	0	0	0	0	0	0	0	0	0	0	0	0	0	0
8	S4	T	4	5	5	5	5	5	4	4	5	5	5	5	5	4
8	S5	F	0	0	0	0	0	0	0	0	0	0	0	0	0	0
8	S6	F	0	0	0	0	4	0	0	0	0	0	0	4	0	0
8	S7	F	5	5	5	5	5	5	5	5	5	5	5	5	5	5
8	S8	F	0	0	5	5	0	0	0	0	0	5	5	0	0	0
9	S1	F	0	0	0	0	0	0	0	0	0	0	0	0	0	0
9	S2	F	0	0	0	0	0	0	0	0	0	0	0	0	0	0
9	S3	F	0	0	0	0	0	0	0	0	0	0	0	0	0	0
9	S4	F	0	0	0	0	0	0	0	0	0	0	0	0	0	0
9	S5	F	0	0	0	0	0	0	0	0	0	0	0	0	0	0
9	S6	F	0	0	0	0	0	0	0	0	0	0	0	0	0	0
9	S7	T	5	5	5	5	5	5	5	5	5	5	5	5	5	5
9	S8	F	0	0	4	0	0	5	4	0	0	4	0	0	5	0
10	S1	F	0	0	5	0	0	0	0	0	0	5	0	0	0	0
10	S2	F	0	0	0	0	3	0	0	0	0	0	0	0	0	0
10	S3	F	4	0	4	0	0	0	0	0	0	0	0	0	0	0
10	S4	F	5	4	5	5	3	0	3	5	4	5	0	0	0	3
10	S5	F	0	0	0	0	0	0	0	0	0	0	0	0	0	0
10	S6	F	0	0	0	0	3	0	0	0	0	0	0	3	0	0
10	S7	F	0	0	5	0	0	5	0	0	0	5	0	0	5	0
10	S8	F	0	0	0	0	0	0	0	0	0	0	0	0	0	0
11	S1	F	0	0	0	0	0	0	0	0	0	0	0	0	0	0
11	S2	F	0	0	0	0	0	0	0	0	0	0	0	0	0	0
11	S3	F	0	0	0	0	0	0	0	0	0	0	0	0	0	0
11	S4	F	0	0	0	0	0	0	3	0	0	0	0	0	0	0
11	S5	F	0	0	0	0	0	0	0	0	0	0	0	0	0	0
11	S6	F	0	0	0	0	0	0	0	0	0	0	0	0	0	0
11	S7	T	5	4	5	5	4	5	5	4	4	5	5	4	5	5
11	S8	F	0	0	0	0	0	0	0	0	0	0	0	0	0	0
12	S1	F	0	0	4	0	0	0	0	0	0	4	0	0	0	0
12	S2	T	5	4	0	0	5	5	0	5	4	0	0	5	5	0
12	S3	F	0	0	4	0	0	0	0	0	0	0	0	0	0	0

12	S4	F	0	0	0	5	5	5	4	0	0	0	0	5	5	4
12	S5	F	4	4	5	0	4	0	5	4	4	5	0	4	0	5
12	S6	F	0	0	0	0	0	0	5	0	0	0	0	0	0	5
12	S7	F	0	0	0	0	0	0	0	0	0	0	0	0	0	0
12	S8	F	0	0	0	0	0	0	0	0	0	0	0	0	0	0
13	S1	F	0	0	0	0	0	0	0	0	0	0	0	0	0	0
13	S2	F	0	0	0	0	0	0	0	0	0	0	0	0	0	0
13	S3	F	0	0	0	0	0	0	0	0	0	0	0	0	0	0
13	S4	F	0	0	0	0	0	0	0	0	0	0	0	0	0	0
13	S5	F	0	0	0	0	0	0	0	0	0	0	0	0	0	0
13	S6	F	0	0	0	0	0	0	0	0	0	0	0	0	0	0
13	S7	F	0	0	5	5	0	0	0	0	0	5	5	0	0	0
13	S8	T	4	5	4	5	4	5	5	4	5	0	5	0	0	0
14	S1	F	3	0	5	0	0	0	4	0	0	5	0	0	0	0
14	S2	F	0	0	5	0	0	0	0	0	0	0	0	0	0	0
14	S3	F	0	0	4	0	0	0	0	0	0	0	0	0	0	0
14	S4	F	0	0	0	5	0	0	0	0	0	0	5	0	0	0
14	S5	F	0	0	0	0	0	0	0	0	0	0	0	0	0	0
14	S6	F	0	0	0	0	0	0	0	0	0	0	0	0	0	0
14	S7	T	5	5	5	5	5	5	5	5	5	5	5	5	5	5
14	S8	F	0	0	0	0	0	0	0	0	0	0	0	0	0	0
15	S1	T	5	5	5	5	5	5	0	5	5	5	5	5	5	0
15	S2	F	0	0	0	0	0	0	0	0	0	0	0	0	0	0
15	S3	F	0	0	0	0	0	0	0	0	0	0	0	0	0	0
15	S4	F	0	0	0	0	0	0	0	0	0	0	0	0	0	0
15	S5	F	0	0	0	0	0	0	0	0	0	0	0	0	0	0
15	S6	F	0	0	0	0	0	0	0	0	0	0	0	0	0	0
15	S7	F	0	0	0	0	0	0	0	0	0	0	0	0	0	0
15	S8	F	0	0	0	0	0	0	0	0	0	0	0	0	0	0
16	S1	F	0	0	0	0	0	0	0	0	0	0	0	0	0	0
16	S2	F	0	0	0	0	0	0	0	0	0	0	0	0	0	0
16	S3	T	0	5	5	5	4	5	0	0	5	5	5	3	5	0
16	S4	T	4	0	4	0	4	0	5	0	0	0	0	0	0	5
16	S5	F	0	0	0	0	0	0	0	0	0	0	0	0	0	0
16	S6	F	0	0	0	0	0	0	0	0	0	0	0	0	0	0
16	S7	T	4	5	4	5	3	0	5	4	5	0	5	3	0	5
16	S8	F	0	5	5	5	5	5	0	0	5	5	0	5	5	0
17	S1	F	0	0	0	0	0	0	0	0	0	0	0	0	0	0
17	S2	F	0	0	0	0	0	0	0	0	0	0	0	0	0	0
17	S3	F	0	0	0	0	0	0	0	0	0	0	0	0	0	0
17	S4	F	0	0	0	0	0	5	4	0	0	0	0	0	5	4
17	S5	F	0	0	0	0	0	0	0	0	0	0	0	0	0	0
17	S6	F	0	0	0	0	0	0	0	0	0	0	0	0	0	0
17	S7	F	0	0	0	0	0	0	0	0	0	0	0	0	0	0
17	S8	F	0	0	5	0	5	5	3	0	0	5	0	5	5	3
18	S1	F	5	4	5	5	5	5	4	5	0	5	5	5	5	4
18	S2	F	0	0	0	0	4	0	0	0	0	0	0	0	0	0

18	S3	F	0	0	0	0	0	0	0	0	0	0	0	0	0	0
18	S4	F	0	0	0	0	0	0	0	0	0	0	0	0	0	0
18	S5	F	0	0	0	0	0	0	0	0	0	0	0	0	0	0
18	S6	F	0	0	0	0	0	0	0	0	0	0	0	0	0	0
18	S7	T	5	4	0	5	4	5	4	5	0	0	5	4	5	0
18	S8	F	0	0	0	0	0	0	0	0	0	0	0	0	0	0
19	S1	F	0	0	0	5	0	0	0	0	0	0	5	0	0	0
19	S2	T	5	5	5	5	5	5	5	5	5	5	5	5	5	5
19	S3	F	0	0	0	0	0	0	0	0	0	0	0	0	0	0
19	S4	F	0	0	0	0	0	0	0	0	0	0	0	0	0	0
19	S5	F	0	0	0	0	0	0	0	0	0	0	0	0	0	0
19	S6	F	4	0	0	0	0	5	4	4	0	0	0	0	5	4
19	S7	F	0	0	0	0	0	0	0	0	0	0	0	0	0	0
19	S8	F	0	0	0	0	0	0	0	0	0	0	0	0	0	0
20	S1	F	0	0	0	0	0	0	0	0	0	0	0	0	0	0
20	S2	F	0	0	0	0	0	0	0	0	0	0	0	0	0	0
20	S3	F	0	0	0	0	0	0	0	0	0	0	0	0	0	0
20	S4	T	5	5	5	5	4	5	5	5	5	5	5	3	5	5
20	S5	F	0	0	0	0	0	0	0	0	0	0	0	0	0	0
20	S6	F	0	0	0	0	0	0	0	0	0	0	0	0	0	0
20	S7	F	0	0	0	0	5	0	0	0	0	0	0	5	0	0
20	S8	F	0	0	0	0	0	0	0	0	0	0	0	0	0	0
21	S1	F	0	0	0	0	0	0	0	0	0	0	0	0	0	0
21	S2	F	0	0	0	0	0	0	0	0	0	0	0	0	0	0
21	S3	F	0	0	0	0	0	0	0	0	0	0	0	0	0	0
21	S4	F	0	0	5	0	4	5	0	0	0	5	0	4	5	0
21	S5	F	0	0	0	0	0	0	0	0	0	0	0	0	0	0
21	S6	F	0	5	5	5	0	0	0	0	5	5	5	0	0	0
21	S7	F	5	5	5	5	5	5	5	5	5	5	5	5	5	5
21	S8	F	0	0	0	0	0	0	0	0	0	0	0	0	0	0
22	S1	F	0	0	4	0	0	0	0	0	0	3	0	0	0	0
22	S2	F	0	0	0	0	0	0	0	0	0	0	0	0	0	0
22	S3	F	0	0	0	0	0	0	5	0	0	0	0	0	0	5
22	S4	F	0	0	0	0	0	0	0	0	0	0	0	0	0	0
22	S5	F	0	0	0	0	0	0	0	0	0	0	0	0	0	0
22	S6	F	0	0	0	0	0	0	0	0	0	0	0	0	0	0
22	S7	T	5	5	5	5	5	5	5	5	5	5	5	5	5	5
22	S8	F	0	0	0	0	0	0	0	0	0	0	0	0	0	0
23	S1	F	5	5	5	5	0	5	5	5	5	5	5	0	5	5
23	S2	F	0	0	0	0	0	0	0	0	0	0	0	0	0	0
23	S3	F	0	0	0	0	0	0	0	0	0	0	0	0	0	0
23	S4	F	0	0	0	0	0	0	0	0	0	0	0	0	0	0
23	S5	F	0	0	0	0	0	0	0	0	0	0	0	0	0	0
23	S6	F	4	0	0	0	3	0	0	4	0	0	0	3	0	0
23	S7	T	5	5	5	5	5	5	3	5	5	5	5	5	5	3
23	S8	F	0	0	0	0	0	0	0	0	0	0	0	0	0	0
24	S1	F	0	0	0	0	0	0	0	0	0	0	0	0	0	0

24	S2	F	0	3	5	0	0	0	0	0	3	5	0	0	0	0
24	S3	F	0	0	5	0	4	5	0	0	0	5	0	4	5	0
24	S4	F	0	0	0	0	0	0	0	0	0	0	0	0	0	0
24	S5	F	0	0	0	0	0	0	0	0	0	0	0	0	0	0
24	S6	F	0	0	0	0	0	0	0	0	0	0	0	0	0	0
24	S7	T	0	3	5	5	5	0	0	0	3	5	5	5	0	0
24	S8	F	0	0	0	0	0	0	0	0	0	0	0	0	0	0
25	S1	F	0	0	0	0	0	0	0	0	0	0	0	0	0	0
25	S2	F	0	0	0	0	0	0	0	0	0	0	0	0	0	0
25	S3	F	0	0	0	0	0	0	0	0	0	0	0	0	0	0
25	S4	F	0	0	0	0	0	0	0	0	0	0	0	0	0	0
25	S5	F	0	0	0	0	0	0	0	0	0	0	0	0	0	0
25	S6	F	0	0	0	0	0	0	0	0	0	0	0	0	0	0
25	S7	T	5	5	5	5	5	5	5	5	5	5	5	5	5	5
25	S8	F	3	0	0	0	3	0	0	3	0	0	0	3	0	0
26	S1	F	0	0	5	5	0	0	0	0	0	5	5	0	0	0
26	S2	F	0	0	0	0	0	0	0	0	0	0	0	0	0	0
26	S3	F	0	0	0	0	0	0	0	0	0	0	0	0	0	0
26	S4	T	5	5	5	5	5	0	4	5	5	5	5	5	0	4
26	S5	F	0	4	0	0	0	0	5	0	4	0	0	0	0	5
26	S6	F	0	0	0	0	0	0	0	0	0	0	0	0	0	0
26	S7	F	0	0	0	0	0	0	0	0	0	0	0	0	0	0
26	S8	F	0	0	0	0	0	0	0	0	0	0	0	0	0	0
27	S1	F	0	0	3	0	0	0	0	0	0	3	0	0	0	0
27	S2	T	5	3	5	5	5	5	5	5	3	0	0	5	5	0
27	S3	F	0	4	0	0	0	0	0	0	4	0	0	0	0	0
27	S4	F	0	0	0	0	0	0	3	0	0	0	0	0	0	3
27	S5	F	0	0	0	0	0	0	0	0	0	0	0	0	0	0
27	S6	F	0	0	0	0	0	0	0	0	0	0	0	0	0	0
27	S7	F	0	3	0	0	0	0	0	0	3	0	0	0	0	0
27	S8	F	0	0	0	0	0	0	0	0	0	0	0	0	0	0
28	S1	F	0	0	5	0	5	5	4	0	0	5	0	5	5	4
28	S2	T	4	3	5	0	5	5	4	0	3	5	0	5	0	4
28	S3	F	5	0	5	0	5	0	0	5	0	5	0	5	0	0
28	S4	F	0	3	4	0	3	3	0	0	3	0	0	0	0	0
28	S5	F	0	0	0	0	0	0	0	0	0	0	0	0	0	0
28	S6	F	0	0	0	0	0	0	0	0	0	0	0	0	0	0
28	S7	F	0	0	0	0	0	0	0	0	0	0	0	0	0	0
28	S8	F	0	0	0	0	0	0	0	0	0	0	0	0	0	0
29	S1	F	0	0	0	0	0	0	0	0	0	0	0	0	0	0
29	S2	F	0	0	0	0	0	0	0	0	0	0	0	0	0	0
29	S3	F	0	0	0	0	0	0	0	0	0	0	0	0	0	0
29	S4	F	0	0	0	0	0	0	0	0	0	0	0	0	0	0
29	S5	F	0	0	0	0	0	0	0	0	0	0	0	0	0	0
29	S6	F	0	0	0	0	0	0	0	0	0	0	0	0	0	0
29	S7	F	0	0	0	0	0	0	0	0	0	0	0	0	0	0
29	S8	F	0	0	0	0	0	0	0	0	0	0	0	0	0	0

30	S1	T	4	5	5	0	3	3	4	4	5	5	0	3	0	4
30	S2	F	0	0	0	0	0	0	0	0	0	0	0	0	0	0
30	S3	F	0	0	0	0	0	0	0	0	0	0	0	0	0	0
30	S4	F	0	0	0	0	0	0	0	0	0	0	0	0	0	0
30	S5	F	0	0	0	0	0	0	0	0	0	0	0	0	0	0
30	S6	F	0	0	0	0	0	0	0	0	0	0	0	0	0	0
30	S7	F	0	0	0	0	0	0	0	0	0	0	0	0	0	0
30	S8	F	0	0	0	0	0	0	0	0	0	0	0	0	0	0

1st column=patient id
2nd column=segment id
3rd column=reference standard diagnosis for the segment (T=contains polyp, F=no polyp)
4th-10nd columns are readers' 1-7 maximum score with CAD
11nd-17th columns are readers' 1-7 maximum score without CAD

3. Carotid Artery Stenosis Data

The data are presented in table A.5. There are 4 rows for each patient (163 patients x 4 = 652 rows). Each row gives the results for one of the four radiologists.

Table A.5   Carotid Artery Stenosis Results for Case Study 3

1	1	0	69	1	2	1	100	1	0	1	100	1	0
1	2	0	69	1	2	1	100	1	0	1	100	1	0
1	3	0	69	1	2	1	100	1	35	1	100	1	0
1	4	0	69	1	2	1	100	1	29	1	100	1	0
2	1	0	64	0	2	1	0	5	99	5	70	5	85
2	2	0	64	0	2	2	40	1	95	4	66	5	86
2	3	0	64	0	2	1	100	5	99	5	66	5	82
2	4	0	64	0	2	2	58	4	77	4	67	5	80
4	1	1	73	0	3	1	10	5	90	1	15	1	66
4	2	1	73	0	3	1	0	5	95	1	0	5	77
4	3	1	73	0	3	5	83	1	20	1	0	5	64
4	4	1	73	0	3	1	5	5	80	1	17	5	71
5	1	1	62	0	4	1	100	5	90	1	100	5	85
5	2	1	62	0	4	1	100	5	95	1	100	5	79
5	3	1	62	0	4	1	100	5	80	1	100	5	72
5	4	1	62	0	4	1	100	5	80	1	100	5	80
6	1	0	82	0	0	5	75	1	33	5	61	1	12
6	2	0	82	0	0	5	90	1	20	5	68	4	67
6	3	0	82	0	0	4	60	1	39	1	55	1	19
6	4	0	82	0	0	4	64	2	43	4	69	1	27
7	1	1	63	1	1	1	0	1	0	1	0	1	0
7	2	1	63	1	1	1	0	1	0	1	0	1	0
7	3	1	63	1	1	1	0	1	0	1	0	1	0
7	4	1	63	1	1	1	0	1	0	1	0	1	0
8	1	0	79	0	3	5	99	1	0	1	0	5	75
8	2	0	79	0	3	5	99	1	20	5	80	1	0
8	3	0	79	0	3	5	95	1	0	5	71	1	0
8	4	0	79	0	3	5	99	1	7	2	83	1	0
9	1	0	64	1	3	1	25	5	80	1	55	5	77
9	2	0	64	1	3	1	25	5	95	2	50	5	71
9	3	0	64	1	3	1	23	5	83	1	38	1	76
9	4	0	64	1	3	2	36	5	80	1	40	5	82
10	1	0	76	0	4	5	99	5	70	5	76	5	71
10	2	0	76	0	4	5	95	4	72	5	76	4	73
10	3	0	76	0	4	5	70	5	90	1	69	2	50
10	4	0	76	0	4	5	90	4	63	5	78	4	56
11	1	0	57	1	3	1	33	1	0	1	51	1	24
11	2	0	57	1	3	2	55	1	0	5	60	1	0
11	3	0	57	1	3	1	29	1	51	1	51	1	10
11	4	0	57	1	3	4	51	1	0	2	54	1	7
12	1	0	68	0	2	2	57	5	70	2	53	5	73
12	2	0	68	0	2	3	58	5	85	2	50	5	75
12	3	0	68	0	2	5	64	5	80	1	50	1	75

12	4	0	68	0	2	4	62	4	77	2	50	2	33
13	1	0	72	1	4	5	90	5	90	1	50	5	79
13	2	0	72	1	4	4	95	5	95	1	65	1	78
13	3	0	72	1	4	5	95	5	84	2	50	5	75
13	4	0	72	1	4	4	54	5	71	4	66	5	85
15	1	1	72	0	0	1	47	5	90	1	50	5	82
15	2	1	72	0	0	2	55	4	95	1	20	5	87
15	3	1	72	0	0	4	64	4	90	1	20	5	84
15	4	1	72	0	0	3	58	5	86	1	38	5	87
16	1	1	67	0	5	5	90	1	25	5	85	1	25
16	2	1	67	0	5	5	80	1	25	5	82	1	14
16	3	1	67	0	5	5	84	1	24	5	75	1	27
16	4	1	67	0	5	5	75	1	29	5	81	1	15
17	1	1	54	1	0	1	50	1	10	1	100	1	100
17	2	1	54	1	0	1	100	2	100	1	100	1	100
17	3	1	54	1	0	1	100	5	99	1	100	1	100
17	4	1	54	1	0	1	100	5	99	1	100	1	100
18	1	1	80	0	1	5	95	1	0	5	85	1	0
18	2	1	80	0	1	5	95	1	0	5	78	1	0
18	3	1	80	0	1	5	99	1	22	1	75	1	0
18	4	1	80	0	1	5	99	1	0	5	80	1	0
19	1	0	70	0	3	5	95	1	10	5	75	1	25
19	2	0	70	0	3	5	95	1	20	5	80	1	27
19	3	0	70	0	3	5	88	1	17	5	66	1	34
19	4	0	70	0	3	5	83	1	17	5	82	1	21
20	1	0	71	1	4	1	52	1	40	1	25	1	50
20	2	0	71	1	4	1	32	3	58	1	17	2	30
20	3	0	71	1	4	4	50	4	50	1	31	1	40
20	4	0	71	1	4	3	51	3	50	1	13	2	45
21	1	1	64	0	2	5	90	1	0	5	74	1	0
21	2	1	64	0	2	5	95	1	0	5	80	1	0
21	3	1	64	0	2	5	95	1	0	5	78	1	0
21	4	1	64	0	2	5	83	1	0	1	0	5	2
22	1	0	60	0	4	1	100	5	90	1	100	5	70
22	2	0	60	0	4	1	100	5	95	1	100	4	66
22	3	0	60	0	4	1	100	5	99	1	100	5	64
22	4	0	60	0	4	1	100	5	88	1	100	5	74
23	1	0	44	0	3	1	0	1	0	1	0	1	0
23	2	0	44	0	3	1	0	2	50	1	0	2	50
23	3	0	44	0	3	1	4	4	99	1	0	1	25
23	4	0	44	0	3	1	24	4	70	1	0	3	36
25	1	1	74	0	4	1	100	1	10	1	100	5	65
25	2	1	74	0	4	1	100	4	90	1	100	4	60
25	3	1	74	0	4	1	100	4	85	1	100	4	61
25	4	1	74	0	4	1	100	3	47	1	100	4	60
26	1	0	56	0	2	1	25	1	30	1	30	1	50

26	2	0	56	0	2	1	0	3	55	1	30	1	44
26	3	0	56	0	2	2	57	1	29	1	10	1	48
26	4	0	56	0	2	2	45	3	35	2	20	2	44
27	1	0	59	1	3	1	0	5	99	1	50	5	90
27	2	0	59	1	3	2	50	5	99	1	25	5	90
27	3	0	59	1	3	1	19	5	99	1	21	5	99
27	4	0	59	1	3	2	43	5	99	1	15	5	88
28	1	0	61	0	4	1	100	1	100	1	100	1	100
28	2	0	61	0	4	1	100	1	100	1	100	1	100
28	3	0	61	0	4	5	99	1	100	1	100	1	100
28	4	0	61	0	4	1	100	1	100	1	100	1	100
29	1	0	70	0	3	1	0	5	65	1	50	5	70
29	2	0	70	0	3	1	0	5	75	2	47	4	63
29	3	0	70	0	3	1	36	5	73	1	47	5	67
29	4	0	70	0	3	2	31	4	73	2	40	4	71
30	1	1	72	1	1	1	40	1	20	1	55	1	50
30	2	1	72	1	1	2	40	2	45	1	0	2	54
30	3	1	72	1	1	1	48	1	35	2	48	2	55
30	4	1	72	1	1	3	45	2	30	2	47	2	46
31	1	0	79	0	1	1	0	5	70	1	35	5	66
31	2	0	79	0	1	1	40	5	80	1	40	2	47
31	3	0	79	0	1	1	0	5	75	1	39	2	50
31	4	0	79	0	1	2	17	5	64	2	29	4	70
32	1	1	78	0	5	1	10	5	85	1	0	5	85
32	2	1	78	0	5	2	40	5	95	1	30	5	75
32	3	1	78	0	5	1	12	5	86	1	27	5	61
32	4	1	78	0	5	2	45	4	73	2	28	4	78
34	1	1	71	0	0	5	99	5	70	5	75	1	40
34	2	1	71	0	0	4	90	5	80	5	78	1	40
34	3	1	71	0	0	5	99	4	78	5	76	1	39
34	4	1	71	0	0	5	99	4	63	5	76	1	0
35	1	1	69	1	1	5	95	1	33	5	85	1	0
35	2	1	69	1	1	5	95	1	45	5	81	1	0
35	3	1	69	1	1	5	88	1	28	5	75	1	8
35	4	1	69	1	1	5	83	2	46	5	89	1	0
36	1	1	53	1	1	1	0	1	0	1	0	1	0
36	2	1	53	1	1	1	0	1	0	1	0	1	0
36	3	1	53	1	1	5	0	5	0	5	63	1	0
36	4	1	53	1	1	2	0	1	0	1	0	1	0
38	1	0	62	0	1	1	100	5	65	1	100	5	63
38	2	0	62	0	1	1	100	5	80	1	100	5	76
38	3	0	62	0	1	1	100	5	68	1	100	1	57
38	4	0	62	0	1	1	100	4	68	1	100	4	63
39	1	1	77	0	3	1	0	5	90	1	2	5	85
39	2	1	77	0	3	1	0	5	90	1	10	5	82
39	3	1	77	0	3	1	17	5	95	1	2	5	85

39	4	1	77	0	3	2	15	5	77	2	12	5	88
40	1	1	60	0	5	1	50	1	100	1	33	1	100
40	2	1	60	0	5	2	54	1	100	1	42	1	100
40	3	1	60	0	5	2	50	.	.	2	31	1	100
40	4	1	60	0	5	3	45	1	100	2	40	1	100
42	1	0	56	1	4	1	0	5	95	1	33	5	86
42	2	0	56	1	4	1	25	5	95	1	20	5	90
42	3	0	56	1	4	1	19	5	95	1	30	1	88
42	4	0	56	1	4	2	13	5	92	1	20	5	88
45	1	0	66	0	1	5	95	1	0	5	85	1	33
45	2	0	66	0	1	5	95	1	0	5	98	1	10
45	3	0	66	0	1	5	99	1	15	5	99	1	5
45	4	0	66	0	1	5	99	1	20	5	84	1	29
46	1	1	64	1	3	5	75	1	40	5	62	1	52
46	2	1	64	1	3	5	85	1	0	5	80	1	0
46	3	1	64	1	3	5	86	1	0	4	59	1	0
46	4	1	64	1	3	5	75	2	57	5	62	2	48
47	1	0	73	0	3	5	99	2	50	2	50	1	38
47	2	0	73	0	3	3	60	2	50	2	50	1	10
47	3	0	73	0	3	4	61	4	60	1	50	1	40
47	4	0	73	0	3	4	70	2	58	4	62	2	35
48	1	0	71	0	3	1	0	1	35	1	0	1	42
48	2	0	71	0	3	1	0	1	40	1	0	1	20
48	3	0	71	0	3	1	0	1	34	1	0	1	42
48	4	0	71	0	3	1	0	2	45	1	0	3	42
49	1	0	70	1	1	1	0	5	65	1	80	5	80
49	2	0	70	1	1	1	0	5	90	1	0	5	78
49	3	0	70	1	1	1	0	5	95	1	0	5	77
49	4	0	70	1	1	1	0	4	63	1	0	5	80
50	1	0	74	0	3	1	25	5	70	1	17	5	72
50	2	0	74	0	3	1	50	5	70	1	20	5	75
50	3	0	74	0	3	1	48	5	72	1	31	5	69
50	4	0	74	0	3	3	42	4	79	2	36	5	73
51	1	0	67	0	3	5	95	4	60	5	85	1	5
51	2	0	67	0	3	5	95	2	54	5	90	1	20
51	3	0	67	0	3	5	99	4	65	5	84	1	22
51	4	0	67	0	3	5	99	5	57	5	88	1	11
53	1	0	54	0	1	1	25	1	100	1	48	1	100
53	2	0	54	0	1	4	70	1	100	1	30	1	100
53	3	0	54	0	1	1	29	1	100	1	26	1	100
53	4	0	54	0	1	4	66	1	100	3	42	1	100
54	1	0	73	0	5	5	90	1	100	1	100	5	81
54	2	0	73	0	5	5	90	1	100	5	80	1	100
54	3	0	73	0	5	5	95	1	100	4	41	1	100
54	4	0	73	0	5	5	99	1	100	5	83	1	100
55	1	0	72	0	1	1	15	4	60	1	9	5	75

55	2	0	72	0	1	1	15	5	75	1	0	5	75
55	3	0	72	0	1	1	5	5	63	1	0	5	67
55	4	0	72	0	1	2	25	5	58	1	15	5	70
60	1	0	60	1	0	1	0	5	65	1	0	1	30
60	2	0	60	1	0	1	0	4	64	1	0	1	34
60	3	0	60	1	0	1	0	2	65	1	0	1	32
60	4	0	60	1	0	2	20	4	57	1	0	1	26
61	1	0	66	0	5	5	95	1	35	5	95	1	45
61	2	0	66	0	5	5	90	4	69	5	85	1	30
61	3	0	66	0	5	5	99	5	64	5	99	1	26
61	4	0	66	0	5	4	88	3	71	5	85	1	33
63	1	1	72	0	3	5	90	5	90	5	90	1	50
63	2	1	72	0	3	5	90	5	90	5	90	2	46
63	3	1	72	0	3	5	95	5	87	5	86	1	54
63	4	1	72	0	3	5	85	4	72	5	90	1	40
64	1	1	49	1	1	4	60	1	35	1	45	1	25
64	2	1	49	1	1	5	75	1	45	2	47	1	25
64	3	1	49	1	1	4	65	1	40	1	40	1	23
64	4	1	49	1	1	4	67	1	27	4	50	2	29
65	1	1	73	0	3	5	90	5	80	5	65	2	58
65	2	1	73	0	3	5	90	5	90	3	58	5	62
65	3	1	73	0	3	5	86	5	85	1	54	1	56
65	4	1	73	0	3	5	71	4	77	4	58	2	34
66	1	1	66	1	0	5	95	5	66	5	90	5	70
66	2	1	66	1	0	4	95	5	80	5	84	5	82
66	3	1	66	1	0	2	99	.	99	5	80	5	76
66	4	1	66	1	0	5	99	4	99	4	80	4	84
67	1	0	67	1	1	1	45	5	90	1	0	5	85
67	2	0	67	1	1	2	58	5	90	1	0	5	86
67	3	0	67	1	1	1	51	5	85	5	84	1	0
67	4	0	67	1	1	3	45	5	88	1	6	5	84
68	1	0	54	0	3	4	60	5	85	1	40	5	66
68	2	0	54	0	3	5	78	5	90	1	43	5	69
68	3	0	54	0	3	3	60	5	86	1	27	5	71
68	4	0	54	0	3	4	64	4	77	2	29	4	75
69	1	0	74	0	3	1	100	5	95	1	100	5	77
69	2	0	74	0	3	1	100	5	95	1	100	5	72
69	3	0	74	0	3	1	100	5	95	4	62	5	73
69	4	0	74	0	3	1	100	5	86	1	100	4	77
71	1	1	69	0	5	5	95	1	30	5	90	1	0
71	2	1	69	0	5	5	99	1	35	5	99	1	0
71	3	1	69	0	5	5	99	1	40	5	99	1	19
71	4	1	69	0	5	5	99	2	45	5	90	1	0
73	1	1	69	1	2	5	66	1	0	2	57	1	0
73	2	1	69	1	2	5	90	1	0	5	75	1	0
73	3	1	69	1	2	1	0	5	75	1	45	1	0

73	4	1	69	1	2	5	67	1	0	4	74	1	0
74	1	0	59	1	3	5	72	5	70	5	65	1	50
74	2	0	59	1	3	5	82	5	85	5	64	1	42
74	3	0	59	1	3	5	85	5	69	1	64	1	45
74	4	0	59	1	3	4	71	4	64	5	73	2	42
75	1	0	70	1	5	5	90	1	25	5	65	1	40
75	2	0	70	1	5	5	90	1	20	4	60	1	45
75	3	0	70	1	5	5	77	1	25	5	69	1	39
75	4	0	70	1	5	5	90	1	33	5	77	2	40
76	1	0	72	1	0	1	30	1	0	2	57	1	0
76	2	0	72	1	0	2	40	1	0	2	50	1	0
76	3	0	72	1	0	2	52	1	0	1	47	1	0
76	4	0	72	1	0	3	36	1	0	4	58	1	0
77	1	1	51	1	3	1	100	1	35	1	100	1	40
77	2	1	51	1	3	1	100	1	40	1	100	1	33
77	3	1	51	1	3	1	100	2	37	1	100	1	39
77	4	1	51	1	3	1	100	2	30	1	100	2	33
78	1	0	69	0	4	1	40	5	80	1	42	5	72
78	2	0	69	0	4	1	40	5	80	1	40	5	86
78	3	0	69	0	4	2	52	5	85	1	37	5	84
78	4	0	69	0	4	3	42	5	78	2	39	4	87
80	1	0	64	0	3	5	90	1	45	5	65	1	30
80	2	0	64	0	3	5	90	1	42	2	55	1	30
80	3	0	64	0	3	5	81	1	40	5	64	1	20
80	4	0	64	0	3	5	83	2	37	4	74	1	28
81	1	0	77	0	5	5	70	5	90	1	33	5	75
81	2	0	77	0	5	5	75	5	88	1	30	5	75
81	3	0	77	0	5	5	74	5	85	1	42	5	71
81	4	0	77	0	5	3	58	5	83	2	35	5	68
82	1	0	70	0	2	1	45	1	30	1	54	1	33
82	2	0	70	0	2	3	58	1	35	4	60	1	17
82	3	0	70	0	2	1	36	1	30	1	37	1	23
82	4	0	70	0	2	1	45	2	25	1	33	1	15
83	1	1	74	1	5	1	25	1	100	1	38	1	100
83	2	1	74	1	5	1	30	1	100	2	40	1	100
83	3	1	74	1	5	1	32	1	100	1	23	1	100
83	4	1	74	1	5	2	46	1	100	5	26	1	100
84	1	0	65	1	4	2	50	5	95	1	35	5	98
84	2	0	65	1	4	4	62	5	99	1	42	5	90
84	3	0	65	1	4	2	53	5	99	1	45	5	99
84	4	0	65	1	4	2	50	5	99	1	36	5	91
85	1	0	60	0	4	5	95	5	75	5	85	5	61
85	2	0	60	0	4	5	95	5	80	5	90	4	60
85	3	0	60	0	4	5	95	5	80	5	84	5	73
85	4	0	60	0	4	5	99	5	79	5	85	2	53
87	1	0	76	1	4	1	40	5	75	1	10	1	38

87	2	0	76	1	4	1	50	5	77	1	20	2	33
87	3	0	76	1	4	1	0	.	65	1	2	1	2
87	4	0	76	1	4	3	20	3	55	1	4	3	45
88	1	0	65	0	2	1	0	5	90	1	0	5	80
88	2	0	65	0	2	1	0	5	90	1	0	5	70
88	3	0	65	0	2	1	0	5	95	1	0	5	65
88	4	0	65	0	2	1	0	5	99	1	0	5	80
89	1	0	58	0	3	5	85	1	35	5	75	1	40
89	2	0	58	0	3	5	90	2	53	5	80	2	45
89	3	0	58	0	3	5	75	1	27	5	76	1	35
89	4	0	58	0	3	5	80	2	14	5	85	3	55
90	1	0	60	0	4	5	90	5	85	5	69	1	54
90	2	0	60	0	4	5	90	5	80	1	64	2	50
90	3	0	60	0	4	5	83	5	84	5	71	1	41
90	4	0	60	0	4	5	88	5	87	4	73	4	64
91	1	1	63	1	2	1	0	5	95	1	0	5	66
91	2	1	63	1	2	1	0	5	95	1	0	5	68
91	3	1	63	1	2	1	15	5	95	1	28	5	63
91	4	1	63	1	2	1	0	5	99	1	0	5	68
92	1	0	70	0	2	1	35	5	99	1	53	1	100
92	2	0	70	0	2	1	40	4	99	4	60	1	100
92	3	0	70	0	2	2	48	5	99	5	70	1	100
92	4	0	70	0	2	4	50	3	99	3	53	1	100
93	1	1	58	0	2	1	10	5	95	1	29	5	84
93	2	1	58	0	2	1	0	5	95	1	0	5	82
93	3	1	58	0	2	1	0	5	95	1	0	1	99
93	4	1	58	0	2	1	0	5	99	1	0	5	84
94	1	0	70	1	3	5	80	1	0	5	68	1	15
94	2	0	70	1	3	5	82	1	30	5	66	1	0
94	3	0	70	1	3	5	87	1	0	5	72	1	0
94	4	0	70	1	3	5	83	1	0	5	80	1	0
95	1	1	60	1	2	1	25	1	30	5	4	5	85
95	2	1	60	1	2	1	0	1	0	1	0	1	0
95	3	1	60	1	2	1	0	1	0	5	84	5	84
95	4	1	60	1	2	2	0	2	0	5	83	5	93
97	1	0	62	0	5	4	64	2	45	1	25	5	68
97	2	0	62	0	5	5	70	5	75	1	25	4	66
97	3	0	62	0	5	5	67	5	70	1	33	5	64
97	4	0	62	0	5	4	75	4	70	2	31	3	62
98	1	0	66	0	5	1	100	1	20	1	100	1	13
98	2	0	66	0	5	1	100	1	46	1	100	1	20
98	3	0	66	0	5	1	100	1	34	1	100	1	26
98	4	0	66	0	5	1	100	2	36	1	100	1	22
99	1	0	80	1	2	1	33	1	45	1	28	1	33
99	2	0	80	1	2	1	0	1	48	1	0	1	27
99	3	0	80	1	2	1	0	1	44	1	0	1	33

99	4	0	80	1	2	1	0	3	36	1	0	2	42
100	1	0	66	0	3	5	70	2	57	1	57	1	30
100	2	0	66	0	3	5	85	2	55	4	60	1	37
100	3	0	66	0	3	5	80	.	52	1	64	1	34
100	4	0	66	0	3	3	77	3	56	4	60	2	44
101	1	0	77	0	1	5	80	1	100	5	65	1	100
101	2	0	77	0	1	5	85	1	100	4	65	1	100
101	3	0	77	0	1	5	85	1	100	3	60	1	100
101	4	0	77	0	1	4	75	1	100	4	73	1	100
102	1	0	62	0	2	5	95	1	0	5	90	1	0
102	2	0	62	0	2	5	99	1	0	5	87	1	0
102	3	0	62	0	2	5	95	1	0	5	73	1	0
102	4	0	62	0	2	4	99	1	0	5	94	1	0
103	1	0	76	0	2	5	82	2	50	5	74	1	27
103	2	0	76	0	2	4	75	2	55	5	71	2	20
103	3	0	76	0	2	1	47	2	50	5	73	1	20
103	4	0	76	0	2	2	50	3	56	4	79	1	27
104	1	0	70	1	4	1	12	5	95	1	17	5	78
104	2	0	70	1	4	1	0	5	95	1	0	5	81
104	3	0	70	1	4	1	0	5	95	1	5	5	99
104	4	0	70	1	4	1	0	5	99	1	8	5	85
105	1	1	35	0	0	5	95	1	20	5	88	1	0
105	2	1	35	0	0	5	90	1	0	5	82	1	.
105	3	1	35	0	0	1	95	1	17	5	79	1	0
105	4	1	35	0	0	1	13	5	99	5	85	1	14
106	1	0	72	0	3	5	95	5	95	5	60	5	85
106	2	0	72	0	3	5	90	5	95	4	64	5	85
106	3	0	72	0	3	5	95	5	95	3	61	5	86
106	4	0	72	0	3	5	82	5	78	3	65	5	85
107	1	0	58	0	5	5	88	1	0	5	85	1	0
107	2	0	58	0	5	5	95	1	0	5	82	1	.
107	3	0	58	0	5	5	90	1	0	5	74	1	0
107	4	0	58	0	5	5	88	1	0	5	76	1	0
108	1	0	62	0	3	5	95	5	90	5	70	5	78
108	2	0	62	0	3	5	95	5	90	5	68	5	85
108	3	0	62	0	3	5	95	5	92	4	62	2	52
108	4	0	62	0	3	5	99	5	90	5	79	5	82
109	1	0	58	1	2	1	49	5	95	1	45	5	63
109	2	0	58	1	2	2	55	5	95	1	47	4	62
109	3	0	58	1	2	2	57	5	95	1	34	3	60
109	4	0	58	1	2	2	20	5	84	2	43	2	58
110	1	0	72	0	3	5	78	1	0	5	75	5	62
110	2	0	72	0	3	5	88	1	0	5	74	2	53
110	3	0	72	0	3	2	86	1	0	5	71	1	25
110	4	0	72	0	3	5	88	1	0	5	73	2	31
111	1	0	74	1	3	4	62	1	50	5	60	5	60

111	2	0	74	1	3	2	54	5	66	1	30	2	40
111	3	0	74	1	3	5	64	5	65	3	58	1	45
111	4	0	74	1	3	3	49	1	31	3	53	3	55
112	1	1	77	0	2	1	0	4	62	1	0	5	72
112	2	1	77	0	2	1	0	4	64	1	0	5	68
112	3	1	77	0	2	1	0	1	63	1	0	4	63
112	4	1	77	0	2	3	54	1	0	1	0	4	70
113	1	0	67	1	1	1	100	1	40	1	100	1	15
113	2	0	67	1	1	1	100	1	35	1	100	1	0
113	3	0	67	1	1	1	100	1	51	1	100	1	13
113	4	0	67	1	1	1	100	3	56	1	100	2	24
116	1	1	60	1	2	4	63	4	61	5	77	1	33
116	2	1	60	1	2	2	55	5	70	5	75	1	42
116	3	1	60	1	2	1	48	4	60	5	73	1	17
116	4	1	60	1	2	3	55	4	71	5	75	2	38
117	1	0	73	1	2	1	20	5	76	1	33	5	70
117	2	0	73	1	2	1	30	5	90	2	40	5	70
117	3	0	73	1	2	1	47	5	75	1	30	3	61
117	4	0	73	1	2	2	30	5	76	2	40	5	77
118	1	0	68	0	4	5	95	1	0	1	0	5	75
118	2	0	68	0	4	5	95	1	0	5	75	1	0
118	3	0	68	0	4	5	95	1	16	5	66	1	0
118	4	0	68	0	4	5	99	1	0	5	83	1	0
119	1	1	67	0	4	5	80	5	90	1	42	5	86
119	2	1	67	0	4	5	85	5	90	2	50	5	85
119	3	1	67	0	4	5	88	5	93	1	43	5	78
119	4	1	67	0	4	4	80	5	92	2	46	5	84
120	1	0	78	1	3	1	50	1	10	1	43	1	0
120	2	0	78	1	3	1	46	1	0	1	37	1	0
120	3	0	78	1	3	1	41	1	0	1	40	1	0
120	4	0	78	1	3	1	0	3	36	2	50	1	0
121	1	0	74	1	3	1	20	5	99	1	0	5	87
121	2	0	74	1	3	1	0	5	90	1	0	5	90
121	3	0	74	1	3	1	0	5	99	1	3	5	99
121	4	0	74	1	3	1	7	5	99	1	21	5	95
122	1	1	67	0	2	1	0	1	0	1	10	1	33
122	2	1	67	0	2	1	0	1	0	1	0	1	36
122	3	1	67	0	2	1	0	1	0	1	0	1	0
122	4	1	67	0	2	1	0	1	0	1	0	1	0
123	1	0	68	0	4	1	0	5	99	1	15	5	91
123	2	0	68	0	4	1	0	5	90	1	0	5	90
123	3	0	68	0	4	1	0	5	99	1	0	5	99
123	4	0	68	0	4	1	0	5	95	1	0	5	93
124	1	0	79	0	2	5	95	1	0	5	82	1	0
124	2	0	79	0	2	5	90	1	0	5	82	1	0
124	3	0	79	0	2	5	89	1	0	5	68	1	0

124	4	0	79	0	2	5	95	1	0	5	82	1	0
125	1	0	63	0	5	5	95	5	63	5	87	1	30
125	2	0	63	0	5	5	90	2	55	5	85	1	36
125	3	0	63	0	5	5	73	3	60	5	80	1	28
125	4	0	63	0	5	4	95	4	67	5	92	2	42
126	1	0	60	1	2	1	0	5	75	1	0	5	63
126	2	0	60	1	2	5	0	1	76	1	10	4	67
126	3	0	60	1	2	1	0	4	63	1	7	3	62
126	4	0	60	1	2	2	7	4	75	1	19	2	60
128	1	0	63	1	4	5	75	1	50	5	68	1	21
128	2	0	63	1	4	5	73	1	40	5	72	1	29
128	3	0	63	1	4	1	47	1	31	2	45	1	13
128	4	0	63	1	4	4	56	2	30	4	67	1	22
129	1	0	75	1	2	1	26	5	99	1	28	5	99
129	2	0	75	1	2	1	25	5	99	1	23	5	99
129	3	0	75	1	2	1	29	5	99	1	40	5	99
129	4	0	75	1	2	2	23	5	99	2	42	5	99
130	1	1	80	1	3	1	30	5	99	1	15	5	67
130	2	1	80	1	3	1	0	5	95	1	10	5	77
130	3	1	80	1	3	1	10	5	88	1	8	5	67
130	4	1	80	1	3	1	20	5	95	1	21	5	82
131	1	0	75	1	3	1	20	1	100	1	31	1	100
131	2	0	75	1	3	1	33	1	100	1	38	1	100
131	3	0	75	1	3	1	37	1	100	1	30	1	100
131	4	0	75	1	3	1	0	1	100	1	39	1	100
133	1	0	67	0	3	1	50	5	99	2	59	5	99
133	2	0	67	0	3	1	30	4	99	4	62	4	99
133	3	0	67	0	3	1	42	4	99	3	58	5	99
133	4	0	67	0	3	3	57	5	99	4	65	1	100
134	1	1	75	0	0	1	20	1	100	1	22	1	100
134	2	1	75	0	0	1	0	1	100	1	22	1	100
134	3	1	75	0	0	1	11	1	100	1	20	1	100
134	4	1	75	0	0	2	23	1	100	1	27	1	100
135	1	0	67	1	5	5	67	5	83	5	77	5	71
135	2	0	67	1	5	5	83	5	76	4	75	4	73
135	3	0	67	1	5	5	66	5	73	5	74	5	80
135	4	0	67	1	5	4	74	5	81	5	77	4	69
136	1	0	49	1	4	1	42	1	100	1	20	1	100
136	2	0	49	1	4	4	64	1	100	2	47	1	100
136	3	0	49	1	4	1	37	5	99	1	10	1	100
136	4	0	49	1	4	4	43	1	100	4	66	1	100
139	1	1	77	1	4	5	95	2	55	5	72	1	35
139	2	1	77	1	4	5	95	1	45	5	66	1	33
139	3	1	77	1	4	5	84	1	30	3	57	1	25
139	4	1	77	1	4	5	88	3	48	4	73	1	33
140	1	0	65	1	2	1	100	1	100	1	100	1	100

140	2	0	65	1	2	1	100	1	100	1	100	1	100
140	3	0	65	1	2	1	100	1	100	1	100	1	100
140	4	0	65	1	2	1	100	1	100	1	100	1	100
141	1	0	72	1	2	1	0	5	65	1	0	5	63
141	2	0	72	1	2	1	0	4	65	1	0	4	61
141	3	0	72	1	2	1	27	5	77	1	0	3	60
141	4	0	72	1	2	1	17	4	83	1	0	4	65
142	1	0	74	1	1	5	95	4	62	2	58	2	52
142	2	0	74	1	1	5	95	5	70	1	46	1	47
142	3	0	74	1	1	5	95	2	54	1	46	1	47
142	4	0	74	1	1	5	72	5	66	4	58	3	57
143	1	0	74	0	4	1	52	1	100	1	45	1	100
143	2	0	74	0	4	5	75	1	100	2	42	1	100
143	3	0	74	0	4	4	60	1	100	2	56	1	100
143	4	0	74	0	4	4	71	1	100	4	61	1	100
144	1	0	70	1	3	1	0	5	71	1	0	1	52
144	2	0	70	1	3	1	0	5	78	1	0	4	60
144	3	0	70	1	3	1	19	5	81	1	0	1	50
144	4	0	70	1	3	1	3	5	83	1	3	2	54
145	1	0	71	0	3	1	39	1	100	1	43	1	100
145	2	0	71	0	3	2	51	1	100	1	39	1	100
145	3	0	71	0	3	1	40	1	100	1	39	1	100
145	4	0	71	0	3	3	49	1	100	3	44	1	100
146	1	0	56	0	2	1	30	5	90	1	32	5	83
146	2	0	56	0	2	1	30	5	95	1	0	5	83
146	3	0	56	0	2	1	36	5	95	2	16	5	79
146	4	0	56	0	2	2	46	5	87	1	25	4	85
147	1	0	74	0	2	4	62	1	26	5	74	1	23
147	2	0	74	0	2	4	64	1	25	4	64	1	0
147	3	0	74	0	2	3	57	1	37	5	73	1	18
147	4	0	74	0	2	4	60	2	42	1	31	4	78
148	1	1	67	0	4	4	60	5	90	1	55	5	67
148	2	1	67	0	4	5	82	5	90	1	44	5	75
148	3	1	67	0	4	4	65	5	84	2	42	5	72
148	4	1	67	0	4	5	80	5	88	2	66	1	76
150	1	0	70	0	3	5	81	5	99	5	85	1	100
150	2	0	70	0	3	5	85	1	100	5	78	1	100
150	3	0	70	0	3	5	83	5	99	5	74	1	100
150	4	0	70	0	3	5	88	1	100	5	80	1	100
151	1	1	54	0	3	1	53	1	21	5	63	5	85
151	2	1	54	0	3	5	90	5	99	4	62	5	88
151	3	1	54	0	3	1	43	1	0	2	53	5	99
151	4	1	54	0	3	4	71	2	32	5	85	5	90
152	1	0	73	1	3	1	51	1	100	2	56	1	100
152	2	0	73	1	3	4	73	1	100	3	58	1	100
152	3	0	73	1	3	1	48	1	100	2	52	1	100

152	4	0	73	1	3	3	53	1	100	3	70	1	100
153	1	0	58	0	3	5	78	5	95	5	72	5	78
153	2	0	58	0	3	5	88	5	90	5	70	5	82
153	3	0	58	0	3	5	70	5	75	5	66	5	76
153	4	0	58	0	3	4	79	5	91	4	73	4	76
154	1	0	53	0	3	5	65	1	14	5	73	1	29
154	2	0	53	0	3	5	70	1	20	4	60	1	25
154	3	0	53	0	3	3	61	1	36	5	71	1	21
154	4	0	53	0	3	4	64	1	14	4	72	1	50
155	1	0	74	0	0	5	95	5	99	5	75	5	82
155	2	0	74	0	0	5	95	5	99	5	80	5	86
155	3	0	74	0	0	5	87	5	95	5	71	5	99
155	4	0	74	0	0	5	92	5	99	5	83	5	88
156	1	1	77	0	1	5	90	5	99	5	72	5	80
156	2	1	77	0	1	5	99	4	99	5	81	5	77
156	3	1	77	0	1	5	99	5	99	5	99	5	99
156	4	1	77	0	1	5	81	5	99	5	71	5	78
158	1	1	74	0	1	1	46	1	40	1	37	1	33
158	2	1	74	0	1	5	77	2	34	1	40	1	30
158	3	1	74	0	1	3	60	1	31	1	41	1	28
158	4	1	74	0	1	4	58	2	45	3	43	3	36
159	1	1	59	1	3	5	80	1	0	5	70	1	0
159	2	1	59	1	3	5	90	1	0	5	70	1	0
159	3	1	59	1	3	5	75	1	0	3	61	1	8
159	4	1	59	1	3	5	80	1	0	5	73	1	30
160	1	0	63	1	2	1	18	5	99	1	28	1	100
160	2	0	63	1	2	1	20	4	99	1	30	1	100
160	3	0	63	1	2	1	0	5	99	1	34	1	100
160	4	0	63	1	2	1	42	1	100	1	30	1	100
163	1	0	57	0	1	1	19	5	95	1	26	3	35
163	2	0	57	0	1	1	0	5	99	1	25	5	95
163	3	0	57	0	1	1	13	5	95	1	24	3	51
163	4	0	57	0	1	1	26	5	99	1	27	5	88
164	1	0	63	1	2	5	94	5	67	5	73	5	65
164	2	0	63	1	2	5	95	5	82	5	75	5	87
164	3	0	63	1	2	5	90	5	82	5	75	3	55
164	4	0	63	1	2	5	91	4	75	5	73	4	68
165	1	1	50	1	2	1	37	1	0	1	51	1	0
165	2	1	50	1	2	4	70	1	0	2	52	1	0
165	3	1	50	1	2	3	0	1	0	3	56	1	0
165	4	1	50	1	2	4	58	1	0	4	63	1	0
166	1	0	66	1	3	1	90	1	100	5	77	1	100
166	2	0	66	1	3	5	85	1	100	5	70	1	100
166	3	0	66	1	3	5	85	1	100	5	73	5	99
166	4	0	66	1	3	5	82	1	100	5	79	1	100
167	1	0	60	1	5	4	61	1	35	1	35	1	0

167	2	0	60	1	5	5	80	1	25	2	44	1	25
167	3	0	60	1	5	3	51	1	43	1	38	1	0
167	4	0	60	1	5	2	38	4	74	2	32	2	0
168	1	0	79	0	1	1	0	5	95	1	0	5	78
168	2	0	79	0	1	1	0	5	97	1	0	5	80
168	3	0	79	0	1	1	0	5	95	1	0	5	77
168	4	0	79	0	1	1	0	5	92	1	0	5	82
169	1	1	77	1	5	5	72	5	69	1	54	4	62
169	2	1	77	1	5	5	75	5	83	2	54	5	70
169	3	1	77	1	5	5	74	5	69	2	53	4	61
169	4	1	77	1	5	4	75	5	83	3	46	3	64
170	1	0	69	0	2	1	100	1	25	1	100	1	33
170	2	0	69	0	2	1	100	1	25	1	100	1	33
170	3	0	69	0	2	1	100	1	45	1	100	1	38
170	4	0	69	0	2	1	100	1	31	1	100	2	33
171	1	0	68	0	2	1	0	5	95	1	36	5	86
171	2	0	68	0	2	1	20	5	99	1	33	5	99
171	3	0	68	0	2	1	0	5	99	1	31	5	99
171	4	0	68	0	2	2	10	5	99	2	40	5	96
172	1	0	78	0	3	5	78	1	15	5	84	1	33
172	2	0	78	0	3	5	80	1	0	5	82	1	33
172	3	0	78	0	3	5	75	1	6	5	73	1	34
172	4	0	78	0	3	5	77	1	0	5	75	1	24
173	1	1	78	1	4	1	39	5	80	1	19	5	76
173	2	1	78	1	4	1	35	5	86	1	15	5	80
173	3	1	78	1	4	1	32	5	81	1	7	5	71
173	4	1	78	1	4	2	42	5	89	2	11	4	80
174	1	0	69	1	5	5	99	5	95	5	89	5	86
174	2	0	69	1	5	5	99	5	95	5	99	5	90
174	3	0	69	1	5	5	99	5	90	5	99	5	83
174	4	0	69	1	5	5	99	5	91	5	88	5	90
175	1	0	71	1	4	5	90	1	49	5	74	1	39
175	2	0	71	1	4	5	90	4	64	2	55	1	33
175	3	0	71	1	4	5	79	5	73	5	67	1	46
175	4	0	71	1	4	5	91	2	50	4	60	2	36
178	1	0	78	0	5	5	84	5	85	5	73	5	70
178	2	0	78	0	5	5	87	5	87	5	70	5	65
178	3	0	78	0	5	5	83	5	87	5	73	5	67
178	4	0	78	0	5	5	82	5	89	4	70	4	67
179	1	1	70	0	3	5	70	1	22	5	65	1	8
179	2	1	70	0	3	5	86	4	66	5	80	1	0
179	3	1	70	0	3	5	65	1	38	4	65	1	6
179	4	1	70	0	3	5	75	2	50	4	70	2	24
180	1	1	70	1	4	1	40	1	0	1	0	1	0
180	2	1	70	1	4	1	0	1	0	1	0	1	0
180	3	1	70	1	4	1	0	1	0	1	0	1	0

180	4	1	70	1	4	4	67	2	0	2	42	2	50
181	1	0	65	1	3	5	83	1	33	5	73	1	0
181	2	0	65	1	3	5	90	1	0	5	78	1	0
181	3	0	65	1	3	5	77	1	46	3	56	1	0
181	4	0	65	1	3	4	75	2	55	4	82	2	29
183	1	1	58	1	4	5	76	1	44	4	60	1	43
183	2	1	58	1	4	5	90	5	85	4	62	2	52
183	3	1	58	1	4	5	87	5	63	3	60	1	45
183	4	1	58	1	4	5	80	4	73	3	53	3	48
184	1	0	73	0	4	5	86	1	31	5	68	1	19
184	2	0	73	0	4	5	90	1	30	5	80	1	20
184	3	0	73	0	4	5	82	1	31	5	65	1	19
184	4	0	73	0	4	5	79	2	23	4	71	2	23
185	1	0	65	1	4	1	0	5	84	1	0	5	89
185	2	0	65	1	4	1	0	5	95	2	0	5	92
185	3	0	65	1	4	1	0	5	95	2	47	5	89
185	4	0	65	1	4	2	13	4	73	1	0	5	93
186	1	1	77	0	5	1	48	5	99	1	33	5	88
186	2	1	77	0	5	4	62	5	99	1	33	5	99
186	3	1	77	0	5	3	64	5	99	1	42	5	99
186	4	1	77	0	5	4	56	5	99	2	33	5	99
187	1	0	72	1	3	4	58	1	0	5	63	5	64
187	2	0	72	1	3	5	70	2	50	5	66	5	72
187	3	0	72	1	3	4	73	1	0	3	55	4	62
187	4	0	72	1	3	4	75	3	67	4	58	4	57
189	1	0	72	1	5	1	0	1	0	1	13	1	0
189	2	0	72	1	5	1	0	1	0	1	16	1	0
189	3	0	72	1	5	1	0	1	0	1	15	1	0
189	4	0	72	1	5	1	0	1	0	1	0	1	0
190	1	0	77	0	5	1	38	5	90	1	33	5	65
190	2	0	77	0	5	2	50	5	90	1	33	5	84
190	3	0	77	0	5	1	45	5	72	1	33	5	99
190	4	0	77	0	5	4	60	5	99	3	42	4	83
192	1	1	72	0	3	5	71	1	0	1	47	1	0
192	2	1	72	0	3	5	66	1	0	1	0	1	100
192	3	1	72	0	3	4	69	1	17	1	33	1	0
192	4	1	72	0	3	5	67	1	8	3	55	2	23
193	1	0	64	1	1	1	20	1	0	1	20	1	9
193	2	0	64	1	1	4	65	1	0	1	25	1	20
193	3	0	64	1	1	1	29	1	0	1	26	1	0
193	4	0	64	1	1	3	60	1	0	2	20	1	0
194	1	0	64	1	4	1	0	5	67	1	0	1	40
194	2	0	64	1	4	1	0	5	68	1	0	4	64
194	3	0	64	1	4	1	0	5	68	1	0	5	78
194	4	0	64	1	4	1	0	4	70	1	0	4	64
195	1	0	71	1	4	1	0	5	90	1	0	4	63

195	2	0	71	1	4	1	0	5	95	1	0	4	63
195	3	0	71	1	4	1	0	5	95	1	0	3	56
195	4	0	71	1	4	2	19	5	99	1	0	4	64
196	1	1	74	1	3	1	18	5	99	1	10	1	100
196	2	1	74	1	3	2	46	1	100	1	47	1	20
196	3	1	74	1	3	1	12	1	100	1	0	1	100
196	4	1	74	1	3	4	84	3	99	2	15	1	100
197	1	0	53	1	2	1	100	5	90	1	100	4	62
197	2	0	53	1	2	1	100	5	95	1	100	4	62
197	3	0	53	1	2	1	100	5	95	5	99	3	58
197	4	0	53	1	2	1	100	5	99	1	100	4	69

1st column=patient ID

2nd column=radiologist ID

3rd column=gender (1=female; 0=male)

4th column=age in years

5th column=symptomatic (1=yes, previous stroke or TIA; 0=no symptoms)

6th column=total number of risk factors (a number between 0 and 5, indicating the number of prominent risk factors the patient has. The risk factors are smoker, high blood pressure, high lipids, diabetes, and/or obesity)

7th column=MRA result, for left carotid artery, indicating the radiologist's confidence that a significant lesion is present (score from 1-5)

8th column=MRA result, for left carotid artery, indicating the % of stenosis measured by the radiologist.

9th column=MRA result, for right carotid artery, indicating the radiologist's confidence that a significant lesion is present (score from 1-5)

10th column=MRA result, for right carotid artery, indicating the % of stenosis measured by the radiologist.

11th column=catheter angiogram result, for left carotid artery, indicating the radiologist's confidence that a significant lesion is present (score from 1-5)

12th column=catheter angiogram result, for left carotid artery, indicating the % of stenosis measured by the radiologist.

13th column=catheter angiogram result, for right carotid artery, indicating the radiologist's confidence that a significant lesion is present (score from 1-5)

14th column=catheter angiogram result, for right carotid artery, indicating the % of stenosis measured by the radiologist.

Table A.6   Biomarker Data for Pancreatic Patients in Chapter 8

Control		Cases		Control		Cases	
CA 19-9	CA125	CA19-9	CA125	CA 19-9	CA125	CA19-9	CA125
28.00	13.30	2.40	79.10	15.50	11.10	719.00	31.40
8.20	16.70	2106.66	15.00	3.40	12.60	24000.00	77.80
17.30	7.40	1715.00	25.70	15.20	5.50	3.60	11.70
32.90	32.10	521.50	8.25	11.10	27.20	1600.00	14.95
87.50	6.60	454.00	8.70	16.20	9.80	109.70	14.10
107.90	10.50	23.70	123.90	5.70	7.80	464.00	12.10
25.60	9.10	9810.00	99.10	31.20	12.30	255.00	18.60
21.60	12.00	58.70	10.50	55.60	42.10	225.00	6.60
8.80	5.90	90.10	74.00	6.50	9.20	50.00	43.90
22.10	7.30	5.60	45.70	14.40	6.80	4070.00	13.00
44.20	10.70	592.00	7.30	3.70	15.70	28.60	8.60
7.80	8.00	6160.00	17.20	8.90	6.80	1090.00	15.40
18.00	47.35	10.40	14.30	6.50	17.90	27.30	93.10
4.90	96.20	162.00	66.30	10.40	108.90	3560.00	26.70
5.00	16.60	14.70	32.40	5.30	9.50	83.30	9.90
6.50	179.00	336.00	30.30	6.90	12.10	55.70	11.20
8.20	35.60	1520.00	202.00	21.80	15.00	3.90	35.70
6.60	12.60	5.80	9.20	7.60	5.90	8.45	103.60
15.40	10.10	361.00	21.40	59.20	8.50	369.00	8.10
5.10	11.40	8230.00	29.90	10.00	54.65	39.30	17.50
5.30	9.70	43.50	30.80	32.60	11.20	361.00	57.30
4.60	35.70	12.80	6.50	6.90	22.50	18.00	33.80
4.00	21.20	9590.00	53.60	3.65	5.60	555.00	17.20
7.8	9.40	60.20	94.20	32.50	12.00	21.80	33.50
11.50	9.80	900.00	3.70	4.00	17.20	6.60	11.70
10.20	10.60	239.00	19.90			3100.00	38.70
		3275.00	27.30			682.00	20.10
		85.40	86.10			10290.00	844.00
		770.00	36.90			247.60	6.90
		12320.00	27.70			113.10	9.90
		1079.00	38.60			45.60	142.60
		1630.00	12.50			79.40	11.60
		508.00	21.20			3190.00	13.20
		542.00	19.20			1021.00	1024.00
		235.00	14.10			251.00	34.80
		3160.00	35.30			479.00	35.00
		222.00	15.50			15.70	12.10
		2540.00	31.60			11630.00	184.80
		1810.00	24.80			6.90	10.40
		4.10	34.50			15.60	19.40
		9820.00	22.20			1490.00	53.90
		15.70	15.40			45.80	17.30
		7.80	36.80			12.80	49.80
		100.53	26.56			227.00	9.70
		70.90	19.20			2500.00	14.20

APPENDIX B

JACKKNIFE AND BOOTSTRAP METHODS OF ESTIMATING VARIANCES AND CONFIDENCE INTERVALS

B4.1 Jackknife Estimator

Jackknife is generally used to reduce bias of parameter estimates and to estimate variance. Let n be the total sample size. The procedure is to estimate a parameter θ for n times, each time deleting one sample data point. The resulting estimator can be denoted by θ_{-i} where the i-th data point has been excluded before calculating the estimate. So-called "pseudovalues" are constructed as

$$\theta_{-i} = n\,\theta_0 - (n-1)\theta_{-i}, \tag{B.1}$$

where θ_0 is the value of the parameter estimated from the entire data set. These pseudovalues act as if they are independent and identically distributed normal random variables. The mean of these pseudovalues is an estimate of

Statistical Methods in Diagnostic Medicine,
Second Edition. By Xiao-Hua Zhou, Nancy A. Obuchowski, Donna K. McClish

the parameter θ:

$$\widehat{\theta} = \widehat{\theta}_n = \frac{1}{n} \sum_{i=1}^{n} \theta_{-i},$$

where the subscript n on $\widehat{\theta}_n$ indicates that θ is based on n values. The variance of these pseudovalues is the estimate of the variance of $\widehat{\theta}$:

$$Var(\widehat{\theta}) = \frac{1}{n-1} \sum_{i=1}^{n} (\widehat{\theta}_{-i} - \theta_0)^2. \tag{B.2}$$

For large n, the jackknife estimate is approximately normally distributed about the true parameter θ. A 95% confidence interval for θ can be estimated as

$$\widehat{\theta} \pm 1.96 \sqrt{Var(\widehat{\theta})}. \tag{B.3}$$

While the usual jackknife creates pseudovalues by excluding data points one at a time from the n total cases, an alternative suggested by Cox and Hinkley (1974) is

$$\widehat{\theta} = (n-1)\widehat{\theta}_n - (n_1 - 1)\bar{\theta}_{n_0-1,n_1} - (n_1 - 1)\bar{\theta}_{n_0,n_1-1}, \tag{B.4}$$

where $\bar{\theta}_{n_0-1,n_1}$ is the average of the n_0 pseudovalues based on deleting one case at a time from the subjects without the condition and $\bar{\theta}_{n_0,n_1-1}$ is the average of the n_1 pseudovalues derived from deleting one case at a time from the subjects with the condition. Song (1997) further discusses grouped jackknife methods that delete more than 1 subject at a time (see article for details).

Some researchers use the pseudo-values themselves in analyses. For example, McClish (1987) used the pseudovalues to compare the area for more than two ROC curves; Dorfman et al. (1992) used pseudovalues to analyze data in the multi-reader case and Song used them for analysis of correlated ROC curve areas.

B4.2 Bootstrap Estimation

The bootstrap method involves drawing samples repeatedly from the empirical distribution. Suppose we have data $X = \{X_1, \ldots, X_n\}$ and have an interest in estimating a parameter θ. First we draw a sample of size n, with replacement, from the data points (called a bootstrap sample). This sample may have some values of X not included at all, while others may be included multiple times. An estimate of θ, denoted $\widehat{\theta}^1$ is calculated. This sampling and estimation procedure is repeated B times. The bootstrap estimate, $\widehat{\theta}^*$ is the mean of these B bootstrap estimates, and the variance is the sample variance of these bootstrap estimates. That is,

$$\widehat{\theta}^* = \frac{1}{B} \sum_{b=1}^{B} \widehat{\theta}^b, \; Var(\widehat{\theta}) = \frac{1}{B-1} \sum_{b=1}^{B} (\widehat{\theta}^b - \widehat{\theta}^*). \tag{B.5}$$

While the usual bootstrap estimator would draw bootstrap samples from the entire dataset, it has been suggested for estimators of diagnostic accuracy that separate bootstrap samples of size n_1 and n_0 be drawn from those with and without the condition respectively. Mossman (1995) indicates that both methods yield similar results. We recommend the separate bootstrap method, as the data may have arisen from different distributions, and also to maintain the same prevalence of the condition (since some ROC curve estimators are dependent on the ratio of the sample sizes). Note that the bootstrap methodology can be used with any of the ROC curve measures, either parametric or nonparametric.

B4.3 Bootstrap Percentile Confidence Interval

To construct a bootstrap percentile confidence interval, we must first generate B bootstrap samples. For the b-th bootstrap sample, we obtain a bootstrap estimate $\widehat{\theta}^b$ for θ. From the distribution of the B $\widehat{\theta}^b$'s, we find its 100α percentile, denoted by $\widehat{\theta}^{*(\alpha)}$. Then a $100(1-\alpha)\%$ 2-sided bootstrap confidence interval for θ is given as

$$\left(\widehat{\theta}^{*(\alpha/2)}, \widehat{\theta}^{*(1-\alpha/2)}\right). \tag{B.6}$$

B4.4 Bias-Corrected-and-Accelerated (BCa) Bootstrap Confidence Interval

The BCa interval is similar to the percentile interval except that they are corrected for bias and for the rate of change of the SE of $\widehat{\theta}$ with respect to the true parameter value θ (Efron and Tibshirani, 1993). The standard normal approximation assumes that the SE of $\widehat{\theta}$ is the same for all values of θ, but this assumption is not correct - at least for the ROC curve area. The BCa interval corrects for this.

The BCa confidence interval for the area is

$$\left(\widehat{\theta}^{b\alpha_1}, \widehat{\theta}^{b\alpha_2}\right), \tag{B.7}$$

where

$$\alpha_1 = \Phi\left\{\widehat{z}_0 + \frac{[\widehat{z}_0 + z_{\alpha/2}]}{1 - \widehat{a}(\widehat{z}_0 + z_{\alpha/2})}\right\}, \tag{B.8}$$

and

$$\alpha_2 = \Phi\left\{\widehat{z}_0 + \frac{[\widehat{z}_0 + z_{1-\alpha/2}]}{1 - \widehat{a}(\widehat{z}_0 + z_{1-\alpha/2})}\right\},$$

where Φ is the standard normal cumulative distribution function and z_α is the $100 \times \alpha$th percentile point of the standard normal distribution. The value of z_0- the bias correction $-$ is estimated from the proportion of bootstrap replications that are less than the original estimate. That is

$$\widehat{z}_0 = \Phi^{-1}\left(\frac{\#\,[\widehat{\theta}^b < \widehat{\theta}]}{n_0 + n_1}\right), \tag{B.9}$$

where $\widehat{\theta}$ is the estimate of θ calculated from the original sample. We compute the acceleration value $\widehat{a}$ by using the jackknife approach:

$$\widehat{a} = \frac{\sum_{k=1}^{n_0+n_1}[\widehat{\theta}_{-k} - \widehat{\theta}_0]^3}{6\left\{\sum_{k=1}^{n_0+n_1}[\widehat{\theta}_{-k} - \widehat{\theta}_0]^2\right\}^{3/2}}, \tag{B.10}$$

where $\widehat{\theta}_0 = \sum_{k=1}^{n}\widehat{\theta}_{-k}$.

B4.5 Bootstrap t Confidence Intervals

For the bootstrap t confidence interval, B bootstrap samples are drawn, and the pivotal t statistic is calculated for each sample

$$R^b = (\widehat{\theta}^b - \widehat{\theta})/\widehat{\sigma}^b, \tag{B.11}$$

where $\widehat{\theta}^b$ and $\widehat{\sigma}^b$ are the estimates calculated from the bth bootstrap sample and $\widehat{\theta}$ is the estimate calculated from the original sample. The confidence interval is then

$$\widehat{\theta} - \widehat{\sigma}G_{boot}^{-1}(1 - \alpha/2), \ \widehat{\theta} + \widehat{\sigma}G_{boot}^{-1}(\alpha/2), \tag{B.12}$$

where $\widehat{\sigma}$ is the standard error of $\widehat{\theta}$ estimated from the original sample and G_{boot} is such that

$$G_{boot}(x) = Prob(R^b < x). \tag{B.13}$$

B4.6 Nonparametric Method of ROC Curve Summary Measure

Wieand et al. (1989) provide a framework for non-parametric estimation of the total area, partial area and sensitivity at a fixed false positive rate, which is based on a weighted average of sensitivities. The general formulation is the following

$$\int_0^1 \bar{F}_1(p)dW(p), \tag{B.14}$$

where $\bar{F}_1$ is the survivor function for test results of a patient with the condition. For $W(p) = p$, $0 < p < 1$, Eq. (B.14) is equivalent to the usual nonparametric estimate of the total area (4.75). If $W(p)$ puts all its mass on one point, then Eq. (B.14) gives the sensitivity for a fixed specificity, which is equivalent to the work by Linnet (1985, 1987) and Greenhouse and Mantel (1950). The work of Wieand et al. (1989) is perhaps most useful in providing a method of non-parametric estimation of the partial area for a continuous scale test. Suppose we want to estimate the partial area between false positive rates e_1 and e_2. If we let $W(p) = 0$ for $0 < p < e_1$, $W(p) = (p - e_1)/(e_2 - e_1)$ for $e_1 < p < e_2$ and $W(p) = 1$ if $e_2 < p < 1$ then we have

$$A_{(e_1 \leq FPR \leq e_2)} = \frac{1}{e_2 - e_1}\int_{e_1}^{e_2} \bar{F}(p)dp. \tag{B.15}$$

REFERENCES

Agresti, A. (1990). *Categorical Data Analysis.* John Wiley & Sons, New York, NY.

Agresti, A. and Coull, B. A. (1998). Approximate is better than 'exact' for interval estimation of binomial proportions. *American Statistician* **52,** 119–126.

Albert, P. S. (2007). Random effects modeling approaches for estimating roc curves from repeated ordinal tests without gold standards. *Biometrics* **63,** 947–957.

Alonzo, T. A. and Pepe, M. S. (2002). Distribution-free ROC analysis using binary regression techniques. *Biostatistics* **3,** 421–432.

Alonzo, T. A. and Pepe, M. S. (2005). Assessing accuracy of a continuous screening test in the presence of verification bias. *Applied Statistics* **54,** 173–190.

Altham, P. M. E. (1973). A non-parametric measure of signal discriminability. *British Journal of Mathematical and Statistical Psychology* **26,** 1–12.

Alvord, W. G., Drummond, J. E., Arthur, L. O., and et al (1988). A method for predicting individual hiv infection status in the absence of clinical information. *Aids Research and Human Retroviruses* **4**, 295–304.

American College of Radiology (1995). *Breast Imaging Reporting and Data Systems.* American College of Radiology, Reston, Virginia.

Arends, L. R., Hamza, T. H., van Houwelingen, J. C., Heijenbrok-Kal, M. H., Hunink, M. G. M., and Stiljnen, T. (2008). Bivariate random effects meta-analysis of ROC curves. *Medical Decision Making* **28**, 621–638.

Arkin, C. F. and Wachtel, M. S. (1990). How many patients are necessary to assess test performance? *Journal of the American Medical Association* **263**, 275–278.

Astin, M. P., Brazzelli, M. G., Fraser, C. M., Counsell, C. E., Needham, G., and Grimshow, J. M. (2008). Developing a sensitive search strategy in medline to retrieve studies on assessment of the diagnostic performance of imaging techniques. *Radiology* **247**, 365–373.

Bachmann, L. M., Coray, R., Estermann, P., and Riet, G. T. (2002). Identifying diagnostic studies in medline: reducing the number needed to read. *Journal of the American Medical Informatics Association* **9**, 653–658.

Bachmann, L. M., Puhan, M. A., ter Riet, G., and Bossuyt, P. M. (2006). Sample sizes of studies on diagnostic accuracy: literature survey. *British Medical Journal* **332**, 1127–1129.

Baker, M. E., Bogoni, L., Obuchowski, N. A., Dass, C., Kendzierski, R., Remer, E. M., Einstein, D. M., Cathier, P., Jerebko, A., Lakare, S., Blum, A., Caroline, D., and Macari, M. (2007). Computer-aided detection of colorectal polyps: can it improve sensitivity of less-experienced readers? *Radiology* **245**, 140–149.

Baker, S. G. (1995). Evaluating multiple diagnostic tests with partial verification. *Biometrics* **51**, 330–337.

Bamber, D. (1975). The area above the ordinal dominance graph and the area below the receiver operating graph. *Journal of Mathematical Psychology* **12**, 387–415.

Bandos, A. I., Rockette, H. E., and Gur, D. (2005a). A conditional nonparametric test for comparing two areas under the ROC curves from a paired design. *Academic Radiology* **12**, 291–297.

Bandos, A. I., Rockette, H. E., and Gur, D. (2005b). A permutation test sensitive to differences in areas for comparing ROC curves from a paired design. *Statistics in Medicine* **24**, 2873–2893.

Bandos, A. I., Rockette, H. E., Song, T., and Gur, D. (2009). Area under the free-response ROC curve (FROC) and a related summary index. *Biometrics* **65**, 247–256.

Bates, A. S., Margolis, P. A., and Evants, A. T. (1993). Verification bias in pediatric studies evaluating diagnostic tests. *Journal of Pediatrics* **122**, 585–590.

Baul, R. A., Rutter, C. M., Sunshine, J. H., Blebea, J. S., Blebea, J., Carpenter, J. P., Dickey, K. W., Quinn, S. F., Gomes, A. S., Grist, T. M., and McNeil, B. J. (1995). Multicenter trial to evaluate vascular magnetic resonance angiography of the lower extremity. *Journal of the American Medical Association* **274**, 875–880.

Bayes, T. (1763). An essay towards solving a problem in the doctrine of chances. *Philos Trans R Soc Lond* **53**, 370–418.

Beam, C. A. (1992). Strategies for improving power in diagnostic radiology research. *American Journal of Roentgenology* **159**, 631–637.

Beam, C. A. (1998). Analysis of clustered data in receiver operating characteristic studies. *Statistical Methods in Medical Research* **7**, 324–336.

Beam, C. A., Baker, M. E., Paine, S. S., Sostman, H. D., and Sullivan, D. C. (1992). Answering unanswered questions: proposal for a shared resource in clinical diagnostic radiology research. *Radiology* **183**, 619–620.

Beam, C. A., Layde, P. M., and Sullivan, D. C. (1996). Variability in the interpretation of screening mammograms by us radiologists: findings from a national sample. *Archives of Internal Medicine* **156**, 209–213.

Beam, C. A., Sullivan, D. C., and Layde, P. M. (1996). Effect of human variability on independent double reading in screening mammography. *Academic Radiology* **3**, 891–897.

Begg, C. B. (1987). Biases in the assessment of diagnostic tests. *Statistics in Medicine* **6**, 411–423.

Begg, C. B. (1989). Experimental design of medical imaging trials: issues and options. *Investigative Radiology* **24**, 934–936.

Begg, C. B. (1994). Publication bias. In Cooper, H. and Hedges, L. V., editors, *The Handbook of Research Synthesis*, pages 399–410, New York. Sage Foundation.

Begg, C. B. and Greenes, R. A. (1983). Assessment of diagnostic tests when disease verification is subject to selection bias. *Biometrics* **39**, 207–215.

Begg, C. B., Greenes, R. A., and Iglewicz, B. (1986). The influence of un-interpretability on the assessment of diagnostic tests. *Journal of Chronic Diseases* **39,** 575–584.

Begg, C. B. and McNeil, B. J. (1988). Assessment of radiologic tests; control of bias and other design considerations. *Radiology* **167,** 565–569.

Begg, C. B. and Metz, C. E. (1990). Consensus diagnoses and "gold standards". *Medical Decision Making* **10,** 29–30.

Beiden, S. V., Wagner, R. F., and Campbell, G. (2000). Components-of-variance models and multiple bootstrap experiments: an alternative method for random-effects, receiver operating characteristic analysis. *Academic Radiology* **7,** 341–349.

Berlin, J. A., Begg, C. B., and Thoma, A. L. (1989). An assessment of publication bias using a sample of published clincal trials. *Journal of the American Statistical Association* **84,** 381–392.

Bhat, B. R. (1962). On the distribution of certain quadratic forms in normal variates. *Royal Statistical Society B* **24,** 148–151.

Black, W. C. (1990). How to evaluate the radiology literature. *American Journal of Roentgenology* **154,** 17–22.

Black, W. C. and Welch, H. G. (1993). Advances in diagnostic imaging and overestimations of disease prevalence and the benefits of therapy. *New England Journal of Medicine* **328,** 1237–1243.

Blackwelder, W. C. (1982). Proving the null hypothesis. *Clinical Trials* **3,** 345–353.

Blume, J. D. (2009). Bounding sample size projections for the area under a roc curve. *Journal of Statistical Planning and Inference* **139,** 711–721.

Bossuyt, P. M., Reitsma, J. B., Bruns, D. E., Gatsonis, C. A., Glasziou, P. P., Irwig, L. M., Lijmer, J. G., Moher, D., Rennie, D., and de Vet, H. C. W. for the STARD Group (2003). Towards complete and accurate reporting of studies of diagnostic accuracy: the STARD initiative. *Annals of Internal Medicine* **138,** 40–44.

Box, G. E. P. and Cox, D. R. (1964). An analysis of transformations. *Journal of the Royal Statistical Society, Series B* **42,** 72–78.

Bozdogan, H. and Ramirez, D. E. (1986). Testing for model fit: assessing the box-cox transformation of multivariate data to "near" normality. *Computation Statistics* **3,** 127–150.

Bradley, J. (1968). *Distribution-free statistical tests.* Prentice-Hall, Englewood Cliffs, NJ, 2nd edition.

Branscum, A. J., Gardner, I. A., and Johnson, W. O. (2005). Estimation of diagnostic-test sensitivity and specificity through bayesian modeling. *Statistics in Medicine* pages 145–163.

Braun, T. and Alonzo, T. A. (2008). A modified sign test for comparing paired ROC curves. *Biostatistics* **9**, 364–372.

Brazma, A., Hingamp, P., Quackenbush, J., and Sherlock, G., et al. (2001). Minimum information about a microarray experiment (MIAME) - toward standards for microarray data. *Nature Genetics* **29**, 365–71.

Broemeling, L. D. (2007). Detection and localization in test accuracy: A bayesian perspective. *Communications in Statistics, Theory and Methods* **36**, 1555–1564.

Brown, L. D., Cai, T. T., and DasGupta, A. (2001). Interval estimation for a binomial proportion. *Statistical Science* **16**, 101–133.

Browner, W. S. and Newman, T. B. (1987). Are all significant p values created equal? the analogy between diagnostic tests and clinical research. *Journal of the American Medical Association* **257**, 2459–2463.

Bunch, P. C., Hamilton, J. F., Sanderson, G. K., and Simmons, A. H. (1978). A free-response approach to the measurement and characterization of radiographic-observer performance. *Journal of Applied Photographic Engineering* **4**, 166–171.

Cai, T. (2004). Semi-parametric ROC regression analysis with placement values. *Biostatistics* **5**, 45–60.

Cai, T. and Moskowitz, C. S. (2004). Semi-parametric estimation of the binormal ROC curve for a continuous diagnostic test. *Biostatistics* **5**, 573–586.

Callaham, M. L., Wear, R. L., Weber, E. J., Barton, C., and Young, G. (1998). Positive-outcome bias and other limitations in the outcome of research abstracts submitted to a scientific meeting. *Journal of the American Medical Association* **280**, 254–257.

Campbell, G. (1994). General methodology i: Advances in statistical methodology for the evaluation of diagnostic and laboratory tests. *Statistics in Medicine* **13**, 499–508.

Chakraborty, D. P. (2006). Analysis of location specific observer performance data: Validated extensions of the jackknife free-response (JAFROC) method. *Academic Radiology* **13**, 1187–1193.

Chakraborty, D. P. and Berbaum, K. (2004). Observer studies involving detection and localization: modeling, analysis, and validation. *Medical Physics* **31**, 2313–2330.

Chakraborty, D. P. and Berbaum, K. S. (1989). Maximum likelihood analysis of free-response receiver operating characteristic (FROC) data. *Medical Physics* **16,** 561–568.

Chalmers, I., Hetherington, J., Newdick, M., Mutch, L., Grant, A., Enkin, M., Enkin, E., and Dickersin, K. (1986). The oxford database of perinatal trials: Developing a register of published reports of controlled trials. *Controlled Clinical Trials* **7,** 306–324.

Chalmers, T. C., Hewett, P., Reitman, D., and Sacks, H. S. (1989). Selection and evaluation of empirical research in technology assessment. *International Journal of Technology Assessment in Health Care* **5,** 521–536.

Chilcote, W. A., Dowden, R. V., Paushter, D. M., Hale, J. C., Desberg, A. L., Singer, A. A., Obuchowski, N. A., and Godec, K. (1994). Ultrasound detection of silicone gel breast implant failure: a prospective analysis. *Breast Disease* **7,** 307–316.

Choi, B. C. K. (1998). Slopes of a receiver operating characteristic curve and likelihood ratios for a diagnostic test. *American Journal of Epidemiology* **148,** 1127–1132.

Choi, Y. K., Johnson, W. O., Collins, M. T., and Gardner, I. A. (2006). Bayesian estimation of roc curves in the absence of a gold standard. *Journal of Agricultural, Biological, and Environment Statistics* **11,** 210–229.

Chu, H. and Cole, S. R. (2006). Bivariate meta-analysis of sensitivity and specificity with sparse data: a generalized linear mixed model approach. *Journal of Clinical Epidemiology* **2006,** 1331–1333.

Claeskens, G., Jing, B., Pend, L., and Zhou, W. (2003). Empirical likelihood confidence regions for comparison distributions and ROC curves. *Canadian Journal of Statistics* **31,** 173–190.

Cochran, W. G. (1977). *Sampling Techniques.* Wiley, New York, 3rd edition.

Coffin, M. and Sukhatme, S. (1997). Receiver operating characteristic studies and measurement errors. *Biometrics* **53,** 823–837.

Cohen, J. (1977). *Statistical Power Analysis for the Behavioral Sciences.* Academic Press, Inc., Orlando, FL.

Connor, R. J. (1987). Sample size for testing differences in proportions for the paired-sample design. *Biometrics* **43,** 207–211.

Cook, N. R. (2007). Use and misuse of the receiver operating characteristic curve in risk prediction. *Circulation* **115,** 928–935.

Cooper, L. S., Chalmers, T. C., McCally, M., Berrier, J., and Sacks, H. S. (1988). The poor quality of early evaluations of magnetic resonance imaging. *Journal of the American Medical Association* **259**, 3277–3280.

Coppus, S. F., van der Veen, F., Bossuyt, P. M., and Mol, B. W. (2006). Quality of reporting of test accuracy studies in reproductive medicine: impact of the Standards for Reporting of Diagnostic Accuracy (STARD) initiative. *Fertility and Sterility* **86**, 1321–1329.

Cox, D. R. (1970). *The Analysis of Binary Data*. Methuen, London.

Cox, D. R. and Hinkley, D. (1974). *Theoretical Statistics*. Chapman and Hall.

Davison, A. C. and Hinkley, D. V. (1997). *Bootstrap Methods and Their Application*. Cambridge University, Cambridge, UK.

Dawid, A. P. and Skene, A. M. (1979). Maximum likelihood estimation of observer error rates using the EM algorithm. *Applied Statistics* **28**, 20–28.

de Graaff, J. C., Ubbink, D. T., Tijssen, J. G. P., and Legemate, D. A. (2004). The diagnostic randomized clinical trial is the best solution for management issues in critical limb ischemia. *Journal of Clinical Epidemiology* **57**, 1111–1118.

Deeks, J. J., Macaskill, P., and Irwig, L. (2005). The performance of tests of publication bias and other sample size effects in systematic reviews of diagnostic test accuracy was assessed. *Journal of Clinical Epidemiology* **58**, 882–893.

DeLong, E. R., DeLong, D. M., and Clarke-Pearson, D. L. (1988). Comparing the areas under two or more correlated receiver operating characteristic curves: A nonparametric approach. *Biometrics* **44**, 837–845.

Dendukuri, N. and Joseph, L. (2001). Bayesian approaches to modeling the conditional dependence between diagnostic tests. *Biometrics* **57**, 158–67.

DerSimonian, R. and Laird, N. M. (1986). Meta-analysis in clinical trials. *Controlled Clinical Trials* **7**, 177–188.

Deville, W. L., Bezemer, P. D., and Bouter, L. M. (2000). Publications on diagnostic test evaluation in family medicine journals: an optimal search strategy. *Journal of Clinical Epidemiology* **53**, 65–69.

DeVille, W. L., Buntinx, F., Bunter, L. M., Montori, V. M., deVet, H. C., van der Windt, D. A., and Bezemer, P. D. (2002). Conductint systematic reviews of diagnostic studies: didactic guidelines. *BMC Medical Research Methodology* **2**, 9.

DeVries, S. O., Hunink, M. G. M., and Polak, J. F. (1996). Summary receiver operating characteristic curves as a technique for meta-analysis of the diagnostic performance of duplex ultrasonography in peripheral arterial disease. *Academic Radiology* **3**, 361–369.

Diamond, G. A. (1991). Affirmative actions. *Medical Decision Making* **11**, 48–59.

Dickersin, K., Chan, S., Chalmers, T. C., Sacks, H. S., and Smith, H. (1987). Publication bias and clinical trials. *Controlled Clinical Trials* **8**, 343–353.

Dickersin, K., Hewitt, P., Mutch, L., Chalmers, I., and Chalmers, T. C. (1985). Purusing the literature: Comparison of MEDLINE searching with a perinatal trials database. *Controlled Clinical Trials* **6**, 306–317.

Dickersin, K., Hewitt, P., Mutch, L., Chalmers, I., and Chalmers, T. C. (1994). Identifying relevant studies for systematic reviews. *British Medical Journal* **309**, 1286–1291.

Dickersin, K., Min, Y. I., and Meinert, C. L. (1992). Factors influencing publication of research results: Follow-up of applications submitted to two institutional review boards. *Journal of the American Medical Association* **267**, 374–378.

Dinnes, J., Deeks, J., Kirby, J., and Roderick, P. (2005). A methodological review of how heterogeneity has been examined in systematic reviews of diagnostic test accuracy. *Health Technology Assessment* **9**, 1–113.

Dodd, L. E. and Pepe, M. S. (2003). Partial AUC estimation and regression. *Biometrics* **59**, 614–623.

Dodd, L. E., Wagner, R. F., Armato, S. G., McNitt-Gray, M. F., Beiden, S., Chan, H. P., Gur, D., McLennan, G., Metz, C. E., Petrick, N., Sahiner, B., Sayre, J., and Lung Image Database Consortium Research Group (2004). Assessment methodologies and statistical issues for computer-aided diagnosis of lung nodules in computed tomography: contemporary research topics relevant to the lung image database consortium. *Academic Radiology* **11**, 462–475.

Dorfman, D. D. and Alf, E. (1968). Maximum-likelihood estimation of parameters of signal-detection theory - a direct solution. *Psychometrika* **33**, 117–124.

Dorfman, D. D. and Alf, E. (1969). Maximum-likelihood estimation of parameters of signal-detection theory and determination of confidence intervals - rating-method data. *Journal of Mathematical Psychology* **6**, 487–496.

Dorfman, D. D. and Berbaum, K. S. (1995). Degeneracy and discrete receiver operating characteristic rating data. *Academic Radiology* **2**, 907–925.

Dorfman, D. D. and Berbaum, K. S. (2000a). A contaminated binormal model for ROC data: Part II. A formal model. *Academic Radiology* **7**, 427–437.

Dorfman, D. D. and Berbaum, K. S. (2000b). A contaminated binormal model for ROC data. Part III. Initial evaluation with detection of ROC data. *Academic Radiology* **7**, 438–447.

Dorfman, D. D., Berbaum, K. S., Lenth, R. V., Chen, Y. F., and Donaghy, B. A. (1998). Monte carlo validation of a multireader method for receiver operating characteristic discrete rating data: factorial experimental design. *Academic Radiology* **5**, 591–602.

Dorfman, D. D., Berbaum, K. S., and Metz, C. E. (1992). Receiver operating characteristic rating analysis: generalization to the population of readers and patients with the jackknife method. *Investigative Radiology* **27**, 723–731.

Dorfman, D. D., Berbaum, K. S., Metz, C. E., Lenth, R. V., and Hanley, J. A. (1997). Proper receiver operating characteristic analysis: The bigamma model. *Academic Radiology* **4**, 138–149.

Doust, J. A., Pietrak, E., Sanders, S., and Glasziou, P. P. (2005). Identifying studies for systematic reviews of diagnostic tests was difficult due to the poor sensitivity and precision of methodologic filters and the lack of information in the abstracts. *Journal of Clinical Epidemiology* **58**, 444–449.

Dreiseitl, S., Ohno-Machado, L., and Binder, M. (2000). Comparing three-class diagnostic tests by three-way ROC analysis. *Medical Decision Making* **20**, 323–331.

Drum, D. and Chrisacopoulos, J. (1972). Hepatic scintigraphy in clinical decision making. *Journal of Nuclear Medicine* **13**, 908–915.

Drummond, M. F., Sculpher, M. J., Torrance, G. W., O'Brien, B. J., and Stoddart, G. L. (2005). *Methods for the Economic Evaluation of Health Care Programmes*. Oxford University Press, Oxford.

Dukic, V. and Gatsonic, C. (2003). Meta-analysis of diagnostic test accuracy assessment studies with varying number of thresholds. *Biometrics* **59**, 936–946.

Dundar, Y., Dodd, S., Williamson, P., Walley, T., and Dickson, R. (2006). Searching for and us of conference abstracts in health technology assessment: policy and practice. *International Journal of Technology Assessment in Health Care* **22**, 283–287.

Dwyer, A. J. (1997). In pursuit of a piece of the ROC. *Radiology* **202**, 621–625.

Easterbrook, P. J., Berlin, J. A., Gopalan, R., and Matthews, D. R. (1991). Publication bias in clinical research. *Lancet* **337**, 867–872.

Edwards, D. C., Metz, C. E., and Kupinski, M. A. (2004). Ideal observers and optimal ROC hypersurfaces in n-class classification. *IEEE Trans. Med. Imaging* **23,** 891–895.

Efron, B. and Tibshirani, R. J. (1993). *An Introduction to the Bootstrap.* Chapman & Hall, 3rd edition.

Egan, J. P. (1975). *Signal Detection Theory and ROC Analysis.* Academic Press, New York, 1st edition.

Egger, M., Smith, G. D., Schneider, M., and Minder, C. (1997). Bias in meta-analysis detected by a simple, graphical test. *British Medical Journal* **315,** 629–634.

Egglin, T. K. P. and Feinstein, A. R. (1996). Context Bias: a problem in diagnostic radiology. *Journal of the American Medical Association* **276,** 1752–1755.

Eisenberg, M. J. (1995). Accuracy and predictive values in clinical decision-making. *Cleveland Clinic Journal of Medicine* **62,** 311–316.

Ellis, W. J., Etzioni, R., Vessella, R. L., Hu, C., and Goodman, G. E. (2001). Serial prostate specific antigen, free-to-total prostate specific antigen ratio annd complexed prostate specific antigen for the diagnosis of prostate cancer. *Journal of Urology* **166,** 93–99.

Eng, J. (2004). Sample size estimation: a glimpse beyond simple formulas. *Radiology* **230,** 606–612.

Espeland, M. A., Platt, O. S., and Gallagher, D. (1989). Joint estimation of incidence and diagnostic error rates from irregular longitudinal data. *Journal of the American Statistical Association* **84,** 972–945.

Faraggi, D. and Reiser, B. (2002). Estimation of the area under the ROC curve. *Statistics in Medicine* **21,** 3093–3106.

Flahault, A., Cadilhac, M., and Thomas, G. (2005). Sample size calculation should be performed for design accuracy in diagnostic test studies. *Journal of Clinical Epidemiology* **58,** 859–862.

Fluss, R., Faraggi, D., and Reisser, B. (2005). Estimation of the youden index and its associated cutoff point. *Biometrical Journal* **47,** 458–472.

Fluss, R., Reiser, B., Faraggi, D., and Rotnitzky, A. (2009). Estimation of the ROC curve under verification bias. *Biometrical Journal* **51,** 475–490.

Freedman, L. S. (1987). *Investigational Techniques in Oncology.* Springer-Verlag, Great Britain.

Fryback, D. G. and Thornbury, J. R. (1991). The efficacy of diagnostic imaging. *Medical Decision Making* **11,** 88–94.

Fultz, P. J., Jacobs, C. V., Hall, W. J., Gottlieb, R., Rubens, D., Totterman, S. M. S., Meyers, S., Angel, C., Priore, G. D., Warshal, D. P., Zou, K. H., and Shapiro, D. E. (1999). Ovarian cancer: comparison of observer performance for four methods of interpreting CT scans. *Radiology* **212,** 401–410.

Gart, J. J. and Nam, J. (1988). Approximate interval estimation of the ratio of binormal parameters: A review and corrections for skewness. *Biometrics* **44,** 323–328.

Gatsonis, C. and Paliwal, P. (2006). Meta-analysis of diagnostic and screening test accuracy evaluations: Methodologic primer. *American Journal of Roentgenology* **187,** 271–281.

Gatsonis, C. A. (1995). Random-effects models for diagnostic accuracy data. *Academic Radiology* **2,** S14–S21.

Gelfand, D. W. and Ott, D. J. (1985). Methodologic considerations in comparing imaging modalities. *American Journal of Roentgenology* **144,** 1117–1121.

Gelman, A., Carlin, J. B., Stern, H. S., and Rubin, D. B. (1995). *Bayesian Data Analysis.* Chapman and Hall, New York, NY.

Gilbert, G. K. (1885). Finley's tornado predictions. *American Meteorological Journal* **1,** 167.

Glass, G. V. (1976). Primary, secondary and meta-analysis of research. *Education Research* **5,** 3–8.

Glick, H. A., Doshi, J. A., Sonnad, S. S., and Polsky, D. (2007). *Economic Evaluation in Clinical Trials.* Oxford University Press, Oxford.

Godambe, V. (1991). *Estimating Functions.* Oxford University Press, Oxford, UK.

Goddard, M. J. and Hinberg, I. (1990). Receiver operating characteristic (ROC) curves and non-normal data: An empirical study. *Statistics in Medicine* **9,** 325–337.

Goetghebeur, E., Eiinev, J., Boelaert, J., and Vander, P. S. (2000). Diagnostic test analyses in search of their gold standard: latent class analyses with random effects. *Statistical Methods in Medical Research* **9,** 231–248.

Gold, M. R., Siegel, J. E., Russell, L. B., and Weinstein, M. C. (1996). *Cost-Effectiveness in Health and Medicine.* Oxford University Press, New York, NY.

Goodman, L. A. (1974). Exploratory latent structure analysis using both identifiable and unidentifiable models. *Biometrika* **61**, 215–231.

Gray, R., Begg, C., and Greenes, R. (1984). Construction of receiver operating characteristic curves when disease verification is subject to selection bias. *Medical Decision Making* **4**, 151–164.

Green, D. M. and Swets, J. A. (1966). *Signal Detection Theory and Psychophysics*. John Wiley & Sons, New York, NY.

Greenes, R. and Begg, C. (1985). Assessment of diagnostic technologies: Methodology for unbiased estimation from samples of selective verified patients. *Investigative Radiology* **20**, 751–756.

Greenhouse, S. and Mantel, N. (1950). The evaluation of diagnostic tests. *Biometrics* **6**, 399–412.

Greenland, S. (2008). The need for reorientation toward cost-effective prediction: Comments on 'Evaluating the added predictive ability of a new marker: From area under the ROC curve to reclassification and beyond'. *Statistics in Medicine* **27**, 199–206.

Gregoire, G., Derderian, F., and LeLoirer, J. (1995). Selecting the language of the publications included in a meta-analysis: is there a Tower of Babel bias? *Journal of Clinical Epidemiology* **48**, 159–163.

Greiner, M., Pfeiffer, D., and Smith, R. D. (2000). Principals and practical application of the receiver operating characteristic analysis for diagnostic tests. *Preventive Veterinary Medicine* **45**, 23–41.

Grey, D. R. (1972). Some aspects of ROC curve-fitting: normal and logistic models. *Journal of Mathematical Psychology* **9**, 128–139.

Griner, P. R., Mayewski, R. J., Mushlin, A. I., and Greenland, P. (1981). Selection and interpretation of diagnostic tests and procedures. *Annals of Internal Medicine* **94**, 553–592.

Gur, D. (2007). Objectively measuring and comparing performance levels of diagnostic imaging systems and practices. *Academic Radiology* **14**, 641–642.

Gur, D., Rockette, H. E., Armfield, D. R., Blachar, A., Bogan, J. K., Brancatelli, G., Britton, C. A., Brown, M. L., Davis, P. L., Ferris, J. V., Fuhrman, C. R., Golla, S. K., Katyal, S., Lacois, J. M., and McCook, B. M. (2003). Prevalence effect in a laboratory environment. *Radiology* **228**, 10–14.

Gur, D., Rockette, H. E., Good, W. F., Slasky, B. S., Cooperstein, L. A., Straub, W. H., Obuchowski, N. A., and Metz, C. E. (1990). Effect of observer instruction on ROC study of chest images. *Investigative Radiology* **25,** 230–234.

Gyorkos, Y. W., Genta, R. M., Viens, P., and et al (1990). Seroepidemiology of *strongyloides* infection in the southeast Asian refugee population in Canada. *American Journal of Epidemiology* **132,** 257–264.

Habord, R. M., Deeks, J. J., Egger, M., Whiting, P., and Sterne, J. A. (2007). A unification of models for meta-analysis of diagnostic accuracy studies. *Biostatistics* **8,** 239–251.

Hajian-Tilaki, K. O., Hanley, J. A., Joseph, L., and Collet, S. (1997). A comparison of parametric and nonparametric approaches to ROC analysis of quantitative diagnostic tests. *Medical Decision Making* **17,** 94–102.

Hall, K., Hendrie, H., Rodgers, D. D., Prince, C., Pillay, N., Blue, A., Brittain, H., Norton, J. A., Kaufert, J. N., Nath, A., Shelton, P., Osuntokun, B., and Postl, B. (1993). The development of a dementia screeing interview in two distinct languages. *International Journal of Methods in Psychiatric Research* **3,** 1–28.

Hall, P. (1998). *The Bootstrap and Edgeworth Expansion.* Springer-Verlag, New York, NY.

Hall, P. and Zhou, X. H. (2003). Nonparametric estimation of component distributions in a multivariate mixture. *Annals of Statistics* **31,** 201–224.

Halpern, E. J., Albert, M., Krieger, A. M., Metz, C. E., and Maidment, A. D. (1996). Comparison of receiver operating characteristic curves on the basis of optimal operating points. *Academic Radiology* **3,** 245–253.

Hamza, T. H., Arends, L. R., van Houwelingen, H. C., and Stinjen, T. (2009). Multivariate random effects meta-analysis of diagnostic tests with multiple thresholds. *BMC Medical Research Methodology* **9,** 73–87.

Hamza, T. H., Reitsma, J. B., and Stijnen, T. (2008). Meta-analysis of diagnostic studies: a comparison of random intercept, normal-normal and binomial-normal bivariate summary ROC approaches. *Medical Decision Making* **28,** 639–649.

Hamza, T. H., van Houwelingen, H. C., and Stijnen, T. (2008). The binomial distribution of meta-analysis was preferred to model within-study variability. *Journal of Clinical Epidemiology* **61,** 41–51.

Hanley, J. A. (1988). The robustness of the binormal assumption used in fitting ROC curves. *Medical Decision Making* **8,** 197–203.

Hanley, J. A. (1989). Receiver operating characteristic (ROC) methodology: the state of the art. *Critical Reviews Diagnostic Imaging* **29,** 307–335.

Hanley, J. A. and Hajian-Tilaki, K. O. (1997). Sampling variability of nonparametric estimates of the areas under receiver operating characteristic curves: An update. *Academic Radiology* **4**, 49–58.

Hanley, J. A. and McNeil, B. J. (1982). The meaning and use of the area under a receiver operating characteristic (ROC) curve. *Radiology* **143**, 29–36.

Hanley, J. A. and McNeil, B. J. (1983). A method of comparing the areas under roc curves derived from same cases. *Radiology* **148**, 839–843.

Hans, O., Albert, A., Born, J., and Chapelle, J. (1985). Derivation of a bioclinical index in severe head trauma. *Intensive Care Medicine* **11**, 186–191.

Harrell, F. E., Lee, K. L., and Mark, D. B. (1996). Tutorial in biostatistics: multivariable prognostic models: issues in developing models, evaluating assumptions and adequacy, and meaning and reducing errors. *Statistics in Medicine* **15**, 361–387.

Harrell, F. R. (2001). *Regression Modeling Strategies*. Springer, New York.

Harter, H. L. (1960). Tables of range and studentized range. *The Annals of Mathematical Statistics* **31**, 1122–1147.

Haynes, R. B. and Wilcynski, N. L. (2004). Optimal search strategies for retrieving scientifically strong studies of diagnosis from Medline: analytic survey. *British Medical Journal* **328**, 1040.

He, H., Lyness, M. L., and McDermott, M. P. (2009). Direct estimation of the area under the receiver operating characteristic curve in the presence of verification bias. *Statistics in Medicine* **28**, 361–376.

He, Y. and Escobar, M. (2008). Nonparametric statistical inference method for partial areas under receiver operating characteristic curves, with applications to genomic studies. *Statistics in Medicine* **27**, 5291–5308.

Heagerty, P. J. and Pepe, M. S. (1999). Semiparametric estimation of regression quantiles with application to standardizing weight for height and age in children. *Applied Statistics* **48**, 533–551.

Hellmich, M., Abrams, K. R., Jones, D. R., and Lambert, P. C. (1988). A bayesian approach to a general regression model for ROC curves. *Medical Decision Making* **18**, 436–443.

Hellmich, M., Abrams, K. R., and Sutton, A. J. (1999). Bayesian approaches to meta-analysis of ROC curves. *Medical Decision Making* **19**, 252–264.

Hendrie, H., Osuntokun, B. O., Hall, K. S., Ogunniyi, A. O., Hui, S. L., Unverzagt, F. W., Gureje, O., Rodenberg, A. C., Baiyewu, O., and Musick, B. S. (1995). The prevalence of Alzheimer's disease and dementia in two communities of Nigerian Africans and African Americans. *American Journal of Geriatric Psychiatry* **152,** 1485–1492.

Henkelman, R. M., Kay, I., and Bronskill, M. J. (1990). Receiver operating characteristic (ROC) analysis without truth. *Medical Decision Making* **10,** 24–29.

Hershey, J. C., Cebul, R. D., and Williams, S. V. (1986). Clinical guidelines for using two dichotomous tests. *Medical Decision Making* **6,** 68–78.

Hilden, J. (1991). The area under the ROC curve and its competitors. *Medical Decision Making* **11,** 95–101.

Hilden, J. (2000). Prevalence-free utility-respecting summary indices of diagnostic power do not exist. *Statistics in Medicine* **19,** 431–440.

Hilden, J. and Glasziou, P. (1996). Regret graphs, diagnostic uncertainty and Youden's index. *Statistics in Medicine* **15,** 969–986.

Hilgers, R. A. (1991). Distribution free confidence bounds for ROC curves. *Methods of Information in Medicine* **30,** 96–101.

Hillis, S. L. (2007). Comparison of denominator degrees of freedom methods for multiple observed ROC analysis. *Statistics in Medicine* **26,** 596–610.

Hillis, S. L. and Berbaum, K. S. (2004). Power estimation for the Dorfman-Berbaum-Metz method. *Academic Radiology* **11,** 1260–1273.

Hillis, S. L., Obuchowski, N. A., Schwarz, K. M., and Berbaum, K. S. (2005). A comparison of the dorfman-berbaum-mets and obuchowswki-rockette methods for receiver operating characteristic (ROC) data. *Statistics in Medicine* **24,** 1579–1609.

Hollingworth, W., Medina, L. S., Lenkinski, R. E., Shibata, D. K., Bernard, B., Zurakowski, D., Comstock, B., and Jarvik, J. G. (2006). Inter-rateer reliability in assessing quality of diagnostic accuracy studies using the QUADAS tool: A preliminary assessment. *Academic Radiology* **13,** 803–810.

Holmquist, N. D., McMahan, C. A., and Williams, O. D. (1967). Variability in classification of carcinoma in situ of the uterien cervix. *Archives of Pathology* **84,** 334–345.

Hosmer, D. W. and Lemeshow, S. (1989). *Applied Logistic Regression.* John Wiley & Sons, Canada.

Hsieh, H. N., Su, H. Y., and Zhou, X. (2009). Interval estimation for the difference in paired areas under the roc curves in the absence of a gold standard test. *Statistics in Medicine* **28,** 3108–3123.

Hui, S. L. and Walter, S. D. (1980). Estimating the error rates of diagnostic tests. *Biometrics* **36**, 167–171.

Hunink, M. G. M., Polak, J., Barlan, M., and O'Leary, D. H. (1993). Detection and quantification of carotid artery stenosis: Efficacy of various doppler velocity parameters. *American Journal of Roentgenology* **160**, 619–625.

Hunink, M. G. M., Richardson, D. K., Doubilet, P. M., and Begg, C. B. (1990). Testing for fetal pulmonay maturity: ROC analysis involving covariates, verification bias, and combination testing. *Medical Decision Making* **10**, 201–211.

Irwig, L. M., Bossuyt, P., Glasziou, P., Gatsonis, C., and Lijmer, J. (2002). Designing studies to ensure that estimates of test accuracy are transferable. *British Medical Journal* **324**, 669–671.

Irwig, L. M., Macaskill, P., Glasziou, P., and Fahey, M. (1995). Meta-analytic methods for diagnostic test accuracy. *Journal of Clinical Epidemiology* **48**, 119–130.

Irwig, L. M., Tosteson, A. N. A., Gatsonis, C., Lau, J., Colditz, G., Chalmers, T. C., and Mosteller, F. (1994). Guidelines for meta-analyses evaluating diagnostic tests. *Annals of Internal Medicine* **120**, 667–676.

Irwig, L. M., Troit, R. S. D., Sluis-Cremer, G. K., and et al (1979). Risk of asbestosis in crocidolite and amosite mines in South Africa. *Annals of the New York Academy of Sciences* **330**, 35–52.

Ishwaran, H. and Gatsonis, C. (2000). A general class of hierarchical ordinal regression models with applications to correlated roc analysis. *Canadian Journal of Statistics* **28**, 731–750.

Janes, H. and Pepe, M. S. (2008a). Adjusting for covariates in studies of diagnostic, screening, or prognostic markers: an old concept in a new setting. *American Journal of Epidemiology* **168**, 89–97.

Janes, H. and Pepe, M. S. (2008b). Matching in studies of classification accuracy: implications for analysis, efficiency, and assessment of incremental value. *Biometrics* **64**, 1–9.

Janes, H. J. and Pepe, M. S. (2009). Adjusting for covariate effects on classification accuracy using the covariate-adjusted receiver operating characteristic curve. *Biometrika* **96**, 371–382.

Jansen, R. C. (1993). Maximum likelihood in a generalized linear finite mixture model by using the EM algorithm. *Biometrics* **49**, 227–231.

Jensen, A., Vejborg, I., Severinsen, N., Nielsen, S., Rank, F., Mikkelsen, G. J., Hilden, J., Vistisen, D., Dyreborg, U., and Lynge, E. (2006). Performance of clinical mammography: a nationwide study from denmark. *International Journal of Cancer* **119,** 183–191.

Jensen, K., Muller, H. H., and Schafer, H. (2000). Regional confidence bands for ROC curves. *Statistics in Medicine* **19,** 493–509.

Jiang, Y., Metz, C. E., and Nishikawa, R. M. (1996). A receiver operating characteristic partial area index for highly sensitive diagnostic tests. *Radiology* **201,** 745–750.

Johnson, W. O. and Gastwirth, J. L. (1991). Bayesian inference for medical screening tests: approximations useful for the analysis of acquired immune deficiency syndrome. *Journal of the Royal Statistical Society, Series B* **2,** 427–439.

Jones, G., Johnson, W. O., Hanson, T. E., and Christensen, R. (2010). Identifiability of models for multiple diagnostic testing in the absence of a gold standard. *Biometrics* **66,** 855–863.

Joseph, L., Gyorkos, T. W., and Coupal, L. (1995). Bayesian estimation of disease prevalence and the parameters of diagnostic tests in the absence of a gold standard. *American Journal of Epidemiology* **3,** 263–272.

Jund, J., Rabilloud, M., Wallon, M., and Ecochard, R. (2005). Methods to estimate the optimal threshold for normally or log-normally distributed biological tests. *Medical Decision Making* **25,** 406–415.

Kardaun, J. W. and Kardaun, O. J. (1990). Comparative diagnostic performance of three radiological procedures for the detection of lumbar disk herniation. *Methods of Informatics in Medicine* **29,** 12–22.

Kastner, M., Wilczynskia, N. L., McKibbona, A. K., Garga, A. X., and Haynes, R. B. (2009). Diagnostic test systematic reviews: Bibliographic search filters ("Clinical Queries") for diagnostic accuracy studies perform well. *Journal of Clinical Epidemiology* **62,** 974–981.

Kester, A. D. M. and Buntinx, F. (2000). Meta-analysis of ROC curves. *Medical Decision Making* **20,** 430–439.

Kijewski, M. F., Swensson, R. G., and Judy, P. F. (1989). Analysis of rating data from multiple-alternative tasks. *Journal of Mathematical Psychology* **33,** 428–451.

Koenker, R. and Basset, G. (1978). Regression quantiles. *Econometrica* **33,** 33–50.

Koepsell, T. D., Chi, Y. Y., Zhou, X., Lee, W. W., Ramos, E. M., and Kukull, W. A. (1978). An alternative method for estimating efficacy of the an1792 vaccine for Alzheimer' disease. *Neurology* **69,** 1868–1872.

Kraemer, H. C. (1992). *Evaluating Medical Tests*. Sage Publications, California.

Kraemer, H. C., Periyakoil, V. S., and Noda, A. (2004). Kappa coefficients in medical research. In *Tutorial in Biostatistics, Volume 1: Statistical Methods in Clinical Studies*, pages 85–105, New York, USA. Wiley & Sons.

L'Abbe, K. A., Detsky, A. S., and O'Rourke, K. (1987). Meta-analysis in clinical research. *Annals of Internal Medicine* **107**, 224–233.

Landis, J. R. and Koch, G. (1977). The measurement of observer agreement for categorical data. *Biometrics* **33**, 159–174.

Leeflang, M. M. G., Deeks, J. J., Gatsonis, C., and Bossuyt, P. M. M. on behalf of the Cochrane Diagnostic Test Accuracy Working Group (2008). Systematic reviews of diagnostic test accuracy. *Annals of Internal Medicine* **149**, 889–897.

Leisenring, W., Alonzo, T. A., and Pepe, M. S. (2000). Comparisons of predictive values of binary diagnostic tests for paired designs. *Biometrics* **56**, 341–351.

Li, G., Tiwari, R. C., and Wells, M. T. (1996). Quantile comparison functions in two-sample problems, with application to comparisons of diagnostic markers. *Journal of the American Statistical Association* **91**, 689–698.

Lijmer, J. G., Bossuyt, P. M. M., and Heisterkamp, S. H. (2002). Exploring sources of heterogeneity in systematic reviews of diagnostic tests. *Statistics in Medicine* **21**, 1525–1537.

Lijmer, J. G., Mol, B. W., Heisterkamp, S., Bonsel, G. J., Prins, M. H., van der Meulen, J. H., and Bossuyt, P. M. (1999). Empirical evidence of design-related bias in studies of diagnostic tests. *Journal of the American Medical Association* **282**, 1061–1066.

Lin, C. and Mudholkar, G. (1980). A simple test for normality against asymmetric alternatives. *Biometrika* **67**, 455–461.

Lin, H., Li, G., and Zhou, X. H. (2011). Direct semiparametric ROC regression with unknown link and baseline functions. Technical report.

Lin, H., Zhou, L., Peng, H., and Zhou, X. H. (2011). Selection and combination of biomarkers using roc method for disease classification and prediction. *Canadian Journal of Statistics* **in press,**.

Linnet, K. (1985). Precision of sensitivity estimations in diagnostic test evaluations. power functions for comparisons of sensitivity of two tests. *Clinical Chemistry* **31**, 573–580.

Linnet, K. (1987). Comparison of quantitative diagnostic test: Type I error, power and sample size. *Statistics in Medicine* **6**, 147–158.

Littenberg, B. and Moses, L. E. (1993). Estimating diagnostic accuracy from multiple conflicting reports - a new meta analytic method. *Medical Decision Making* **13**, 313–321.

Little, R. and Rubin, D. (1987). *Statistical Analysis with Missing Data.* John Wiley & Sons, New York. NY.

Liu, A., Schisterman, E. F., Mazumdar, M., and Hu, J. (2005). Power and sample size calculations of comparative diagnostic accuracy studies with multiple correlated test results. *Biometrical Journal* **47**, 140–150.

Liu, D. and Zhou, X. H. (2011a). A model for adjusting for nonignorable verification bias in estimation of ROC curve and its area with likelihood based approach. *Biometrics* **in press**,.

Liu, D. and Zhou, X. H. (2011b). Nonparametric estimation of the covariate-specific ROC curve in presence of ignorable verification bias. *Biometrics* **in press**,.

Lloyd, C. and Yong, Z. (1999). Kernel estimators of the ROC curve are better than empirical. *Statistics and Probability Letters* **44**, 221–228.

Lloyd, C. J. (1998). Using smooth receiver operating characteristic curves to summarize and compare diagnostic systems. *Journal of the American Statistical Association* **93**, 1356–1364.

Loy, C. T., Irwig, L. M., Katelaris, P. H., and Talley, N. J. (1996). Do commercial serological kits for helicobacter pylori infection differ in accuracy? a meta-analysis. *American Journal of Gastroenterology* **91**, 1138–1142.

Lumbreras, B., Porta, M., Marquez, S., Pollan, M., Parker, L. A., and Hernandez-Aguado, I. (2008). QUADOMICS: an adaptation of the Quality Assessment of Diagnostic Accuracy Assessment (QUADAS) for the evaluation of the methodological quality of studies on the diagnostic accuracy of '-omics'-based technologies. *Clinical Biochemistry* **41**, 1316–1325.

Lumley, T. (1998). Marginal regression modelling of weakly dependent data. Technical report, Department of statistics, University of Washington, Seattle, Washington.

Lumley, T. (2005). An empirical process central limit theroem for sparsely correlated data. Technical Report 255, Department of Biostatistics, University of Washington, Seattle, Washington.

Lusted, L. B. (1971). Signal detectability and medical decision-making. *Science* **171**, 1217–1219.

Ma, G. and Hall, W. J. (1993). Confidence bands for receiver operating characteristic curves. *Medical Decision Making* **13,** 191–197.

Macaskill, P. (2004). Empirical Bayes estimates generated in a hierarchical summary ROC analysis agreed closely with those of a full bayesian analysis. *Journal of Clinical Epidemiology* **57,** 925–932.

Macaskill, P., Walter, S. D., and Irwig, L. (2001). A comparison of methods to detect publication bias in meta-analysis. *Statistics in Medicine* **20,** 641–654.

McClish, D. K. (1987). Comparing the area under more than two ROC curves. *Medical Decision Making* **7,** 149–155.

McClish, D. K. (1989). Analyzing a portion of the ROC curve. *Medical Decision Making* **9,** 190–195.

McClish, D. K. (1990). Determining a range of false positives for which ROC curves differ. *Medical Decision Making* **10,** 283–287.

McClish, D. K. (1992). Combining and comparing area estimates across studies or strata. *Medical Decision Making* **12,** 274–279.

McCullagh, P. (1980). Regression models for ordinal data. *Journal of the Royal Statistical Society, Series B* **42,** 109–142.

McCullagh, P. and Nelder, J. A. (1989). *Generalized Linear Models.* Chapman and Hall, Boca Raton, Fl.

McNeil, B. J. and Adelstein, S. J. (1976). Determining the value of diagnostic and screening tests. *Journal of Nuclear Medicine* **17,** 439–448.

McNeil, B. J. and Hanley, J. A. (1984). Statistical approaches to the analysis of receiver operating characteristic (ROC) curves. *Medical Decision Making* **4,** 137–150.

Megibow, A., Zhou, X., Rotterdam, H., Francis, I. R., Zerhouni, E. A., Balfe, D. M., Weinreb, J. C., Aisen, A., Kuhlman, J., and Heiken, J. P. (1995). Computed tomography vs magnetic resonance imaging in evaluation of resectability of pancreatic adenocarcinoma. *Radiology* **195,** 327–332.

Mercaldo, N. D., Lau, K. F., and Zhou, X. H. (2007). Confidence intervals for predictive values with an emphasis to case-control studies. *Statistics in Medicine* **26,** 2170–2183.

Metz, C. E. (1978). Basic principles of ROC analysis. *Seminars in Nuclear Medicine* **8,** 283–298.

Metz, C. E. (1986). ROC methodology in radiologic imaging. *Investigative Radiology* **21,** 720–733.

Metz, C. E. (1989). Some practical issues of experimental design and data analysis in radiologic ROC studies. *Investigative Radiology* **24**, 234–245.

Metz, C. E., Herman, B. A., and Roe, C. A. (1998). Statistical comparison of two ROC curve estimates obtained from partially paired datasets. *Medical Decision Making* **18**, 110–121.

Metz, C. E., Herman, B. A., and Shen, J. (1998). Maximum likelihood estimation of receiver operating characteristic (ROC) curves from continuously distributed data. *Statistics in Medicine* **17**, 1033–1053.

Metz, C. E. and Kronman, H. B. (1980). Statistical significance tests for binormal ROC curves. *Journal of Mathematical Psychology* **22**, 218–243.

Metz, C. E., Wang, P., and Kronman, H. B. (1984). A new approach for testing the significant differences between roc curves measured from correlated data. In Deconinck, F., editor, *Information processing in medical imaging*, The Hague, The Netherlands. Nijihoff.

Moher, D., Cook, D. J., Eastwood, S., Olkin, I., Rennie, D., and Stroup, D. R. (1999). Improving the quality of reports of meta-analyses of randomized controlled trials: the QUOROM statement. *Lancet* **354**, 1896–1900.

Moher, D., Fortin, P., Jadad, A. R., Juni, P., Klassen, T., Lorier, J. L., Liberati, A., Linde, K., and Penne, A. (1996). Completeness of reporting of trials published in languages other than English; implications for conduct and reporting of systematic reviews. *Lancet* **347**, 363–366.

Molodianovitch, K., Faraggi, D., and Reiser, B. (2006). Comparing the areas under two correlated ROC curves: parametric and non-parametric approaches. *Biometrical Journal* **48**, 745–757.

Mooney, C., Phelps, C. E., and Mushlin, A. I. (1990). Targeting assessments of magnetic resonance imaging in suspected multiple sclerosis. *Medical Decision Making* **10**, 77–94.

Moses, L. E., Shapiro, D., and Littenberg, B. (1993). Combining independent studies of a diagnostic test in to a summary ROC curve: Data-analytic approaches and some additional considerations. *Statistics in Medicine* **12**, 1293–1316.

Moskowitz, C. S. and Pepe, M. S. (2006). Comparing the predictive values of diagnostic tests: sample size and analysis for paired study designs. *Clinical Trials* **3**, 272–279.

Mossman, D. (1995). Resampling techniques in the analysis of non-binormal ROC data. *Medical Decision Making* **15**, 358–366.

Mossman, D. (1999). Three-way ROCS. *Medical Decision Making* **19**, 78–89.

Mossman, D. (2001). Intervals for posttest probabilities: A comparison of 5 methods. *Medical Decision Making* **21,** 498–507.

Mossman, D. and Somoza, E. (1989). Maximizing diagnostic information from the dexamethasone suppression test. *Archives of General Psychiatry* **46,** 653–660.

Murden, R. A., McRae, T. D., Kaner, S., and Bucknam, M. E. (1991). Mini-mental state exam scores vary with education in blacks and whites. *Journal of American Geriatrics Society* **39,** 149–155.

Mushlin, A. I., Detsky, A. S., Phelps, C. E., O'Connor, P. W., Kido, D. K., Kucharczyk, W., Giang, D. W., Mooney, C., Tansey, C. M., and Hall, W. J. (1993). The accuracy of magnetic resonance imaging in patients with suspected multiple sclerosis. *Journal of the American Medical Association* **269,** 3146–3151.

Nadaraya, E. A. (1964). Some new estimates for distribution functions. *Theory of Probability and its Applications* **9,** 497–500.

Nelson, L. S. (1975). Use of the range to estimate variability. *Journal of Quality Technology* **7,** 46–48.

Nierenberg, A. A. and Feinstein, A. R. (1988). How to evaluate a diagnostic marker test: lessons from the rise and fall of dexamethasone suppression test. *Journal of the American Medical Association* **259,** 1699–1702.

Obuchowski, N. A. (1994). Computing sample size for receiver operating characteristic studies. *Investigative Radiology* **29,** 238–243.

Obuchowski, N. A. (1995). Multireader receiver operating characteristic studies: a comparison of study designs. *Academic Radiology* **2,** 709–716.

Obuchowski, N. A. (1997a). Nonparametric analysis of clustered ROC curve data. *Biometrics* **53,** 567–578.

Obuchowski, N. A. (1997b). Testing for equivalence of diagnostic tests. *American Journal of Roentgenology* **168,** 13–17.

Obuchowski, N. A. (2003). Determining sample size for ROC studies: what is reasonable for the expected difference in tests' ROC areas? *Academic Radiology* **10,** 1327–1328.

Obuchowski, N. A. (2005). Estimating and comparing diagnostic tests' accuracy when the gold standard is not binary. *Academic Radiology* **12,** 1198–1204.

Obuchowski, N. A. (2006). An ROC-type measure of diagnostic accuracy when the gold standard is continuous-scale. *Statistics in Medicine* **8,** 481–493.

Obuchowski, N. A. (2009). Reducing the number of reader interpretations in MRMC studies. *Academic Radiology* **16**, 209–217.

Obuchowski, N. A., Applegate, K. E., Goske, M. J., Arheart, K. L., Myers, M. T., and Morrison, S. (2001). The differential diagnosis for multiple diseases: comparison with the binary-truth state experiment in two empirical studies. *Academic Radiology* **8**, 947–954.

Obuchowski, N. A., Beiden, S., Berbaum, K. S., Hillis, S. L., Ishwaran, H., Song, H. H., and Wagner, R. F. (2004). Multireader, multicase receiver operating characteristic analysis: an empirical comparison of five methods. *Academic Radiology* **11**, 980–995.

Obuchowski, N. A., Hazzone, P. J., and Dachman, A. H. (2010). Bias, underestimation of risk, and loss of statistical power in patient-level analyses of lesion detection. *European Radiology* **20**, 584–594.

Obuchowski, N. A. and Lieber, M. L. (1998). Confidence intervals for the receiver operating characteristic area in studies with small samples. *Academic Radiology* **5**, 561–571.

Obuchowski, N. A. and Lieber, M. L. (2002). Confidence bounds when the estimated ROC area is 1.0. *Academic Radiology* **9**, 526–530.

Obuchowski, N. A., Lieber, M. L., and Powell, K. A. (2000). Statistical analysis for detecting and locating multiple abnormalities with application to mammography. *Academic Radiology* **7**, 516–525.

Obuchowski, N. A., Lieber, M. L., and Wians, F. H. (2004). ROC curves in clinical chemistry: uses, misuses, and possible solutions. *Clinical Chemistry* **50**, 1118–1125.

Obuchowski, N. A. and McClish, D. K. (1997). Sample size determination for diagnostic accuracy studies involving binormal ROC curve indices. *Statistics in Medicine* **16**, 1529–1542.

Obuchowski, N. A. and Rockette, H. E. (1995). Hypothesis testing of diagnostic accuracy for multiple readers and multiple tests: an ANOVA approach with dependent observations. *Commuications in Statistics - Simulation* **24**, 285–308.

Obuchowski, N. A. and Zepp, R. C. (1996). Simple steps for improving multiple-reader studies in radiology: perspective. *American Journal of Roentgenology* **166**, 517–521.

Ogilvie, J. and Creelman, C. D. (1968). Maximum-likelihood estimation of receiver operating characteristic curve parameters. *Journal of Mathematical Psychology* **5**, 377–391.

Olson, C. M., Rennie, D., Cook, D., Dickersin, K., Flannagin, A., Hogan, J. W., Zhu, Q., Reilig, J., and Pace, B. (2002). Publication bias in editorial decision making. *Journal of the American Medical Association* **287**, 2825–2828.

O'Malley, A. J. and Zou, K. H. (2001). Bayesian multivariate hierarchical transformation models for ROC analysis. *Statistics in Medicine* **25**, 459–479.

Omenn, G., Goodman, G. E., Thornquist, M., Balmes, J., Cullen, M. R., Glass, A., Keogh, K. P., Meyskens, F. L., Valanis, B., Williams, J. H., Barnhart, S., and Hammar, S. (1996). Effects of a combination of beta carotene and vitamin a on lung cancer and cardiovascular disease. *New England Journal of Medicine* **334**, 1150–1155.

Pan, X. and Metz, C. E. (1997). The "proper" binormal model: parametric receiver operating characteristic curve estimation with degenerate data. *Academic Radiology* **4**, 380–389.

Pauker, S. G. and Kassirer, J. P. (1975). Therapeutic decision making: A cost-benefit analysis. *New England Journal of Medicine* **293**, 229–234.

Pavur, R. (1984). Exact F tests in an ANOVA procedure for dependent observations. *Multivariate Behavioral Research* **19**, 408–420.

Pencina, M. J., D'AgostinoSr., R. B., D'AgostinoJr., R. B., and Vasan, R. S. (2008). Evaluating the added predictive ability of a new marker: From area under the ROC curve to reclassification and beyond. *Statistics in Medicine* **27**, 157–172.

Penedo, M., Souto, M., Tahoces, P. G., Carreira, J. M., Villalon, J., Porto, G., Seoane, C., Vidal, J. J., Berbaum, K. S., Chakraborty, D. P., and Fajardo, L. L. (2005). Free-response receiver operating characteristic evaluation of lossy JPEG2000 and object-based set partitioning in hierarchical trees compression of digitized mammogram. *Radiology* **237**, 450–457.

Peng, F. and Hall, W. J. (1996). Bayesian analysis of ROC curves using Markov-chain Monte Carlo methods. *Medical Decision Making* **16**, 404–411.

Pepe, M. S. (1998). Three approaches for regression analysis of receiver operating characteristic curves for continuous test results. *Biometrics* **54**, 124–135.

Pepe, M. S. (2000). An interpretation for the ROC curve and inference using GLM procedures. *Biometrics* **56**, 352–359.

Pepe, M. S. (2003). *The Statistical Evaluation of Medical Tests for Classification and Prediction.* Oxford University Press, New York.

Pepe, M. S. and Cai, T. (2004). The analysis of placement values for evaluating discriminatory measures. *Biometrics* **60,** 528–535.

Pepe, M. S., Cai, T., and Longton, G. (2006). Combining predictors for classification using the area under the receiver operating characteristic curve. *Biometrics* **62,** 221–229.

Pepe, M. S. and Thompson, M. L. (2000). Combining diagnostic test results to increase accuracy. *Biostatistics* **1,** 123–140.

Pepe, M. S., Urban, N., Rutter, C., and Longton, G. (1997). Design of a study to improve accuracy in reading mammograms. *Journal of Clinical Epidemiology* **50,** 1327–1338.

Perkins, N. J. and Schisterman, E. F. (2006). The inconsistency of "optimal" cutpoints obtained using two criteria based on the receiver operating characteristic curve. *American Journal of Epidemiology* **163,** 670–675.

Pesce, L. L. and Metz, C. E. (2007). Reliable and computationally efficient maximum likelihood estimation of "proper" binormal ROC curves. *Academic Radiology* **14,** 814–829.

Phelps, C. E. and Mushlin, A. I. (1988). Focusing technology assessment using medical decision theory. *Medical Decision Making* **8,** 279–289.

Philbrick, J. T., Howritz, R. I., and Feinstein, A. R. (1980). Methodologic problems of exercise testing for coronary artery disease. *American Journal of Cardiology* **46,** 807–8212.

PIOPED Investigators (1990). Value of the ventilation/perfusion scan in acute pulmonary embolism: results of the prospective investigation of pulmonary embolism diagnosis (pioped). *Journal of the American Medical Association* **263,** 2753–2759.

Platt, R. W., Hanley, J. A., and Yang, H. (2000). Bootstrap confidence intervals for the sensitivity of a quantitative diagnostic test. *Statistics in Medicine* **19,** 313–322.

Polistser, P. (1982). Reliability, decision rules, and the value of repeated tests. *Medical Decision Making* **2,** 47–69.

Popescu, L. M. (2007). Nonparametric ROC and LROC analysis. *Medical Physics* **34,** 1556–1564.

Pouchot, J., Grasland, A., Collet, C., Coste, J., Esdaile, J. M., and Vinceneux, P. (1997). Reliability of tuberculin skin test measurement. *Annals of Internal Medicine* **126,** 210–214.

Powell, K., Obuchowski, N. A., Chilcote, W. A., Barry, M., Ganobcik, S. N., and Cardenosa, G. (1999). Film-screen versus digitized mammography:

assessment of clinical equivalence. *American Journal of Roentgenology* **173,** 889–894.

Powell, K., Obuchowski, N. A., Mueller, K., Hwang, C., Ganobcik, S., Strum, B., LaPresto, E., Hirsch, J., Selzer, R., Nissen, J., and Cornhill, J. F. (1996). Quantitative detection and classification of single-leg fractures in the outlet struts of bjork-shiley convex-concave heart valves. *Circulation* **94,** 3251–3256.

Poynard, T., Chaput, J. C., and Etienne, J. P. (1982). Relations between effectiveness of a diagnostic test, prevalence of the disease, and percentages of uninterpretable results: an example in the diagnosis of jaundice. *Medical Decision Making* **2,** 285–297.

Punglia, R. S., DAmicoa, A. V., Catalona, W. J., Roehl, K. A., and Kuntz, K. M. (2003). Effect of verification bias on screening for prostate cancer by measurement of prostate specific antigen. *New England Journal of Medicine* **349,** 335–342.

Qin, G. and Hotiloac, L. (2008). Comparison of non-parametric confidence intervals for the area under the ROC curve of a continuous-scale diagnostic test. *Statistical Methods in Medical Research* **17,** 272–221.

Qin, G. and Zhou, X. H. (2006). Empirical likelihood inference for the area under the ROC curve. *Biometrics* **62,** 613–622.

Qu, Y., Tang, M., and Kutner, M. H. (1996). Random effects models in latent class analysis for evaluating accuracy of diagnostic tests. *Biometrics* **52,** 797–810.

Radack, K. L., Rouan, G., and Hedges, J. (1986). The likelihood ratio: an improved measure for reporting and evaluating diagnostic test results. *Archives of Pathology and Laboratory Medicine* **110,** 689–693.

Ransohoff, D. J. and Feinstein, A. R. (1978). Problems of spectrum and bias in evaluating the efficacy of diagnostic tests. *New England Journal of Medicine* **299,** 926–930.

Rao, J. N. K. and Scott, A. J. (1992). A simple method for the analysis of clustered binary data. *Biometrics* **48,** 577–585.

Redelmeier, D. A., Bloch, D. A., and Hickam, D. H. (1991). Assessing predictive accuracy: how to compare brier scores. *Journal of Clinical Epidemiology* **44,** 1141–1146.

Reid, M. C., Lachs, M. S., and Feinstein, A. R. (1995). Use of methodologic standards in diagnostic test research: getting better but still not good. *Journal of the American Medical Association* **274,** 645–651.

Reitsma, J. B., Glas, A. S., Rutjes, A. W. S., Scholten, R. S. P. M., Bossuyt, P. M., and Zwinderman, A. H. (2005). Bivariate analysis of sensitivity and specificity produces informative summary measures in diagnostic reviews. *Journal of Clinical Epidemiology* **58**, 982–990.

Remer, E. M., Obuchowski, N. A., Ellis, J. D., Rice, T. W., Adelstein, D. J., and Baker, M. E. (2000). Adrenal mass evaluation in patients with lung carcinoma: a cost-effectiveness analysis. *American Journal of Roentgenology* **174**, 1033–1039.

Ridker, P. M. and Cook, N. (2004). Clinical usefulness of very high and very low levels of c-reactive protein across the full range of Framingham risk scores. *Circulation* **109**, 1955–1959.

Rifkin, M. D., Zerhouni, E. A., Gatsonis, C. A., Quint, L. E., Paushter, D. M., Epstein, J. I., Hamper, U., Walsh, P. C., and McNeil, B. J. (1990). Comparison of magnetic resonance imaging and ultrasonography in staging early prostate cancer. *New England Journal of Medicine* **323**, 621–626.

Riley, R. D., Abrams, K. R., Sutton, A. J., Lambert, P. C., and Thompson, J. R. (2007). Bivariate random-effects meta-analysis and the estimation of between-study correlation. *BMC Medical Research Methodology* **7**, 1–15.

Rindskopf, D. and Rindskopf, W. (1986). The value of latent class analysis in medical diagnosis. *Statistics in Medicine* **5**, 21–28.

Robertson, E. A., Zweig, M. H., and Van Steirteghem, A. C. (1983). Evaluating the clinical efficacy of laboratory tests. *American Journal of Clinical Pathology* **79**, 78–86.

Robins, J. M., Rotnitzky, A., and Zhao, L. P. (1994). Estimation of regression coefficient when some regressors are not always observed. *Journal of the American Statistical Association* **89**, 826–866.

Rockette, H. E. (1994). An index of diagnostic accuracy in the multiple disease setting. *Academic Radiology* **1**, 283–286.

Rockette, H. E., Campbell, W. L., Britton, C. A., Holbert, J. M., King, J. L., and Gur, D. (1999). Empiric assessment of parameters that affect the design of multireader receiver operating characteristic studies. *Academic Radiology* **6**, 723–729.

Rockette, H. E., Gur, D., and Metz, C. E. (1992). The use of continuous and discrete confidence judgments in receiver operating characteristic studies of diagnostic imaging techniques. *Investigative Radiology* **27**, 169–172.

Rockette, H. E., King, J. L., Medina, J. L., Eisen, H. B., Brown, M. L., and Gur, D. (1995). Imaging systems evaluation: effect of subtle cases on the design and analysis of receiver operating characteristic studies. *American Journal of Roentgenology* **165,** 679–683.

Rockette, H. E., Obuchowski, N. A., and Gur, D. (1990). Nonparametric estimation of degenerate ROC data sets used for comparing imaging systems. *Investigative Radiology* **25,** 835–837.

Rockette, H. E., Obuchowski, N. A., Gur, D., and Good, W. F. (1991). Effect of experimental design on sample size. *SPIE* **1446,** 276–283.

Rodenberg, C. and Zhou, X. H. (2000). ROC curve estimation when covariates affect the verification process. *Biometrics* **56,** 131–136.

Rodenberg, C. A. (1996). *Correcting for verification bias in ROC estimation with covariates.* PhD thesis, Department of Statistics, Purdue University, West Layafette, Indiana.

Roe, C. A. and Metz, C. E. (1997). Dorfman-berbaum-metz method for statistical analysis of multireader, multimodality receiver operating characteristic data: validation with computer simulation. *Academic Radiology* **4,** 298–303.

Rotnitzky, A., Faraggi, D., and Schisterman, E. (2006). Doubly robust estimation of the area under the receiver-operating characteristic curve in the presence of verification bias. *Journal of the American Statistical Association* **101,** 1276–1288.

Russell, L. B., Gold, M. R., Siegel, J. E., Daniels, N., and Weinstein, M. C. (1996). The role of cost-effectiveness analysis in health and medicine. *Journal of the American Medical Association* **276,** 1172–1177.

Rutjes, A. W. S., Reitsma, J. B., Di Nisio, M., Smidt, N., van Rijn, J. C., and Bossuyt, P. M. M. (2006). Evidence of bias and variation in diagnostic accuracy studies. *Canadian Medical Association Journal* **174,** 469–476.

Rutter, C. M. (2000). Bootstrap estimation of diagnostic accuracy with patient-clustered data. *Academic Radiology* **7,** 413–419.

Rutter, C. M. and Gatsonis, C. A. (1995). Regression methods for meta-analysis of diagnostic test data. *Academic Radiology* **2,** S46–S56.

Rutter, C. M. and Gatsonis, C. A. (2001). A hierarchical regression approach to meta-analysis of diagnostic test accuracy evaluations. *Statisitcs in Medicine* **20,** 2865–2884.

Rutter, C. M. and Taplin, S. (2000). Assessing mammographers' accuracy. a comparison of clinical and test performance. *Journal of Clinical Epidemiology* **53,** 443–450.

Sacks, H. S., Berrier, J., Reitman, D., Angona-berk, V. A., and Chalmers, T. C. (1987). Meta-analyses of randomized controlled trials. *New England Journal of Medicine* **316,** 450–455.

Sacks, H. S., Reitman, D., Pagano, D., and Kupelnick, B. (1996). Meta-analysis: An update. *Mt Sinai Journal of Medicine* **63,** 216–224.

Schafer, H. (1989). Constructing a cut-off point for a quantitative diagnostic test. *Statistics in Medicine* **8,** 1381–1391.

Schafer, H. (1994). Efficient confidence bounds for ROC curves. *Statistics in Medicine* **13,** 1551–1561.

Schapira, R. M., Schapira, M. M., Funahashi, A., McAuliffe, T. L., and Varkey, B. (1993). The value of the forced expiratory time in the physical diagnnosis of obstructive airways disease. *Journal of the American Medical Association* **270,** 731–736.

Scheidler, J., Hricak, H., Yu, K. K., Subak, L., and Segal, M. R. (1997). Radiological evaluation of lymph node metastases in patients with cervical cancer: A meta-analysis. *Journal of the American Medical Association* **278,** 1096–1101.

Schisterman, E. F. and Perkins, N. (2007). Confidence intervals for the youden index and corresponding optimal cut-point. *Communications in Statistics - Simulation and Computation* **36,** 549–563.

Schisterman, E. F., Perkins, N. J., and et al, L. A. L. (2005). Optimal cutpoint and its corresponding Youden index to discriminate individuals using pooled blood samples. *Epidemiology* **16,** 73–81.

Schuirmann, D. U. J. (1987). A comparison of the two 1-sided tests procedure and the power approach for assessing the equivalence of average bioavailability. *Journal of Pharmacokinetic Biopharmacy* **15,** 657–680.

Scott, A., Greenberg, P. B., and Poole, P. J. (2008). Cautionary tales in the clinical interpretation of studies of diagnostic tests. *International Medicine Journal* **38,** 120–129.

Sen, P. K. and Singer, J. M. (1993). *Large Sample Methods in Statistics.* Chapman & Hall, New York, NY.

Shapiro, D. E. (1995). Issues in combining independent estimates of the sensitivity and specificity of a diagnostic test. *Academic Radiology* **2,** S37–S47.

Simel, D. L., Samsa, G. P., and Matchar, D. B. (1991). Likelihood ratios with confidence: sample size estimation for diagnostic test studies. *Journal of Clinical Epidemiology* **44,** 763–770.

Sinclair, M. D. (1989). *Evaluating Reinterview Survey Methods for Measuring Response Errors.* PhD thesis, George Washington University, Washington, DC.

Skaltsa, K., Jover, L., and Carrasco, J. L. (2010). Estimation of the diagnostic threshold accounting for decision costs and sampling uncertainty. *Biometrical Journal* **52,** 676–697.

Slasky, B. S., Gur, D., Good, W. F., Costa-Greco, M. A., Harris, K. M., Cooperstein, L. A., and Rockette, H. E. (1990). Receiver operating characteristic analysis of chest image interpretation with conventional, laser-printed, and high-resolution workstation images. *Radiology* **174,** 775–780.

Smidt, N., Rutjes, A. W., van der Windt, D. A., Ostelo, R. W., Reitsma, J. B., Bossuyt, P. M., Outer, L. M., and de Vet, H. C. (2005). Quality of reporting of diagnostic accuracy studies. *Radiology* **235,** 347–53.

Somoza, E. and Mossman, D. (1991). Biological markers and psychiatric diagnosis: Risk-benefit balancing using ROC analysis. *Biological Psychiatry* **29,** 811–826.

Song, F., Eastwood, A. J., Gilbody, S., Duley, L., and Sutton, A. J. (2004). Publication and related biases. *Health Technology Assessment* **4,** 1–115.

Song, F., Khan, K. S., Dinnes, J., and Sutton, A. J. (2002). Asymmetric funnel plots and publication bias in meta-analysis of diagnostic accuracy. *International Journal of Epidemiology* **31,** 88–95.

Song, H. (1997). Analysis of correlated ROC areas in diagnostic testing. *Biometrics* **53,** 370–382.

Song, X. and Zhou, X. H. (2005). A marginal model approach for analysis of multi-reader multi-test receiver operating characteristic (ROC) data. *Biostatistics* **6,** 303–312.

Sox, H., Stern, S., Owens, D., and Abrams, H. L. (1989). *Assessment of Diagnostic Technology in Health Care: Rationale, Methods, Problems, and Directions.* National Academy Press, Washington, DC.

Sox, H. C., Blatt, M. A., Higgins, M. C., and Marton, K. I. (1989). *Medical Decision Making.* Butterworths-Heinemann, Boston, MA.

Spiegalhalter, D., Thomas, A., Best, N., and Gilks, W. (1996). *Bayesian Inference Using Gibbs Sampling, Version 0.5.* Medical Research Council Biostatistics Unit, Cambridge, UK.

Starr, S. J., Metz, C. E., and Lusted, L. B. (1977). Comments on generalization of receiver operating characteristic analysis to detection and localization tasks. *Physics and Medical Biology* **22,** 376–379.

Starr, S. J., Metz, C. E., Lusted, L. B., and Goodenough, D. J. (1975). Visual detection and localization of radiographic images. *Radiology* **116,** 533–538.

Steen, F. H. (1982). *Elements of Probability and Mathematical Statistics.* Duxbury Press, Boston, MA.

Stover, L., M. P, G., and Neely, T. (1996). Towards optimizing the clinical utility of distortion product otoacoustic emission measurements. *Journal of the Acoustical Society of America* **100,** 956–967.

Straub, W. H., Rockette, H., King, J. L., Obuchowski, N. A., Good, W. F., Feist, J. H., Good, B. C., and Metz, C. E. (1990). Training observers for receiver operating characteristic (ROC) studies. *SPIE* **1234,** 126–130.

Stroup, D. F., Berlin, J. A., Morton, S. C., Olkin, I., Williamson, G. D., Rennie, D., Moher, D., Becker, B. J., Sipe, T. A., and Thacker, S. B. (2000). Meta-analysis of observational studies in epidemiology: a proposal for reporting. *Journal of the American Medical Association* **283,** 2008–2012.

Stuart, A., Ord, J. K., and Arnold, S. (1999). *Kendall's Advanced Theory of Statistics, Classical Inference and Linear Models.* Chapman and Hall, New York, 6th edition.

Sukhatme, S. and Beam, C. A. (1994). Stratification in nonparametric ROC studies. *Biometrics* **50,** 149–163.

Swensson, R. G. (1996). Unified measurements of observer performance in detecting and localizing target objects on images. *Medical Physics* **23,** 1709–1725.

Swensson, R. G. (2000). Using localization data from image interpretations to improve estimates of performance accuracy. *Medical Decision Making* **20,** 170–185.

Swensson, R. G. and Judy, P. F. (1981). Detection of noisy visual targets: Models for the effects of spatial uncertainty and signal-to-noise ratio. *Perception and Psychophysics* **29,** 521–534.

Swets, J. A. (1986a). Empirical ROCs in discrimination and diagnostic tasks: Implications for theory and measurement of performance. *Psychological Bulletin* **99,** 181–198.

Swets, J. A. (1986b). Indices of discrimination or diagnostic accuracy: their ROCs and implied models. *Psychological Bulletin* **99,** 100–107.

Swets, J. A. (1988). Measuring the accuracy of diagnostic systems. *Science* **240,** 1285–1293.

Swets, J. A., Getty, D. J., Pickett, R. M., D'Orsi, C. J., Seltzer, S. E., and Mc-Neil, B. J. (1991). Enhancing and evaluating diagnostic accuracy. *Medical Decision Making* **11,** 9–18.

Tanimoto, S., Ikari, Y., Tanabe, K., Yachi, S., Nakajima, H., Nakayama, T., Hastori, M., Nakazawa, G., Onuma, Y., Higashikuni, Y., Yamamoto, H., Tooda, E., and Hara, K. (2005). Prevalence of carotid artery stenosis in patients with coronary artery disease in Japanese population. *Stroke* **36,** 2094–2098.

Tanner, M. A. (1993). *Tools for Statistical Inference.* Springer-Verlag, New York, NY.

Tavel, M. E., Enas, N. H., and Woods, J. R. (1987). Sensitivity and specificity of tests: can the "silent majority" speak? *American Journal of Cardiology* **60,** 1167–1169.

Taylor, C. F. (2006). Minimum reporting requirements for proteomics: a MIAPE primer. *Proteomics* **6(Suppl 2),** 39–44.

Tempany, C. M., Zhou, X., Zerhouni, E. A., Rifkin, M. D., Quint, L. A., Picoli, C., Ellis, J., J., and McNeil, B. J. (1994). Staging of prostate cancer with MRI - the results of Rradiology Diagnostic Oncology Group project: Comparison of three MR imaging techniques. *Radiology* **192,** 47–54.

Thompson, M. L. (2003). Assessing the diagnostic accuracy of a sequence of tests. *Biostatistics* **4,** 341–351.

Thompson, M. L. and Zucchini, W. (1989). On the statistical analysis of ROC curves. *Statistics in Medicine* **8,** 1277–1290.

Thornbury, J. R., Fryback, D. G., Turski, P. A., Javid, M. J., McDonald, J. V., Bemlieh, B. R., Gentry, L. R., Sackett, J. F., Dasbach, E. J., and Martin, P. A. (1993). Disk-caused nerve compression in patients with acute low-back pain: diagnosis with MR, CT myelography and plain CT. *Radiology* **186,** 731–738.

Thornbury, J. R., Kido, D. K., Mushlin, A. I., Phelps, C. E., Mooney, C., and Fryback, D. G. (1991). Increasing the scientific quality of clinical efficacy studies of magnetic resonance imaging. *Investigative Radiology* **26,** 829–835.

Toledano, A. Y. and Gatsonis, C. (1996). Ordinal regression methodology for ROC curves derived from correlated data. *Statistics in Medicine* **15,** 1807–1826.

Toledano, A. Y. and Gatsonis, C. A. (1999). Gees for ordinal categorical data: arbitrary patterns of missing responses and missingness in a key covariate. *Biometrics* **55,** 488–496.

Torrance-Rynard, V. L. and Walter, S. D. (1997). Effects of dependent errors in the assessment of diagnostic tests performance. *Statistics in Medicine* **16,** 2157–2175.

Tosteson, A. A. N. and Begg, C. B. (1988). A general regression methodology for ROC curve estimation. *Medical Decision Making* **8,** 204–215.

Tu, D. (1997). Two one-sided tests procedures in establishing therapeutic equivalence with binary clinical endpoints: fixed sample performances and sample size determination. *Journal of Statistical Computation and Simulation* **59,** 271–290.

Turner, D. A. (1978). An intuitive approach to receiver operating characteristic curve analysis. *Journal of Nuclear Medicine* **19,** 213–220.

Uebersax, J. S. (1999). Probit latent class analysis: conditional independence and conditional dependence models. *Applied Psychological Measurement* **23,** 283–297.

Vacek, P. M. (1985). The effect of conditional dependence on the evaluation of diagnostic tests. *Biometrics* **41,** 959–968.

Valenstein, P. N. (1990). Evaluating diagnostic tests with imperfect standards. *American Journal of Clinical Pathology* **93,** 252–258.

Vamvakas, E. C. (1998). Meta-analyses of studies of the diagnostic accuracy of laboratory tests. a review of the concepts and methods. *Archives of Pathology and Laboratory Medicine* **122,** 675–686.

Van den Bruel, A., Aertgeerts, B., and Buntinx, F. (2006). Results of diagnostic accuracy studies are not always validated. *Journal of Clinical Epidemiology* **59,** 559–566.

van Houwelingen, H. C., Arends, L. R., and Stignen, T. (2002). Advanced methods in meta-analysis: Multivariate approach and meta-regression. *Statistics in Medicine* **21,**.

Venkatraman, E. S. (2000). A permutation test to compare receiver operating characteristic curves. *Biometrics* **56,** 1134–1138.

Venkatraman, E. S. and Begg, C. (1996). A distribution-free procedure for comparing receiver operating characteristic curves from a paired experiment. *Biometrika* **83,** 835–848.

Vickers, A. J. and Elkin, E. B. (2006). Decision curve analysis: a novel method for evaluating prediction models. *Medical Decision Making* **26,** 565–574.

Wagner, R. F., Metz, C. E., and Campbell, G. (2007). Assessment of medical imaging systems and computer aids: a tutorial review. *Academic Radiology* **14,** 723–748.

Walsh, S. J. (1997). Limitation to the robustness of binormality of ROC curves: Effects of model misspecification and location of decision thresholds on bias, precision, size and power. *Statistics in Medicine* **16,** 669–679.

Walsh, S. J. (1999). Goodness-of-fit issues in ROC curve estimation. *Medical Decision Making* **19,** 193–201.

Walter, S. D. (2002). Properties of the summary receiver operating characteristic (SROC) curve for diagnostic test data. *Statistics in Medicine* **21,** 1236–1256.

Walter, S. D. (2005). The partial area under the summary ROC curve. *Statistics in Medicine* **24,** 2025–2040.

Walter, S. D. and Irwig, L. M. (1988). Estimation of test error rates, disease prevalence and relative risk from misclassified data: a review. *Journal of Clinical Epidemiology* **41,** 923–937.

Ware, J. H. and Cai, T. (2008). Comments on 'evaluating the added predictive ability of a new marker: From area under the ROC curve to reclassification and beyond'. *Statistics in Medicine* **27,** 185–187.

Webb, W. R., Gatsonis, C., Zerhouni, E. A., Heelan, R. T., Glazer, G. M., Francis, I. R., and McNeil, B. J. (1991). CT and MR imaging in staging non-small cell bronchogenic carcinoma: report of the Radiologic Diagnostic Oncology Group. *Radiology* **178,** 705–713.

Weinstein, M. C., Berwick, D. M., Goldman, P. A., Murphy, J. M., and Barsky, A. J. (1989). A comparison of three psychiatric screening tests using receiver operating characteristic (ROC) analysis. *Medical Care* **27,** 593–607.

Weinstein, M. C., Siegel, J. E., Gold, M. R., Kamlet, M. S., and Russell, L. B. (1996). Recommendations of the panel on cost-effectiveness in health and medicine. *Journal of the American Medical Association* **276,** 1253–1258.

West, S. G., Emden, W., Werner, M. H., and Kotzin, B. L. (1995). Neuropsychiatric lupus erythematosus: a 10-year prospective study on the value of diagnostic tests. *American Journal of Medicine* **99,** 153–163.

Westwood, M. E., Whiting, P. F., and Kleijnen, J. (2005). How does study quality effect the results of a diagnostic meta-analysis? *BMC Medical Research Methodology* **5,** 20.

Whiting, P., Rutjes, A. W., Reitsma, J. B., Bossuyt, P. M., and Kleijnen, J. (2003). The development of quadas: a tool for the quality assessment of studies of diagnostic accuracy included in systematic reviews. *BMC Medical Research Methodology* **3,** 25.

Whiting, P., Rutjes, A. W. S., Dinnes, J., Reitsma, J. B., Bossuyt, P. M. M., and Kleijnen, J. A. (2005). A systematic review finds that diagnostic reviews fail to incorporate quality despite available tools. *Journal of Clinical Epidemiology* **58**, 1–12.

Whiting, P., Rutjes, A. W. S., Reitsma, J. B., Glas, A. S., Bossuyt, P. M., and Kleijnen, J. (2004). Sources of variation and bias in studies of diagnostic accuracy. a systematic review. *Annals of Internal Medicine* **140**, 189–202.

Whiting, P., Westwood, M., Burke, H., Stern, J., and Glanville, J. (2008). Systematic reviews of test accuracy should search a range of databases to identify primary studies. *Journal of Clinical Epidemiology* **61**, 357–364.

Wieand, S., Gail, M. H., James, B. R., and James, K. L. (1989). A family of nonparametric statistics for comparing diagnostic markers with paired or unpaired data. *Biometrika* **76**, 585–592.

Willan, A. R. and Briggs, A. H. (2006). *Statistical Analysis of Cost-Effectiveness Data*. Wiley, New York.

Winer, B. J., Brown, D. R., and Michels, K. M. (1991). *Statistical Principles in Experimental Design*. McGraw-Hill, New York, 3rd edition.

Wortman, P. M. and Yeaton, W. H. (1987). Using research synthesis in medical technology assessment. *International Journal of Technology Assessment in Health Care* **3**, 309–522.

Yang, I. and Becker, M. P. (1997). Latent variable modeling of diagnostic accuracy. *Biometrics* **53**, 948–958.

Zafar, A., Khan, G. I., and Siddiqui, M. A. (2008). The quality of reporting of diagnostic accuracy studies in diabetic retinopathy screening: a systematic review. *Clinical Experimental Ophthalmology* **36**, 537–542.

Zhang, D. D., Zhou, X. H., Freeman, D. H., and Freeman, J. L. (2002). A nonparametric method for the comparison of partial areas under ROC curves and its application to large health care data sets. *Statistics in Medicine* **21**, 701–715.

Zheng, Y., Barlow, W. E., and Cutter, G. (2005). Assessing accuracy of mammography in the presence of verification bias and intrareader correlation. *Biometrics* **61**, 259–268.

Zhou, X. H. (1993). Maximum likelihood estimators of sensitivity and specificity corrected for verification bias. *Communications in Statistics - Theory and Methods* **22**, 3177–3198.

Zhou, X. H. (1995). Testing an underlying assumption on a ROC curve based on rating data. *Medical Decision Making* **15**, 276–282.

Zhou, X. H. (1996a). Empirical bayes combination of estimated areas under ROC curves using estimating equations. *Medical Decision Making* **16**, 24–28.

Zhou, X. H. (1996b). Nonparametric ML estimate of an ROC area corrected for verification bias. *Biometrics* **52**, 310–316.

Zhou, X. H. (1998a). Comparing accuracies of two screening tests in a two-phase study for dementia. *Journal of the Royal Statistical Society, Series C* **47**, 135–147.

Zhou, X. H. (1998b). Comparing the correlated areas under the ROC curves of two diagnostic tests in the presence of verification bias. *Biometrics* **54**, 349–366.

Zhou, X. H. and Castelluccio, P. (2003). Nonparametric analysis for the ROC curve areas of two diagnostic tests in the presence of nonignorable verification bias. *Journal of Statistical Planning and Inference* **115**, 193–213.

Zhou, X. H., Castelluccio, P., and Zhou, C. (2005). Nonparametric estimation of roc curves in the absence of a gold standard. *Biometrics* **61**, 600–609.

Zhou, X. H., Chen, B., Xie, Y. M., Tian, F., Liu, H., and Liang, X. (2011). Variable selection using the optimal roc curve: An application to a Traditional Chinese Medicine study on osteoporosis disease. *Statistics in Medicine* **in press,**.

Zhou, X. H. and Gatsonis, C. A. (1996). A simple method for comparing correlated ROC curves using incomplete data. *Statistics in Medicine* **15**, 1687–1693.

Zhou, X. H. and Harezlak, J. (2002). Comparison of bandwidth selection methods for kernel smoothing of ROC curves. *Statistics in Medicine* **21**, 2045–2055.

Zhou, X. H., Li, C. M., and Yang, Z. (2008). Improving interval estimation of binomial proportions. *Philosophical Transactions of the Royal Society, A* **366**, 2405–2419.

Zhou, X. H. and Lin, H. (2008). Semi-parametric maximum likelihood estimates for ROC curves of continuous-scale data. *Statistics in Medicine* **27**, 5271–5290.

Zhou, X. H. and Qin, G. (2005). Improved confidence intervals for the sensitivity at a fixed level of specificity of a continuous scale diagnostic test. *Statistics in Medicine* **24**, 465–477.

Zhou, X. H. and Rodenberg, C. A. (1997). Estimating an ROC curve in the presence of non-ignorable verification bias. *Communications in Statistics - Theory and Methods* **27**, 635–657.

Zou, K. and Hall, W. J. (2000a). Semiparametric and parametric transformation models for comparing diagnostic markers with paired design. *Journal of Applied Statistics* **29**, 803–816.

Zou, K. and Hall, W. J. (2000b). Two transformation models for estimating an ROC curve derived from continuous data. *Journal of Applied Statistics* **27**, 621–633.

Zou, K. H. (2001). Comparison of correlated receiver operating characteristic curves derived from repeated diagnostic test data. *Academic Radiology* **8**, 225–233.

Zou, K. H., Hall, W. J., and Shapiro, D. E. (1997). Smooth nonparametric receiver operating characteristic (ROC) curves for continuous diagnostic tests. *Statistics in Medicine* **16**, 2143–2156.

Zou, K. H., Tempany, C. M., Fielding, J. R., and Silverman, S. G. (1998). Original smooth receiver operating characteristic curve estimation from continuous data: Statistical methods for analyzing the predictive value of spiral CT of ureteral stones. *Academic Radiology* **5**, 680–687.

Zweig, M. H. and Campbell, G. (1993). Receiver-Operating Characteristic (ROC) Plots: a fundamental evaluation tool in clinical medicine. *Clinical Chemistry* **39**, 561–577.

Zweig, M. H. and Robertson, E. A. (1982). Why we need better test evaluations. *Clinical Chemistry* **28**, 1272–1276.

INDEX

Statistical Methods in Diagnostic Medicine,
Second Edition. By Xiao-Hua Zhou, Nancy A. Obuchowski, Donna K. McClish
Copyright © 2011 by John Wiley & Sons, Inc.

WILEY SERIES IN PROBABILITY AND STATISTICS
ESTABLISHED BY WALTER A. SHEWHART AND SAMUEL S. WILKS

Editors: *David J. Balding, Noel A. C. Cressie, Garrett M. Fitzmaurice, Iain M. Johnstone, Geert Molenberghs, David W. Scott, Adrian F. M. Smith, Ruey S. Tsay, Sanford Weisberg*
Editors Emeriti: *Vic Barnett, J. Stuart Hunter, Joseph B. Kadane, Jozef L. Teugels*

The *Wiley Series in Probability and Statistics* is well established and authoritative. It covers many topics of current research interest in both pure and applied statistics and probability theory. Written by leading statisticians and institutions, the titles span both state-of-the-art developments in the field and classical methods.

Reflecting the wide range of current research in statistics, the series encompasses applied, methodological and theoretical statistics, ranging from applications and new techniques made possible by advances in computerized practice to rigorous treatment of theoretical approaches.

This series provides essential and invaluable reading for all statisticians, whether in academia, industry, government, or research.

*Now available in a lower priced paperback edition in the Wiley Classics Library.
†Now available in a lower priced paperback edition in the Wiley–Interscience Paperback Series.

BECHHOFER, SANTNER, and GOLDSMAN · Design and Analysis of Experiments for Statistical Selection, Screening, and Multiple Comparisons

BELSLEY · Conditioning Diagnostics: Collinearity and Weak Data in Regression

† BELSLEY, KUH, and WELSCH · Regression Diagnostics: Identifying Influential Data and Sources of Collinearity

BENDAT and PIERSOL · Random Data: Analysis and Measurement Procedures, *Fourth Edition*

BERRY, CHALONER, and GEWEKE · Bayesian Analysis in Statistics and Econometrics: Essays in Honor of Arnold Zellner

BERNARDO and SMITH · Bayesian Theory

BHAT and MILLER · Elements of Applied Stochastic Processes, *Third Edition*

BHATTACHARYA and WAYMIRE · Stochastic Processes with Applications

BILLINGSLEY · Convergence of Probability Measures, *Second Edition*

BILLINGSLEY · Probability and Measure, *Third Edition*

BIRKES and DODGE · Alternative Methods of Regression

BISGAARD and KULAHCI · Time Series Analysis and Forecasting by Example

BISWAS, DATTA, FINE, and SEGAL · Statistical Advances in the Biomedical Sciences: Clinical Trials, Epidemiology, Survival Analysis, and Bioinformatics

BLISCHKE AND MURTHY (editors) · Case Studies in Reliability and Maintenance

BLISCHKE AND MURTHY · Reliability: Modeling, Prediction, and Optimization

BLOOMFIELD · Fourier Analysis of Time Series: An Introduction, *Second Edition*

BOLLEN · Structural Equations with Latent Variables

BOLLEN and CURRAN · Latent Curve Models: A Structural Equation Perspective

BOROVKOV · Ergodicity and Stability of Stochastic Processes

BOULEAU · Numerical Methods for Stochastic Processes

BOX · Bayesian Inference in Statistical Analysis

BOX · R. A. Fisher, the Life of a Scientist

BOX and DRAPER · Response Surfaces, Mixtures, and Ridge Analyses, *Second Edition*

* BOX and DRAPER · Evolutionary Operation: A Statistical Method for Process Improvement

BOX and FRIENDS · Improving Almost Anything, *Revised Edition*

BOX, HUNTER, and HUNTER · Statistics for Experimenters: Design, Innovation, and Discovery, *Second Editon*

BOX, JENKINS, and REINSEL · Time Series Analysis: Forcasting and Control, *Fourth Edition*

BOX, LUCEÑO, and PANIAGUA-QUIÑONES · Statistical Control by Monitoring and Adjustment, *Second Edition*

BRANDIMARTE · Numerical Methods in Finance: A MATLAB-Based Introduction

† BROWN and HOLLANDER · Statistics: A Biomedical Introduction

BRUNNER, DOMHOF, and LANGER · Nonparametric Analysis of Longitudinal Data in Factorial Experiments

BUCKLEW · Large Deviation Techniques in Decision, Simulation, and Estimation

CAIROLI and DALANG · Sequential Stochastic Optimization

CASTILLO, HADI, BALAKRISHNAN, and SARABIA · Extreme Value and Related Models with Applications in Engineering and Science

CHAN · Time Series: Applications to Finance with R and S-Plus®, *Second Edition*

CHARALAMBIDES · Combinatorial Methods in Discrete Distributions

CHATTERJEE and HADI · Regression Analysis by Example, *Fourth Edition*

CHATTERJEE and HADI · Sensitivity Analysis in Linear Regression

CHERNICK · Bootstrap Methods: A Guide for Practitioners and Researchers, *Second Edition*

CHERNICK and FRIIS · Introductory Biostatistics for the Health Sciences

CHILÈS and DELFINER · Geostatistics: Modeling Spatial Uncertainty

---

*Now available in a lower priced paperback edition in the Wiley Classics Library.
†Now available in a lower priced paperback edition in the Wiley–Interscience Paperback Series.

---

*Now available in a lower priced paperback edition in the Wiley Classics Library.

†Now available in a lower priced paperback edition in the Wiley–Interscience Paperback Series.

† ETHIER and KURTZ · Markov Processes: Characterization and Convergence

EVANS, HASTINGS, and PEACOCK · Statistical Distributions, *Third Edition*

FELLER · An Introduction to Probability Theory and Its Applications, Volume I, *Third Edition,* Revised; Volume II, *Second Edition*

FISHER and VAN BELLE · Biostatistics: A Methodology for the Health Sciences

FITZMAURICE, LAIRD, and WARE · Applied Longitudinal Analysis

* FLEISS · The Design and Analysis of Clinical Experiments

FLEISS · Statistical Methods for Rates and Proportions, *Third Edition*

† FLEMING and HARRINGTON · Counting Processes and Survival Analysis

FUJIKOSHI, ULYANOV, and SHIMIZU · Multivariate Statistics: High-Dimensional and Large-Sample Approximations

FULLER · Introduction to Statistical Time Series, *Second Edition*

† FULLER · Measurement Error Models

GALLANT · Nonlinear Statistical Models

GEISSER · Modes of Parametric Statistical Inference

GELMAN and MENG · Applied Bayesian Modeling and Causal Inference from Incomplete-Data Perspectives

GEWEKE · Contemporary Bayesian Econometrics and Statistics

GHOSH, MUKHOPADHYAY, and SEN · Sequential Estimation

GIESBRECHT and GUMPERTZ · Planning, Construction, and Statistical Analysis of Comparative Experiments

GIFI · Nonlinear Multivariate Analysis

GIVENS and HOETING · Computational Statistics

GLASSERMAN and YAO · Monotone Structure in Discrete-Event Systems

GNANADESIKAN · Methods for Statistical Data Analysis of Multivariate Observations, *Second Edition*

GOLDSTEIN and LEWIS · Assessment: Problems, Development, and Statistical Issues

GREENWOOD and NIKULIN · A Guide to Chi-Squared Testing

GROSS, SHORTLE, THOMPSON, and HARRIS · Fundamentals of Queueing Theory, *Fourth Edition*

GROSS, SHORTLE, THOMPSON, and HARRIS · Solutions Manual to Accompany Fundamentals of Queueing Theory, *Fourth Edition*

* HAHN and SHAPIRO · Statistical Models in Engineering

HAHN and MEEKER · Statistical Intervals: A Guide for Practitioners

HALD · A History of Probability and Statistics and their Applications Before 1750

HALD · A History of Mathematical Statistics from 1750 to 1930

† HAMPEL · Robust Statistics: The Approach Based on Influence Functions

HANNAN and DEISTLER · The Statistical Theory of Linear Systems

HARTUNG, KNAPP, and SINHA · Statistical Meta-Analysis with Applications

HEIBERGER · Computation for the Analysis of Designed Experiments

HEDAYAT and SINHA · Design and Inference in Finite Population Sampling

HEDEKER and GIBBONS · Longitudinal Data Analysis

HELLER · MACSYMA for Statisticians

HINKELMANN and KEMPTHORNE · Design and Analysis of Experiments, Volume 1: Introduction to Experimental Design, *Second Edition*

HINKELMANN and KEMPTHORNE · Design and Analysis of Experiments, Volume 2: Advanced Experimental Design

HOAGLIN, MOSTELLER, and TUKEY · Fundamentals of Exploratory Analysis of Variance

* HOAGLIN, MOSTELLER, and TUKEY · Exploring Data Tables, Trends and Shapes

* HOAGLIN, MOSTELLER, and TUKEY · Understanding Robust and Exploratory Data Analysis

HOCHBERG and TAMHANE · Multiple Comparison Procedures

*Now available in a lower priced paperback edition in the Wiley Classics Library.

†Now available in a lower priced paperback edition in the Wiley–Interscience Paperback Series.

*Now available in a lower priced paperback edition in the Wiley Classics Library.

†Now available in a lower priced paperback edition in the Wiley–Interscience Paperback Series.

MEEKER and ESCOBAR · Statistical Methods for Reliability Data
MEERSCHAERT and SCHEFFLER · Limit Distributions for Sums of Independent
  Random Vectors: Heavy Tails in Theory and Practice
MICKEY, DUNN, and CLARK · Applied Statistics: Analysis of Variance and
  Regression, *Third Edition*
* MILLER · Survival Analysis, *Second Edition*
MONTGOMERY, JENNINGS, and KULAHCI · Introduction to Time Series Analysis
  and Forecasting
MONTGOMERY, PECK, and VINING · Introduction to Linear Regression Analysis,
  Fourth Edition
MORGENTHALER and TUKEY · Configural Polysampling: A Route to Practical
  Robustness
MUIRHEAD · Aspects of Multivariate Statistical Theory
MULLER and STOYAN · Comparison Methods for Stochastic Models and Risks
MURRAY · X-STAT 2.0 Statistical Experimentation, Design Data Analysis, and
  Nonlinear Optimization
MURTHY, XIE, and JIANG · Weibull Models
MYERS, MONTGOMERY, and ANDERSON-COOK · Response Surface Methodology:
  Process and Product Optimization Using Designed Experiments, *Third Edition*
MYERS, MONTGOMERY, VINING, and ROBINSON · Generalized Linear Models.
  With Applications in Engineering and the Sciences, *Second Edition*
† NELSON · Accelerated Testing, Statistical Models, Test Plans, and Data Analyses
† NELSON · Applied Life Data Analysis
NEWMAN · Biostatistical Methods in Epidemiology
OCHI · Applied Probability and Stochastic Processes in Engineering and Physical
  Sciences
OKABE, BOOTS, SUGIHARA, and CHIU · Spatial Tesselations: Concepts and
  Applications of Voronoi Diagrams, *Second Edition*
OLIVER and SMITH · Influence Diagrams, Belief Nets and Decision Analysis
PALTA · Quantitative Methods in Population Health: Extensions of Ordinary Regressions
PANJER · Operational Risk: Modeling and Analytics
PANKRATZ · Forecasting with Dynamic Regression Models
PANKRATZ · Forecasting with Univariate Box-Jenkins Models: Concepts and Cases
* PARZEN · Modern Probability Theory and Its Applications
PEÑA, TIAO, and TSAY · A Course in Time Series Analysis
PIANTADOSI · Clinical Trials: A Methodologic Perspective
PORT · Theoretical Probability for Applications
POURAHMADI · Foundations of Time Series Analysis and Prediction Theory
POWELL · Approximate Dynamic Programming: Solving the Curses of Dimensionality
PRESS · Bayesian Statistics: Principles, Models, and Applications
PRESS · Subjective and Objective Bayesian Statistics, *Second Edition*
PRESS and TANUR · The Subjectivity of Scientists and the Bayesian Approach
PUKELSHEIM · Optimal Experimental Design
PURI, VILAPLANA, and WERTZ · New Perspectives in Theoretical and Applied
  Statistics
† PUTERMAN · Markov Decision Processes: Discrete Stochastic Dynamic Programming
QIU · Image Processing and Jump Regression Analysis
* RAO · Linear Statistical Inference and Its Applications, *Second Edition*
RAUSAND and HØYLAND · System Reliability Theory: Models, Statistical Methods,
  and Applications, *Second Edition*
RENCHER · Linear Models in Statistics
RENCHER · Methods of Multivariate Analysis, *Second Edition*
RENCHER · Multivariate Statistical Inference with Applications

---

*Now available in a lower priced paperback edition in the Wiley Classics Library.
†Now available in a lower priced paperback edition in the Wiley–Interscience Paperback Series.

* RIPLEY · Spatial Statistics
* RIPLEY · Stochastic Simulation
ROBINSON · Practical Strategies for Experimenting
ROHATGI and SALEH · An Introduction to Probability and Statistics, *Second Edition*
ROLSKI, SCHMIDLI, SCHMIDT, and TEUGELS · Stochastic Processes for Insurance and Finance
ROSENBERGER and LACHIN · Randomization in Clinical Trials: Theory and Practice
ROSS · Introduction to Probability and Statistics for Engineers and Scientists
ROSSI, ALLENBY, and McCULLOCH · Bayesian Statistics and Marketing
† ROUSSEEUW and LEROY · Robust Regression and Outlier Detection
* RUBIN · Multiple Imputation for Nonresponse in Surveys
RUBINSTEIN and KROESE · Simulation and the Monte Carlo Method, *Second Edition*
RUBINSTEIN and MELAMED · Modern Simulation and Modeling
RYAN · Modern Engineering Statistics
RYAN · Modern Experimental Design
RYAN · Modern Regression Methods, *Second Edition*
RYAN · Statistical Methods for Quality Improvement, *Second Edition*
SALEH · Theory of Preliminary Test and Stein-Type Estimation with Applications
* SCHEFFE · The Analysis of Variance
SCHIMEK · Smoothing and Regression: Approaches, Computation, and Application
SCHOTT · Matrix Analysis for Statistics, *Second Edition*
SCHOUTENS · Levy Processes in Finance: Pricing Financial Derivatives
SCHUSS · Theory and Applications of Stochastic Differential Equations
SCOTT · Multivariate Density Estimation: Theory, Practice, and Visualization
† SEARLE · Linear Models for Unbalanced Data
† SEARLE · Matrix Algebra Useful for Statistics
† SEARLE, CASELLA, and McCULLOCH · Variance Components
SEARLE and WILLETT · Matrix Algebra for Applied Economics
SEBER · A Matrix Handbook For Statisticians
† SEBER · Multivariate Observations
SEBER and LEE · Linear Regression Analysis, *Second Edition*
† SEBER and WILD · Nonlinear Regression
SENNOTT · Stochastic Dynamic Programming and the Control of Queueing Systems
* SERFLING · Approximation Theorems of Mathematical Statistics
SHAFER and VOVK · Probability and Finance: It's Only a Game!
SILVAPULLE and SEN · Constrained Statistical Inference: Inequality, Order, and Shape Restrictions
SMALL and McLEISH · Hilbert Space Methods in Probability and Statistical Inference
SRIVASTAVA · Methods of Multivariate Statistics
STAPLETON · Linear Statistical Models, *Second Edition*
STAPLETON · Models for Probability and Statistical Inference: Theory and Applications
STAUDTE and SHEATHER · Robust Estimation and Testing
STOYAN, KENDALL, and MECKE · Stochastic Geometry and Its Applications, *Second Edition*
STOYAN and STOYAN · Fractals, Random Shapes and Point Fields: Methods of Geometrical Statistics
STREET and BURGESS · The Construction of Optimal Stated Choice Experiments: Theory and Methods
STYAN · The Collected Papers of T. W. Anderson: 1943–1985
SUTTON, ABRAMS, JONES, SHELDON, and SONG · Methods for Meta-Analysis in Medical Research
TAKEZAWA · Introduction to Nonparametric Regression
TAMHANE · Statistical Analysis of Designed Experiments: Theory and Applications
TANAKA · Time Series Analysis: Nonstationary and Noninvertible Distribution Theory

*Now available in a lower priced paperback edition in the Wiley Classics Library.
†Now available in a lower priced paperback edition in the Wiley–Interscience Paperback Series.

THOMPSON · Empirical Model Building
THOMPSON · Sampling, *Second Edition*
THOMPSON · Simulation: A Modeler's Approach
THOMPSON and SEBER · Adaptive Sampling
THOMPSON, WILLIAMS, and FINDLAY · Models for Investors in Real World Markets
TIAO, BISGAARD, HILL, PEÑA, and STIGLER (editors) · Box on Quality and Discovery: with Design, Control, and Robustness
TIERNEY · LISP-STAT: An Object-Oriented Environment for Statistical Computing and Dynamic Graphics
TSAY · Analysis of Financial Time Series, *Third Edition*
UPTON and FINGLETON · Spatial Data Analysis by Example, Volume II: Categorical and Directional Data
† VAN BELLE · Statistical Rules of Thumb, *Second Edition*
VAN BELLE, FISHER, HEAGERTY, and LUMLEY · Biostatistics: A Methodology for the Health Sciences, *Second Edition*
VESTRUP · The Theory of Measures and Integration
VIDAKOVIC · Statistical Modeling by Wavelets
VINOD and REAGLE · Preparing for the Worst: Incorporating Downside Risk in Stock Market Investments
WALLER and GOTWAY · Applied Spatial Statistics for Public Health Data
WEERAHANDI · Generalized Inference in Repeated Measures: Exact Methods in MANOVA and Mixed Models
WEISBERG · Applied Linear Regression, *Third Edition*
WEISBERG · Bias and Causation: Models and Judgment for Valid Comparisons
WELSH · Aspects of Statistical Inference
WESTFALL and YOUNG · Resampling-Based Multiple Testing: Examples and Methods for *p*-Value Adjustment
WHITTAKER · Graphical Models in Applied Multivariate Statistics
WINKER · Optimization Heuristics in Economics: Applications of Threshold Accepting
WONNACOTT and WONNACOTT · Econometrics, *Second Edition*
WOODING · Planning Pharmaceutical Clinical Trials: Basic Statistical Principles
WOODWORTH · Biostatistics: A Bayesian Introduction
WOOLSON and CLARKE · Statistical Methods for the Analysis of Biomedical Data, *Second Edition*
WU and HAMADA · Experiments: Planning, Analysis, and Parameter Design Optimization, *Second Edition*
WU and ZHANG · Nonparametric Regression Methods for Longitudinal Data Analysis
YANG · The Construction Theory of Denumerable Markov Processes
YOUNG, VALERO-MORA, and FRIENDLY · Visual Statistics: Seeing Data with Dynamic Interactive Graphics
ZACKS · Stage-Wise Adaptive Designs
ZELTERMAN · Discrete Distributions—Applications in the Health Sciences
* ZELLNER · An Introduction to Bayesian Inference in Econometrics
ZHOU, OBUCHOWSKI, and McCLISH · Statistical Methods in Diagnostic Medicine, *Second Edition*

*Now available in a lower priced paperback edition in the Wiley Classics Library.
†Now available in a lower priced paperback edition in the Wiley–Interscience Paperback Series.